Nursing Procedures

made Incredibly Easy!®

Second edition

Nursing Procedures

made Incredibly *Easy!*®

Second edition

Clinical Editor
Adele Webb, PhD, RN, FNAP, FAAN
Campus President
Chamberlain College of Nursing
Cleveland, Ohio

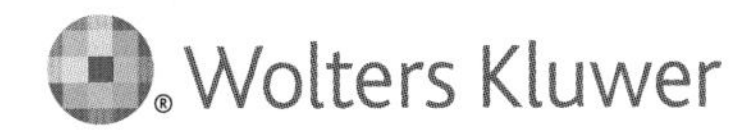

Philadelphia • Baltimore • New York • London
Buenos Aires • Hong Kong • Sydney • Tokyo

Executive Editor: Shannon W. Magee
Product Development Editor: Maria M. McAvey
Senior Marketing Manager: Mark Wiragh
Editorial Assistant: Kathryn Leyendecker
Senior Production Project Manager: Cynthia Rudy
Design Coordinator: Elaine Kasmer
Manufacturing Coordinator: Kathleen Brown
Prepress Vendor: Absolute Service, Inc.

9 8 7 6 5 4 3 2 1

Printed in China

Library of Congress Cataloging-in-Publication Data

Nursing procedures made incredibly easy! / edited by Adele Webb. — 2nd edition (r).
p. ; cm.
Includes bibliographical references (p. 628) and index.
ISBN 978-1-4963-0041-6
I. Webb, Adele A.
[DNLM: 1. Nursing Care—methods—Handbooks. WY 49]
RT51
610.73—dc23

2015023708

LWW.com

CCS0915

Contributors

Valerie Becker, MSN, RN
Manager
Center for Academic Success
Chamberlain College of Nursing
Cleveland, Ohio

Darlene Cantu, RNC-NIC, C-EFM, MSN
Associate Professor
San Antonio College ADN Program
Chamberlain College of Nursing RN to BSN Program
University of Phoenix Online Faculty
San Antonio, Texas

Sandra M. Costello, RN
Clinical Nurse
Orthopaedic Triage Service
University Hospitals Case Medical Center
Cleveland, Ohio

Cindy Ebner, RN, MSN, CPHRM, FASHRM
VP Ambulatory Care Management, Interim CQO/PSO Springfield Market
Population Health Services Organization
Mercy Health
Cincinnati, Ohio

Colleen M. Fries, CRNP
Family Nurse Practitioner
Churchville, Pennsylvania

Nicole Goetz, DNP, MS, BSN, BS, RN, FNP-C
Visiting Professor
Chamberlain College of Nursing
Miramar, Florida

Celeste M. Grossi, RN, MSN, CRRN, CWON
Nursing Instructor
Chamberlain College of Nursing
Addison, Illinois

Heike K. Huchler, ARNP
Nurse Practitioner
Internal Medicine Department
Cleveland Clinic Hospital
Weston, Florida

Kathryn Kay, MSN, RN, PCCN-CMC
Instructor
Chamberlain College of Nursing
Cleveland, Ohio

Susan Leininger, RN, MSN
Advanced Practice Nurse
Performance Improvement Quality Department
Allegheny Health Network
Allegheny General Hospital
Pittsburgh, Pennsylvania

Geri Pallija, ARNP
Nurse Practitioner
North Florida Pediatrics
Lake City, Florida

Mary Judith Yoho, PhD, RN, CNE
Senior Director Pre-licensure BSN Programs
Chamberlain College of Nursing
Houston, Texas

Previous edition contributors

Susan E. Appling, RN, MS, CRNP

Deborah Becker, RN, MSN, CCRN, CRNP, CS

Darlene Nebel Cantu, RN,C, MSN

Janice T. Chussil, RN,C, MSN, ANP

Jean Sheerin Coffey, RN, MS, PNP

Colleen M. Fries, RN, MSN, CCRN, CRNP

Rebecca Crews Gruener, RN, MS

Sandra Hamilton, RN, MED, CRNI

Dr. Joyce Lyne Heise, MSN, EdD

Lucy J. Hood, RN, DNSC

Mary Ellen Kelly, RN, BSN

Susan M. Leininger, RN, MSN

Catherine Todd Magel, RN,C, EdD

Donna Nielsen, RN, MSN, CCRN, CEN, MICN

Ruthie Robinson, RN, MSN, CCRN, CEN

Lisa Salamon, RN,C, MSN, CNS

Cynthia C. Small, RN, MSN

Foreword

Nurses at all skill levels need clear and concise evidence-based information to assist them in the performance of nursing procedures. Although there are a variety of sources that provide this information at varying levels of complexity, the need remains for a one-stop, "go-to" reference for instruction and assistance.

The implementation and refinement of technology in health care can lead to changes in technical aspects of nursing procedures. The development and revision of guidelines and professional standards can contribute as well. *Nursing Procedures Made Incredibly Easy!* provides the most up-to-date information about the performance of nursing procedures. You will find this book comprehensive yet concise, enjoyable yet educational. Its light-hearted approach will assist you as you attain procedural perfection.

The book begins with four chapters that encompass broad nursing topics. "Fundamental procedures" covers the entire journey of the patient's hospital stay, from admission to assessment; it includes such essentials as ensuring patient safety and comfort and caring for the surgical patient. "Specimen collection" explains the procedures for collecting blood, urine, stool, and other specimens. "Physical treatments" describes the nursing procedures for such techniques as heat and cold application, baths, support devices, and wound care. "Drug administration and I.V. therapy" covers drug delivery procedures ranging from simple to complex.

The next seven chapters focus on nursing procedures related to the care of specific body systems—cardiovascular, respiratory, neurologic, gastrointestinal, renal and urologic, orthopedic, and integumentary. The last two chapters detail the special needs of maternal, neonatal, and pediatric patients.

To help you use this book, each nursing procedure appears in the same easy-to-follow format, with short paragraphs and bulleted lists that let you quickly skim an entire entry to instantly pinpoint the specific information you need.

Throughout the book, a playful cast of cartoon characters takes the tedium out of learning. Within each chapter, special features enhance your understanding. Each chapter starts with a summary of key topics and ends with a quick quiz (which includes answers and rationales) to reinforce learning. Special logos highlight important points:

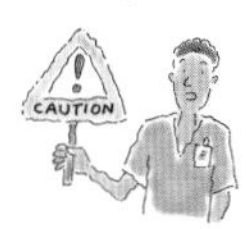

Warning alerts you to possible dangers, risks, complications, or contraindications associated with a specific procedure.

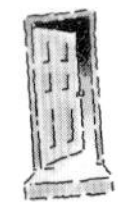

Home care connection gives tips for adapting a procedure to the home care setting.

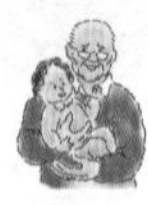

Ages and stages highlights important age-related variations in performing a particular procedure.

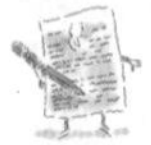

Write it down features essential points to document for each procedure.

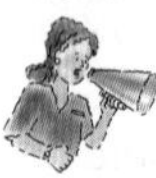

Listen up provides quick hints for performing skills and procedures.

Please take the time to fully acquaint yourself with *Nursing Procedures Made Incredibly Easy.* The more you familiarize yourself with the content, the more confident you'll be when performing procedures. Your patients, sensing your confidence and expertise, will feel more confident and comfortable, too.

Adele Webb, PhD, RN, FNAP, FAAN
Campus President
Chamberlain College of Nursing
Cleveland, Ohio

Contents

Chapter 1

Fundamental procedures

Just the facts

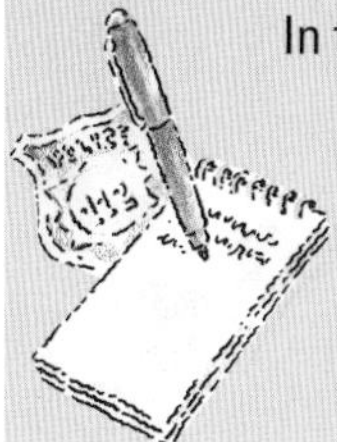

In this chapter, you'll learn:

- about fundamental procedures and how to perform them
- what patient care, complications, and patient teaching are associated with each procedure
- about essential documentation for each procedure.

Hand hygiene

Clean hands are the single most important factor for preventing the transfer of pathogens, which can lead to hospital-associated infections (HAIs). Hospital patients in the United States get an estimated 722,000 infections each year or about 1 infection for every 25 patients. To protect patients from HAIs, hand hygiene must be performed routinely and thoroughly.

What you need

Soap and water, antiseptic handwash, or alcohol-based handrub ✱ disposable towels ✱ optional: fingernail brush, plastic sponge brush, or plastic cuticle stick.

How you do it

Hand hygiene generally refers to performing hand washing with soap and water, antiseptic handwash, alcohol-based handrub, or surgical antiseptic handwash/handrub. The general guidelines for which method to use are as follows:

- When hands are visibly dirty, contaminated, or soiled, wash with non-antimicrobial or antimicrobial soap and water.
- If hands are not visibly soiled, use an alcohol-based handrub for routinely decontaminating hands.

How to Handwash?

WASH HANDS WHEN VISIBLY SOILED! OTHERWISE, USE HANDRUB

Duration of the entire procedure: 40-60 seconds

0

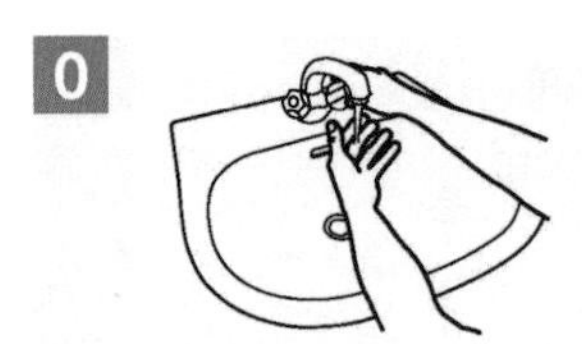

Wet hands with water;

1

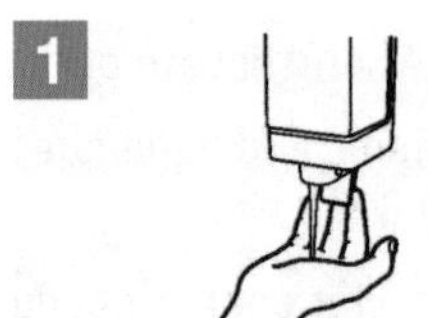

Apply enough soap to cover all hand surfaces;

2

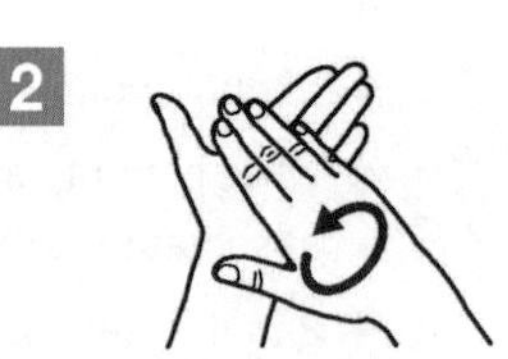

Rub hands palm to palm;

3

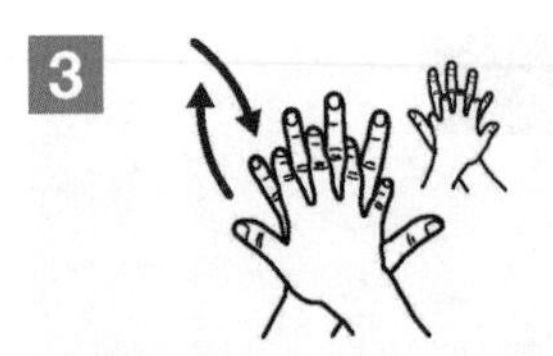

Right palm over left dorsum with interlaced fingers and vice versa;

4

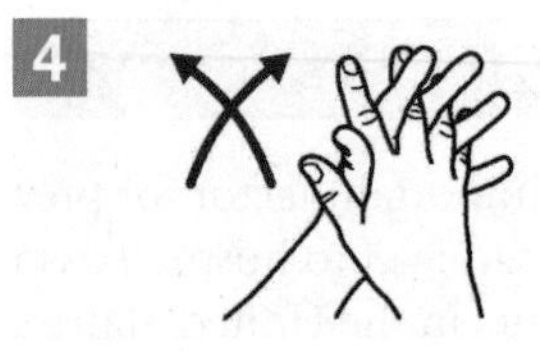

Palm to palm with fingers interlaced;

5

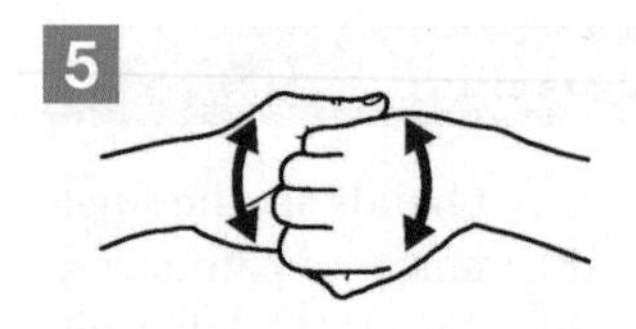

Backs of fingers to opposing palms with fingers interlocked;

6

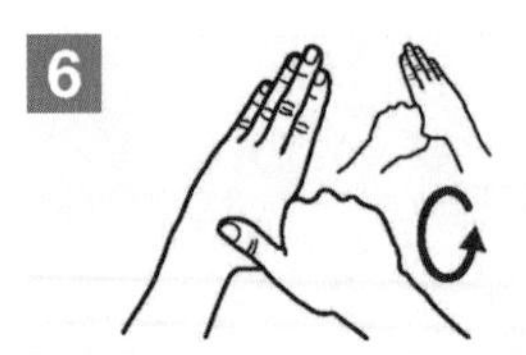

Rotational rubbing of left thumb clasped in right palm and vice versa;

7

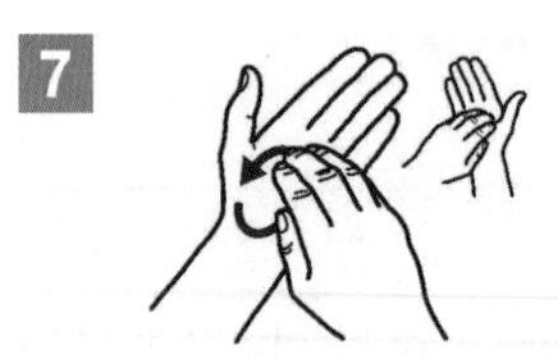

Rotational rubbing, backwards and forwards with clasped fingers of right hand in left palm and vice versa;

8

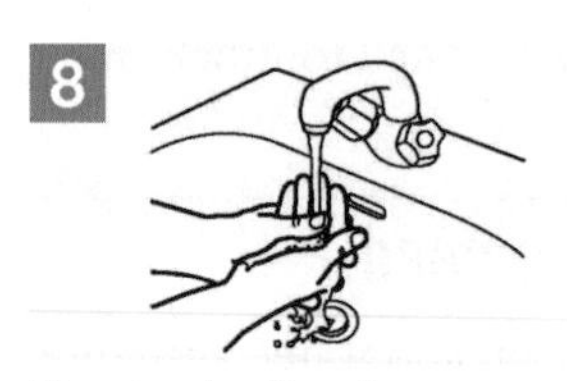

Rinse hands with water;

9

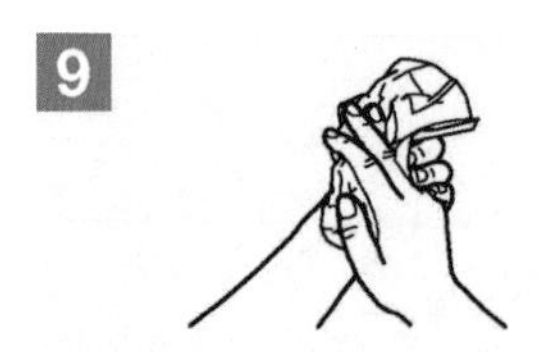

Dry hands thoroughly with a single use towel;

10

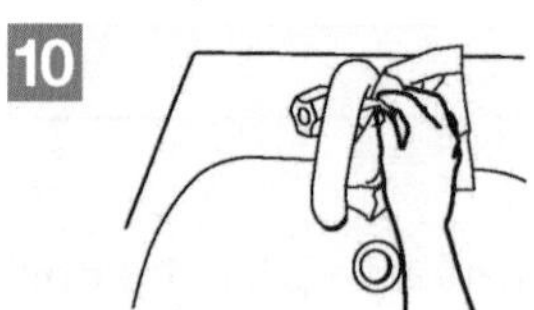

Use towel to turn off faucet;

11

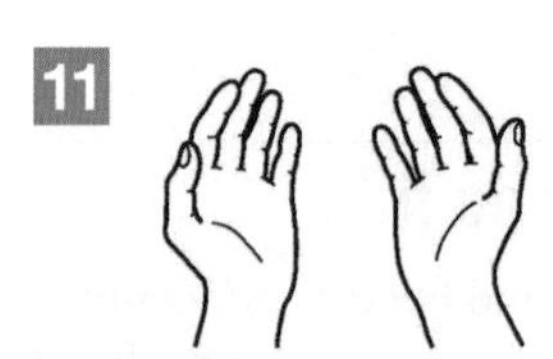

Your hands are now safe.

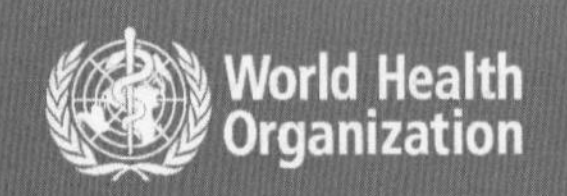

Patient Safety

A World Alliance for Safer Health Care

SAVE LIVES

Clean Your Hands

WHO acknowledges the Hôpitaux Universitaires de Genève (HUG), in particular the members of the Infection Control Programme, for their active participation in developing this material.

How to Handrub?

RUB HANDS FOR HAND HYGIENE! WASH HANDS WHEN VISIBLY SOILED

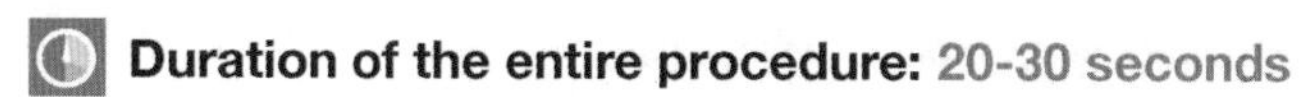

Duration of the entire procedure: 20-30 seconds

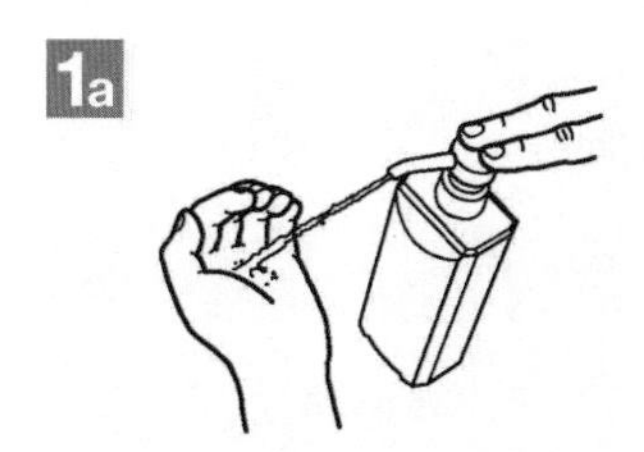

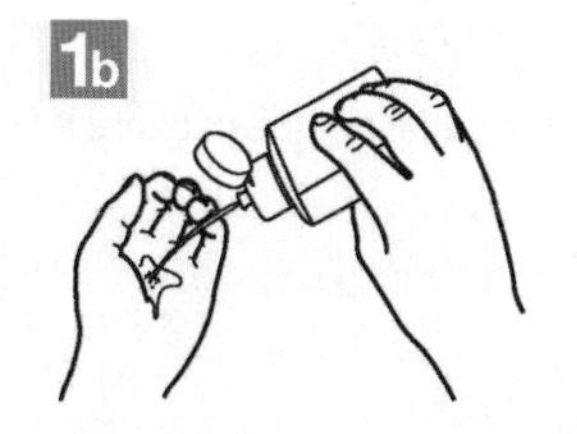

Apply a palmful of the product in a cupped hand, covering all surfaces;

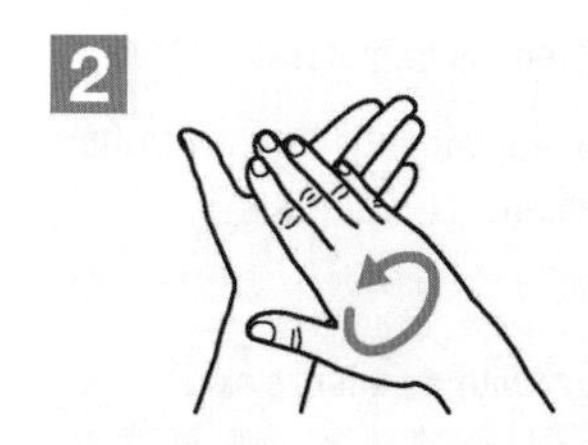

Rub hands palm to palm;

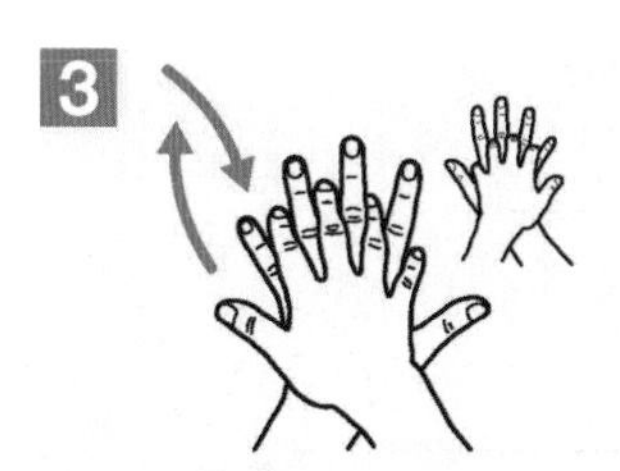

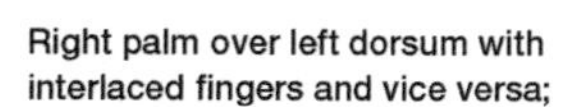

Right palm over left dorsum with interlaced fingers and vice versa;

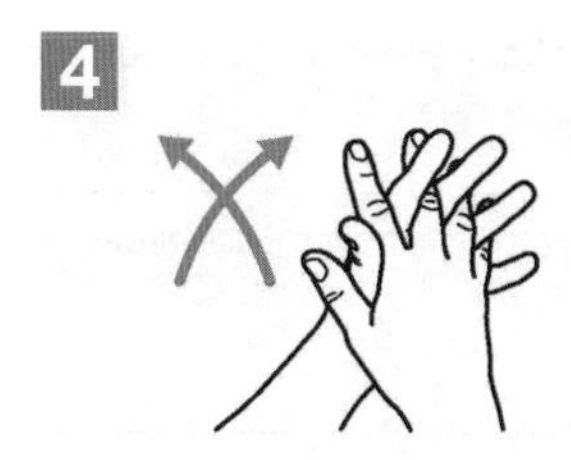

Palm to palm with fingers interlaced;

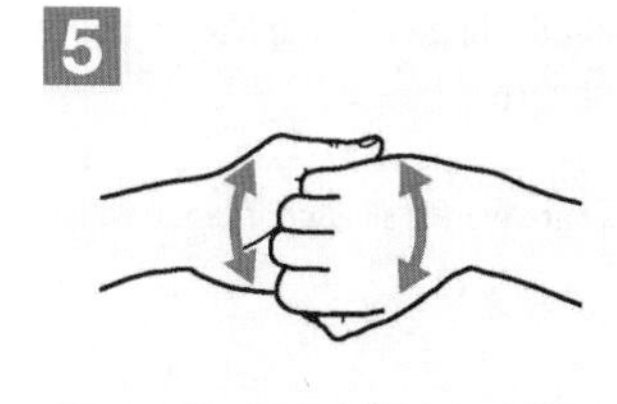

Backs of fingers to opposing palms with fingers interlocked;

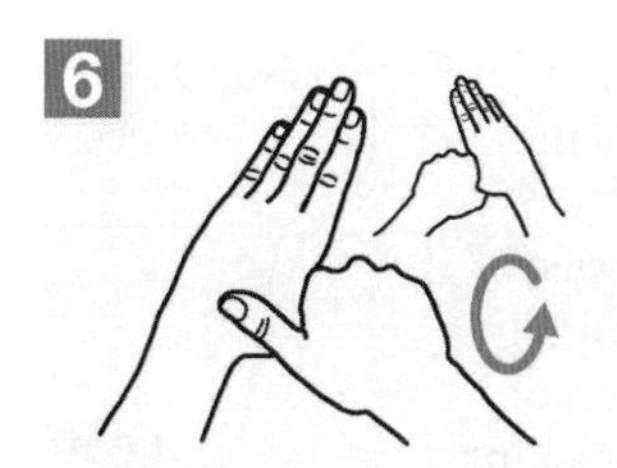

Rotational rubbing of left thumb clasped in right palm and vice versa;

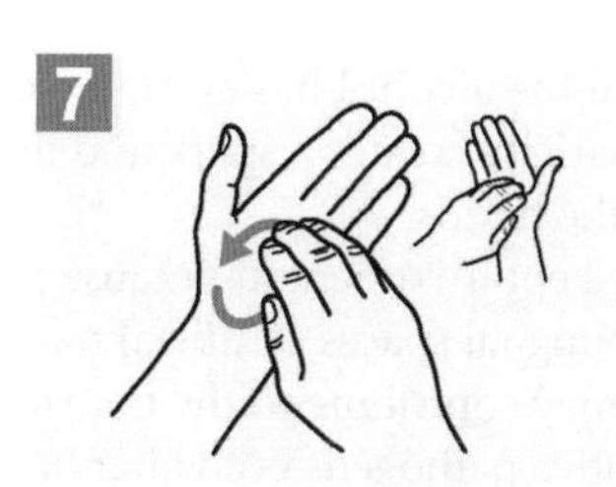

Rotational rubbing, backwards and forwards with clasped fingers of right hand in left palm and vice versa;

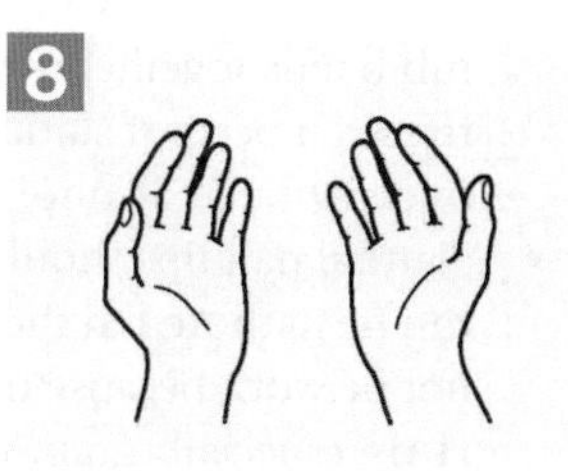

Once dry, your hands are safe.

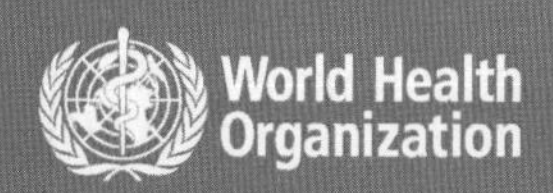

Patient Safety

A World Alliance for Safer Health Care

SAVE LIVES

Clean **Your** Hands

WHO acknowledges the Hôpitaux Universitaires de Genève (HUG), in particular the members of the Infection Control Programme, for their active participation in developing this material.

Indications for hand hygiene

Always perform hand hygiene in the following situations:

Before:

- Patient contact, even if wearing gloves
- Prior to performing aseptic task (e.g., accessing a port, preparing an injection)
- Invasive procedures (inserting urinary catheters, peripheral vascular catheters, central venous catheters)
- Exiting the patient's care area after touching the patient or the patient's immediate environment

After:

- Contact with a patient's skin
- Contact with body fluids or excretions, nonintact skin, or wound dressings or contaminated surfaces even if gloves were used
- Removing gloves
- If hands will be moving from a contaminated body site to a clean body site during patient care

Health care workers in accordance with universal precautions should use gloves.

Practice pointers

- Follow facility policies and procedures for hand hygiene.
- WARNING: Following the application of alcohol-based handrub, rub hands together until all the alcohol has evaporated. **Flash fires** can occur if static electricity creates a spark and ignites the unevaporated alcohol on the hands.
- Natural nail tips should be kept to ¼″ length because pathogens can be harbored in the subungual spaces. Artificial nails should not be worn because they may contribute to the transmission of HAIs, especially gram-negative pathogens even after hand washing.
- Remember to use hand lotions or creams to reduce the occurrence of irritation contact dermatitis associated with hand washing.
- Gloves should be removed after caring for a patient. The same pair of gloves should not be worn to care for another patient. Do not wash gloves.
- Encourage patients and families to remind health care workers to use hand hygiene.
- Encourage families to do hand hygiene when entering and leaving the patient's room.

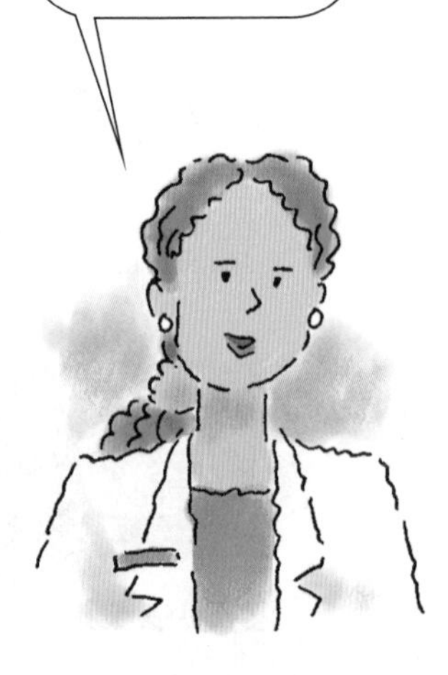
Hint: Singing Happy Birthday twice will equal the length of time needed to properly rub your hands during hand washing.

- Home health care workers should carry a supply of soap and disposable paper towels because they may not be available. If there's no running water, disinfect your hands with an antiseptic cleaner.

Isolation precautions

- Isolation precautions are implemented to prevent the spread of infection in the hospital.
- Different types of isolation precautions are needed depending on the type of germs (pathogens) involved.

Standard precautions

- You should follow standard precautions with all patients.
- When you are close to or in contact with blood or bodily fluids, tissues, mucous membranes, or open areas of skin, you must use personal protective equipment (PPE).
- Based on the anticipated level of exposure, types of PPE required include:
    - gloves
    - masks and goggles
    - aprons, gowns, and shoe covers
- It is also important to follow the hand hygiene guidelines afterward.

Transmission-based precautions

Transmission-based precautions (TBPs) are steps taken in addition to the standard precautions for certain pathogens. Some infections may also require more than one type of TBP.

- Follow TBPs as soon as infectious illness is first suspected.
- Patients should stay in their rooms as much as possible while these precautions are in place.
- Follow the policies and procedures at your facility.

Types of TBP:

- **Airborne precautions** are necessary for pathogens that are so small they float in the air and can travel long distances.
    - Some common illnesses that warrant airborne precautions are chicken pox, measles, and tuberculosis (TB).
    - They may require a negative pressure room that pulls air in so the germs do not escape the room.
    - A special respirator mask will be required for those entering the room so they don't inhale the small pathogens.
- **Contact precautions** are necessary for pathogens that are spread by touching an object or the patient has touched.
    - Some common illnesses that warrant contact precautions are *Clostridium difficile* and *Norovirus* infections.
    - Anyone entering the room must wear a gown and gloves.

- **Droplet precautions** are to prevent contact with secretions from the respiratory tract.
  - Common illnesses that warrant droplet precautions are influenza, pertussis, and mumps.
  - When a person talks, coughs, or sneezes, the droplets can travel 3′ (0.91 m) and expose a person to the illness.
  - A surgical mask is required for anyone who goes into the room.

Using PPE

What you need

Gowns ✳ gloves ✳ goggles ✳ masks ✳ specially marked laundry bags (and water-soluble laundry bags, if used) ✳ plastic trash bags.

An isolation cart may be used when the patient's room has no anteroom. It should include a work area (such as a pull-out shelf), drawers or a cabinet area for holding isolation supplies, and, possibly, a pole on which to hang coats or jackets. A door card announcing that isolation precautions are in effect should also be posted.

Getting ready

Remove the cover from the isolation cart if necessary and set up the work area. Check the cart or anteroom to ensure that correct and sufficient supplies are in place for the designated isolation category.

How you do it

- Wash your hands with an antiseptic cleaner to prevent the growth of microorganisms under gloves.

Putting on PPE

- Put the gown on and wrap it around the back of your uniform. Tie the strings or fasten the snaps or pressure-sensitive tabs at the neck. Make sure your uniform is completely covered and secure the gown at the waist.
- Place the mask snugly over your nose and mouth. Secure ear loops around your ears or tie the strings behind your head high enough so the mask won't slip off. If the mask has a metal strip, squeeze it to fit your nose firmly but comfortably. (See *Putting on a face mask*.) If you wear eyeglasses, tuck the mask under their lower edge.
- Put on goggles, if necessary.
- Put on the gloves. Pull the gloves over the cuffs to cover the edges of the gown's sleeves.

Putting on a face mask

To avoid spreading airborne particles, wear a sterile or nonsterile face mask as indicated. Position the mask to cover your nose and mouth and secure it high enough to ensure stability.

Get all tied up

Tie the top strings at the back of your head above the ears. Then tie the bottom strings at the base of your neck. Adjust the metal nose strip if the mask has one.

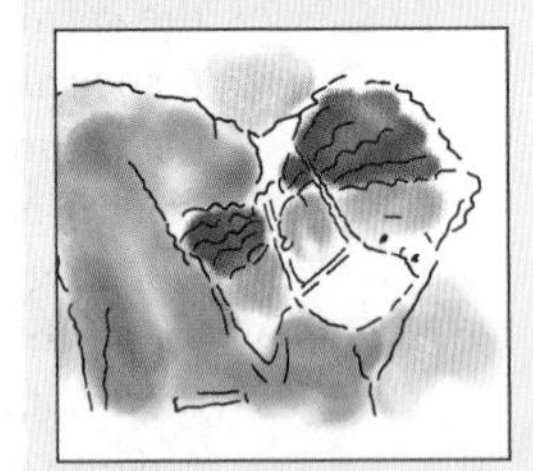

Removing PPE

- Remember that the outside surfaces of your barrier clothes are contaminated.
- Untie the gown's waist strings with gloves still on.
- With your gloved left hand, remove the right glove by pulling on the cuff, turning the glove inside out as you pull. Don't touch any skin with the outside of either glove. (See *Removing contaminated gloves*.) Then remove the left glove by wedging one or two fingers of your right hand inside the glove and pulling it off, turning it inside out as you remove it. Discard the gloves in the trash container.

Mask can be last

- Untie your mask, holding it only by the strings. Discard the mask in the trash container. If the patient has a disease that's spread by airborne pathogens, you may prefer to remove the mask last.
- Untie the neck straps of your gown. Grasp the outside of the gown at the back of the shoulders and pull it down over your arms, turning it inside out as you remove it to avoid spreading the pathogens.
- Holding the gown well away from your uniform, fold it inside out. Discard it in the laundry or trash container as necessary.

Hand hygiene

- If the sink is inside the patient's room, wash your hands according to the hand hygiene guidelines before leaving the room. Turn off the faucet using a paper towel and discard the towel in the room. Grasp the door handle with a clean paper towel to open it and discard the towel in a trash container inside the room. Close the door from the outside with your bare hand.
- If the sink is in an anteroom, wash your hands and forearms following the hand hygiene guidelines after leaving the room.
- A poster illustrating donning PPE is available from the CDC at http://www.cdc.gov/HAI/pdfs/ppe/ppeposter148.pdf or a video, CNA Skill #8 Donning and Doffing PPE, is available from the ACLS Certification Center at http://www.youtube.com/watch?v=urKd0Up_yao.

Practice pointers

- Use gowns, gloves, goggles, and masks only once and discard them in the appropriate container before leaving a contaminated area. If your mask is reusable, retain it for further use unless it's damaged or damp. Be aware that PPE loses its effectiveness when wet because moisture permits organisms to seep through the material. Change masks and gowns as soon as moisture is noticeable or according to manufacturer recommendations or facility policy.

Removing contaminated gloves

Proper removal techniques are essential for preventing the spread of pathogens from gloves to your skin surface. Follow these steps carefully:

Using your left hand, pinch the right glove near the top. Avoid allowing the glove's outer surface to buckle inward against your wrist.

Pull downward, allowing the glove to turn inside out as it comes off. Keep the right glove in your left hand after removing it.

Now insert the first two fingers of your ungloved right hand under the edge of the left glove. Avoid touching the glove's outer surface or folding it against your left wrist.

Pull downward so that the glove turns inside out as it comes off. Continue pulling until the left glove completely encloses the right one and its uncontaminated inner surface is facing out.

Fill 'er up

- After patient transfer or discharge, return the isolation cart to the appropriate area for cleaning and restocking of supplies. An isolation room and all equipment in it such as intravenous (I.V.) pumps, monitors, and so forth must be thoroughly cleaned and disinfected before use by another patient. Special cleaning agents may be required to eliminate the pathogens and prevent the spread of infection. Refer to policies and procedures at your facility.
- Restock items at the end of your shift so PPE is readily available for the next shift. (See *Documenting isolation precautions*.)

Write it down

Documenting isolation precautions

Record any special needs for isolation precautions on the nursing plan of care and as otherwise indicated by your facility.

Temperature

Body temperature represents the balance between heat that metabolism, muscular activity, and other factors produce and heat that's lost through the skin, lungs, and body wastes. A stable temperature pattern promotes proper function of cells, tissues, and organs; a change in this pattern may signal the onset of illness.

Choose one of two

Temperature can be measured with one of two types of thermometers: electronic digital (includes temporal artery and tympanic thermometers) or chemical-dot. Oral temperature in adults normally ranges from 97° to 99.5° F (36.1° to 37.5° C). Rectal temperature, the most accurate reading, is usually 1° F (0.6° C) higher. Axillary temperature, the least accurate reading, is usually 1° to 2° F (0.6° to 1.1° C) lower. Tympanic temperature reads 0.5° to 1° F higher. (See *Types of thermometers*.) Temperature changes outside the usual range are related to changes in heat loss or production.

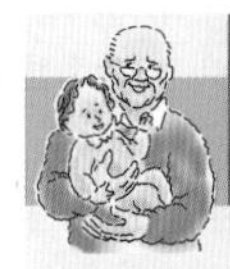

Ages and stages

Differences in temperature

Besides activity level, other factors that influence temperature include sex, age, emotional conditions, stress, exercise, hormone levels, and environment. Keep these principles in mind:

- Women normally have higher temperatures than men, especially during ovulation.
- Normal temperature is highest in neonates and lowest in elderly persons.
- A hot external environment can raise temperature; a cold environment lowers it.

Normal ups and downs

Temperature is controlled by the hypothalamus. Temperature normally fluctuates with rest and activity (circadian rhythm). Lowest readings typically occur between 1 and 4 a.m. and the highest readings between 4 and 8 p.m. Other factors also influence temperature. (See *Differences in temperature*.)

What you need

Electronic thermometer, chemical-dot thermometer, temporal artery thermometer, or tympanic thermometer ✱ water-soluble lubricant or petroleum jelly (for rectal temperature) ✱ facial tissue ✱ disposable thermometer sheath or probe cover (except for chemical-dot thermometer) ✱ alcohol pad ✱ gloves (for rectal temperature).

Types of thermometers

You can take a patient's oral, rectal, or axillary temperature with a chemical-dot device or an electronic digital thermometer. The temporal artery and tympanic membrane are other sites that can be used for temperature measurement and require special electronic thermometers.

Oral, tympanic, and temporal thermometers are the most frequently used in adults and pediatrics. Which type you choose will depend on the condition of the patient. Here are some site tips:

1. **Do not** use an oral thermometer in infants; small children; or patients who are confused, unconscious, or uncooperative. Also, do not use with a history of epilepsy or oral surgery.
2. In newborns, tympanic and temporal artery sites conserve heat because there is less temperature loss from unbundling and handling the baby.
3. Temporal artery site gives a rapid measurement and reflects rapid change in core temperature.
4. Tympanic site requires careful positioning in neonates, infants, and children under 3 years because the anatomy of the ear canal makes it difficult to position.

Tympanic thermometer

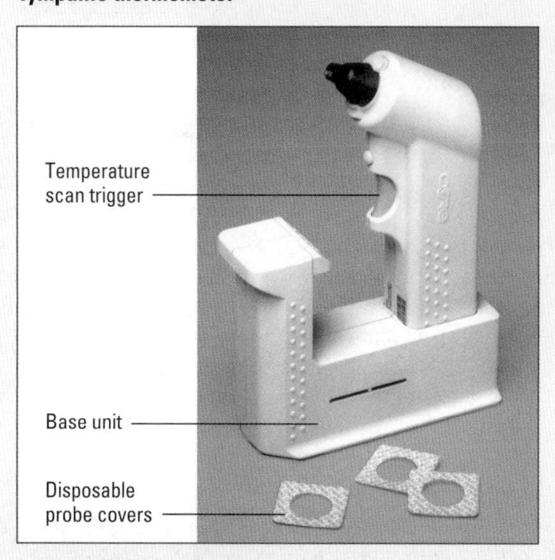

Individual electronic digital thermometer

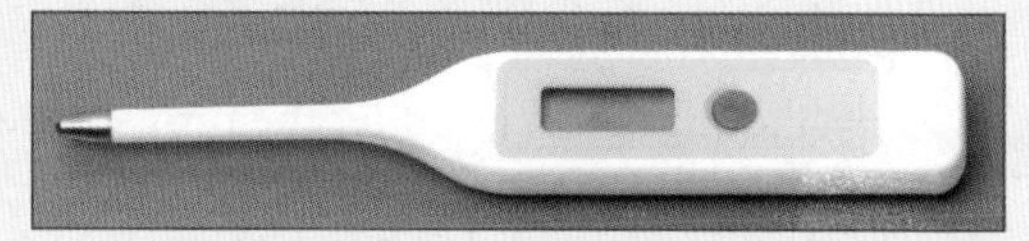

Institutional electronic digital thermometer

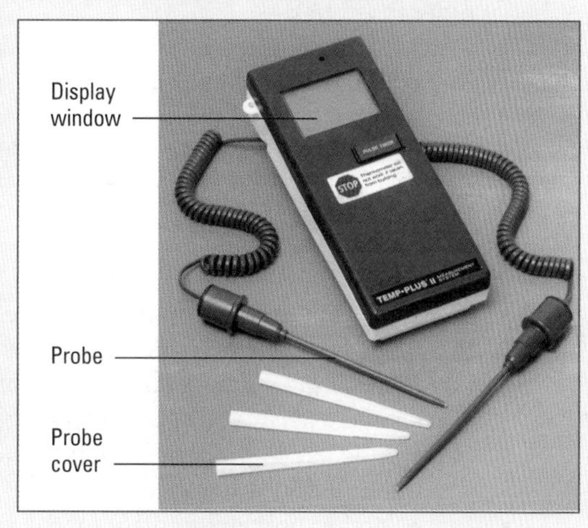

Chemical-dot thermometer

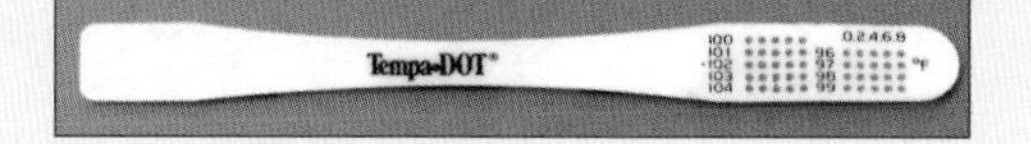

How you do it

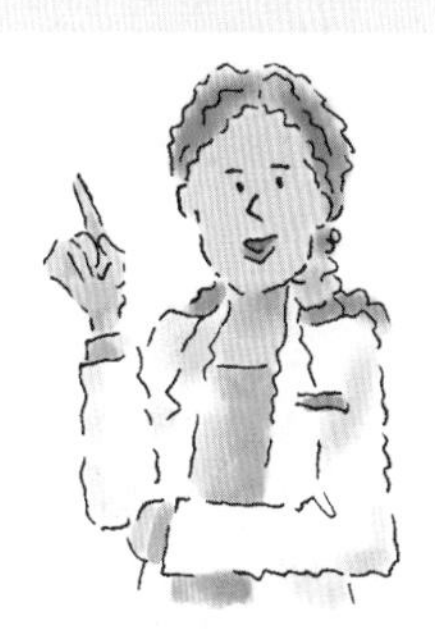

- Identify the patient with two identifiers per facility policy.
- Perform hand hygiene.
- Explain the procedure to the patient. If you're taking an oral temperature and the patient had hot or cold liquids, chewed gum, or smoked, wait 15 minutes before getting started.

With an electronic thermometer

- Insert the probe into a disposable probe cover. If taking a rectal temperature, lubricate the probe cover *to reduce friction and ease insertion*. Leave the probe in place until the maximum temperature appears on the digital display. Then remove the probe and note the temperature.

With a chemical-dot thermometer

- Remove the thermometer from its protective case by grasping the handle end with your thumb and forefinger, moving the handle up and down to break the seal, and pulling the handle straight out. Leave the chemical-dot thermometer in place for 45 seconds.
- Read the temperature as the last dye dot that has changed color, or fired, then discard the thermometer and its dispenser case.

With a tympanic thermometer

- Make sure the lens under the probe is clean and shiny. Attach a disposable probe cover.
- Stabilize the patient's head, then gently pull his ear straight back (for children up to age 1) or up and back (for children age 1 and older to adults).
- Insert the thermometer until the entire ear canal is sealed. The thermometer should be inserted toward the tympanic membrane in the same way that an otoscope is inserted.
- Press the activation button and hold it for 1 second. The temperature will appear on the display. (See *Taking an infant's temperature.*)

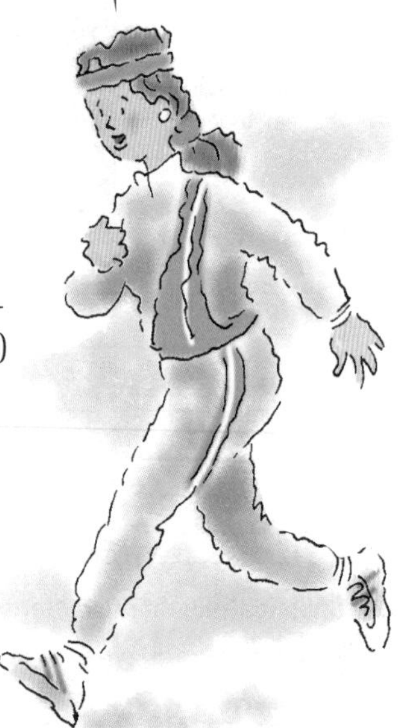
Lowest body temperature typically occurs in the early morning, after a night of rest. Highest occurs in the late afternoon or early evening, after a day of activity. Phew!

Taking an oral temperature

- Put on gloves and position the tip of the thermometer under the patient's tongue on either side of the frenulum as far back as possible. *Placing the tip in this area promotes contact with superficial blood vessels and ensures a more accurate reading.*
- Instruct the patient to close his lips but to not bite down with his teeth *to avoid breaking the thermometer in his mouth.*
- Leave the thermometer in place for the appropriate length of time, depending on which thermometer was used.

Taking a rectal temperature

- Position the patient on his side with his top leg flexed and drape him *to provide privacy*. Then fold back the bed linens *to expose his anus.*
- Squeeze the lubricant onto a facial tissue *to avoid contaminating the lubricant supply.*

- Lubricate about ½″ (1 cm) of the thermometer tip for an infant, 1″ (2.5 cm) for a child, and 1½″ (3.8 cm) for an adult *to reduce friction and ease insertion.* This step may be unnecessary when using disposable rectal sheaths *because they're prelubricated.*
- Put on gloves, lift the patient's upper buttock, and insert the thermometer about ½″ (1 cm) for an infant and 1½″ (3.8 cm) for an adult.
- Gently direct the thermometer along the rectal wall toward the umbilicus *to avoid perforating the anus or rectum or breaking the thermometer and to help ensure an accurate reading.* (The thermometer will register hemorrhoidal artery temperature instead of fecal temperature.)
- Hold the thermometer in place for the appropriate length of time *to prevent damage to rectal tissues caused by displacement.*
- Carefully remove the thermometer, wiping it as necessary. Then wipe the patient's anal area *to remove any lubricant or feces.*
- Remove your gloves and wash your hands.

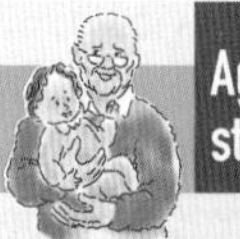

Ages and stages

Taking an infant's temperature

For infants under age 3 months, take three readings and use the highest.

Taking an axillary temperature

- Position the patient with the axilla exposed.
- Put on gloves and gently pat the axilla dry with a facial tissue *because moisture conducts heat.* Avoid harsh rubbing, *which generates heat.*
- Ask the patient to reach across his chest and grasp his opposite shoulder, lifting his elbow.
- Position the thermometer in the center of the axilla, with the tip pointing toward the patient's head.
- Tell him to keep grasping his shoulder and to lower his elbow and hold it against his chest *to promote skin contact with the thermometer.*
- Leave the thermometer in place for the appropriate length of time, depending on which thermometer you're using. Axillary temperature takes longer to register than oral or rectal temperature *because the thermometer isn't enclosed in a body cavity.*
- Grasp the end of the thermometer and remove it from the axilla. Remove your gloves and wash your hands.

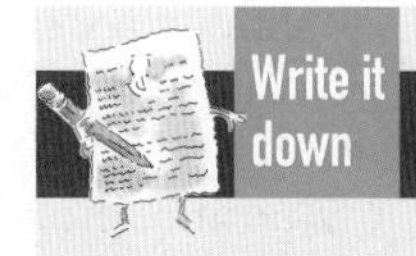

Write it down

Documenting temperature

Record the time, route, and temperature on the patient's chart. Compare measurement with baseline and acceptable values and review trends.

Practice pointers

- Oral measurement is contraindicated in young children and infants and in patients who are unconscious or disoriented or who must breathe through their mouth or are prone to seizures.
- Rectal measurement is contraindicated in patients with diarrhea, recent rectal or prostatic surgery or injury *because it may injure inflamed tissue,* or recent myocardial infarction *because anal manipulation may stimulate the vagus nerve, causing bradycardia or another rhythm disturbance.*

- Use the same thermometer for repeat temperature taking *to ensure more consistent results.*
- Store chemical-dot thermometers in a cool area *because exposure to heat activates the dye dots.*
- If your patient is receiving nasal oxygen, know that you can still measure his temperature orally because oxygen administration raises oral temperature by only about 0.3° F (0.2° C). (See *Documenting temperature,* page 11.)

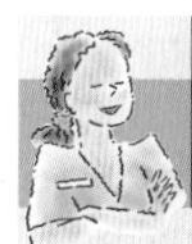

Peak technique

Pinpointing pulse sites

You can assess your patient's pulse rate at several sites, including those shown in the illustration below.

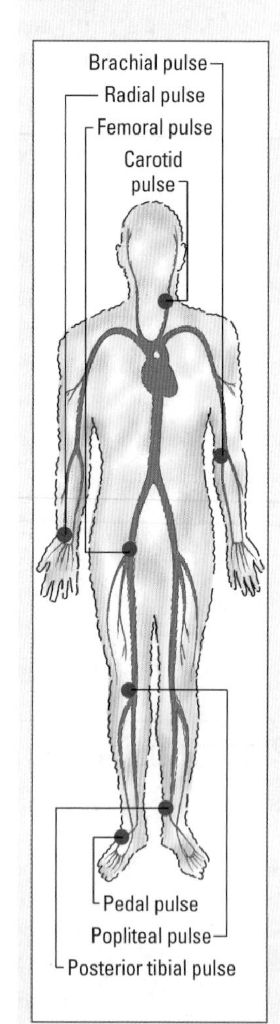

Measuring a pulse

Blood pumped into an already full aorta during ventricular contraction creates a fluid wave that travels from the heart to the peripheral arteries. This recurring wave—called a *pulse*—can be palpated at locations on the body where an artery crosses over bone or firm tissue. (See *Pinpointing pulse sites.*) The pulse is an indicator of how well the blood is circulating. An abnormally slow, rapid, or irregular pulse alters the amount of blood the heart pumps and can affect the ability to meet the tissues' demand for nutrients.

Rate, rhythm, and volume (character of the pulse)

Taking a patient's pulse involves determining the number of beats per minute (the pulse rate), the pattern or regularity of the beats (the rhythm), and the volume of blood pumped (strength) with each beat. (See *Choosing the best site.*)

Practice pointers

- Always review the patient's baseline pulse rate for comparison.
- You will only measure rate and rhythm with an apical pulse.
- The heart rate will increase temporarily when a person changes position from lying to sitting or standing because the movement alters the blood volume and sympathetic activity.
- If the pulse is faint or weak, consider using a Doppler ultrasound blood flow detector. (See *Using a Doppler device.*)

What you need

Watch with a second hand ✳ stethoscope (for auscultating apical pulse) ✳ Doppler ultrasound blood flow detector if necessary.

Using a Doppler device

More sensitive than palpation for determining pulse rate, the Doppler ultrasound blood flow detector is especially useful when a pulse is faint or weak. Unlike palpation, which detects arterial wall expansion and retraction, this instrument detects the movement of red blood cells. Here's how you use it.

- Apply a small amount of transmission gel to the ultrasound probe.
- Position the probe on the skin directly over the selected artery. In the illustration below, the probe is over the posterior tibial artery.
- When using a Doppler probe with an amplifier (as shown below), turn the instrument on and, moving counterclockwise, set the volume control to the lowest setting. If your model doesn't have a speaker, plug in the earphones and slowly raise the volume.
- To obtain the best signals, put gel between the skin and the probe and tilt the probe 45 degrees from the artery. Slowly move the probe in a circular motion to locate the center of the artery and the Doppler signal—a hissing noise at the heartbeat. Avoid moving the probe rapidly because this distorts the signal.
- Count the signals for 60 seconds to determine the pulse rate.
- After you have measured the pulse rate, clean the probe with a soft cloth soaked in antiseptic solution or soapy water. Don't immerse the probe.

Doppler probe with an amplifier

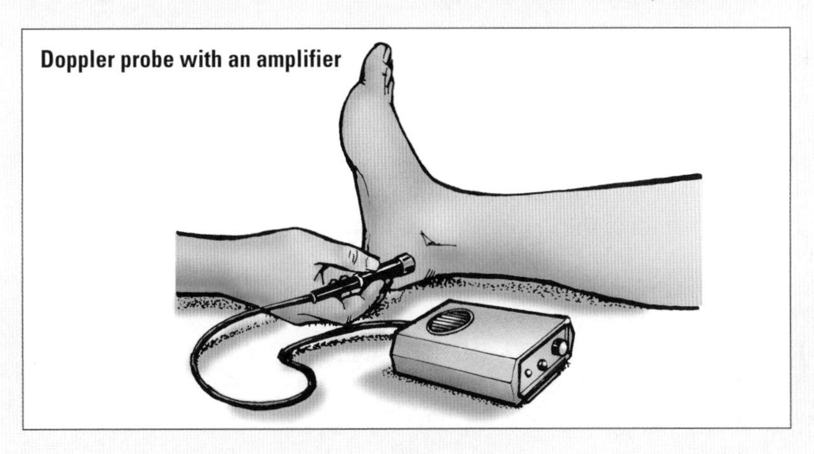

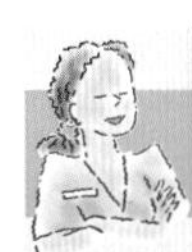

Peak technique

Choosing the best site

- Any artery can be used to assess a pulse rate, but the radial and apical locations are the most common. If the radial pulse is abnormal or the patient takes medication that affects the heart rate, use the apical pulse for a more accurate assessment of heart function.
- In infants and young children, the brachial or apical pulse is the best site to measure the pulse because the other peripheral pulses are deep and difficult to palpate accurately. The apical pulse is the preferred site in children less than 3 years old.
- When a patient's condition rapidly deteriorates, the carotid site is recommended because the heart continues to pump blood through the carotid artery to the brain.

How you do it

- Use proper hand hygiene and tell the patient that you're going to check his pulse.
- Make sure the patient is comfortable and relaxed *because an awkward, uncomfortable position may affect his heart rate.*

Taking a radial pulse

- Place the patient in a sitting or supine position, with his arm at his side or across his chest.

Keep the thumb out of it

- Gently press your index, middle, and ring fingers on the radial artery, inside the patient's wrist. You should feel a pulse with only moderate pressure; *excessive pressure may obstruct blood flow distal to the pulse site.* Don't use your thumb to take the patient's pulse; *the thumb has a strong pulse of its own and may easily be confused with the patient's pulse.*

One, two, three . . . sixty

- After locating the pulse, count the beats for 60 seconds, or count for 30 seconds and multiply by 2. *Counting for a full minute provides a more accurate picture of irregularities.*
- While counting the rate, assess pulse rhythm and volume by noting the pattern and strength of the beats. If you detect an irregularity, repeat the count and note whether the irregularity occurs in a pattern or randomly. If you're still in doubt, take an apical pulse. (See *Identifying pulse patterns.*)

Taking an apical pulse

- Help the patient to a supine position and drape him if necessary.

Warm the 'scope first, please

- Keeping in mind that the bell of the stethoscope transmits low-pitched sounds more effectively than the diaphragm, warm the bell or diaphragm in your hand. *Placing a cold stethoscope against the patient's skin may startle him and momentarily increase his heart rate.*
- Place the warmed bell or diaphragm over the apex of the heart (normally located at the fifth intercostal space, left of the midclavicular line) and insert the earpieces into your ears.
- Count the beats for 60 seconds and note their rhythm, volume, and intensity.
- Remove the stethoscope, and make the patient comfortable.

Taking an apical-radial pulse

An apical-radial pulse is measured if it is suspected that the patient's heart is not effectively pumping blood. If the apical rate is different than the radial rate, a pulse deficit exists, which is usually caused by an abnormal heart rhythm (dysrhythmia). If the apical rate is 84 and the radial rate is 76, there is a pulse deficit of 8 beats where a pulse wave does not reach the periphery. This can affect the ability to supply nutrients to the bodily tissues and membranes.

Identifying pulse patterns

Type	Rate (beats/min)	Rhythm	Causes and incidence
Normal	Infant: 120 to 160 Toddler: 90 to 140 Preschooler: 80 to 110 School-age child: 75 to 100 Adolescent: 60 to 90 Adult: 60 to 100	● ● ● ●	• Varies with such factors as age, physical activity, and gender (infants and children have higher pulse rates than adults and older adults who have lower pulse rates)
Tachycardia	More than 100 in adults	●●●●●●●	• Accompanies stimulation of the sympathetic nervous system resulting from emotional stress (such as anger, fear, or anxiety) or the use of certain drugs (such as caffeine) • May result from exercise or such health conditions as heart failure, chronic obstructive pulmonary disease (COPD), anemia, and fever, which increase oxygen requirements and thus pulse rate
Bradycardia	Less than 60 in adults	● ● ●	• Accompanies stimulation of the parasympathetic nervous system resulting from drug use, especially cardiac glycosides, and such conditions as cerebral hemorrhage, hypothermia, and heart block • May also be present in fit athletes and persons with hypothyroidism
Irregular	Uneven time intervals between beats (for example, periods of regular rhythm interrupted by pauses or premature beats)	●●●● ●●●	• May indicate cardiac irritability, hypoxia, digoxin toxicity, potassium imbalance, or a more serious arrhythmia if premature beats occur frequently (occasional premature beats are normal)

How you do it

- One nurse counts the apical pulse rate simultaneously with a second nurse who counts the radial pulse rate. The nurse counting the radial pulse uses his watch and calls the time for both nurses.
- Please note the apical pulse cannot be less than the radial pulse. If this occurs, you must take both pulses again.

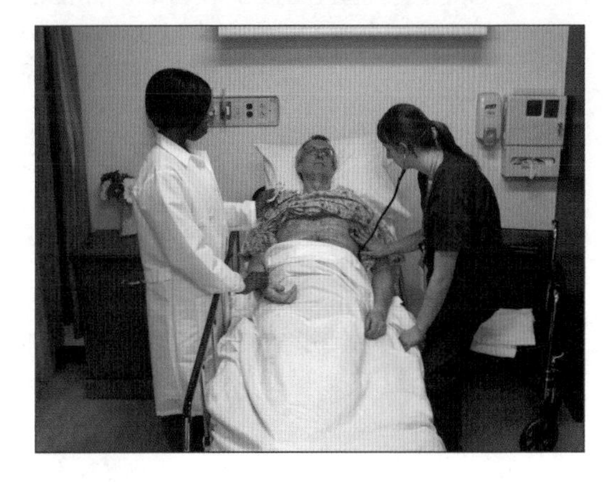

Practice pointers

- When the patient's peripheral pulse is irregular, take an apical pulse *to measure the heartbeat more directly*. (See *Documenting pulse*.)

Documenting pulse

1. Record the pulse rate and the site (example: rate 98, apical).
2. Record the rhythm as regular or irregular.
3. Record the strength as bounding (4+), full or strong (3+), normal and expected (2+), diminished or barely palpable (1+), or absent (0).

Blood pressure

The force of ventricular contractions, arterial wall elasticity, peripheral vascular resistance, and blood volume and viscosity affects blood pressure, which is the lateral force that blood exerts on arterial walls. Blood pressure measurements consist of systolic pressure and diastolic pressure readings. (See *Effects of age on blood pressure*.)

Systolic (contract) vs. diastolic (relax)

Systolic pressure occurs when the left ventricle contracts. It reflects the integrity of the heart, arteries, and arterioles. *Diastolic pressure* occurs when the left ventricle relaxes. It indicates blood vessel resistance. Both pressures are measured in millimeters of mercury with a sphygmomanometer (aneroid or mercury) and a stethoscope, usually at the brachial artery.

Systolic pressure − diastolic pressure = pulse pressure

Pulse pressure, or the difference between systolic and diastolic pressures, varies inversely with arterial elasticity. Normally, systolic pressure exceeds diastolic pressure by about 40 mm Hg. Narrowed pulse pressure, or a difference of less than 30 mm Hg, occurs when systolic pressure falls and diastolic pressure rises. These changes reflect reduced stroke volume, increased peripheral resistance, or both.

Widened pulse pressure, or a difference of more than 50 mm Hg between systolic and diastolic pressures, occurs when systolic pressure rises and diastolic pressure remains constant or when systolic pressure rises and diastolic pressure falls. These changes reflect increased stroke volume, decreased peripheral resistance, or both.

What you need

Sphygmomanometer ✻ stethoscope ✻ automated vital signs monitor (if available) ✻ cuff.

Cuffs come in six standard sizes, ranging from newborn to extra-large adult. Disposable cuffs are available. (See *Selecting the right cuff size*.)

Selecting the right cuff size

The "ideal" cuff should have a bladder length that is 80% and a width that is at least 40% of arm circumference (a length-to-width ratio of 2:1). A recent study comparing intra-arterial and auscultatory blood pressure concluded that the error is minimized with a cuff width of 46% of the arm circumference. The recommended cuff sizes are as follows:

- For arm circumference of 22 to 26 cm, the cuff should be "small adult" size: 12 × 22 cm.
- For arm circumference of 27 to 34 cm, the cuff should be "adult" size: 16 × 30 cm.
- For arm circumference of 35 to 44 cm, the cuff should be "large adult" size: 16 × 36 cm.
- For arm circumference of 45 to 52 cm, the cuff should be "adult thigh" size: 16 × 42 cm.
- There are also sizes for infants and children.

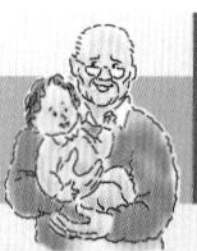

Ages and stages

Effects of age on blood pressure

Blood pressure changes with age. Below are normal blood pressure values, measured in millimeters of mercury (mm Hg), at different ages.

Neonate
- Systolic: 50 to 52
- Diastolic: 25 to 30
- Mean: 35 to 40

3 years
- Systolic: 78 to 114
- Diastolic: 46 to 78

10 years
- Systolic: 90 to 132
- Diastolic: 56 to 86

16 years
- Systolic: 104 to 108
- Diastolic: 60 to 92

Adult
- Systolic: 90 to 130
- Diastolic: 60 to 85

Older adult
- Systolic: 140 to 160
- Diastolic: 70 to 90

The automated vital signs monitor is a noninvasive device that measures pulse rate, systolic and diastolic pressures, and mean arterial pressure at preset intervals. (See *Using an electronic vital signs monitor*, page 18.)

Getting ready

Size matters

Carefully choose a cuff of appropriate size for the patient. *An excessively narrow cuff may cause a false-high reading; an excessively wide one, a false-low reading.* This is one of the most important steps to getting an accurate blood pressure measurement.

To use an automated vital signs monitor, collect the monitor, dual air hose, and pressure cuff. Then make sure the monitor unit is firmly positioned near the patient's bed.

How you do it

- Wash your hands and tell the patient that you're going to take his blood pressure.
- Position the patient:
  - Blood pressure measurement is most commonly done in the supine or sitting position.
  - The arm should be at the level of the right atrium and supported in that position to avoid muscle tension that will alter the measurement. In the supine position, the arm should be supported with a pillow to elevate the arm to the right atrium that is halfway between the bed and the sternum. In the sitting position, the right atrium is at the fourth intercostal space or the midpoint of the sternum.

Using an electronic vital signs monitor

An electronic vital signs monitor allows you to continually track a patient's vital signs, without having to reapply a blood pressure cuff each time. What's more, the patient won't need an invasive arterial line to gather similar data. The machine shown here is a Dinamap VS Monitor 8100, but the steps below can be followed with most other monitors.

Some automated vital signs monitors, such as the Dinamap, are lightweight and battery-operated and can be attached to an I.V. pole for continual monitoring, even during patient transfers. Make sure you know the capacity of the monitor's battery, and plug the machine in whenever possible to keep it charged.

Before using any monitor, check its accuracy. Determine the patient's pulse rate and blood pressure manually using the same arm you'll use for the monitor cuff. Compare your results when you get initial readings from the monitor. If the results differ, call your supply department or the manufacturer's representative.

Preparing the device

- Explain the procedure to the patient. Describe the alarm system so he won't be frightened if it's triggered.
- Make sure the power switch is off. Then plug the monitor into a properly grounded wall outlet. Secure the dual air hose to the front of the monitor.
- Connect the pressure cuff's tubing into the other ends of the dual air hose and tighten the connections to prevent air leaks. Keep the air hose away from the patient so that it isn't accidentally dislodged.
- Squeeze all air from the cuff and wrap the cuff loosely around the patient's arm or leg, allowing two fingerbreadths between the cuff and the arm or leg. Never apply the cuff to a limb that has an I.V. line in place or to an individual who has had breast or lymph node excision on that side or has an arteriovenous graft, shunt, or fistula. Position the cuff's "artery" arrow over the palpated brachial artery. Then secure the cuff for a snug fit.

Selecting parameters

- When you turn on the monitor, it will default to a manual mode. (In this mode, you can obtain vital signs yourself before switching to the automatic mode.) Press the AUTO/MANUAL button to select the automatic mode. The monitor will give you baseline data for the pulse rate, systolic and diastolic pressures, and mean arterial pressure.
- Compare your previous manual results with these baseline data. If they match, you're ready to set the alarm parameters. Press the SELECT button to blank out all displays except systolic pressure.
- Use the HIGH and LOW limit buttons to set the specific parameters for systolic pressure. (These limits range from a high of 240 to a low of 0.) You'll also do this three more times for mean arterial pressure, pulse rate, and diastolic pressure. After you have set the parameters for diastolic pressure, press the SELECT button again to display all current data. If you forget to do this last step, the monitor will automatically display current data 10 seconds after you set the last parameters.

Collecting data

- You also need to tell the monitor how often to obtain data. Press the SET button until you reach the desired time interval in minutes. If you have chosen the automatic mode, the monitor will display a default cycle time of 3 minutes. You can override the default cycle time to set the interval you prefer.
- You can obtain a set of vital signs any time by pressing the START button. Also, pressing the CANCEL button will stop the interval and deflate the cuff. You can retrieve stored data by pressing the PRIOR DATA button. The monitor will display the last data obtained along with the time elapsed since then. Scrolling backward, you can retrieve data from the previous 99 minutes.

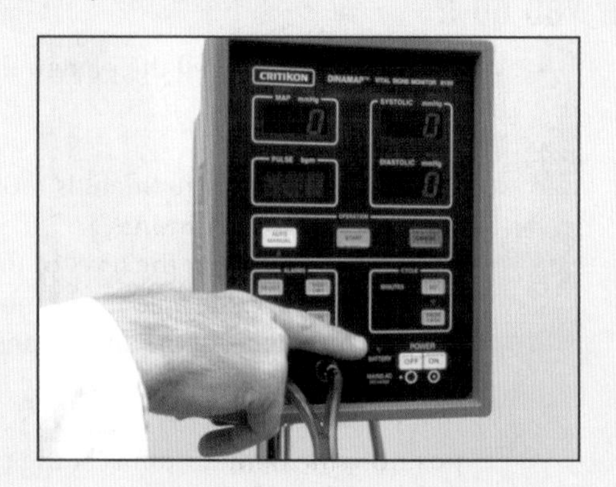

  - In the sitting position, the back should be supported and the feet should be flat on the floor; legs/ankles uncrossed. Crossing the legs can raise the systolic pressure by 2 to 8 mm Hg.
  - Neither the patient nor observer should talk during the blood pressure measurement.
- WARNING: Don't take a blood pressure measurement on the same arm of an arteriovenous fistula or hemodialysis shunt *because blood flow through the device may be compromised*. Don't take a blood pressure measurement on the affected side of a mastectomy *because it may compromise lymphatic circulation, worsen edema, and damage the arm*. Also, don't take blood pressure on the same arm as a peripherally inserted central catheter *because it may damage the device*.
- Select the appropriate cuff size. (See *Selecting the right cuff size*, page 17.)
- Palpate the brachial artery and place the midline of the bladder of the cuff (commonly marked on the cuff by the manufacturer) over the arterial pulsation on a *bare* arm if possible. Clothing can constrict the arm and alter the measurement.
  - The lower end of the cuff should be approximately 1″ (2.5 cm) above the antecubital fossa to allow for proper placement of the stethoscope.
  - For more information see "Choosing & Positioning a Blood Pressure Cuff" (http://www.youtube.com/watch?v=II0ioJNLnyg)

Go with the bell

- Palpate the brachial artery. Center the bell of the stethoscope over the part of the artery where you detect the strongest beats and hold it in place with one hand. *The bell of the stethoscope transmits low-pitched arterial blood sounds more effectively than does the diaphragm.*
- Using the thumb and index finger of your other hand, turn the thumbscrew on the rubber bulb of the air pump clockwise to close the valve.
- Pump air into the cuff while auscultating for the sound over the brachial artery *to compress and, eventually, occlude arterial blood flow*. Continue pumping air until the mercury column or aneroid gauge registers 160 mm Hg or at least 30 mm Hg above the level of the last audible sound.
- Carefully open the valve of the air pump. Then deflate the cuff no faster than 5 mm Hg/second while watching the mercury column or aneroid gauge and auscultating for the sound over the artery.

Tune in to the five sounds

- When you hear the first beat or clear tapping sound, note the pressure on the column or gauge—that is, the systolic pressure.

(The beat or tapping sound is the first of five Korotkoff sounds. The second sound resembles a murmur or swish; the third, crisp tapping; the fourth, a soft, muffled tone; and the fifth, the last sound heard.)

- Continue to release air gradually while auscultating for the sound over the artery.
- Note the diastolic pressure—the fifth Korotkoff sound. If you continue to hear sounds as the column or gauge falls to zero (common in children), record the pressure at the beginning of the fourth sound. *This step is important because, in some patients, a distinct fifth sound is absent.* (See *Korotkoff phases.*) (For information on situations that can cause false-high or false-low readings, see *Correcting problems of blood pressure measurement.*)
- http://www.youtube.com/watch?v=VJrLHePNDQ4— It is excellent!

Correcting problems of blood pressure measurement

Causes	Nursing actions
False-high reading	
• Cuff too small	• Make sure the cuff bladder is 20% wider than the circumference of the arm or leg being used for measurement.
• Cuff wrapped too loosely, reducing its effective width	• Tighten the cuff.
• Cuff deflated too slowly, causing venous congestion in the arm or leg	• Never deflate the cuff more slowly than 2 mm Hg per heartbeat.
• Mercury column tilted	• Read pressures with the mercury column vertical.
• Measurement poorly timed (for example, after the patient has eaten, ambulated, appeared anxious, or flexed his arm muscles)	• Postpone the blood pressure measurement or help the patient relax before measuring his blood pressure.
False-low reading	
• Arm or leg positioned incorrectly	• Make sure the patient's arm or leg is level with his heart.
• Mercury column below eye level	• Read the mercury column at eye level.
• Auscultatory gap (sound fades out for 10 to 15 mm Hg and then returns) unnoticed	• Estimate systolic pressure by palpation before measuring it. Then check this pressure against measured pressure.
• Low-volume sounds inaudible	• Before reinflating the cuff, instruct the patient to raise his arm or leg to decrease venous pressure and amplify low-volume sounds. After inflating the cuff, tell him to lower his arm or leg. Then deflate the cuff and listen. If you still fail to detect low-volume sounds, chart palpated systolic pressure.

Korotkoff phases

Phase	Sound	Cuff pressure (mm Hg)
Phase 1	Sharp thudding sound	120 to 100
Phase 2	Blowing or whooshing sound	110 to 100
Phase 3	Softer thump (softer than phase 1)	100 to 90
Phase 4	Softer blowing sound that fades	80 to 90
Phase 5	Silence	80 and below

- Do not round up the numbers when recording blood pressure measurements. Record the actual numbers you auscultate. Rounding up can lead to false-high readings and affect clinical decision making.

One mo' time

- Rapidly deflate the cuff. Record the pressure, wait 30 seconds, and then repeat the procedure and record the pressures *to confirm your original findings*. After doing so, remove and fold the cuff and return it to storage.

Practice pointers

- If you can't auscultate the patient's blood pressure, you can estimate systolic pressure. To do this, first palpate the brachial or radial pulse. Then inflate the cuff until you no longer detect the pulse. Slowly deflate the cuff and when you detect the pulse again, record the pressure as the palpated systolic pressure.
- Palpation of systolic blood pressure may also be important *to avoid underestimating results in patients with an auscultatory gap*. This gap is a loss of sound between the first and second Korotkoff sounds and may be as great as 40 mm Hg. You may find this in patients with venous congestion or hypertension.
- Clinical setting
  - If you obtain a blood pressure measurement greater than 140/90 mm Hg, repeat the blood pressure prior to the patient leaving the office. If the second reading remains greater than 140/90 mm Hg, notify the provider. Document both readings and the site.

- There is something known as a white coat effect when the medical office blood pressure is higher than the average daytime ambulatory blood pressure. It is thought to be caused by the presence of the physician. It can be minimized, but not always eliminated, by taking a series of five automated blood pressures over 15 to 20 minutes in the clinic/office.
- When rooming a patient, have the patient sit quietly for 5 minutes before taking the blood pressure to decrease anxiety and reduce the effects of exercise from walking into the room.
- If the patient is on antihypertensive medications, always ask and document if the medicine was taken that day and when.
- Elderly patients should have their blood pressure taken sitting and standing because they commonly have postural hypotension. Record both readings and the position.

Write it down

Documenting blood pressure

On the patient's chart, record systolic pressure over diastolic pressure (for example, 120/78 mm Hg); if necessary, record systolic pressure over two diastolic pressures (for example, 120/78/20 mm Hg). Chart an auscultatory gap, if present. If your facility requires you to chart blood pressures on a graph, use dots or check marks. Also, document the extremity used and the patient's position.

Make adjustments for special circumstances

- If your patient is crying or anxious, delay measuring his blood pressure, if possible, until he calms down *to avoid falsely elevated readings.*
- If your patient is taking an antihypertensive, measure his blood pressure while he's in a sitting position *to ensure accurate results.*
- When hypertension is suspected, single readings of blood pressure aren't as significant as are patterns of blood pressure over a period of time. (See *Documenting blood pressure*.)
- If a patient has an abnormally large arm circumference and the arm length is short, place a proper fitting cuff on the forearm, support the arm at the heart level, and feel for the appearance of the radial pulse. This will provide at least a general estimate of the systolic blood pressure.

Respiration

Respiration is the exchange of oxygen and carbon dioxide between the atmosphere and the body. External respiration, or breathing, occurs through the work of the diaphragm and chest muscles and delivers oxygen to the lower respiratory tract and alveoli.

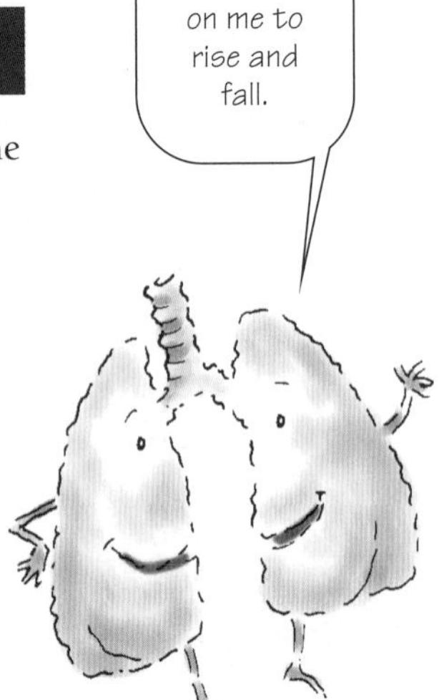
Count on me to rise and fall.

Rate, rhythm, depth, and sound

Respiration can be measured according to rate, rhythm, depth, and sound. These measurements reflect the body's metabolic state, diaphragm and chest muscle condition, and airway patency.

Respiratory rate is recorded as the number of cycles per minute, with inspiration and expiration making up one cycle. Rhythm is the regularity of these cycles. Depth is recorded as the volume of air inhaled and exhaled with each respiration and sound as the audible digression from normal, effortless breathing.

What you need

A watch with a second hand and a stethoscope.

How you do it

- The best time to assess your patient's respirations is immediately after taking his pulse rate. Keep your fingertips over his radial artery and don't tell him that you're counting respirations; *otherwise, he'll become conscious of them and the rate may change.*

Watch the movement

- Count respirations by observing the rise and fall of the patient's chest as he breathes. Alternatively, position the patient's opposite arm across his chest and count respirations by feeling its rise and fall. Consider one rise and one fall one respiration.
- Count respirations for 30 seconds and multiply by 2 or count for 60 seconds if respirations are irregular *to account for variations in respiratory rate and pattern.*
- Observe chest movements for depth of respirations. If the patient inhales a small volume of air, record the depth as shallow; if he inhales a large volume, deep.
- Observe the patient for use of accessory muscles, such as the scalene, sternocleidomastoid, trapezius, and latissimus dorsi. Such use indicates weakness of the diaphragm and the external intercostal muscles—the major muscles of respiration.
- Adults with COPD will often lean forward and rest their hands on the bed or chair to improve their breathing (tripod position). This helps increase lung expansion.

Listen to the sounds

- As you count respirations, watch for and record such breath sounds as stertor, stridor, wheezing, and expiratory grunting.
- *Stertor* is a snoring sound resulting from secretions in the trachea and large bronchi. Listen for it in comatose patients and in patients with a neurologic disorder.
- *Stridor* is an inspiratory crowing sound that occurs in patients with laryngitis, croup, or upper respiratory tract obstruction with a foreign body. (See *How age affects respiration.*)

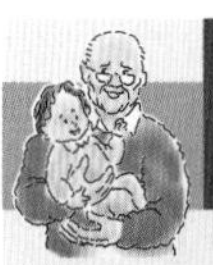

Ages and stages

How age affects respiration

When assessing respirations in pediatric and older patients, keep these points in mind:

- When listening for stridor in infants and children with croup or asthma, check for sternal, substernal, and intercostal retractions.
- In infants, an expiratory grunt indicates imminent respiratory distress.
- In older patients, an expiratory grunt indicates partial airway obstruction.
- A child's respiratory rate may double in response to exercise, illness, or emotion.
- Normally, the rate for newborns is 30 to 80 breaths/minute; for toddlers, 20 to 40 breaths/minute; and for children of school age and older, 15 to 25 breaths/minute.
- Children usually reach the adult rate (12 to 20 breaths/minute) at about age 15.

- *Wheezing* is caused by partial obstruction in the smaller bronchi and bronchioles. This high-pitched, musical sound is common in patients with emphysema or asthma.
- To detect other breath sounds—such as crackles and rhonchi—or the lack of them, you'll need a stethoscope.
- Watch the patient's chest movements and listen to breathing to determine the rhythm and sound of respirations. (See *Identifying respiratory patterns*.)

Identifying respiratory patterns

Type	Characteristics	Pattern	Possible causes
Apnea	Periodic absence of breathing		• Mechanical airway obstruction • Conditions affecting the brain's respiratory center in lateral medulla oblongata
Apneustic	Prolonged, gasping inspiration followed by extremely short, inefficient expiration		• Lesions of respiratory center
Bradypnea	Slow, regular respirations of equal depth		• Normal pattern during sleep • Conditions affecting respiratory center: tumors, metabolic disorders, respiratory decompensation, and use of opiates or alcohol
Cheyne-Stokes	Fast, deep respirations of 30 to 170 seconds punctuated by periods of apnea lasting 20 to 60 seconds		• Increased intracranial pressure, severe heart failure, renal failure, meningitis, drug overdose, and cerebral anoxia
Eupnea	Normal rate and rhythm		• Normal respiration
Kussmaul	Fast (over 20 breaths/minute), deep (resembling sighs), labored respirations without pause		• Renal failure and metabolic acidosis, particularly diabetic ketoacidosis
Tachypnea	Rapid respirations, rate rises with body temperature at about 4 breaths/minute for each degree Fahrenheit above normal		• Pneumonia, compensatory respiratory alkalosis, respiratory insufficiency, lesions of the respiratory center, and salicylate poisoning

Practice pointers

- Respiratory rates of less than 8 breaths/minute or more than 40 breaths/minute are usually considered abnormal and should be reported promptly.
- Observe the patient for signs of dyspnea, such as an anxious facial expression, flaring nostrils, a heaving chest wall, and cyanosis. To detect cyanosis, look for the characteristic bluish discoloration of the nail beds and lips, under the tongue, in the buccal mucosa, and in the conjunctiva.
- When assessing a patient's respiratory status, consider personal and family history. Ask if he smokes and, if he does, the number of years and the number of packs per day. (See *Documenting respirations*.)

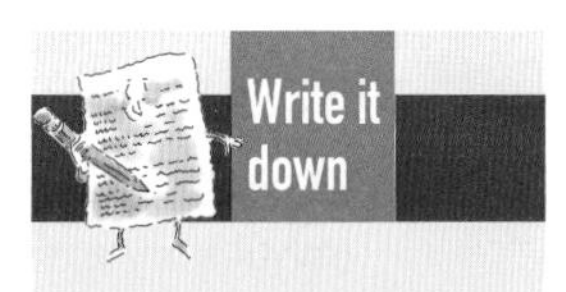
Write it down

Documenting respirations

Record the rate, depth, rhythm, and sound of the patient's respirations.

Height and weight

Height and weight are routinely measured when a patient is admitted to a health care facility. An accurate record of the patient's height and weight is essential for calculating dosages of drugs and contrast agents, assessing the patient's nutritional status, and determining the height-to-weight ratio.

What weight tells you

Because body weight is the best overall indicator of fluid status, daily monitoring is important for patients receiving a diuretic or a medication that causes sodium retention. Rapid weight gain may signal fluid retention; rapid weight loss, diuresis.

Scales for every position

Weight can be measured with a standing scale, chair scale, or bed scale. Height can be measured with the measuring bar on a standing scale or with a tape measure for a patient confined to a supine position.

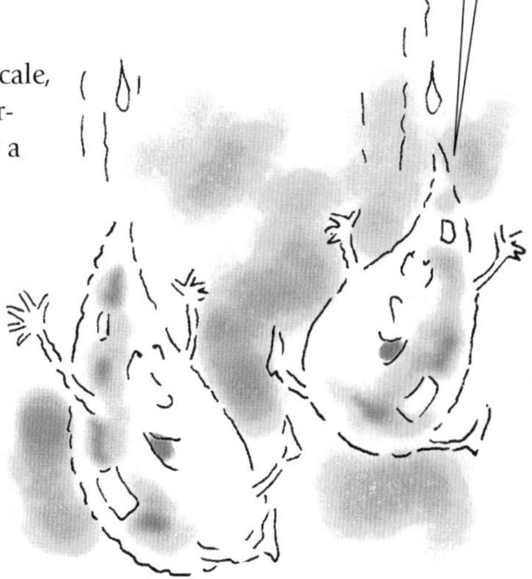
Body weight is the best indicator of fluid status.

What you need

Standing scale with measuring bar or chair or bed scale ✱ wheelchair if needed (to transport patient) ✱ tape measure if needed.

Getting ready

Select the appropriate scale—usually, a standing scale for an ambulatory patient or a chair or bed scale for an acutely ill or debilitated patient. Then make sure the scale is balanced. Standing scales and, to a lesser extent, bed scales may become unbalanced when transported.

How you do it

- Tell the patient that you're going to measure his height and weight. Explain the procedure to him, depending on which type of scale you'll use: standing, chair, or bed.

Using a standing scale

- Place a paper towel on the scale's platform.
- Tell the patient to remove his robe and slippers or shoes. If the scale has wheels, lock them before the patient steps on. Assist the patient onto the scale and remain close to him *to prevent falls*.

That's upright balance

- If you're using an upright balance scale, slide the lower rider to the groove representing the largest increment below the patient's estimated weight. Grooves represent 50, 100, 150, and 200 lb.
- Slide the small upper rider until the beam balances. Add the upper and lower rider figures to determine the weight.

That's multiple weight

- If using a multiple-weight scale, move the appropriate ratio weights onto the weight holder to balance the scale; ratio weights are labeled 50, 100, and 200 lb.
- Add ratio weights until the next weight causes the main beam to fall.
- Adjust the main beam poise until the scale balances.
- To obtain the weight, add the sum of the ratio weights to the figure on the main beam.
- Return ratio weights to their rack and the weight holder to its proper place.

That's digital

- If you're using a digital scale, make sure the display reads 0 before use.
- Read the display with the patient standing as still as possible.

Raising the bar

- If you're measuring height, tell the patient to stand erect on the scale's platform. Raise the measuring bar above the patient's head, extend the horizontal arm and lower the bar until it touches the top of the patient's head. Then read the patient's height.
- Help the patient off the scale and give him his robe and slippers or shoes. Then return the measuring bar to its initial position.

Using a chair scale

- Transport the patient to the weighing area or the scale to the patient's bedside.
- Lock the scale in place *to prevent it from moving accidentally.*
- If you're using a scale with a swing-away chair arm, unlock the arm. When unlocked, the arm swings back 180 degrees *to permit easy access.*
- Position the scale beside the patient's bed or wheelchair with the chair arm open. Transfer the patient onto the scale, swing the chair arm to the front of the scale and lock it in place.
- Weigh the patient by adding ratio weights and adjusting the main beam poise. Then unlock the swing-away chair arm as before and transfer the patient back to his bed or wheelchair.
- Lock the main beam *to avoid damaging the scale during transport.* Then unlock the wheels and remove the scale from the patient's room.

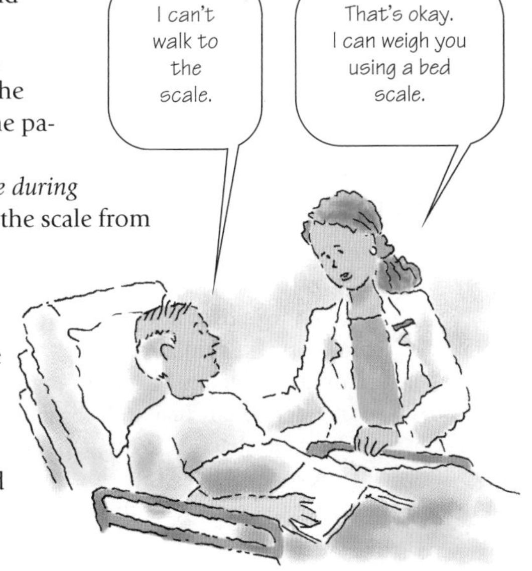
I can't walk to the scale.
That's okay. I can weigh you using a bed scale.

Using a bed scale

- Provide privacy and tell the patient that you're going to weigh him on a special bed scale.

That's multiple weight

- Position the scale next to the patient's bed and lock the scale's wheels. Then turn the patient on his side, facing away from the scale.
- Release the stretcher frame to the horizontal position and pump the hand lever until the stretcher is positioned over the mattress. Lower the stretcher onto the mattress and roll the patient onto the stretcher.
- Raise the stretcher 2" (5.1 cm) above the mattress. Then add ratio weights and adjust the main beam poise as for the standing and chair scales.
- After weighing the patient, lower the stretcher onto the mattress, turn the patient on his side, and remove the stretcher. Be sure to leave the patient in a comfortable position.

That's digital

- Release the stretcher to the horizontal position, then lock it in place. Turn the patient on his side, facing away from the scale.
- Roll the base of the scale under the patient's bed. Adjust the lever *to widen the base of the scale, providing stability*. Then lock the scale's wheels.
- Center the stretcher above the bed, lower it onto the mattress, and roll the patient onto the stretcher. Then position the circular weighing arms of the scale over the patient and attach them securely to the stretcher bars.
- Pump the handle with long, slow strokes *to raise the patient a few inches off the bed*. Make sure that he doesn't lean on or touch the headboard, side rails, or other bed equipment *because doing so will affect weight measurement.*
- Depress the OPERATE button and read the patient's weight on the digital display panel. Then press in the scale's handle *to lower the patient.*
- Detach the circular weighing arms from the stretcher bars, roll the patient off the stretcher and remove it, and position him comfortably in bed.
- Release the wheel lock and withdraw the scale. Return the stretcher to its vertical position.

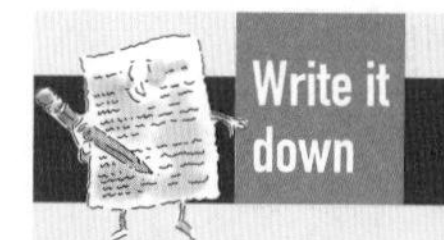

Documenting height and weight

Record the patient's height and weight on the nursing assessment form and other medical records, as required by your facility.

Practice pointers

- Reassure and steady patients who are at risk for losing their balance on a scale.
- Weigh the patient at the same time each day (usually before breakfast), in similar clothing, and using the same scale. If the patient uses crutches, weigh him with the crutches. Then weigh the crutches and any heavy clothing and subtract their weight from the total to determine the patient's weight.
- Before using a bed scale, cover its stretcher with a drawsheet. Balance the scale with the drawsheet in place *to ensure an accurate measurement.*
- When rolling the patient onto the stretcher, be careful not to dislodge I.V. lines, indwelling catheters, and other supportive equipment. (See *Documenting height and weight.*)

Restraint-free environment

The use of restraints was one strategy used to prevent patients at risk for falling, wandering, and pulling out peripheral lines and tubes from injury. The Centers for Medicare and Medicaid Services (CMS) and Joint Commission has made a concerted effort to reduce the use of restraints and to only use them when all other efforts fail.

A restraint-free environment should be the goal for all patients because of the risks associated with physical restraints. There are many alternatives such as sitters, bed alarms, telesitters, and frequent rounding that should be tried before using physical restraints.

How you do it

- Assess the patient's mental status, falls risk, and medications that can put the patient at risk for injury.
- Orient patient and family to surroundings to promote patient understanding and enlist cooperation.
- Use consistent caregivers when possible to increase familiarity and reduce anxiety.
- Place in a room close to the nurse's station and use hourly rounding to reduce the risk of falls in a high-risk patient.
- Make sure the patient has glasses, hearing aids, and any other sensory devices on.
- Keep the patient oriented by providing visual cues; sensory stimuli such as calendar, music, and television; and natural lighting when possible.
- Meet patient's basic needs such as toileting, pain control, meals, and so forth in a timely manner.
- Ambulate patient or turn him on a regular schedule and allow him times of uninterrupted rest.
- Position catheters and tubes out of the patient's reach and/or view by wrapping them with dressings or using undergarments as appropriate.
- Provide a wedge cushion when a patient is in the chair to make it difficult for the patient to get up.
- Use pressure-sensitive bed or chair alarms to alert you to the patient getting up to prevent falls.

Practice pointers

- Telesitters use cameras to monitor several patients at once at a central monitoring station. The observer monitors the patients and can use the audio device to instruct the patient, for example, to lay back down; orient them to their surroundings; or reassure them.
- CAUTION: Family members are helpful in watching these patients; however, please note the patient is still the hospital's responsibility and is liable for the patient. They are not a substitute for the staff monitoring and assessing the patient.

- Home care patients who are at risk for falls and injury or have alterations in their mental status may need close supervision. Caregivers need to be aware of this and be able to provide the necessary supervision. Consult with case management/social workers if the caregivers are not able to provide this level of supervision. They will research alternatives such as home health care or possibly an extended care facility.

Documentation

- All alternatives to restraints that are attempted
- Patient behaviors and responses to interventions
- Patient and family education
- Referral to case management as appropriate

Restraint application

A physical restraint is defined by CMS as any manual method, physical or mechanical device, material, or equipment that immobilizes or reduces the ability of a patient to move his or her extremities, body, or head freely. A restraint or seclusion can only be imposed to ensure the immediate physical safety of the patient, a staff member, or others and must be discontinued at the earliest time possible based on individual assessment and reevaluation. However, the decision to discontinue the intervention should be based on the determination that the need for restraint or seclusion is no longer present or that the patient's needs can be addressed using less restrictive methods. Review the hospital policies and procedures regarding restraints and seclusion.

Soft restraints limit movement to prevent the confused, disoriented, or combative patient from injuring himself or others. Vest and belt restraints, which permit full movement of arms and legs, are used to prevent falls from a bed or a chair. Limb restraints, which allow only slight limb motion, are used to prevent the patient from removing supportive equipment (such as I.V. lines, indwelling catheters, and nasogastric tubes). Mitts prevent the patient from removing supportive equipment, scratching rashes or sores, and injuring himself or others. Body restraints, which immobilize all or most of the body, are used to control the combative or hysterical patient.

When you need something a little stronger

When soft restraints aren't sufficient and sedation is dangerous or ineffective, use leather restraints, which may be applied to all limbs (four-point restraints) or to one arm and one leg (two-point restraints) depending on the patient's behavior. The duration of such restraint is governed by state law and facility policy.

A note of caution

Because restraints increase the risk of fracture and trauma, they must be used cautiously in patients prone to seizures. Restraints can cause skin irritation and restrict blood flow, so they shouldn't be applied directly over wounds or I.V. catheters. Vest restraints should be used with caution in patients with heart failure or a respiratory disorder. Such restraints can tighten with movement, further limiting circulation and respiratory function.

Know your law. The duration of leather restraint use is governed by state law and facility policy.

What you need

For soft restraints

Vest, belt, limb, or body restraints or mitts, as needed ✳ gauze pads or washcloth if needed.

For leather restraints

Two wrist and two ankle leather restraints ✳ four straps ✳ key ✳ large gauze pads to cushion each extremity.

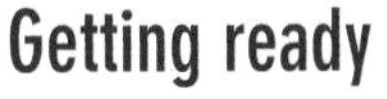

Getting ready

Before entering the patient's room, make sure the restraints are the correct size using the patient's build and weight as a guide. If you use leather restraints, make sure the straps are unlocked and the key fits the locks.

For a child, who may be too small for standard restraints, use child restraints. (See *Types of child restraints*, page 32.)

How you do it

- Obtain a doctor's order for the restraint. Keep in mind that the doctor's order must be time limited—4 hours for adults, 2 hours for children and adolescents ages 9 to 17, and 1 hour for patients under age 9. The original order may be renewed only for a total of 24 hours. After the original order expires, the doctor must see and evaluate the patient before a new order can be written.

Make it a team effort

- If necessary, enlist the help of several coworkers and organize their effort before entering the patient's room, giving each person a specific task; for example, one person explains the procedure to the patient and applies the restraints while the others immobilize the arms and legs.

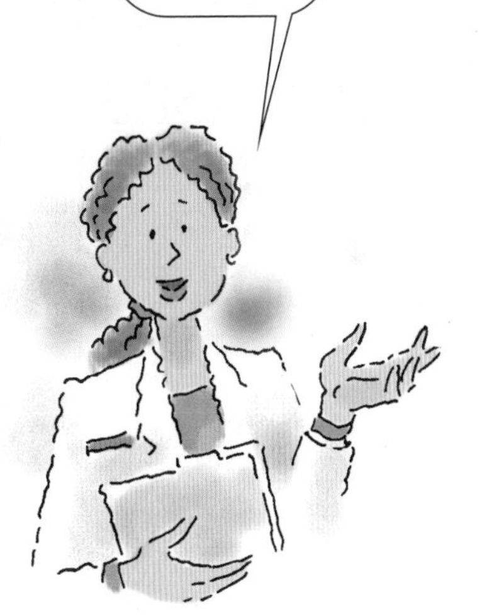
A restraint order must have a time limit.

Types of child restraints

You may need to restrain an infant or a child to prevent injury or to facilitate examination, diagnostic tests, or treatment. If so, follow these steps:

- Provide a simple explanation, reassurance, and constant observation to minimize the child's fear.
- Explain the restraint to the parents and enlist their help.
- Reassure them that the restraints won't hurt the child.
- Make sure restraint ties or safety pins are secured outside the child's reach to prevent injury.
- When using a mummy restraint, secure the infant's arms in proper alignment with the body to avoid dislocation and other injuries.

Vest

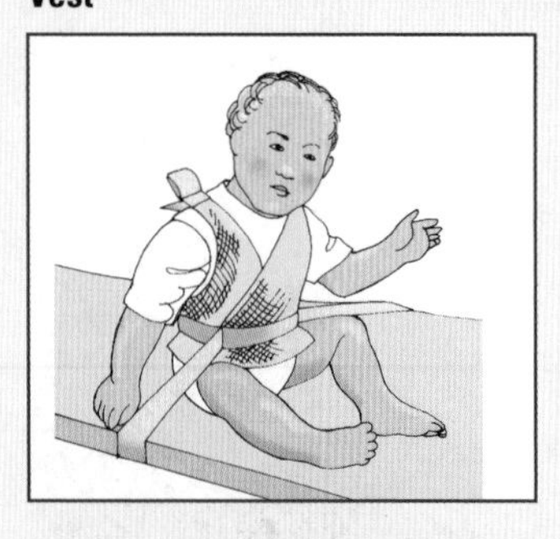

Elbow

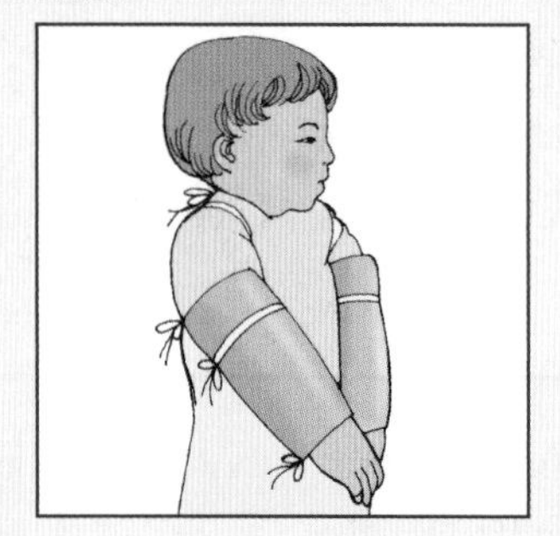

Mummy

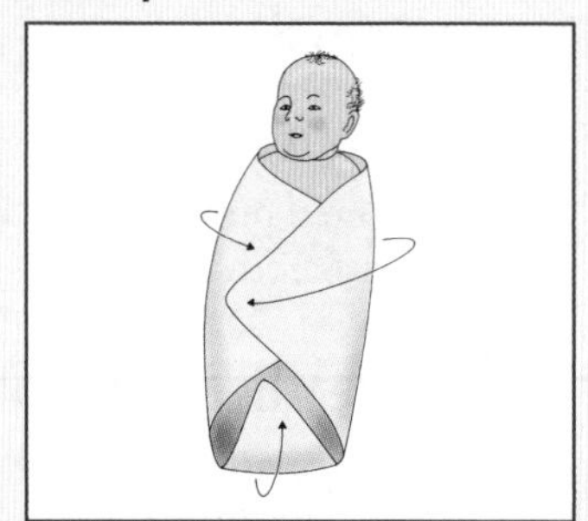

Belt

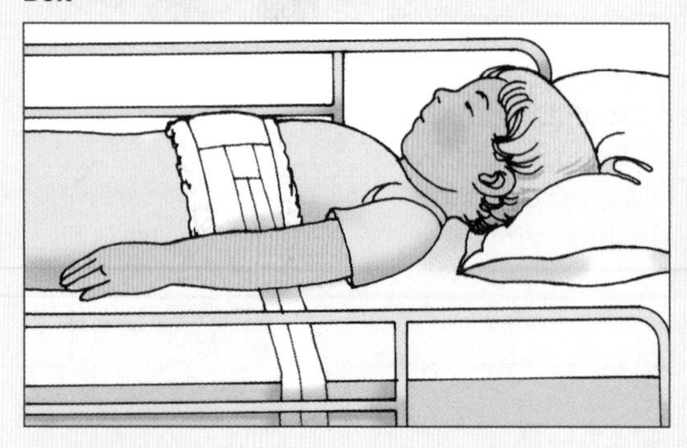

Limb

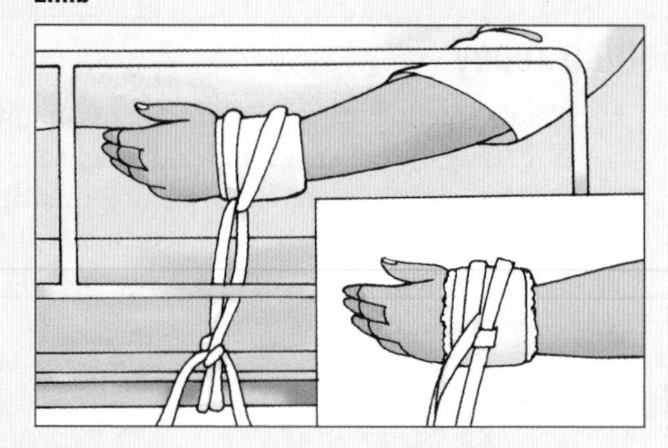

Crib with net

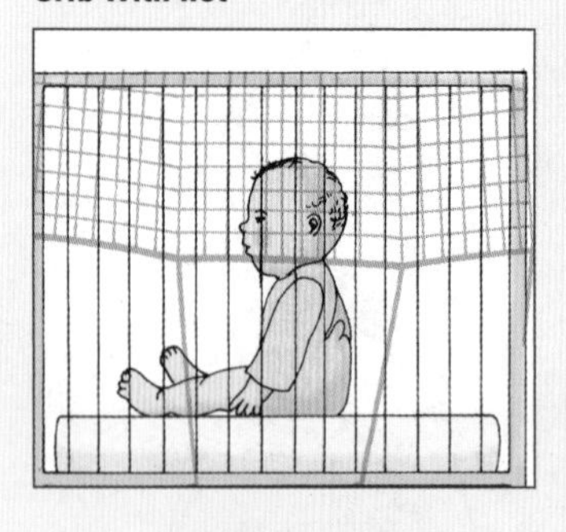

Mitt

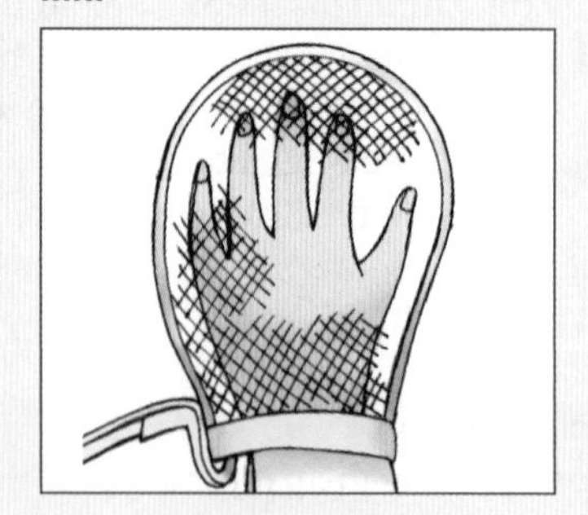

Restraining board

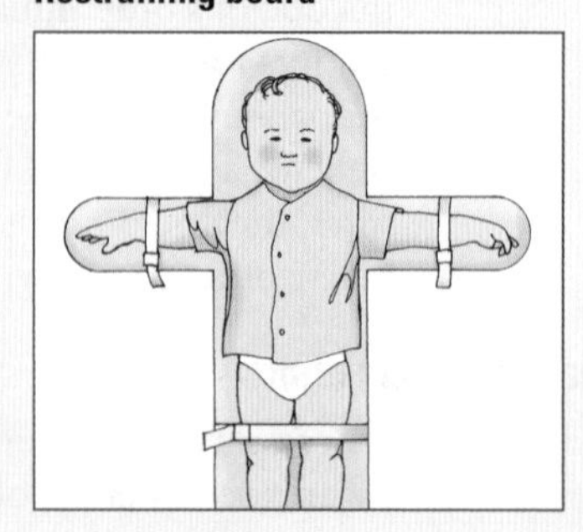

Keep the patient informed

- Tell the patient what you're about to do and describe the restraints to him. Assure him that they're being used to protect him from injury rather than to punish him.

Applying a vest restraint

- Assist the patient to a sitting position if his condition permits.

Cross in front for safety

- Slip the vest over the patient's gown. Crisscross the cloth flaps at the front, placing the V-shaped opening at his throat. Never crisscross the flaps at the back *because this may cause him to choke if he tries to squirm out of the vest.*

Keep it a little loose

- Pass the tab on one flap through the slot on the opposite flap and adjust the vest for the patient's comfort. You should be able to slip your fist between the vest and the patient. Avoid wrapping the vest too tightly *because doing so may restrict his breathing.*

It's all in the knot

- Tie all restraints securely to the frame of the bed, chair, or wheelchair, out of the patient's reach, using a bow or a knot that can be released quickly and easily in an emergency. (See *Knots for securing soft restraints,* page 34.) Never tie a regular knot to secure the straps.
- Leave 1″ to 2″ (2.5 to 5 cm) of slack in the straps *to allow room for movement.*

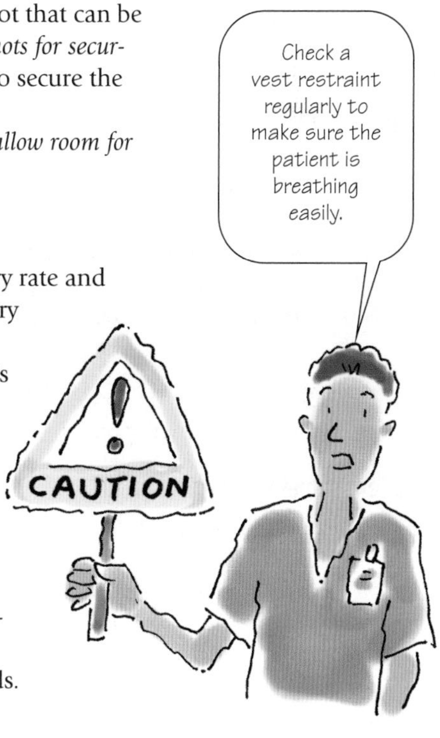

Check a vest restraint regularly to make sure the patient is breathing easily.

Watch the breathing

- After applying the vest, check the patient's respiratory rate and breath sounds regularly. Watch for signs of respiratory distress.
- Make sure the vest hasn't tightened with the patient's movement. Loosen the vest frequently, if possible, so the patient can stretch, turn, and breathe deeply.

CAUTION

Applying a limb restraint

- Wrap the patient's wrist or ankle with gauze pads to reduce friction between the patient's skin and the restraint, helping to prevent irritation and skin breakdown. Then wrap the restraint around the gauze pads.

Knots for securing soft restraints

When securing soft restraints, use knots that can be released quickly and easily, such as those shown below. Remember, never secure restraints to the bed's side rails.

Magnus hitch

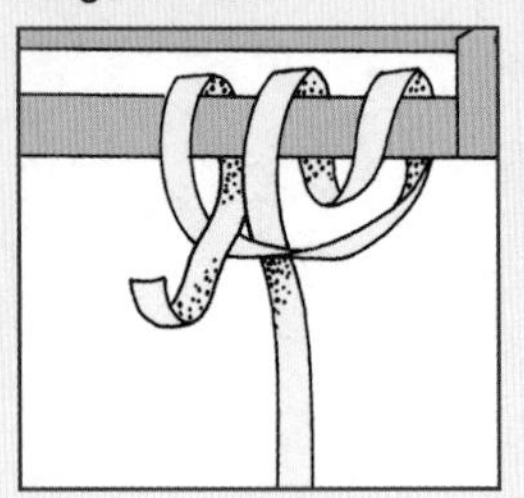

Clove hitch

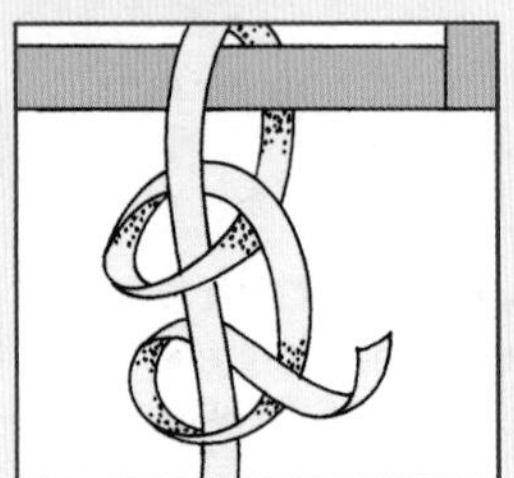

Loop

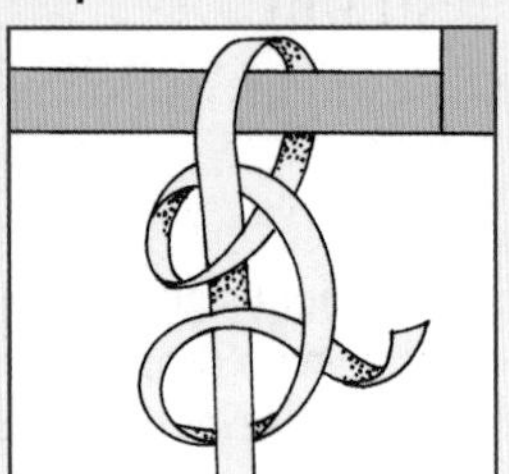

Reverse clove hitch

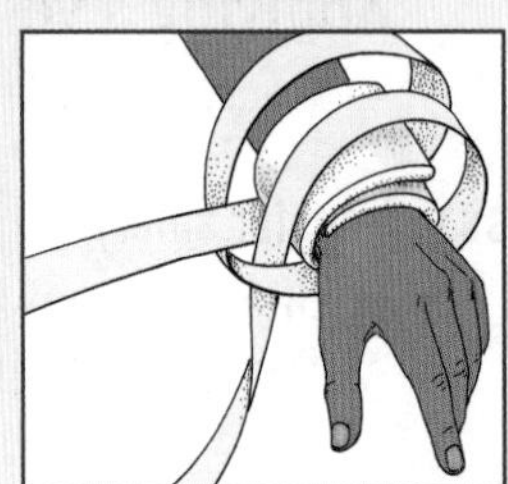

Not too tight

- Pass the strap on the narrow end of the restraint through the slot in the broad end and adjust for a snug fit. Or fasten the buckle or Velcro cuffs to fit the restraint. You should be able to slip one or two fingers between the restraint and the patient's skin. Avoid applying the restraint too tightly *because it may impair circulation distal to the restraint.*
- Tie the restraint as you would a vest restraint using a bow or a knot that can be released quickly and easily in an emergency.

Keep 'em moving

- After applying limb restraints, watch for signs of impaired circulation in the extremity distal to the restraint. If the skin appears blue or feels cold, or if the patient complains of a tingling sensation or numbness, loosen the restraint.
- Perform range-of-motion (ROM) exercises regularly *to stimulate circulation and prevent contractures and loss of mobility.*

Applying a mitt restraint

- Wash and dry the patient's hands.

Give 'em something to hold on to

- Roll up a washcloth or gauze pad and place it in the patient's palm. Have him form a loose fist, if possible, then pull the mitt over it and secure the closure.
- *To restrict the patient's arm movement,* attach the strap to the mitt and tie it securely using a bow or a knot that can be released quickly and easily in an emergency.

Make sure the blood keeps moving

- When using mitts made of transparent mesh, check hand movement and skin color frequently *to assess circulation.*
- Remove the mitts regularly *to stimulate circulation* and perform passive ROM exercises *to prevent contractures.*

Applying a belt restraint

- Center the flannel pad of the belt on the bed. Then wrap the short strap of the belt around the bed frame and fasten it under the bed.
- Position the patient on the pad. Then have him roll slightly to one side while you guide the long strap around his waist and through the slot in the pad.
- Wrap the long strap around the bed frame and fasten it under the bed.

Getting the right fit

- After applying the belt, slip your hand between the patient and the belt *to ensure a secure but comfortable fit.* A loose belt can be raised to chest level; a tight one can cause abdominal discomfort.

Applying a body (Posey net) restraint

- Place the restraint flat on the bed, with arm and wrist cuffs facing down and the V at the head of the bed.
- Place the patient in the prone position on top of the restraint.
- Lift the V over the patient's head. Thread the chest belt through one of the loops in the V *to ensure a snug fit.*
- Secure the straps around the patient's chest, thighs, and legs. Then turn the patient on his back.
- Secure the straps to the bed frame *to anchor the restraint.* Then secure the straps around the patient's arms and wrists.

Applying leather restraints

- Place the patient in a supine position on the bed, with each arm and leg securely held down *to minimize combative behavior and to prevent injury.*

Keep 'em at the joints

- Immobilize the patient's arms and legs at the knees, ankles, shoulders, and wrists *to minimize his movement without exerting excessive force.*
- Apply gauze pads to the patient's wrists and ankles *to reduce friction between his skin and the leather and prevent skin irritation and breakdown.*

Not too tight, but not too loose

- Wrap the restraint around the gauze pads and insert the metal loop through the hole that gives the best fit.
- Apply the restraints securely but not too tightly. You should be able to slip one or two fingers between the restraint and the patient's skin. *A tight restraint can compromise circulation; a loose one can slip off or move up the patient's arm or leg and cause skin irritation and breakdown.*
- Thread the strap through the metal loop on the restraint, close the metal loop, and secure the strap to the bed frame, out of the patient's reach.

Flex, lock, and release

- Flex the patient's arm or leg slightly before locking the strap *to allow room for movement and to prevent joints from locking in place or dislocating.*
- Lock the restraint by pushing in the button on the side of the metal loop and tug it gently *to make sure it's secure.* After it's secure, a coworker can release the arm or leg.
- Place the key in an accessible location at the nurse's station.

Give 'em a break

- Check the patient's pulse rate and vital signs at least every 2 hours.
- Remove or loosen the restraints one at a time, every 2 hours, and perform passive ROM exercises if possible. To unlock the restraint, insert the key into the metal loop, opposite the locking button. This releases the lock, and the metal loop can be opened.
- Watch for signs of impaired peripheral circulation such as cool, cyanotic skin.
- Observe the patient regularly and offer emotional support.

Don't restrain a patient in the prone position. Doing so intensifies feelings of helplessness and can even impair respiration.

Practice pointers

- Know facility policy on using restraints. You may be able to apply them in an emergency without a doctor's order or you may need the family to sign a consent form first.
- Know state regulations on using restraints. Some states prohibit the use of four-point restraints.

Positioning the patient and the restraints

- Don't restrain a patient in the prone position. This position limits his field of vision,

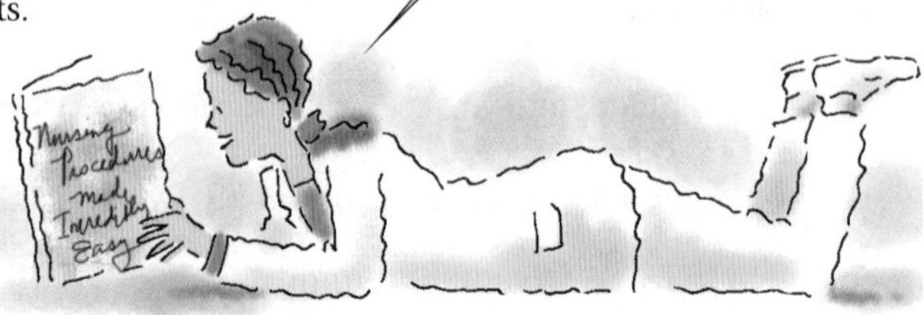

intensifies feelings of helplessness and vulnerability, and impairs respiration.

- When the patient is at high risk for aspiration, restrain him on his side. Never secure all four restraints to one side of the bed *because the patient may fall out of bed.*
- Never secure restraints to the side rails *because someone might inadvertently lower the rail and cause the patient discomfort and trauma.*
- Never secure restraints to the fixed frame of the bed if his position is to be changed.
- After assessing the patient's behavior and condition, you may decide to use a two-point restraint, which should restrain an arm and the opposite leg—for example, the right arm and the left leg. Never restrain an arm and leg on the same side *because the patient may fall out of bed.*
- Don't apply a limb restraint above an I.V. site *because the constriction may occlude the infusion or cause infiltration into surrounding tissue.*
- Nursing assistive personnel (NAP) are only permitted to apply and routinely check a restraint. Only licensed personnel can assess the patient's behavior, level of orientation, the need for restraint, they type of restraint, and ongoing assessments. You can instruct the NAP by:
  - Reviewing correct placement of the restraint; checking the patient's circulation, skin condition, and breathing
  - Reviewing how to routinely toilet, providing ROM exercises, changing the patient's position, and providing skin care
  - Instruct to notify you immediately of behavior changes, skin integrity, difficulty breathing, and decreased circulation to extremities
  - Please refer to your facilities policies and procedures.
- There are regulations from the CMS and state laws that have specific requirements for ordering restraints that should be reflected in your facility's policies.
  - CMS also cautions that restraints should not be considered as part of a falls prevention program because there is no evidence to support they reduce falls and often cause more serious injury during a fall.

Check in regularly

- Because the restrained patient has limited mobility, his nutrition, elimination, and positioning become your responsibility. *To prevent pressure ulcers,* reposition the patient regularly and massage and pad bony prominences and other vulnerable areas.
- Inspect the patient and the restraints every 15 to 30 minutes. Release the restraints every 2 hours, with a coworker on hand to

help restrain him if necessary. Assess the patient's pulse and skin condition and perform ROM exercises. Document all assessments and findings and evaluate the continued need for the restraints.
- Provide regular toileting. (See *Documenting restraint use.*)

Documenting restraint use

Document restraint use hourly on a restraint flow sheet. Record:
- behavior that necessitated restraints
- when the restraints were applied and removed
- type of restraints used
- routine observations usually over 15 minutes: patient's vital signs, skin condition, respiratory status, peripheral circulation, and mental status.

Passive range-of-motion exercises

Passive ROM exercises improve or maintain joint mobility and help prevent contractures. Performed by a nurse, a physical therapist, or a caregiver of the patient's choosing, these exercises are indicated for the patient with temporary or permanent loss of mobility, sensation, or consciousness. Passive ROM exercises require recognition of the patient's limits of motion and support of all joints during movement.

Passive ROM exercises are contraindicated in patients with septic joints, acute thrombophlebitis, severe arthritic joint inflammation, or recent trauma with possible hidden fractures or internal injuries.

How you do it

- Determine the joints that need ROM exercises and consult the doctor or physical therapist about limitations or precautions for specific exercises.
- The exercises discussed here treat all joints, but they don't have to be performed in the order given or all at once. You can schedule them over the course of a day, whenever the patient is in the most convenient position. Remember to perform all exercises slowly, gently, and to the end of the normal ROM or to the point of pain but no further. (See *Types of joint motion.*)
- Before you begin, raise the bed to a comfortable working height.

Exercising the neck

- Support the patient's head with your hands and extend his neck, flex his chin to his chest, and tilt his head laterally toward each shoulder.
- Rotate his head from right to left.

Exercising the shoulder

- Support the patient's arm in an extended, neutral position; extend his forearm and flex it back. Abduct his arm outward from the side of his body and adduct it back to his side.

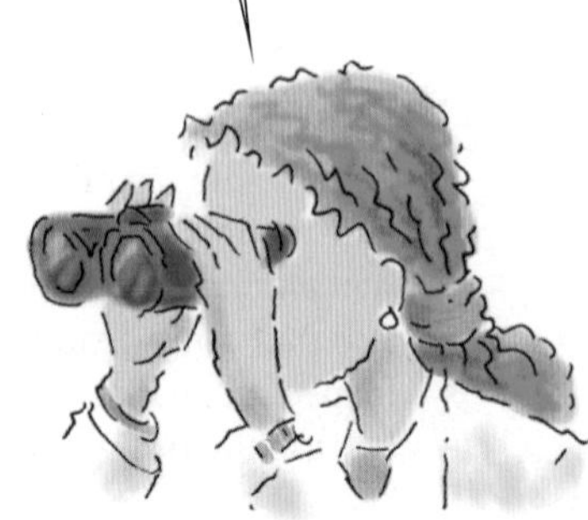
Before performing ROM exercises, be on the lookout for hidden fractures or internal injuries.

Types of joint motion

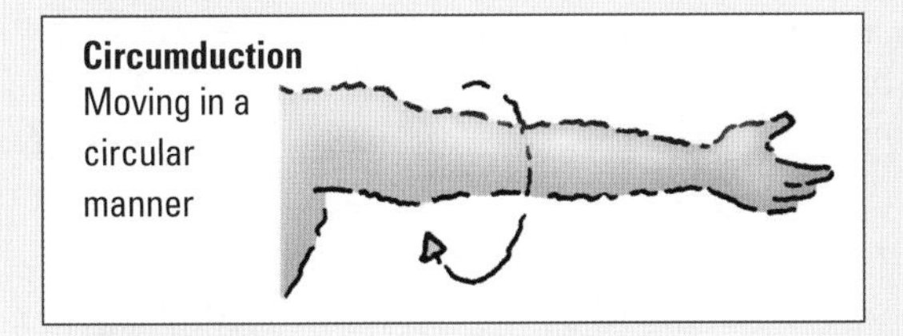

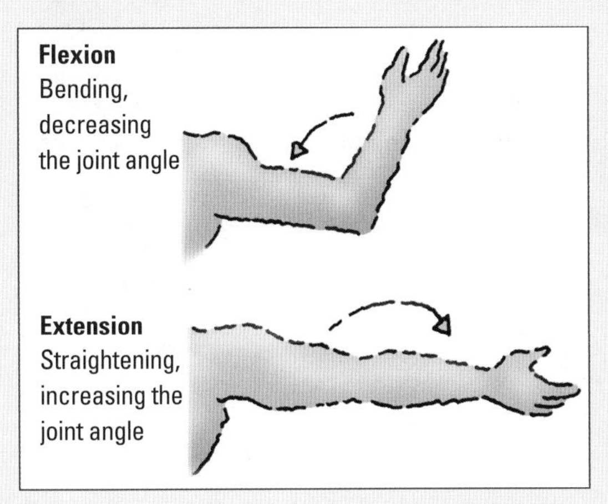

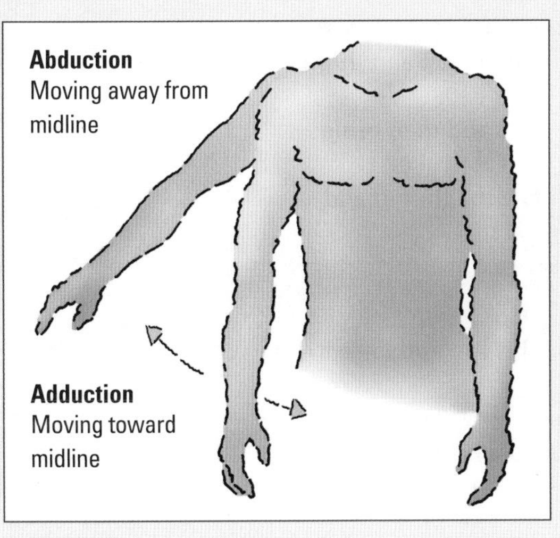

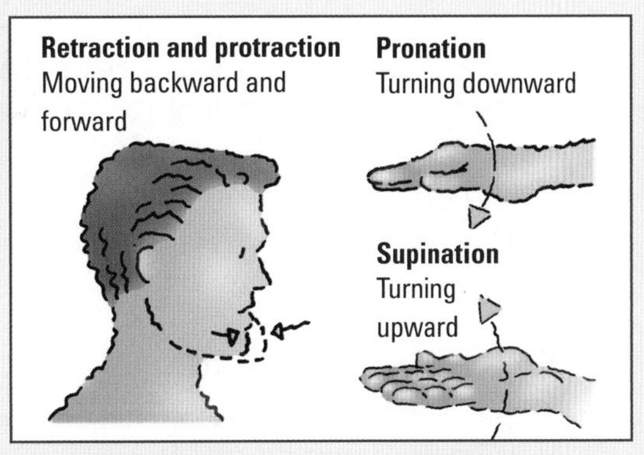

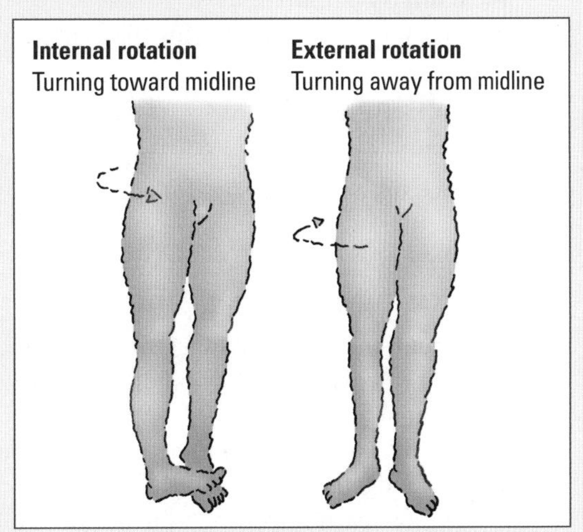

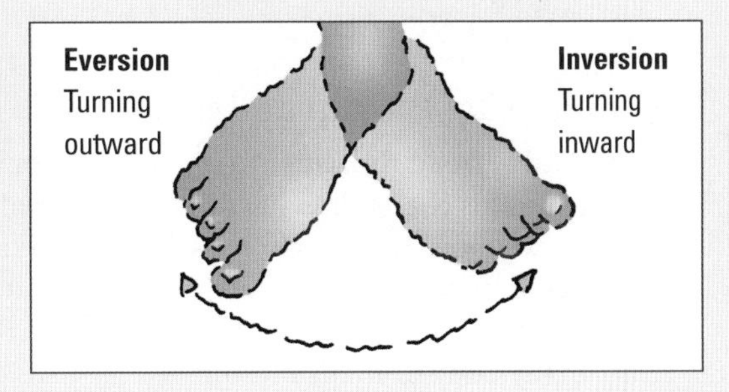

- Rotate his shoulder so that his arm crosses his midline and bend his elbow so that his hand touches his opposite shoulder then touches the mattress of the bed for complete internal rotation.
- Return his shoulder to a neutral position and, with his elbow bent, push his arm backward so that the back of his hand touches the mattress for complete external rotation.

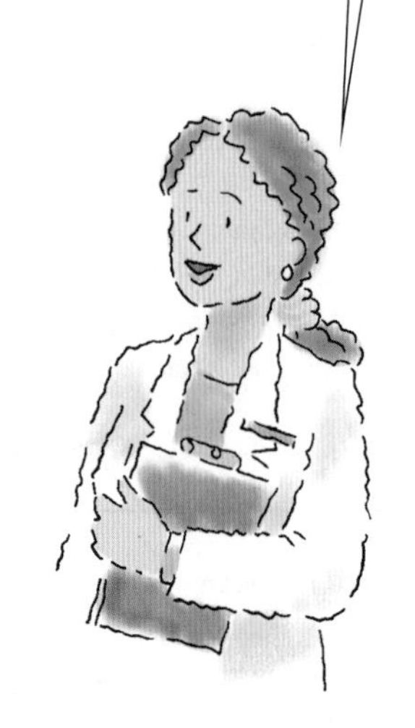
Support is the key to passive ROM exercises.

Exercising the elbow

- Place the patient's arm at his side with his palm facing up.
- Flex and extend his arm at the elbow.

Exercising the forearm

- Stabilize the patient's elbow and then twist his hand to bring his palm up (supination).
- Twist it back again to bring his palm down (pronation).

Exercising the wrist

- Stabilize the patient's forearm and flex and extend his wrist. Then rock his hand sideways for lateral flexion and rotate his hand in a circular motion.

Exercising the fingers and thumb

- Extend the patient's fingers and then flex the hand into a fist; repeat extension and flexion of each joint of each finger and thumb separately.
- Spread two adjoining fingers apart (abduction) and then bring them together (adduction).
- Oppose each fingertip to the thumb and rotate the thumb and each finger in a circle.

Exercising the hip and knee

- Fully extend the patient's leg and then bend his hip and knee toward his chest, allowing full joint flexion.
- Next, move his straight leg sideways, out and away from his other leg (abduction), and then back, over, and across it (adduction).
- Rotate his straight leg internally toward his midline then externally away from his midline.

Exercising the ankle

- Bend the patient's foot so that the toes push upward (dorsiflexion) and then bend the foot so that the toes push downward (plantar flexion).
- Rotate his ankle in a circular motion.

- Invert his ankle so that the sole of his foot faces his midline and then evert his ankle so that the sole faces away from his midline.

Exercising the toes

- Flex the patient's toes toward the sole and then extend them back toward the top of his foot.
- Spread two adjoining toes apart (abduction) and bring them together (adduction).

Practice pointers

- Because joints begin to stiffen within 24 hours of disuse, start passive ROM exercises as soon as possible and perform them at least once per shift, particularly while bathing or turning the patient. Use proper body mechanics, and repeat each exercise at least three times.

Get the family involved

- If the disabled patient requires long-term rehabilitation after discharge, consult with a physical therapist and teach a family member or caregiver to perform passive ROM exercises.

Introduce active ROM

- Patients on prolonged bed rest or with limited activity without profound weakness can also be taught to perform ROM exercises independently (called active ROM). (See *Documenting passive ROM exercises*.)

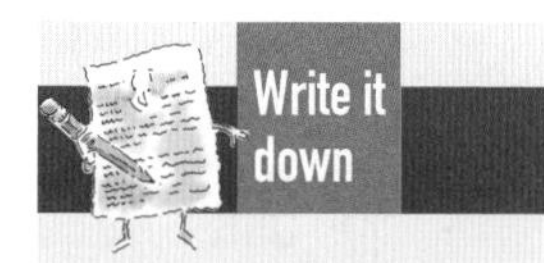

Documenting passive ROM exercises

In your notes, record:
- which joints were exercised
- patient's tolerance of the exercises
- any edema or pressure areas
- pain from the exercises
- ROM limitation.

Latex allergy management

Latex allergy is an immunologic reaction to proteins present in natural rubber latex that come from the milky fluid of the Brazilian rubber tree. Many medical or dental supplies and devices such as catheters, gloves, and syringes are made from latex and can trigger an allergic reaction in sensitive individuals.

Groups at risk for latex allergy:
- health care workers who frequently wear gloves
- workers with occupational exposure to latex such as hairdressers, latex glove manufacturers, or housekeeping personnel
- patients with a history of asthma, dermatitis, or eczema
- patient exposed to repeated bladder catheterization such as those with spinal cord trauma and children with spina bifida
- patients with food allergy, especially kiwi, bananas, avocados, or chestnuts

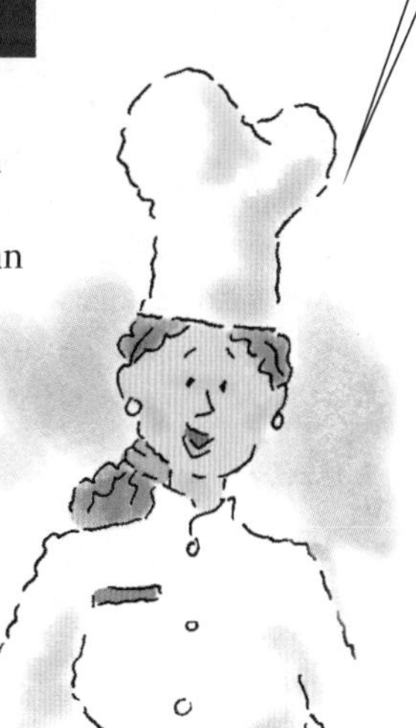
Allergies to certain foods—such as avocado, kiwis, bananas, or chestnuts—may indicate latex allergy.

- patients with a history of anaphylaxis of unknown etiology especially with past procedures or dental visits
- patients with a history of multiple surgeries or medical procedures during childhood
- Female patients are at greater risk because of gynecologic exams, contact with contraceptives, and obstetric procedures.

Telltale foods

There are some foods that have a common allergen with latex that produces a cross-sensitivity reaction in latex-sensitive individuals. Foods with the highest allergen similarities to latex include, avocado, banana, chestnut, and kiwi. Moderate immunologic cross-reactive sensitivity is seen with apples, carrots, celery, melons, papaya, potatoes, and tomatoes. Please note that the foods listed may not produce a clinically significant reaction in latex-sensitive individuals. However, it is important for families to recognize these foods and minimize exposures.

Visit the American Latex Allergy Association (http://latexallergyresources.org/latex-cross-reactive-foods-fact-sheet) for a complete listing.

Itching, sneezing, coughing

Latex allergy can cause various signs and symptoms, including generalized itching (on the hands and arms, for example); itchy, watery, and burning eyes; sneezing and coughing (hay fever–type signs); rash; hives; bronchial asthma, scratchy throat, and difficulty breathing; edema of the face, hands, and neck; and anaphylaxis.

Letting history speak for itself

To help identify people at risk for latex allergy, ask latex allergy–specific questions during the health history. (See *Latex allergy screening*.)

If the patient's history reveals a latex sensitivity, the doctor assigns him to one of three categories based on the extent of his sensitization. Group 1 patients have a history of anaphylaxis or a systemic reaction when exposed to a natural latex product. Group 2 patients have a clear history of a nonsystemic allergic reaction. Group 3 patients don't have a previous history of latex hypersensitivity but are designated as high risk because of an associated medical condition, occupation, or "crossover" allergy.

Going latex-free

If your patient is sensitive to latex, make sure that he does not come in contact with latex *because such contact could result in a life-threatening hypersensitivity reaction*. Creating a latex-free environment is the only way to safeguard your patient. Many facilities now designate

Latex allergy screening

To determine if your patient has a latex sensitivity or allergy, ask the following screening questions:

- Do you have a history of allergies, dermatitis, or asthma? If so, what type of reaction do you have?
- Do you have any congenital abnormalities? If yes, explain.
- Do you have any food allergies? If so, what specific allergies do you have? Ask specifically about the high to moderate cross-sensitivity foods. Describe your reaction.
- Do you experience shortness of breath or wheezing when blowing up latex balloons? If so, describe your reaction.
- Have you had previous surgical procedures? How about as a child? Did you experience associated complications? If so, describe them.
- Have you had previous dental procedures? Did complications result? If so, describe them.
- Are you exposed to latex in your work? Have you experienced a reaction to latex products at work? If so, describe your reaction.

latex-free equipment, which is usually kept on a cart that can be moved into the patient's room. (See *Choosing the right glove.*) Updated lists of nonlatex products are available at the Spina Bifida Association of America (www.sbaa.org) and American Latex Allergy Association (http://latexallergyresources.org/medical-products).

What you need

Latex allergy patient identification wristband ✳ latex-free equipment, including room contents ✳ anaphylaxis kit.

Getting ready

After you've determined that the patient has a latex allergy or is sensitive to latex, arrange for him to be placed in a private room. If that isn't possible, make the room latex-free *to prevent the spread of airborne particles from latex products used on the other patient.*

Choosing the right glove

Health care workers may develop allergic reactions as a result of their exposure to latex gloves and other products containing natural rubber latex. Patients may also have latex sensitivity.

General precautions

Take the following steps to protect yourself and your patient from allergic reactions to latex:

- Use nonlatex (for example, vinyl or synthetic) gloves for activities that aren't likely to involve contact with infectious materials (food preparation, routine cleaning, and so forth).
- Use appropriate barrier protection when handling infectious materials. If you choose latex gloves, use powder-free gloves with reduced protein content. The powder can aerosolize and elicit a reaction in a sensitive patient from breathing in the airborne protein particles.
- After wearing and removing gloves, wash your hands with soap and dry them thoroughly.
- When wearing latex gloves, don't use oil-based hand creams or lotions (which can cause gloves to deteriorate) unless they've been shown to maintain glove barrier protection.
- Refer to the material safety data sheet for the appropriate glove to wear when handling chemicals.
- Learn procedures for preventing latex allergy, and learn how to recognize the signs and symptoms of latex allergy: skin rashes; hives; flushing; itching; nasal, eye, or sinus symptoms; asthma; and shock.
- If you have (or suspect you have) a latex sensitivity, use nonlatex gloves, avoid contact with latex gloves and other latex-containing products, and consult a doctor experienced in treating latex allergy.

If you know you're allergic

If you have latex allergy, consider these precautions:

- Avoid contact with latex gloves and other products that contain latex.
- Avoid areas where you might inhale the powder from latex gloves worn by other workers.
- Inform your employers and your health care providers (doctors, nurses, dentists, and others).
- Wear a medical identification bracelet.
- Follow your doctor's instructions for dealing with allergic reactions to latex.

How you do it

- Check for latex allergy in all patients being admitted to the delivery room or short procedure unit or having a surgical procedure.
- If a patient has a latex allergy, bring a cart with latex-free supplies into his room.
- Document the allergy on the patient's chart according to facility policy. If policy requires the patient to wear a latex allergy identification wristband, place it on him.

Write big

- If the patient will be receiving anesthesia, make sure that "LATEX ALLERGY" is clearly visible on the front of his chart. (See *Anesthesia induction and latex allergy*.) Notify the circulating nurse in the surgical unit, the postanesthesia care unit nurses, and any other team members that the patient has a latex allergy.
- If the patient must be transported to another area of the facility, make certain that the latex-free cart accompanies him and that all health care workers who come in contact with him are wearing nonlatex gloves. The patient should wear a mask with cloth ties when leaving his room *to protect him from inhaling airborne latex particles.*
- If the patient is to have an I.V. line, make sure that it's inserted using latex-free products. Post a LATEX ALLERGY sign on the I.V. tubing *to prevent access of the line with latex products.*

Protect the patient

- Flush I.V. tubing with 50 mL of I.V. solution *because of latex ports in the I.V. tubing.*
- Place a warning label on I.V. bags that says "Don't use latex injection ports."
- Use a stopcock as alternative for giving medications through a running IV.
- Use a nonlatex tourniquet. If none are available, use a latex tourniquet over clothing.
- Remove the vial stopper to mix and draw medications.
- Use latex-free oxygen administration equipment. Remove the elastic and tie equipment on with gauze.
- Use nonlatex tape to secure lines and dressings.
- Wrap your stethoscope with a nonlatex product *to protect the patient from latex contact.* Use a nonlatex stethoscope if available.
- Wrap Tegaderm over the patient's finger before using pulse oximetry.
- Use latex-free syringes when administering medication through a syringe. Also note that some prefilled medication syringes contain latex. Make sure to read the syringe before using it.
- Keep an anaphylaxis kit nearby. If the patient has an allergic reaction to latex, treat him immediately.

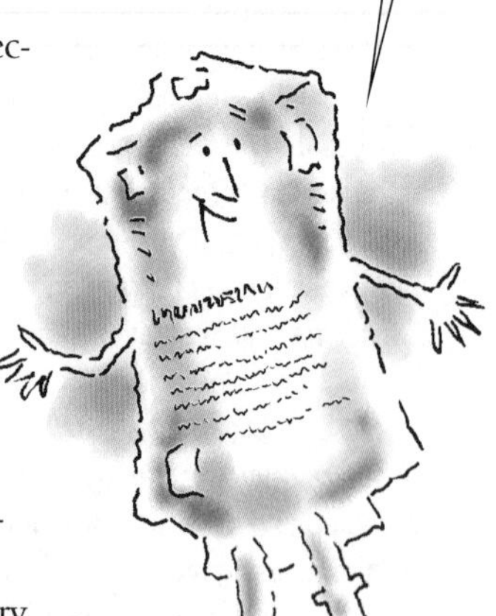
I need a warning label that says "Don't use latex injection ports."

Practice pointers

- Remember that signs and symptoms of latex allergy usually occur within 30 minutes of anesthesia induction. However, the time of onset can range from 10 minutes to 5 hours.
- Don't forget that, as a health care worker, you can develop a latex hypersensitivity. If you suspect that you're sensitive to latex, contact the employee health services department concerning facility protocol for latex-sensitive employees. Use latex-free products whenever possible *to help reduce your exposure to latex.*

Looks can deceive

- Don't assume that if something doesn't look like rubber, it isn't latex. Latex can be found, for example, in electrocardiograph leads, oral and nasal airway tubing, tourniquets, nerve stimulation pads, temperature strips, and blood pressure cuffs.

Anesthesia induction and latex allergy

Intraoperative latex reaction may be caused by contact with the mucous membrane or intraperitoneal serosal lining, inhalation of particles during anesthesia, or injection through latex ports. Here are signs and symptoms in conscious and anesthetized patients.

Conscious patient

- Abdominal cramping
- Anxiety
- Bronchoconstriction
- Diarrhea
- Feeling of faintness
- Pruritus
- Itchy eyes
- Nausea
- Shortness of breath
- Swelling of soft tissue
- Vomiting

Anesthetized patient

- Bronchospasm
- Cardiopulmonary arrest
- Facial edema
- Flushing
- Hypotension
- Laryngeal edema
- Tachycardia
- Urticaria
- Wheezing

Transfer from bed to stretcher

Transfer from bed to stretcher, one of the most common transfers, can require the help of one or more coworkers depending on the patient's size and condition and the primary nurse's physical abilities. Techniques for achieving this transfer include the straight lift, carry lift, lift sheet, and sliding board. The nurse must prevent self-injury by using correct posture, good body mechanics, lifting techniques, and appropriate lift devices. Consider the patient's condition (cognitive status, physiologic status, presence of weakness, etc.) prior to transferring and assess if an assistive device is needed. Refer to an algorithm such as *Safe patient handling and movement algorithms* (http://www.visn8.va.gov).

What you need

Stretcher ✱ sliding board or lift sheet if necessary.

Getting ready

- Adjust the bed to the same height as the stretcher.
- Move any obstacles out of the way.
- If a caregiver needs to lift any more than 35 lb, use assistive devices for the transfer.

How you do it

- Tell the patient that you're going to move him from the bed to the stretcher and place him in the supine position.
- Ask team members to remove watches and rings *to avoid scratching the patient during transfer.*

Even with this kind of strength, moving a patient from a bed to a stretcher is a team job!
500
LBS

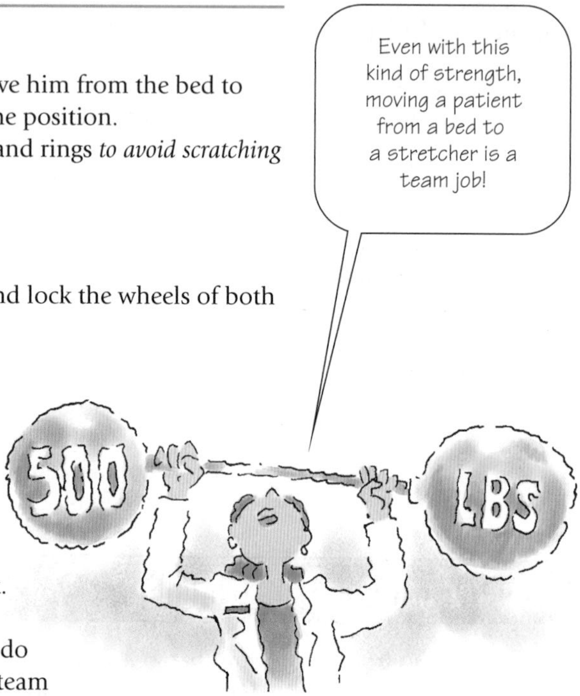

Four-person straight lift

- Place the stretcher parallel to the bed and lock the wheels of both *to ensure patient safety.*

Get into position

- Stand at the center of the stretcher and have another team member stand at the patient's head. The two other team members should stand next to the bed, on the other side—one at the center and the other at the patient's feet.
- Slide your arms, palms up, under the patient, while the other team members do the same. In this position, you and the team member directly opposite to you support the patient's buttocks and hips; the team member at the head of the bed supports the patient's head and shoulders; and the one at the foot supports the patient's legs and feet.

One, two, three

- On a count of three, you and your team members lift the patient several inches, move him onto the stretcher, and slide your arms out from under him. Keep movements smooth *to minimize patient discomfort and avoid muscle strain by team members.*
- Position the patient comfortably on the stretcher, apply safety straps, and raise and secure the side rails.

Four-person carry lift

- Place the stretcher perpendicular to the bed, with the head of the stretcher at the foot of the bed. Lock the bed and stretcher wheels *to ensure patient safety.*
- Raise the bed to a comfortable working height.

Top to bottom, tallest to shortest

- Line up all four team members on the same side of the bed as the stretcher, with the tallest member at the patient's head and the shortest at his feet. The member at the patient's head is the team leader and gives the lift signals.

- Assuming you're the team leader, tell the team members to flex their knees and slide their hands, palms up, under the patient until he rests securely on their upper arms.
- Make sure the patient is adequately supported at the head and shoulders, buttocks and hips, and legs and feet.

Reduce the strain

- On a count of three, the team members straighten their knees and roll the patient onto his side, against their chests. *This reduces strain on the team members and allows them to hold the patient for several minutes if necessary.*
- Together, the team members step back, with the member supporting the feet moving the farthest.

On the count of three

- The team members move forward to the stretcher's edge and, on a count of three, lower the patient onto the stretcher by bending at the knees and sliding their arms out from under the patient.
- Position the patient comfortably on the stretcher, apply safety straps, and raise and secure the side rails.

Four-person lift sheet transfer

- Position the bed, stretcher, and team members for the straight lift.

Make it close to the patient

- Instruct the team to hold the edges of the sheet under the patient, grasping them close to the patient *to obtain a firm grip, provide stability, and spare the patient feelings of instability.*

One smooth, continuous motion

- On a count of three, the team members lift or slide the patient onto the stretcher in one smooth, continuous motion *to avoid muscle strain and minimize patient discomfort.*
- Position the patient comfortably on the stretcher, apply safety straps, and raise and secure the side rails.

Sliding board transfer

- Place the stretcher parallel to the bed and lock the wheels of both *to ensure patient safety.*
- Stand next to the bed and instruct a coworker to stand next to the stretcher.
- Reach over the patient and pull the far side of the bedsheet toward you to turn the patient slightly on his side.

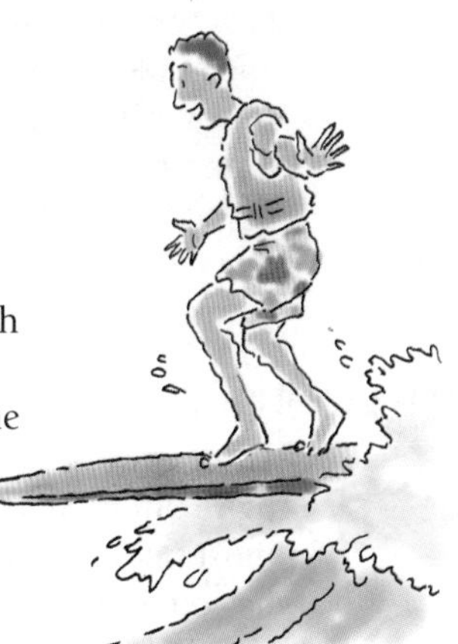
A sliding board can make a bed-to-stretcher transfer easier. This board, not so much.

Bridging the gap

- Instruct your coworker to place the sliding board beneath the patient, making sure the board bridges the gap between stretcher and bed.
- Ease the patient onto the sliding board and release the sheet.

Making the transfer

- Instruct your coworker to grasp the near side of the sheet at the patient's hips and shoulders and to pull him onto the stretcher in a smooth, continuous motion. Then have her reach over the patient, grasp the far side of the sheet, and logroll the patient toward her.

Getting him settled

- Remove the sliding board as your coworker returns the patient to the supine position.
- Position the patient comfortably on the stretcher, apply safety straps, and raise and secure the side rails.

Practice pointers

Use these pointers for patients in special circumstances.

If the patient is obese

- When transferring from bed to stretcher, lift and move the obese patient, in increments, to the edge of the bed. Then rest for a few seconds and lift him onto the stretcher.
- Depending on the patient's size and condition, lift sheet transfer can require two to seven people.

If the patient can bear weight on his arms or legs

- Two or three coworkers can perform a transfer if the patient can bear weight on his arms or legs. One can support the buttocks and guide the patient, another can stabilize the stretcher by leaning over it and guiding the patient into position, and a third can transfer any attached equipment. If a team member isn't available to guide equipment, move I.V. lines and other tubing first *to make sure they're out of the way and not in danger of pulling loose* or disconnect tubes if possible.

If the patient is light

- Three coworkers can perform the carry lift if the patient is light, but no matter how many team members are present, one must stabilize the patient's head if he can't support it himself, has cervical instability or injury, or has undergone surgery. (See *Documenting bed-stretcher transfer*.)

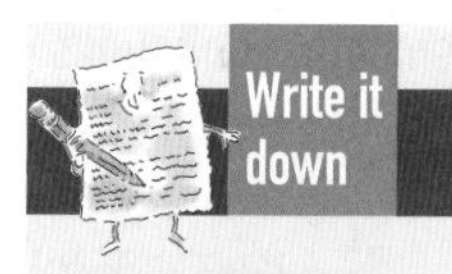

Documenting bed-stretcher transfer

Record the time and the type of transfer, number of assistants, and how well the patient tolerated it in your notes. Complete other required forms as necessary.

Transfer from bed to wheelchair

For a patient with diminished or absent lower body sensation or one-sided weakness, immobility, or injury, transfer from bed to wheelchair may require partial support to full assistance—initially by at least two persons. After transfer, proper positioning helps prevent excessive pressure on bony prominences, which predisposes the patient to skin breakdown.

What you need

Wheelchair with locks (or sturdy chair) ✳ a gait or transfer belt ✳ pajama bottoms (or robe) ✳ shoes or slippers with nonslip soles ✳ optional: transfer board if appropriate. A mechanical lift can also be used to assist patients to a standing position if the patient has limited mobility. (See *Need a lift?*)

How you do it

- Assess the patient's ability to assist with the transfer. Refer to an algorithm such as *Safe patient handling and movement algorithms* (http://www.visn8.va.gov).
- Move any obstacles out of the way.
- Explain the procedure to the patient and demonstrate his role. (See *Teaching the patient to use a transfer board,* page 50.)

Need a lift? (Using a mechanical lift)

Patient is able to walk

- Ensure safety straps are secured when helping a patient to a standing position.
- Patient grasps handles as the motorized lift is started.
- Patient will come to a standing position with feet on the floor and is ready to ambulate to chair with the caregiver's assistance.

Patient is unable to walk

- Secure safety straps and use platform of motorized lift.
- Patient is sitting on the edge of the bed facing the lift grasping the handles with his feet on the platform.
- Patient moves to an upright position when the lift is activated by the caregiver.
- Caregiver positions the patient in front of the chair.
- Instruct the patient to continue to grasp the handles as the lift lowers him into the chair along with guidance from the caregiver.

Teaching the patient to use a transfer board

For the patient who can't stand, a transfer board allows safe transfer from bed to wheelchair. To help the patient perform this transfer, take the following steps:

Explain the procedure to the patient and then demonstrate it. He may eventually become proficient enough to transfer himself with or without supervision.

Help the patient put on pajama bottoms or a robe and shoes or slippers.

Angle the wheelchair slightly facing the foot of the bed. Lock the wheels and remove the armrest closest to the patient. Make sure the bed is flat and adjust its height so that it's level with the wheelchair seat.

Assist the patient to a sitting position on the edge of the bed, with his feet resting on the floor. Make sure the front edge of the wheelchair seat is aligned with the back of the patient's knees (as shown below left). Depending on the patient, he may find it easier to transfer to an even surface or to a slightly lower surface.

Ask the patient to lean away from the wheelchair while you slide one end of the transfer board under him.

Now place the other end of the transfer board on the wheelchair seat and help the patient return to the upright position.

Stand in front of the patient to prevent him from sliding forward. Tell him to push down with both arms, lifting his buttocks up and onto the transfer board. He then repeats this maneuver, edging along the board, until he's seated in the wheelchair. If he can't use his arms to help with the transfer, stand in front of him, put your arms around him, and—if he can—have him put his arms around you. Gradually slide him across the board until he's safely in the chair (as shown below right).

When the patient is in the chair, fasten a seat belt, if necessary, to prevent falls.

Then remove the transfer board, replace the wheelchair armrest, and reposition the patient in the chair.

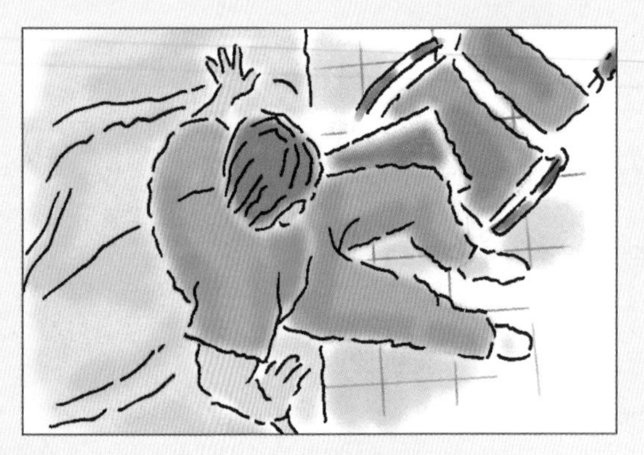

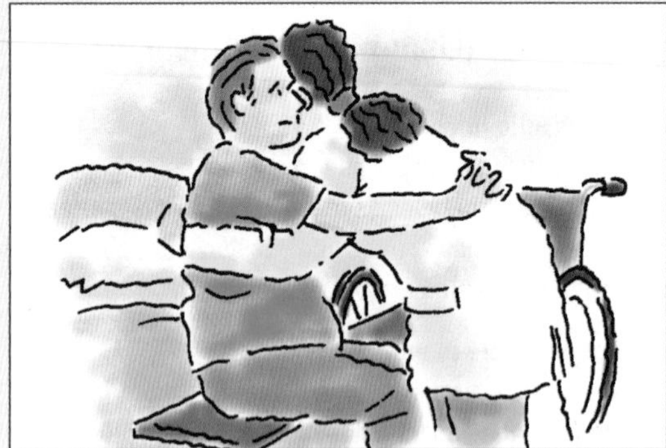

- Apply a gait or transfer belt to the patient according to the manufacturer's recommendations.
- Place the wheelchair parallel to the bed, facing the foot of the bed, and lock its wheels. Make sure the bed wheels are also locked. Raise the footrests *to avoid interfering with the transfer.*

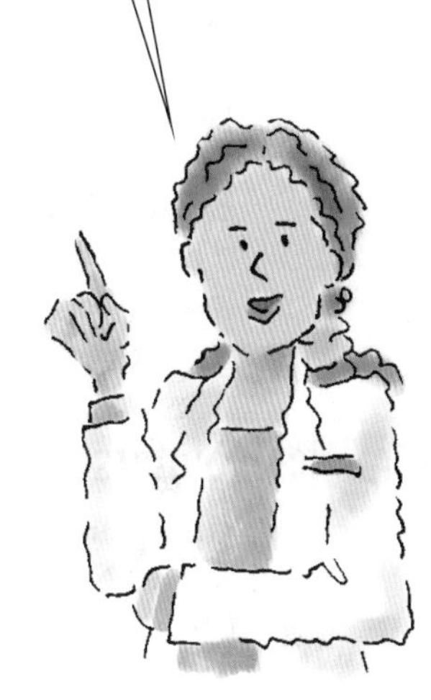
I know it's basic, but remember to lock the wheels of the chair and the bed.

Check the vitals . . .

- Check the patient's pulse rate and blood pressure when he's in a supine position *to obtain a baseline.* Then help him put on the pajama bottoms and slippers or shoes with nonslip soles *to prevent falls.*

. . . and make sure they're stable

- Raise the head of the bed and allow the patient to rest briefly *to adjust to posture changes.* Then bring him to the dangling position. Recheck his pulse rate and blood pressure if you suspect cardiovascular instability and don't proceed until they're stabilized *to prevent falls.*

Out of the bed . . .

- Tell the patient to move toward the edge of the bed and, if possible, to place his feet flat on the floor. Stand in front of the patient, blocking his toes with your feet and his knees with yours *to prevent his knees from buckling.*
- Flex your knees slightly, place your arms around the patient's waist and hold onto the transfer/gait belt, and tell him to place his hands on the edge of the bed. Avoid bending at your waist *to prevent back strain.*
- Ask the patient to push himself off the bed and to support as much of his own weight as possible. At the same time, straighten your knees and hips; using the transfer/gait belt, raise him as you straighten your body.
- Supporting the patient with the transfer/gait belt, pivot toward the wheelchair, keeping your knees next to his. Tell him to grasp the farthest armrest of the wheelchair with his closest hand.

. . . and into the chair

- Help the patient lower himself into the wheelchair by flexing your hips and knees, but not your back, while supporting the patient with the transfer/gait belt. Instruct him to reach back and grasp the other wheelchair armrest as he sits *to avoid abrupt contact with the seat.* Fasten the seat belt *to prevent falls* and, if necessary, check pulse rate and blood pressure *to assess cardiovascular stability.* If his pulse rate is 20 beats or more above baseline, stay with him and monitor him closely until the rate returns to normal *because he's experiencing orthostatic hypotension.*
- Remove the transfer/gait belt.

Position, position, position

- If the patient can't position himself correctly, help him move his buttocks against the back of the chair *so that the ischial tuberosities, not the sacrum, provide the base of support.*
- Place the patient's feet flat on the footrests, pointed straight ahead.
- Position the knees and hips with the correct amount of flexion and in appropriate alignment.
- If appropriate, use elevating leg rests to flex the patient's hips at more than 90 degrees; *this position relieves pressure on the popliteal space and places more weight on the ischial tuberosities.*
- Position the patient's arms on the wheelchair's armrests with shoulders abducted, elbows slightly flexed, forearms pronated, and wrists and hands in the neutral position.
- If necessary, support or elevate his hands and forearms with a pillow *to prevent dependent edema.*

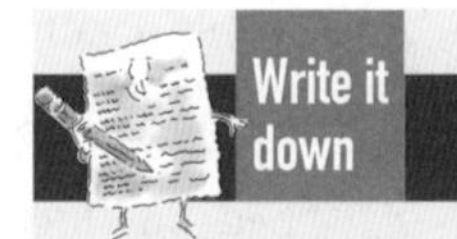

Documenting bed-wheelchair transfer

Record the time of transfer, use of assistive devices, number of personnel to assist, and any pertinent observations (muscle weakness, weight-bearing ability, etc.). Note how the patient tolerated the transfer.

Practice pointers

- If the patient starts to fall during transfer, ease him to the closest surface. Never stretch to finish the transfer. *Doing so can cause loss of balance, falls, muscle strain, and other injuries to you and the patient.*

Compensating for weakness

- If the patient has one-sided weakness, follow the preceding steps, but place the wheelchair on his unaffected side. Instruct him to pivot and bear as much weight as possible on the unaffected side. Support the affected side *because he'll tend to lean to this side.* If the patient is hemiplegic, use pillows to support his affected side *to prevent slumping in the wheelchair.* (See *Documenting bed-wheelchair transfer.*)

Eye care

When paralysis or coma impairs or eliminates the corneal reflex, frequent eye care aims to keep the exposed cornea moist, preventing ulceration and inflammation. Application of saline-saturated gauze pads over the eyelids moistens the eyes. Commercially available eye ointments and artificial tears also lubricate the corneas, but a doctor's order is required for their use.

Although eye care isn't a sterile procedure, maintain asepsis as much as possible.

What you need

Sterile basin ✳ gloves ✳ sterile towel ✳ sterile normal saline solution ✳ sterile cotton balls ✳ mineral oil ✳ artificial tears or eye ointment (if ordered) ✳ gauze or eye pads ✳ hypoallergenic tape.

Getting ready

Assemble the equipment at the patient's bedside. Pour a small amount of saline solution into the basin.

How you do it

- Wash your hands thoroughly, put on gloves, and tell the patient what you're about to do, even if he's comatose or appears unresponsive.

Clean . . .

- To remove secretions or crusts adhering to the eyelids and eyelashes, first soak a cotton ball in sterile normal saline solution. Then gently wipe the patient's eye with the moistened cotton ball, working from the inner canthus to the outer canthus *to prevent debris and fluid from entering the nasolacrimal duct.*
- *To prevent cross-contamination,* use a fresh cotton ball for each wipe until the eye is clean. *To prevent irritation,* avoid using soap to clean the eyes. Repeat the procedure for the other eye.

. . . and lubricate

- After cleaning the eyes, instill artificial tears or apply eye ointment, as ordered, *to keep them moist.*
- Close the patient's eyelids. Dab a small amount of mineral oil on each lid *to lubricate and protect fragile skin.*
- Soak gauze or eye pads in sterile normal saline solution, place them over the eyelids, and secure with hypoallergenic tape. Change gauze pads, as necessary, *to keep them well saturated.*

Finishing up

- After giving eye care, cover the basin with a sterile towel and dispose of the gloves. Change the basin, towel, and normal saline solution at least daily. (See *Documenting eye care.*)

Documenting eye care

Record the time and type of eye care in your notes. If applicable, chart administration of eyedrops or ointment in the patient's medication record. Document unusual crusting or excessive or colored drainage.

Mouth care

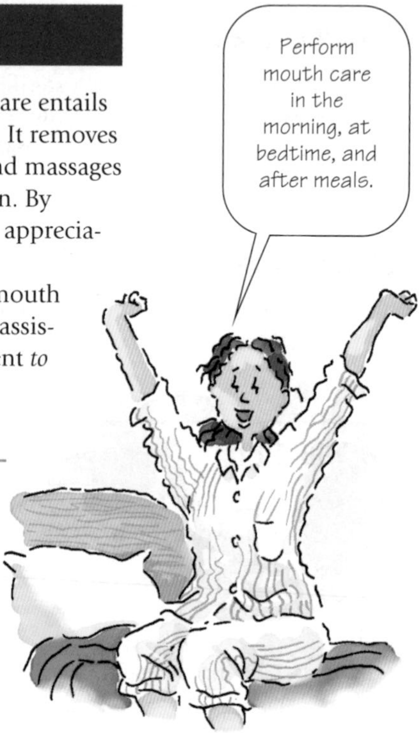

Perform mouth care in the morning, at bedtime, and after meals.

Given in the morning, at bedtime, or after meals, mouth care entails brushing and flossing the teeth and inspecting the mouth. It removes soft plaque deposits and calculus from the teeth, cleans and massages the gums, reduces mouth odor, and helps prevent infection. By freshening the patient's mouth, mouth care also enhances appreciation of food, thereby aiding appetite and nutrition.

Although an ambulatory patient can usually perform mouth care alone, a bedridden patient may require partial or full assistance. A comatose patient requires use of suction equipment *to prevent aspiration during oral care.*

What you need

Towel or facial tissues ✳ emesis basin ✳ trash bag ✳ mouthwash ✳ toothbrush and toothpaste ✳ pitcher and glass ✳ drinking straw ✳ dental floss ✳ gloves ✳ dental floss holder, if available ✳ small mirror, if necessary ✳ optional: oral irrigating device.

For the comatose or debilitated patient as needed

Linen-saver pad ✳ bite block ✳ petroleum jelly ✳ hydrogen peroxide ✳ mineral oil ✳ cotton-tipped mouth swab ✳ oral suction equipment or gauze pads ✳ optional: mouth care kit, tongue blade, 4″ × 4″ gauze pads, adhesive tape.

Getting ready

Fill a pitcher with water and bring it and other equipment to the patient's bedside. If you'll be using oral suction equipment, connect the tubing to the suction bottle and suction catheter, insert the plug into an outlet, and check for correct operation. If necessary, devise a bite block to protect yourself from being bitten during the procedure: Wrap a gauze pad over the end of a tongue blade, fold the edge in, and secure it with adhesive tape.

How you do it

- Wash your hands thoroughly, put on gloves, explain the procedure to the patient, and provide privacy.

Supervising mouth care

- If the patient is bedridden but capable of self-care, encourage him to perform his own mouth care.
- If allowed, place the patient in Fowler's position. Place the overbed table in front of him and arrange the equipment on it. Open the table and set up the built-in mirror, if available, or position a small mirror on the table.
- Drape a towel over the patient's chest to protect his gown. Tell him to floss his teeth while looking into the mirror.

Inspecting the technique

- Observe the patient *to make sure he's flossing correctly* and correct him if necessary.
- Tell him to wrap the floss around the second or third finger of each hand. Starting with his back teeth and without injuring the gums, he should insert the floss as far as possible into the space between each pair of teeth. Then he should clean the surfaces of adjacent teeth by pulling the floss up and down against the side of each tooth. After the patient flosses a pair of teeth, remind him to use a clean 1" (2.5 cm) section of floss for the next pair.

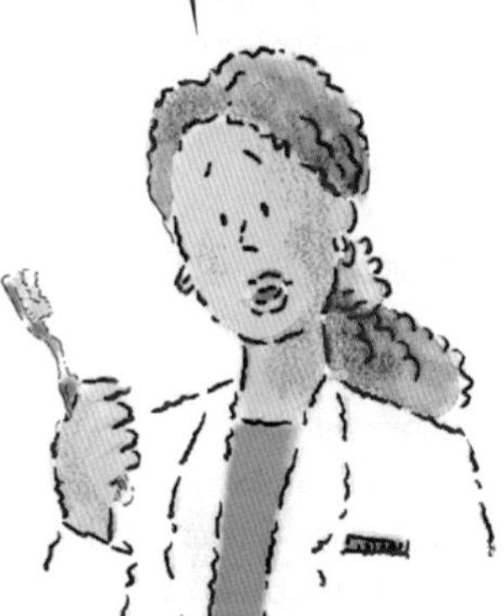
Like the dentist says, don't forget the gums!

After the floss

- After the patient flosses, mix mouthwash and water in a glass (or a mixture of half peroxide and half water), place a straw in it, and position the emesis basin nearby.
- Instruct him to brush his teeth and gums while looking into the mirror. Encourage him to rinse frequently during brushing and provide facial tissues for him to wipe his mouth.

Performing mouth care

- If the patient is comatose or conscious but incapable of self-care, perform mouth care on him. If he wears dentures, clean them thoroughly. (See *Dealing with dentures*, page 56.) Some patients may benefit from using an oral irrigating device. (See *Using an oral irrigating device*, page 57.)

Prepping the patient

- Raise the bed to a comfortable working height *to prevent back strain*. Then lower the head of the bed and position the patient on his side, with his face extended over the edge of the pillow *to facilitate drainage and prevent fluid aspiration*.
- Arrange the equipment on the overbed table or bedside stand, including the oral suction equipment, if necessary. Turn on the machine. If a suction machine isn't available, wipe the inside of the patient's mouth frequently with a gauze pad.

Dealing with dentures

Dentures require proper care to remove soft plaque deposits and calculus and to reduce mouth odor. Such care involves removing and rinsing dentures after meals, daily brushing and removal of tenacious deposits, and soaking in a commercial denture cleaner. Dentures must be removed from the comatose or presurgical patient to prevent possible airway obstruction.

Equipment and preparation

Start by assembling the following equipment at the patient's bedside: emesis basin ✳ labeled denture cup ✳ toothbrush or denture brush ✳ gloves ✳ toothpaste ✳ commercial denture cleaner ✳ paper towel ✳ cotton-tipped mouth swab ✳ mouthwash ✳ gauze ✳ optional: adhesive denture liner.

Wash your hands and put on gloves.

Removing dentures

- To remove a full upper denture, grasp the front and palatal surfaces of the denture with your thumb and forefinger. Position the index finger of your opposite hand over the upper border of the denture and press to break the seal between denture and palate. Grasp the denture with gauze because saliva can make it slippery.
- To remove a full lower denture, grasp the front and lingual surfaces of the denture with your thumb and index finger and gently lift up.
- To remove partial dentures, first ask the patient or caregiver how the prosthesis is retained and how to remove it. If the partial denture is held in place with clips or snaps, then exert equal pressure on the border of each side of the denture. Avoid lifting the clasps, which can easily bend or break.

Oral and denture care

- After removing dentures, place them in a properly labeled denture cup. Add warm water and a commercial denture cleaner to remove stains and hardened deposits. Follow package directions. Avoid soaking dentures in mouthwash containing alcohol because it may damage a soft liner.
- Instruct the patient to rinse with mouthwash to remove food particles and reduce mouth odor. Then stroke the palate, buccal surfaces, gums, and tongue with a soft toothbrush or cotton-tipped mouth swab to clean the mucosa and stimulate circulation. Check for irritated areas or sores because they may indicate a poorly fitting denture.
- Carry the denture cup, emesis basin, toothbrush, and toothpaste to the sink. After lining the basin with a paper towel, fill it with water to cushion the dentures in case you drop them. Hold the dentures over the basin, wet them with warm water, and apply toothpaste to a denture brush or long-bristled toothbrush. Clean the dentures using only moderate pressure to prevent scratches and warm water to prevent distortion.
- Clean the denture cup and place the dentures in it. Rinse the brush and clean and dry the emesis basin. Return all equipment to the patient's bedside stand.

Wearing dentures

- If the patient desires, apply adhesive liner to the dentures. Moisten them with water, if necessary, to reduce friction and ease insertion.
- Encourage the patient to wear his dentures to enhance his appearance, facilitate eating and speaking, and prevent changes in the gum line that may affect denture fit.

- Place a linen-saver pad under the patient's chin and an emesis basin near his cheek *to absorb or catch drainage.*
- Lubricate the patient's lips with petroleum jelly *to prevent dryness and cracking*. Reapply lubricant, as needed, during oral care.
- If necessary, insert the bite block to hold the patient's mouth open during oral care.

Using an oral irrigating device

An oral irrigating device, such as the Waterpik, directs a pulsating jet of water around the teeth to massage gums and remove debris and food particles. It's especially useful for cleaning areas missed by brushing, such as around bridgework, crowns, and dental wires. Because this device enhances oral hygiene, it benefits patients undergoing head and neck irradiation, which can damage teeth and cause severe caries. The device also maintains oral hygiene in a patient with a fractured jaw or with mouth injuries that limit standard mouth care.

Equipment and preparation

To use the device, first assemble the following equipment: oral irrigating device ✳ gloves ✳ towel ✳ emesis basin ✳ pharyngeal suction apparatus ✳ salt solution or mouthwash, if ordered ✳ soap.

Implementation

- Wash your hands and put on gloves.
- Turn the patient to his side to prevent aspiration of water. Then place a towel under his chin and an emesis basin next to his cheek to absorb or catch drainage.
- Insert the oral irrigating device's plug into a nearby electrical outlet. Remove the device's cover, turn it upside down, and fill it with lukewarm water or with a mouthwash or salt solution, as ordered. When using a salt solution, dissolve the salt beforehand in a separate container. Then pour the solution into the cover.
- Secure the cover to the base of the device. Remove the water hose handle from the base and snap the jet tip into place. If necessary, wet the grooved end of the tip to ease insertion. Adjust the pressure dial to the setting most comfortable for the patient. If his gums are tender and prone to bleed, choose a low setting.
- Adjust the knurled knob on the handle to direct the water jet, place the jet tip in the patient's mouth, and turn on the device. Instruct the patient to keep his lips partially closed to avoid spraying water.
- Direct the water at a right angle to the gum line of each tooth and between teeth. Avoid directing water under the patient's tongue because this may injure sensitive tissue.
- After irrigating each tooth, pause briefly and instruct the patient to expectorate the water or solution into the emesis basin. If he can't do so, suction it from the sides of the mouth with the pharyngeal suction apparatus. After irrigating all teeth, turn off the device and remove the jet tip from his mouth.
- Empty the remaining water or solution from the cover, remove the jet tip from the handle, and return the handle to the base. Clean the jet tip with soap and water, rinse the cover, dry them, and return them to storage.

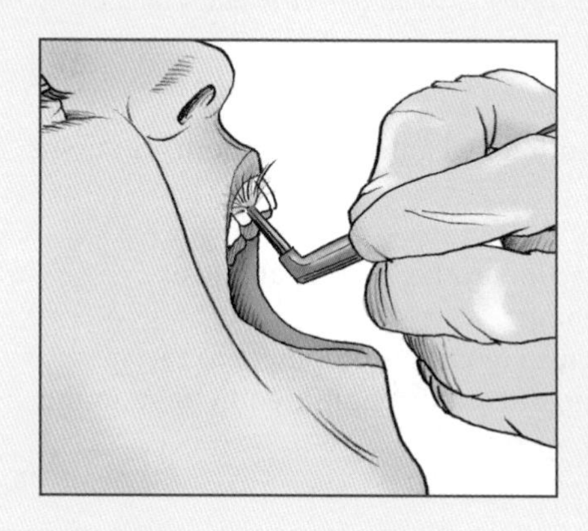

Flossing and rinsing

- Using a dental floss holder, hold the floss against each tooth and direct it as close to the gum as possible without injuring the sensitive tissues around the tooth.
- After flossing the patient's teeth, mix mouthwash and water in a glass and place the straw in it.

Brushing them clean

- Wet the toothbrush with water. If necessary, use hot water *to soften the bristles*. Apply toothpaste.
- Brush the patient's lower teeth from the gum line up; the upper teeth, from the gum line down.
- Place the brush at a 45-degree angle to the gum line and press the bristles gently into the gingival sulcus. Using short, gentle strokes *to prevent gum damage*, brush the buccal surfaces (toward the cheek) and the lingual surfaces (toward the tongue) of the bottom teeth; use just the tip of the brush for the lingual surfaces of the front teeth. Using the same technique, brush the buccal and lingual surfaces of the top teeth. Brush the biting surfaces of the bottom and top teeth using a back and forth motion.
- Hold the emesis basin steady under the patient's cheek and wipe his mouth and cheeks with facial tissues as needed.

Follow up with a swab

- After brushing the patient's teeth, dip a cotton-tipped mouth swab into the mouthwash solution (or a mixture of half peroxide and half water). Press the swab against the side of the glass to remove excess moisture. Gently stroke the gums, buccal surfaces, palate, and tongue *to clean the mucosa and stimulate circulation*.

After mouth care

- Assess the patient's mouth for cleanliness and tooth and tissue condition.
- Rinse the toothbrush and clean the emesis basin and glass.
- Empty and clean the suction bottle, if used, and place a clean suction catheter on the tubing.
- Remove your gloves, return reusable equipment to the appropriate storage location, and discard disposable equipment in the trash bag.

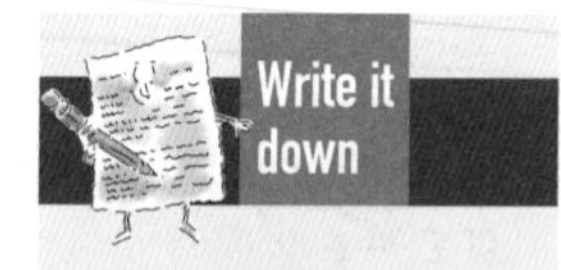

Documenting mouth care

In your notes, record:
- date and time of mouth care
- unusual conditions, such as bleeding, edema, mouth odor, excessive secretions, or plaque on the tongue.

Practice pointers

- Use cotton-tipped mouth swabs to clean the teeth of a patient with sensitive gums. *These swabs produce less friction than a toothbrush but don't clean as well.*
- If your patient is breathing through his mouth or receiving oxygen therapy, moisten his mouth and lips regularly with mineral oil or water. (See *Documenting mouth care*.)
- Always keep dentures in a denture container that is clearly labeled with the patient's name and medical record number. It should be documented on the list of patient items and should be transferred

with the patient and noted they were received at each handoff. Dentures are frequently lost in facilities and can take several weeks to replace so it is important to keep track of them.

Back care

Good thing I'm learning about back care!

Regular bathing and massage of the neck, back, buttocks, and upper arms promotes patient relaxation and allows assessment of skin condition. Particularly important for the bedridden patient, massage causes cutaneous vasodilation, helping to prevent pressure ulcers caused by prolonged pressure on bony prominences or by perspiration. Although you can perform gentle back massage after a patient has a myocardial infarction, it may be contraindicated in those with rib fractures, surgical incisions, or other recent traumatic injury to the back.

What you need

Basin ✱ soap ✱ bath blanket ✱ bath towel ✱ washcloth ✱ back lotion with lanolin base ✱ gloves, if the patient has open lesions or has been incontinent ✱ optional: talcum powder.

Getting ready

Fill the basin two-thirds full with warm water. Place the lotion bottle in the basin to warm it. *Application of warmed lotion prevents chilling or startling the patient, thereby reducing muscle tension and vasoconstriction.*

How you do it

- Assemble the equipment at the patient's bedside.
- Explain the procedure to the patient and provide privacy. Ask him to tell you if you're applying too much or too little pressure.
- Adjust the bed to a comfortable working height and lower the head of the bed, if allowed. Wash your hands and put on gloves, if applicable.
- Place the patient in the prone position, if possible, or on his side. Position him along the edge of the bed nearest you *to prevent back strain.*
- Untie the patient's gown and expose his back, shoulders, and buttocks. Then drape the patient with a bath blanket *to prevent chills and minimize exposure.* Place a bath towel next to or under his side *to protect bed linens from moisture.*

Make it into a mitt

- Fold the washcloth around your hand to form a mitt. This prevents the loose ends of the cloth from dripping water onto the patient and keeps the cloth warm longer.
- Work up a lather with soap. Using long, firm strokes, bathe the patient's back, beginning at the neck and shoulders and moving downward to the buttocks.

Dry well because trapped moisture can cause chafing.

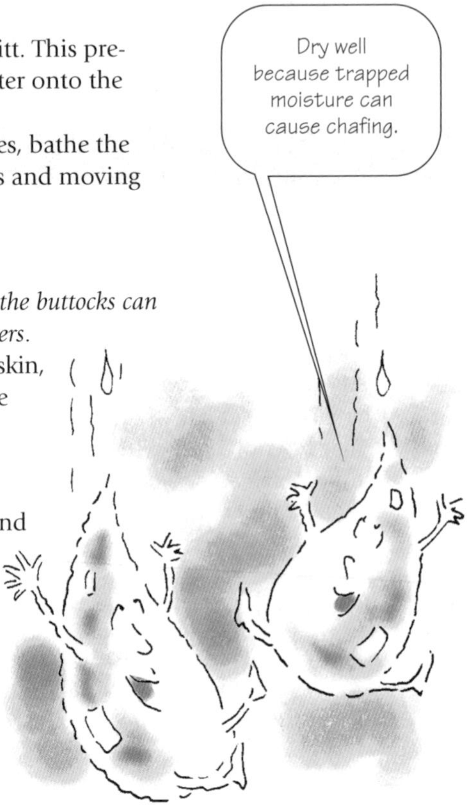

Rinse and dry

- Rinse and dry well *because moisture trapped between the buttocks can cause chafing and predispose the patient to pressure ulcers.*
- While giving back care, closely examine the patient's skin, especially the bony prominences of the shoulders, the scapulae, and the coccyx, for redness or abrasions.

Moisturize first, then massage

- Remove the warmed lotion bottle from the basin and pour a small amount of lotion into your palm. Rub your hands together *to distribute the lotion.*
- Apply the lotion to the patient's back using long, firm strokes. *The lotion reduces friction, making back massage easier.*
- Massage the patient's back, beginning at the base of the spine and moving upward to the shoulders. For a relaxing effect, massage slowly; for a stimulating effect, massage quickly. Alternate the three basic strokes: effleurage, friction, and pétrissage. (See *How to give a back massage.*) Add lotion as needed, keeping one hand on the patient's back *to avoid interrupting the massage.*
- Compress, squeeze, and lift the trapezius muscle *to help relax the patient.*
- Finish the massage by using long, firm strokes and blot any excess lotion from the patient's back with a towel. Then retie the patient's gown and straighten or change the bed linens, as necessary.

When you're done

- Return the bed to its original position and make the patient comfortable. Empty and clean the basin.
- Dispose of gloves, if used, and return equipment to the appropriate storage area.

Practice pointers

- Before giving back care, assess the patient's body structure and skin condition and tailor the duration and intensity of the massage accordingly.

How to give a back massage

Three strokes commonly used during back massage are effleurage, friction, and pétrissage. Start with effleurage, and then go on to friction and pétrissage. Perform each stroke at least six times before moving on to the next, and then repeat the whole series if desired.

When performing effleurage and friction, keep your hands parallel to the vertebrae to avoid tickling the patient. For all three strokes, maintain a regular rhythm and steady contact with the patient's back to help him relax.

Effleurage

Using your palm, stroke from the buttocks up to the shoulders, over the upper arms, and back to the buttocks (as shown below). Use slightly less pressure on the downward strokes.

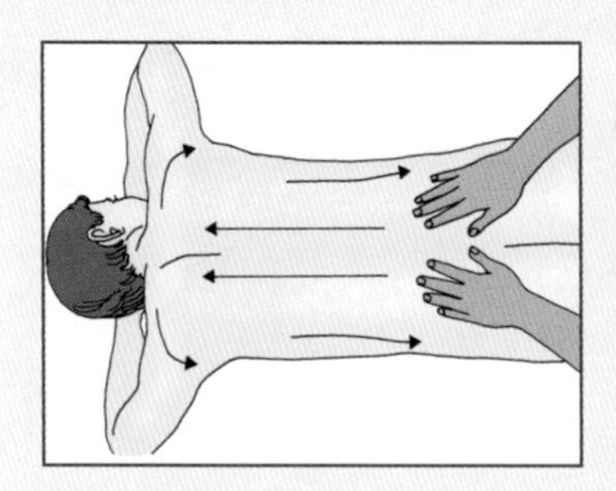

Friction

Use circular thumb strokes to move from buttocks to shoulders; then, using a smooth stroke, return to the buttocks (as shown below).

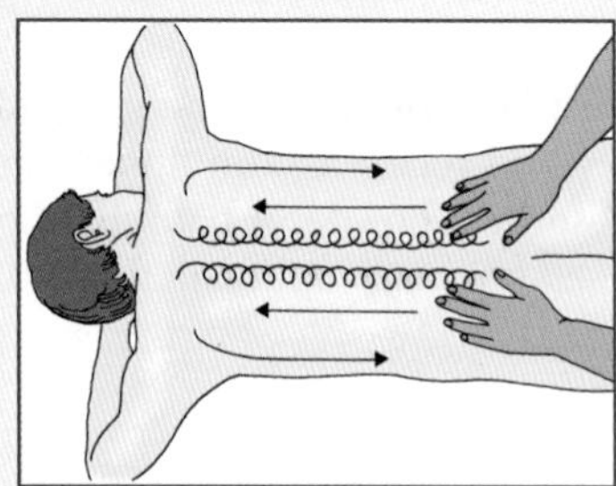

Pétrissage

Using your thumb to oppose your fingers, knead and stroke half the back and upper arms, starting at the buttocks and moving toward the shoulder (as shown below). Then knead and stroke the other half of the back, rhythmically alternating your hands.

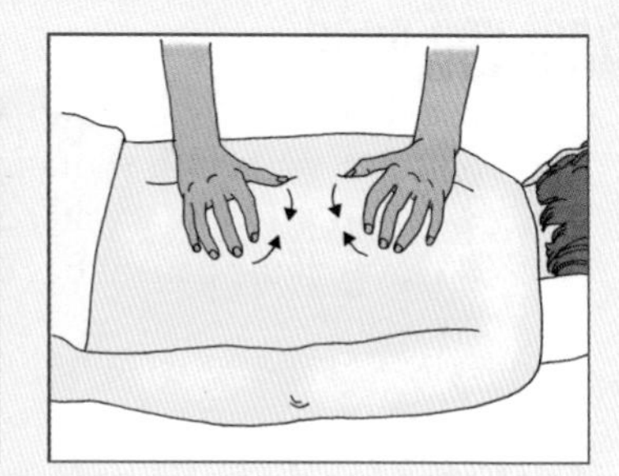

- If the patient has oily skin, substitute a talcum powder or lotion of the patient's choice. However, don't use powder if the patient has an endotracheal or tracheal tube in place *to avoid aspiration.*
- Don't massage the patient's legs unless ordered *because reddened legs can signal clot formation and massage can dislodge the clot, causing an embolus.*
- Give special attention to bony prominences *because pressure ulcers are common in these areas.*

Keep the powder and the lotion separate

- Avoid using powder and lotion together *because this may lead to skin maceration.*
- If you're giving back care at bedtime, have the patient ready for bed beforehand so the massage can help him fall asleep.
- Develop a turning schedule and give back care at each position change. (See *Documenting back care.*)

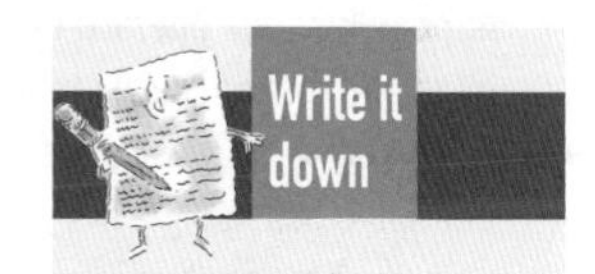

Documenting back care

Chart back care on the flowchart. Record redness, abrasion, or changes in skin condition in your notes.

Foot care

Daily bathing of feet and regular trimming of toenails promotes cleanliness, prevents infection, stimulates peripheral circulation, and controls odor by removing debris from between toes and under toenails.

This type of care is particularly important for bedridden patients and those especially susceptible to foot infection, such as patients with peripheral vascular disease, diabetes mellitus, poor nutritional status, arthritis, or a condition that impairs peripheral circulation. In such patients, proper foot care should include meticulous cleanliness and regular observation for signs of skin breakdown. (See *Foot care for diabetic patients.*)

What you need

Bath blanket ✻ large basin ✻ soap ✻ towel ✻ linen-saver pad ✻ pillow ✻ washcloth ✻ orangewood stick ✻ cotton-tipped applicator ✻ cotton ✻ lotion ✻ water-absorbent powder ✻ bath thermometer ✻ gloves, if the patient has open lesions ✻ optional: gauze pads, heel protectors.

Foot care for diabetic patients

Because diabetes mellitus can reduce blood supply to the feet, normally, minor foot injuries can lead to dangerous infection. When caring for a diabetic patient, keep these foot care guidelines in mind:

- Exercising the feet daily can help improve circulation. While the patient is sitting on the edge of the bed, ask him to point his toes upward then downward 10 times. Then have him make a circle with each foot 10 times.
- A diabetic patient's shoes must fit properly. Instruct the patient to break in new shoes gradually by increasing wearing time by 30 minutes each day. Also, tell him to check old shoes frequently in case they develop rough spots in the lining.
- Tell the patient to wear clean socks daily and to avoid socks with holes; darned spots; or rough, irritating seams.
- Advise the patient to see a doctor if he has corns or calluses.
- Tell the patient to wear warm socks or slippers and use extra blankets *to avoid cold feet.* The patient shouldn't use heating pads and hot water bottles because these can cause burns.
- Teach the patient to regularly inspect the skin on the feet for cuts; cracks; blisters; and red, swollen areas. Even slight cuts on the feet should receive a doctor's attention. As a first-aid measure, tell him to wash the cut thoroughly and apply a mild antiseptic. Urge the patient to avoid harsh antiseptics, such as iodine, because they can damage tissue.
- Advise the diabetic patient to avoid tight-fitting garments or activities that can decrease circulation. He should especially avoid sitting with his knees crossed, picking at sores or rough spots on his feet, walking barefoot, or applying adhesive tape to the skin on his feet.

Getting ready

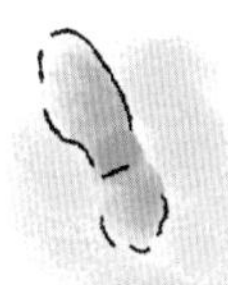

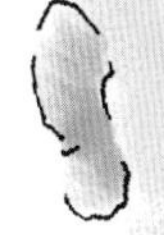

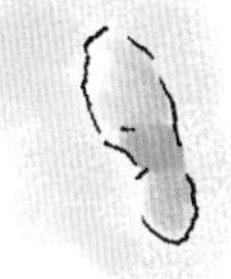

Fill the basin halfway with warm water. Test water temperature with a bath thermometer *because patients with diminished peripheral sensation could burn their feet in excessively hot water (over 105° F [40.6° C]) without feeling any warning pain.* If a bath thermometer isn't available, test the water by inserting your elbow. The water temperature should feel comfortably warm.

WARNING: Patients who have diabetes mellitus, peripheral neuropathy, or peripheral vascular disease should not soak their feet or hands because of the risk of injury from an inability to sense the water temperature and increased risk for infection.

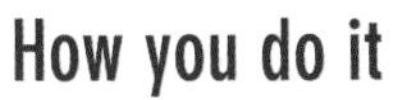

How you do it

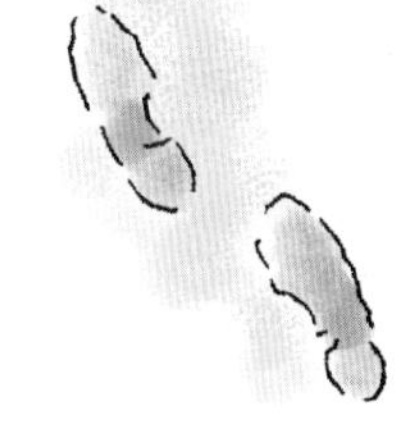

- Assemble equipment at the patient's bedside. Wash your hands and put on gloves if necessary.
- Tell the patient that you'll wash his feet and provide foot and toenail care.
- Cover the patient with a bath blanket. Fanfold the top linen to the foot of the bed.
- Place a linen-saver pad and a towel under the patient's feet *to keep the bottom linen dry.* Then position the basin on the pad.
- Insert a pillow beneath the patient's knee *to provide support* and cushion the rim of the basin with the edge of the towel *to prevent pressure.*

Soak, rinse, dry, detail, and moisturize

- Immerse one foot in the basin and wash it with soap and then allow the foot to soak for about 10 minutes. *Soaking softens the skin and toenails, loosens debris under toenails, and comforts and refreshes the patient.*
- After soaking the foot, rinse it with a washcloth, remove it from the basin, and place it on the towel.
- Dry the foot thoroughly, especially between the toes, *to prevent skin breakdown.* Blot gently to dry *because harsh rubbing may damage the skin.*
- Empty the basin, refill it with warm water, and clean and soak the other foot.

Soak one foot, clean the other

- Check facility policy regarding trimming, cleaning underneath, and filing nails.
  - Trim nails straight across at level of finger or follow curve of finger, ensuring that you do not cut down into nail grooves.

  - Use disposable emery board to file the nails, leaving no sharp corners.
  - Use a plastic applicator stick to clean beneath nails. Do not use an orange stick or end of cotton swab to clean beneath nails; these splinter and can cause injury.
- Consult a podiatrist if the patient has diabetes or circulatory problems.
- Rinse the foot that has been soaking, dry it thoroughly, and repeat the process.
- Apply lotion *to moisten dry skin* or lightly dust water-absorbent powder between the toes *to absorb moisture.*
- Remove and clean all equipment and dispose of gloves.

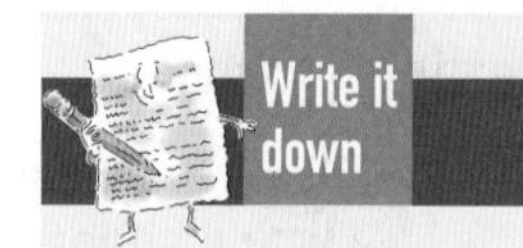

Documenting foot care

Record the date and time of foot care in your notes. Record and report abnormal findings and nursing actions you take.

Practice pointers

- While providing foot care, observe the color, shape, and texture of the toenails. If you see redness, drying, cracking, blisters, discoloration, or other signs of traumatic injury, especially in patients with impaired peripheral circulation, notify the doctor. *Because such patients are vulnerable to infection and gangrene,* they need prompt treatment.

Handling ingrown nails

- If a patient's toenail grows inward at the corners, tuck a wisp of cotton under it *to relieve pressure on the toe.*

Tailoring care to the bedridden patient

- When giving the bedridden patient foot care, perform ROM exercises unless contraindicated *to stimulate circulation and prevent foot contractures and muscle atrophy.* Tuck folded 2″ × 2″ gauze pads between overlapping toes *to protect the skin from the toenails.* Apply heel protectors *to prevent skin breakdown.* (See *Documenting foot care.*)

Perineal care

Perineal care, which includes care of the external genitalia and the anal area, should be performed during the daily bath and, if necessary, at bedtime and after urination and bowel movements. The procedure promotes cleanliness and prevents infection. It also removes irritating and odorous secretions, such as smegma, a cheese-like substance that collects under the foreskin of the penis and on the inner surface of the labia.

For the patient with perineal skin breakdown, frequent bathing followed by application of an ointment or cream aids healing. Always follow standard precautions when providing perineal care.

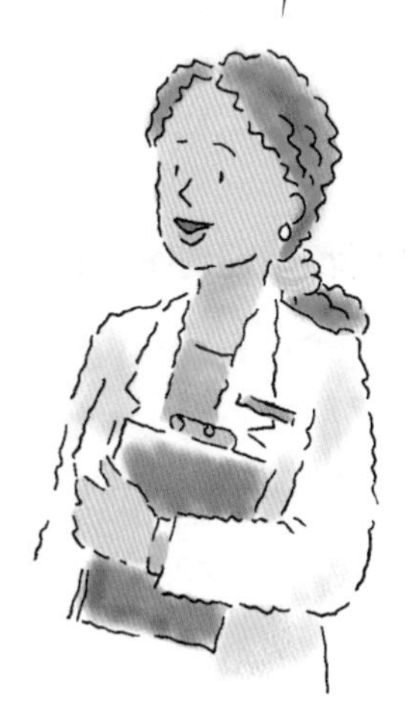
Always follow standard precautions when providing perineal care.

What you need

Gloves ✳ washcloths ✳ clean basin ✳ mild soap ✳ bath towel ✳ bath blanket ✳ toilet tissue ✳ linen-saver pad ✳ trash bag ✳ optional: bedpan, peri bottle, antiseptic soap, petroleum jelly, zinc oxide cream, vitamin A and D ointment, and an ABD pad.

Following genital or rectal surgery, you may need to use sterile supplies, including sterile gloves, gauze, and cotton balls.

Getting ready

Obtain ointment or cream as needed. Fill the basin two-thirds full with warm water. Also, fill the peri bottle with warm water if needed.

How you do it

- Assemble equipment at the patient's bedside and provide privacy.
- Wash your hands thoroughly, put on gloves, and explain to the patient what you're about to do.
- Adjust the bed to a comfortable working height *to prevent back strain* and lower the head of the bed, if allowed.
- Provide privacy and help the patient to a supine position. Place a linen-saver pad under the patient's buttocks *to protect the bed from stains and moisture.*

Caring for the female patient

- To minimize the patient's exposure and embarrassment, place the bath blanket over her with corners head to foot and side to side. Wrap each leg with a side corner, tucking it under the hip. Then fold back the corner between the legs to expose the perineum.

Front to back

- Ask the patient to bend her knees slightly and to spread her legs. Separate her labia with one hand and wash with the other using gentle downward strokes from front to back of the perineum *to prevent intestinal organisms from contaminating the urethra or vagina.* Avoid the area around the anus and use a clean section of washcloth for each stroke *to prevent the spread of contaminated secretions or discharge.*

- Using a clean washcloth, rinse thoroughly from front to back and then pat the area dry with a bath towel *to prevent soap residue and moisture from irritating the skin.* Apply ordered ointments or creams.
- Turn the patient on her side to Sims' position, if possible, *to expose the anal area.*
- Clean, rinse, and dry the anal area, starting at the posterior vaginal opening and wiping from front to back.

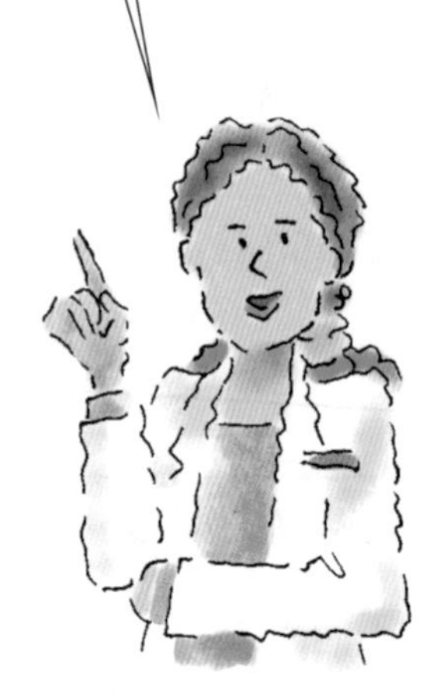
When performing perineal care, minimizing exposure and embarrassment is very important.

Caring for the male patient

- Drape the patient's legs to minimize exposure and embarrassment and to expose the genital area.

Make it a circular motion

- Hold the shaft of the penis with one hand and wash with the other, beginning at the tip and working in a circular motion from the center to the periphery *to avoid introducing microorganisms into the urethra.* Use a clean section of washcloth for each *stroke to prevent the spread of contaminated secretions or discharge.*
- For the uncircumcised patient, gently retract the foreskin and clean beneath it. Rinse well but don't dry *because moisture provides lubrication and prevents friction when replacing the foreskin.* Replace the foreskin *to avoid constriction of the penis, which causes edema and tissue damage.*
- Rinse thoroughly using the same circular motion.

Hitting all the necessary spots

- Wash the rest of the penis using downward strokes toward the scrotum. Rinse well and pat dry with a towel.
- Clean the top and sides of the scrotum. Rinse well and pat dry. Handle the scrotum gently *to avoid causing discomfort.*
- Turn the patient on his side. Clean the bottom of the scrotum and the anal area. Rinse well and pat dry.

After perineal care

- Reposition the patient and make him comfortable. Remove the bath blanket and linen-saver pad and then replace the bed linens.
- Clean and return the basin and dispose of soiled articles including gloves in the trash bag.

Practice pointers

- Give perineal care to all patients in a matter-of-fact way *to minimize embarrassment.*
- Offer patients the option of having someone of the same gender provide the care. Some patients are uncomfortable if someone of the opposite gender performs this care and don't always express their concerns to caregivers. Offering a chaperone is another alternative.

When incontinence is a factor

- If the patient is incontinent, first remove excess feces with toilet tissue. Then position him on a bedpan and add a small amount of antiseptic soap to a peri bottle to eliminate odor. Irrigate the perineal area *to remove any remaining fecal matter.*
- To reduce the number of linen changes, tuck an ABD pad between the patient's buttocks *to absorb oozing feces.* (See *Documenting perineal care.*)

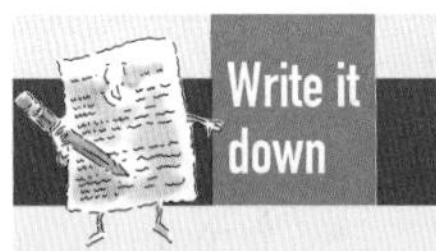

Documenting perineal care

Record perineal care and special treatment in your notes. Document the need for continued treatment, if necessary, in your plan of care. Describe perineal skin condition and odor or discharge.

Male incontinence device

Many patients don't require an indwelling urinary catheter to manage their incontinence. For male patients, a male incontinence device reduces the risk of urinary tract infection (UTI) from catheterization, promotes bladder retraining when possible, helps prevent skin breakdown, and improves the patient's self-image.

The device consists of a condom catheter secured to the shaft of the penis and connected to a leg bag or drainage bag. It has no contraindications, but it can cause skin irritation and edema. Most are made of soft silicone, but there are still latex catheters available.

What you need

Condom catheter kit (condom sheath of appropriate size) ✻ drainage bag or leg bag and straps ✻ extension tubing ✻ hypoallergenic tape or incontinence sheath holder ✻ commercial adhesive strip or skin-bond cement ✻ elastic adhesive or Velcro, if needed ✻ gloves ✻ scissors, if needed ✻ basin ✻ soap ✻ washcloth ✻ towel ✻ optional: solvent.

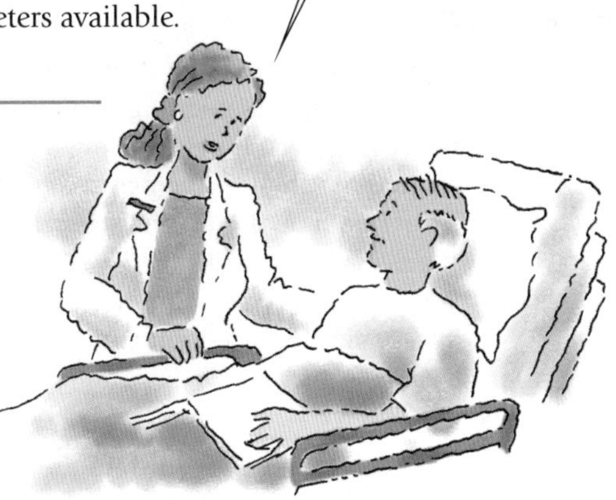
I'm going to apply a simple device to manage your incontinence.

Getting ready

- Fill the basin with lukewarm water. Then bring the basin and the remaining equipment to the patient's bedside.
- Assess the condition of the skin of the patient's penile shaft.
- Determine if there is a latex allergy.
- If a female nurse is responsible for the patient, consider asking if the patient would prefer having a male nurse or NAP perform the procedure.

How you do it

- Explain the procedure to the patient, wash your hands thoroughly, put on gloves, and provide privacy.

Applying the device

- Follow the manufacturer's directions for applying and securing the condom catheter.
- If the patient is circumcised, wash the penis with soap and water, rinse well, and pat dry with a towel. If the patient isn't circumcised, gently retract the foreskin and clean beneath it. Rinse well but don't dry *because moisture provides lubrication and prevents friction during foreskin replacement.* Replace the foreskin *to avoid penile constriction.*
- If necessary, clip the pubic hair at the base of the penis *to prevent the adhesive strip or skin-bond cement from pulling pubic hair.* Some manufacturers provide a hair guard that is placed over the penis before applying the catheter. It is removed once the catheter is placed.

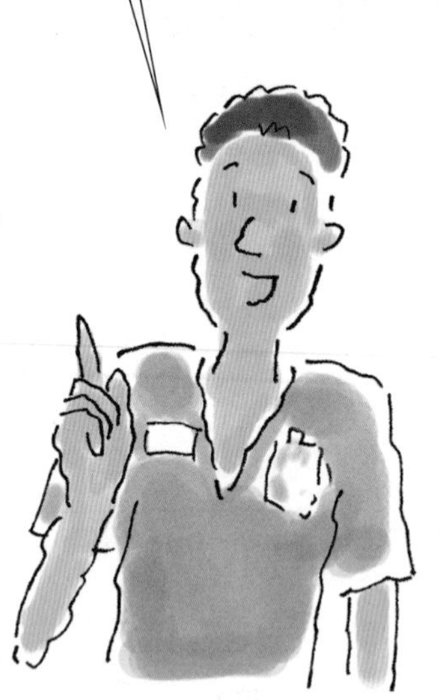
Pubic hair should not be shaved because it poses an increased risk for skin irritation.

Making it stick

- If you're using a precut commercial adhesive strip, insert the glans penis through its opening and position the strip 1″ (2.5 cm) from the scrotal area. If you're using uncut adhesive, cut a strip to fit around the shaft of the penis. Remove the protective covering from one side of the adhesive strip and press this side firmly to the penis *to enhance adhesion.* Remove the covering from the other side of the strip. If a commercial adhesive strip isn't available, apply skin-bond cement and let it dry for a few minutes.

Positioning the catheter

- Position the rolled condom catheter at the tip of the penis, with its drainage opening at the urinary meatus. Allow 1″ to 2″ (2.5 to 5 cm) of space at the tip of the penis *to prevent erosion and to allow for expansion when the patient voids.*

- Unroll the catheter upward, past the adhesive strip on the shaft of the penis. Then gently press the sheath against the strip until it adheres. (See *How to apply a condom catheter.*)
- After the condom catheter is in place, secure it with hypoallergenic tape or an incontinence sheath holder.
- Using extension tubing, connect the condom catheter to the leg bag or drainage bag. Remove and discard your gloves.

How to apply a condom catheter

Apply an adhesive strip to the shaft of the penis about 1" (2.5 cm) from the scrotal area.

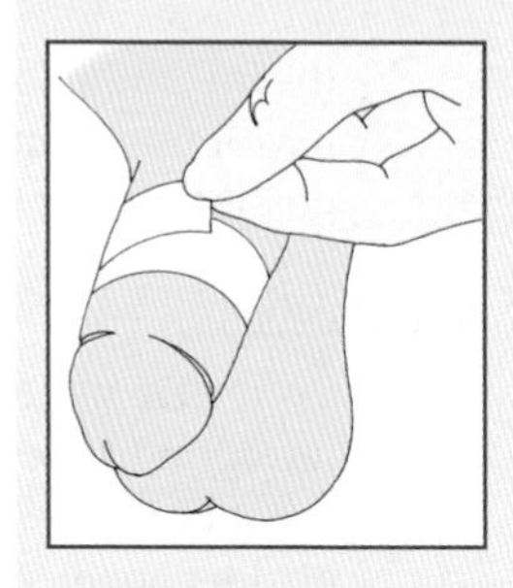

Then roll the condom catheter on to the penis past the adhesive strip, leaving about ½" (1 cm) clearance at the end. Press the sheath gently against the strip until it adheres.

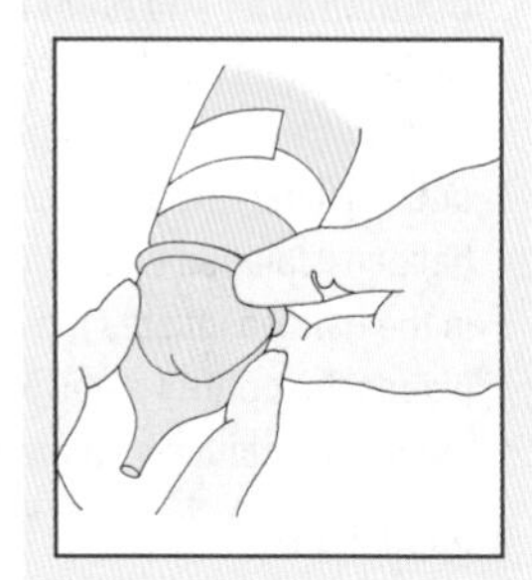

Removing the device

- Put on gloves and simultaneously roll the condom catheter and adhesive strip off the penis and then discard them. If you've used skin-bond cement rather than an adhesive strip, remove it with solvent. Also remove and discard the hypoallergenic tape or incontinence sheath holder.
- Clean the penis with lukewarm water, rinse thoroughly, and dry. Check for swelling or signs of skin breakdown.
- Remove the leg bag by closing the drain clamp, unlatching the leg straps, and disconnecting the extension tubing at the top of the bag. Discard your gloves.

Practice pointers

- If hypoallergenic tape or an incontinence sheath holder isn't available, secure the condom with a strip of elastic adhesive or Velcro. Apply the strip snugly—but not too tightly—*to prevent circulatory constriction.*
- Inspect the condom catheter for twists and the extension tubing for kinks *to prevent obstruction of urine flow, which could cause the condom to balloon and eventually dislodge.* (See *Documenting use of a male incontinence device.*)

Write it down

Documenting use of a male incontinence device

Record the date and time that the incontinence device was applied and removed. Also, note skin condition and the patient's response to the device, including voiding pattern, to assist with bladder retraining. Record urinary output. Report penile erythema, rashes, and/or skin breakdown to the physician.

Incontinence management

In elderly patients, incontinence commonly follows loss of urinary or anal sphincter control or impairment of it. The incontinence can be transient or permanent depending on the cause of the problem and the success of the treatment.

When treating a patient with urinary or fecal incontinence, carefully assess him for underlying disorders. Treatment aims to control the incontinence through bladder or bowel retraining or other behavior management techniques, diet modification, drug therapy, and possibly surgery.

Surgical options

Corrective surgery for urinary incontinence includes transurethral resection of the prostate in men, repair of the anterior vaginal wall or retropelvic suspension of the bladder in women, urethral sling, and bladder augmentation. (See *Artificial urinary sphincter implant* and *Correcting urinary incontinence with bladder retraining*.)

Artificial urinary sphincter implant

An artificial urinary sphincter implant helps restore continence to a patient with a neurogenic bladder.

Configuration and placement

An implant has a control pump, an occlusive cuff, and a pressure-regulating balloon. The cuff is placed around the bladder neck and the balloon is placed under the rectus muscle. Fluid in the balloon inflates the cuff. The surgeon places the control pump in the scrotum in men and in the labium in women.

Implant use

To void, the patient squeezes the bulb to deflate the cuff, which opens the urethra by returning fluid to the balloon. After voiding, the cuff reinflates automatically, sealing the urethra until he needs to void again.

Implant position in a man

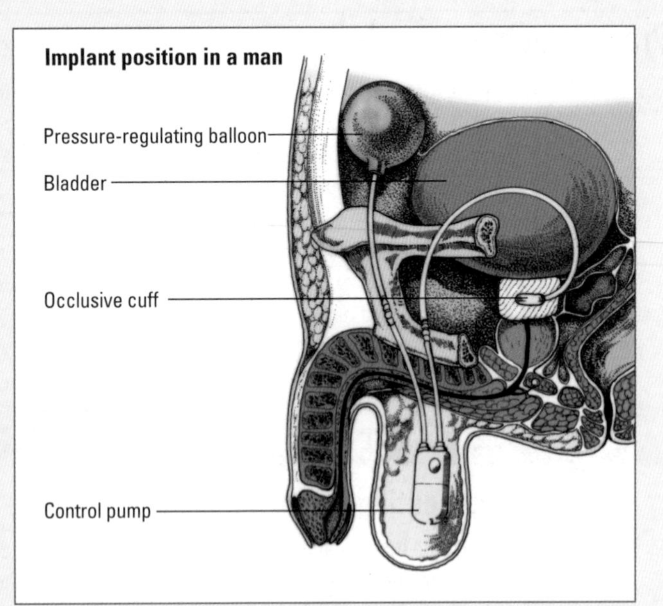

Correcting urinary incontinence with bladder retraining

The incontinent patient typically feels frustrated, embarrassed, and hopeless. Fortunately, he can correct the problem by retraining his bladder—a program that aims to establish a regular voiding pattern. Follow these guidelines.

Assess elimination patterns

First, assess the patient's intake and voiding patterns and reason for each accidental voiding (such as a coughing spell). Use an incontinence monitoring record.

Establish a voiding schedule

Encourage the patient to void regularly, for example, every 2 hours. When he can stay dry for 2 hours, increase the interval by 30 minutes every day until he achieves a 3- to 4-hour voiding schedule. Teach the patient to practice relaxation techniques, such as deep breathing, which help decrease the sense of urgency.

Record results and remain positive

Keep a record of continence and incontinence on a bladder retraining sheet for about 5 days. This may reinforce the patient's efforts to remain continent. Remember, your own and your patient's positive attitudes are crucial to his successful bladder retraining.

Take steps for success

Here are some additional tips to boost the patient's success:

- Locate the patient's bed near a bathroom or portable toilet. Leave a light on at night. If he needs assistance getting out of bed or a chair, promptly answer the call for help.
- Teach him how to prevent UTIs—for example, by drinking plenty of fluids (at least 2 qt [2 L]/day, unless contraindicated), drinking cranberry juice to acidify urine, wearing cotton underpants, and bathing with nonirritating soaps.
- Encourage him to empty his bladder completely before and after meals and at bedtime.
- Advise him to urinate whenever the urge arises and never to ignore it.
- Instruct him to take prescribed diuretics when he gets up in the morning.
- Advise him to limit the use of sleeping aids, sedatives, and alcohol; they decrease the urge to urinate and can increase incontinence, especially at night.
- If he's overweight, encourage him to lose weight.
- Suggest exercises to strengthen pelvic muscles.
- Instruct him to increase dietary fiber to decrease constipation and incontinence.
- Monitor him for signs of anxiety and depression.
- Reassure him that periodic incontinent episodes don't mean that the program has failed. Encourage persistence, tolerance, and a positive attitude.

What you need

Bladder retraining record sheet ✱ gloves ✱ stethoscope (to assess bowel sounds) ✱ moisture barrier cream ✱ incontinence pads ✱ bedpan ✱ specimen container ✱ label ✱ laboratory request form ✱ optional: stool collection kit, urinary catheter.

How you do it

- Whether the patient reports urinary or fecal incontinence or both, you'll need to perform initial and continuing assessments to plan effective interventions.

For urinary incontinence

- Ask the patient when he first noticed urine leakage and whether it began suddenly or gradually. Have him describe his typical urinary pattern: Does he usually experience incontinence during the day or at night? Ask him to rate his urinary control: Does he have moderate control or is he completely incontinent? If he sometimes urinates with control, ask him to identify when and how much he usually urinates.
- Evaluate related problems such as urinary hesitancy, frequency, and urgency; nocturia; and decreased force or interrupted urine stream.
- Ask the patient to describe treatment he has used for incontinence, whether doctor prescribed or self-prescribed.

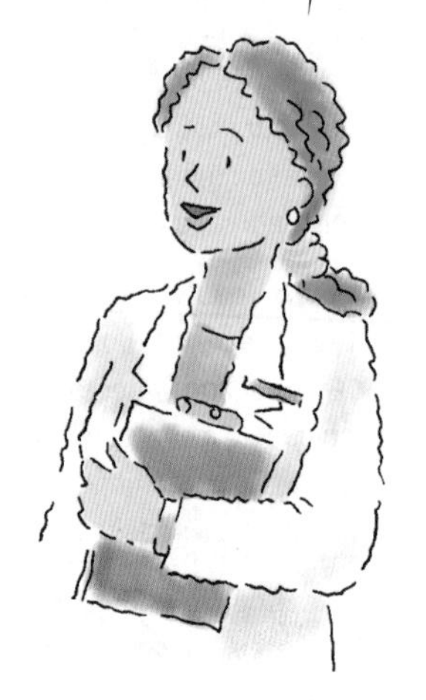
Note the onset, duration, severity and pattern of urinary incontinence.

Know the environment

- Assess the patient's environment. Is a toilet, commode, or bedpan readily available, and how long does the patient take to reach it? After he's in the bathroom, assess his manual dexterity—for example, how easily does he manipulate his clothes?
- Evaluate the patient's mental status and cognitive function.
- Quantify the patient's normal daily fluid intake.
- Review the patient's medication and diet history for drugs and foods that affect digestion and elimination.
- Review or obtain the patient's medical history, noting especially the number and route of births and incidence of UTI; prostate disorders; spinal injury or tumor; cerebrovascular accident; and bladder, prostate, or pelvic surgery. Also check for signs and symptoms of delirium, dehydration, urine retention, restricted mobility, fecal impaction, infection, inflammation, and polyuria.

Doing the inspection

- Put on gloves.
- Inspect the urethral meatus for obvious inflammation or anatomic defects. Have the female patient bear down while you note any urine leakage. Gently palpate the abdomen for bladder distention, which signals urine retention. If possible, have a urologist examine the patient.
- Obtain specimens for appropriate laboratory tests as ordered. Remove gloves and wash your hands. Label each specimen container and send it to the laboratory with a request form.

Retraining the bladder

- Begin incontinence management by implementing an appropriate bladder retraining program.
- Make sure the patient drinks plenty of fluids (six to eight 8-oz glasses) *to ensure adequate hydration and to prevent UTIs*. Restrict fluid intake after 6 p.m.

- Begin an exercise program *to strengthen the pelvic floor muscles and to help manage stress incontinence.* (See *Strengthening pelvic floor muscles.*)
- *To manage functional incontinence,* frequently assess the patient's mental and functional status. Regularly remind him to void. Respond to his calls promptly and help him get to the bathroom quickly. Provide positive reinforcement.

For fecal incontinence

- Ask the patient with fecal incontinence to identify its onset, duration, severity, and pattern (for instance, determine whether it occurs at night or with diarrhea). Focus the history on gastrointestinal (GI), neurologic, and psychological disorders.
- Note the frequency, consistency, and volume of stool passed in the past 24 hours. Obtain a stool specimen if ordered. Protect the patient's bed with an incontinence pad.
- Assess the patient for chronic constipation, GI and neurologic disorders, and laxative abuse.
- Assess the patient's medication regimen. Check for drugs that affect bowel activity, such as aspirin, some anticholinergic antiparkinsonians, aluminum hydroxide, calcium carbonate antacids, diuretics, iron preparations, opiates, tranquilizers, tricyclic antidepressants, and phenothiazines.

Doing the inspection

- Check whether his abdomen is distended and auscultate for bowel sounds. If not contraindicated, check for fecal impaction, which can contribute to overflow incontinence.

Retraining the bowel

- If the patient is neurologically capable, provide bowel retraining *to control chronic incontinence.*
- Advise the patient to eat plenty of fiber-rich foods, including lots of raw, leafy vegetables (such as carrots and lettuce); unpeeled fruits (such as apples); and whole grains (such as wheat or rye breads and cereals).
- Encourage adequate fluid intake.
- Teach the elderly patient to gradually stop using laxatives. Point out that using laxatives to promote regular bowel movement may have the opposite effect, producing either constipation or incontinence over time. Suggest natural laxatives, such as prunes and prune juice, instead.
- Promote regular exercise by explaining how it helps to regulate bowel motility. Even a nonambulatory patient can perform some exercises while sitting or lying in bed.

Strengthening pelvic floor muscles

Stress incontinence usually results from weakening of the urethral sphincter. Teach Kegel exercises to help a patient prevent or minimize stress incontinence.

Teaching Kegel exercises

Explain how to locate pelvic floor muscles by tensing the muscles around the anus, as if to retain stool, and then tightening the muscles of the pelvic floor, as if to stop the flow of urine. When learned, these exercises can be done—10 seconds tensed and 10 seconds relaxed—anywhere, anytime.

Establishing a regimen

A typical regimen starts with 15 contractions in the morning and afternoon and 20 at night. An alternative would be 10 minutes three times per day, working up to 25 contractions as strength improves.

Practice pointers

- To rid the bladder of residual urine, teach the patient to perform Valsalva's or Credé's maneuver or institute clean intermittent catheterization. Use an indwelling urinary catheter only as a last resort *because of the risk of UTI.*

Keeping it clean

- For fecal incontinence, provide proper hygienic care *to increase the patient's comfort and prevent skin breakdown and infection.* Clean the perineal area frequently and apply a moisture barrier cream. Control foul odors as well.

Boost his self-esteem

- Schedule extra time to provide encouragement and support for the patient, who may feel shame, embarrassment, and powerlessness from loss of control. (See *Documenting incontinence management.*)

Documenting incontinence management

In your notes, record:
- all bladder and bowel retraining efforts, noting scheduled bathroom times, food and fluid intake, and elimination amounts, as appropriate
- duration of the patient's continent periods
- complications, including emotional problems and signs of skin breakdown and infection as well as the treatments given for them.

Digital removal of fecal impaction

Fecal impaction is a large, hard, dry mass of stool in the folds of the rectum and, at times, in the sigmoid colon. The impaction results from prolonged retention and accumulation of stool. Common causes include poor bowel habits, inactivity, dehydration, improper diet (especially inadequate fluid intake), the use of constipation-inducing drugs, and incomplete bowel cleaning after a barium enema or barium swallow. Digital removal of fecal impaction is used when oil retention and cleansing enemas, suppositories, and laxatives fail to clear the impaction.

Avoid digital removal of fecal impaction in pregnant patients; in patients who have had rectal, genitourinary, abdominal, perineal, or gynecologic surgery; in patients with heart disease; and in patients with GI or vaginal bleeding, hemorrhoids, rectal polyps, or blood dyscrasias.

What you need

Gloves (two pairs) ✳ linen-saver pad ✳ bedpan ✳ plastic disposal bag ✳ soap ✳ water-filled basin ✳ towel ✳ water-soluble lubricant ✳ washcloth.

How you do it

- Explain the procedure to the patient and provide privacy.
- Position the patient on his left side and flex his knees *to allow easier access to the sigmoid colon and rectum.*

- Drape the patient and place a linen-saver pad beneath his buttocks to prevent soiling of the bed linens.
- Put on gloves and moisten an index finger with water-soluble lubricant *to reduce friction during insertion, thereby avoiding injury to sensitive tissue.*
- Instruct the patient to breathe deeply *to promote relaxation*. Then gently insert your lubricated index finger beyond the anal sphincter until you touch the impaction. Rotate your finger gently around the stool *to dislodge and break it into small fragments*. Then work the fragments downward to the end of the rectum and remove each one separately.

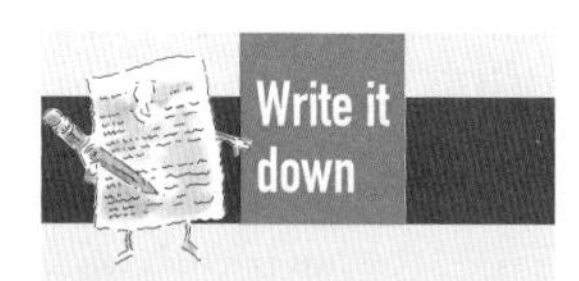

Documenting digital removal of fecal impaction

In your notes, record:
- time and date of the procedure
- patient's response
- color, consistency, and odor of the stool.

Getting the sphincter going

- Before removing your finger, gently stimulate the anal sphincter with a circular motion two or three times *to increase peristalsis and encourage evacuation*.
- Remove your finger and change your gloves. Then clean the anal area with soap and water and lightly pat it dry with a towel.
- Offer the patient the bedpan or commode *because digital manipulation stimulates the urge to defecate.*

Finishing up

- Place disposable items in the plastic bag and discard the bag properly. If necessary, clean the bedpan and return it to the bedside stand.
- Wash your hands.

Practice pointers

- If the patient experiences pain, nausea, rectal bleeding, changes in pulse rate or skin color, diaphoresis, or syncope, stop the procedure immediately and notify the doctor. *Digital removal of fecal impaction can stimulate the vagus nerve and may decrease heart rate and cause syncope.* (See *Documenting digital removal of fecal impaction*.)

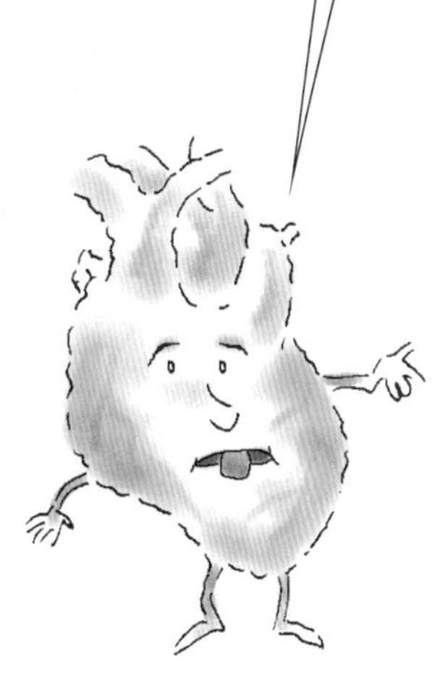
Be aware that digital removal of fecal impaction can decrease the patient's heart rate.

Preoperative care

Preoperative care begins when surgery is first planned and ends when anesthesia is administered. This type of care includes a preoperative interview and assessment to collect baseline subjective and objective data from the patient and his family; diagnostic tests, such as urinalysis, electrocardiogram, and chest radiography; preoperative teaching; securing informed consent from the patient; and physical preparation.

What you need

Gloves ✻ thermometer ✻ sphygmomanometer ✻ stethoscope ✻ watch with second hand ✻ weight scale ✻ tape measure.

Getting ready

Assemble all equipment needed at the patient's bedside or in the admission area.

How you do it

- Obtain a health history and assess the patient's knowledge, perceptions, and expectations about his surgery.
- Measure the patient's height, weight, and vital signs.
- Identify risk factors that may interfere with a positive expected outcome. Assess him for latex allergy.

Getting the patient up to speed

- If the patient is having same-day surgery, make sure he knows ahead of time not to eat or drink anything for 8 hours before surgery. Make sure that he knows the time he's scheduled to arrive at the facility and that he has arranged for someone to take him home afterward. Also, instruct him to leave all jewelry and valuables at home.
- Explain preoperative procedures to the patient. Include typical events that he can expect. Discuss equipment that may be used postoperatively, such as nasogastric tubes and I.V. equipment. Explain the typical incision, dressings, and staples or sutures that will be used. *Preoperative teaching can help reduce postoperative anxiety and pain, increase patient compliance, hasten recovery, and decrease the length of stay.*

Tell the patient he'll feel a drowsy, floating sensation as the anesthesia takes effect.

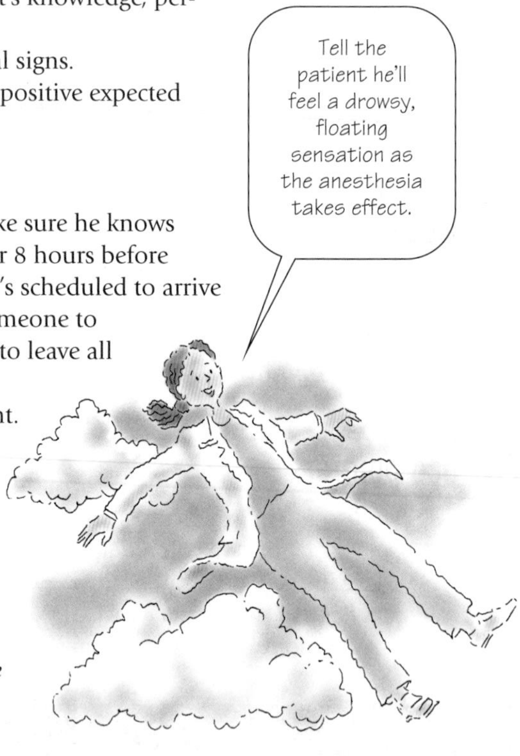

Transferring to the OR

- When discussing transfer procedures and techniques, describe sensations that the patient will experience. Also, inform him that he may have to wait a short time in the holding area before going into the operating room.
- Tell him that he'll be taken to the operating room on a stretcher and transferred from the stretcher to the operating room table.

For his own safety, he'll be held securely to the table with soft restraints. The operating room nurses will check his vital signs frequently.
- Warn the patient that the operating room may feel cool.
- Explain that even though the doctors and nurses will be observing him closely, they won't talk to him much *so that the preoperative medication can take effect.* Describe the drowsy floating sensation he'll feel as the anesthetic takes effect. Tell him it's important that he relax at this time.
- Electrodes may be put on his chest *to monitor his heart rate during surgery.*

Exercising afterward

- Tell the patient about exercises that he may have to perform after surgery—such as deep-breathing, coughing (while splinting the incision if necessary), extremity exercises, and movement and ambulation—*to minimize respiratory and circulatory complications.* If the patient will undergo ophthalmic or neurologic surgery, he won't be asked to cough *because coughing increases intraocular and intracranial pressures.*

Above and beyond preoperative teaching

- On the day of surgery, provide morning care and verify that the patient has signed an informed consent form. (See *Understanding informed consent.*) Administer ordered preoperative medications, complete the preoperative checklist and chart, and provide support to the patient and his family.

Getting the GI tract in order

- Other immediate preoperative interventions include preparing the GI tract (restricting food and fluids for about 8 hours before surgery) *to reduce vomiting and the risk of aspiration,* cleaning the lower GI tract of fecal material with an enema before abdominal or GI surgery, and giving antibiotics for 2 to 3 days preoperatively *to prevent GI bacteria from contaminating the peritoneal cavity.*

The final checklist

- Just before the patient is moved to the surgical area, make sure he's wearing a hospital gown, has his identification band in place, and has his vital signs recorded. Check to see that hairpins, nail polish, and jewelry have been removed. Note whether dentures, contact lenses, or prosthetic devices have been removed or left in place.

Understanding informed consent

Informed consent means that the patient has consented to a procedure after receiving a full explanation of it and its risks and complications. Although obtaining informed consent is the doctor's responsibility, the nurse is responsible for verifying that this step has been taken.

Sign what you witness
If you're asked to witness a patient's authorization but you didn't hear the doctor explain the procedure to the patient, you must sign that you're witnessing only his signature.

No meds before signing
The patient must sign a consent form before receiving preoperative medication. Forms signed after sedatives are given are legally invalid. Emancipated minors can sign their own consent forms; however, a parent or guardian must sign a consent form for a child or adult with impaired mental status.

Practice pointers

- Make sure that preoperative medications are given on time *to enhance the effect of the anesthesia* and that the patient takes nothing by mouth preoperatively, including oral medications, unless ordered.
- Raise the bed's side rails immediately after preoperative medications are given.

In the waiting area

- If family members or others are present, direct them to the appropriate waiting area and offer support as needed. (See *Documenting preoperative care.*)

Write it down

Documenting preoperative care

Complete the preoperative checklist used by your facility. Chart all nursing care measures, preoperative medications, results of diagnostic tests, and the time the patient is transferred to the surgical area. The checklist and chart must accompany the patient to surgery.

Postoperative care

Postoperative care begins when the patient arrives in the postanesthesia care unit (PACU) and continues as he moves on to the short procedure unit, medical-surgical unit, or critical care area. Postoperative care aims to minimize postoperative complications by early detection and prompt treatment. After anesthesia, a patient may experience pain, inadequate oxygenation, or adverse physiologic effects of sudden movement.

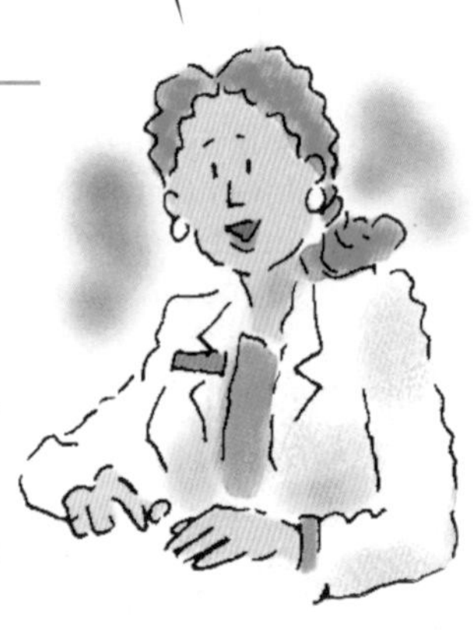
Minimizing complications—that's the goal of postop care.

What you need

Thermometer * watch with second hand * stethoscope * sphygmomanometer * postoperative flowchart or other documentation tool * optional: blankets.

How you do it

- Assemble the equipment at the patient's bedside.
- Obtain the patient's record from the PACU nurse.

Making transfers

- Transfer the patient from the PACU stretcher to the bed and position him properly. Get a coworker to help if necessary.
- When moving the patient, keep transfer movements smooth *to minimize pain and postoperative complications and avoid back strain among team members.*
- If the patient has had orthopedic surgery, get a coworker to help transfer him. Ask the coworker to move only the affected extremity.

- If the patient is in skeletal traction, you may receive special orders for moving him. If you must move him, have a coworker move the weights as you and another coworker move the patient.
- Make the patient comfortable and raise the bed's side rails *to ensure the patient's safety.*

Vital facts

- Assess the patient's level of consciousness (LOC), skin color, and mucous membranes.
- Monitor the patient's respiratory status by assessing his airway. Note breathing rate and depth and auscultate for breath sounds. Administer oxygen and initiate oximetry *to monitor oxygen saturation,* if ordered.
- Monitor the patient's pulse rate. It should be strong and easily palpable. The heart rate should be within 20% of the preoperative heart rate.
- Compare postoperative blood pressure to preoperative blood pressure. It should be within 20% of the preoperative level unless the patient suffered a hypotensive episode during surgery.
- Assess the patient's temperature *because anesthesia lowers body temperature.* Body temperature should be at least 95° F (35° C). If it's lower, apply blankets *to warm the patient.*

Other areas to watch

- Check the patient's infusion sites for redness, pain, swelling, or drainage.
- The patient's surgical wound dressings should be clean and dry. If they're soiled, assess the characteristics of the drainage and outline the soiled area. Note the date and time of assessment on the dressing. Check the soiled area frequently; if it enlarges, reinforce the dressing and alert the doctor.
- Note the presence and condition of drains and tubes. Note the color, type, odor, and amount of drainage. Make sure all drains are properly connected and free from kinks and obstructions.
- If the patient has had vascular or orthopedic surgery, assess the appropriate extremity—or all extremities, depending on the surgical procedure. Evaluate color, temperature, sensation, movement, and presence and quality of pulses and notify the doctor of abnormalities.

When the anesthesia wears off

- As the patient recovers from anesthesia, monitor his respiratory and cardiovascular status closely. Watch for signs of airway obstruction and hypoventilation caused by laryngospasm or for sedation, which can lead to hypoxemia. Cardiovascular complications—such as arrhythmias and hypotension—may result from the anesthetic or the operation.

- Encourage coughing and deep-breathing exercises. Don't encourage them if the patient has just had nasal, ophthalmic, or neurologic surgery *to avoid increasing intraocular and intracranial pressures.*
- Administer postoperative medications, such as antibiotics, analgesics, antiemetics, or reversal agents, as ordered.
- Remove all fluids from the patient's bedside until he's alert enough to eat and drink. Before giving him liquids, assess his gag reflex *to prevent aspiration.* To do this, lightly touch the back of his throat with a cotton swab—the patient will gag if the reflex has returned. Do this test quickly *to prevent a vagal reaction.*

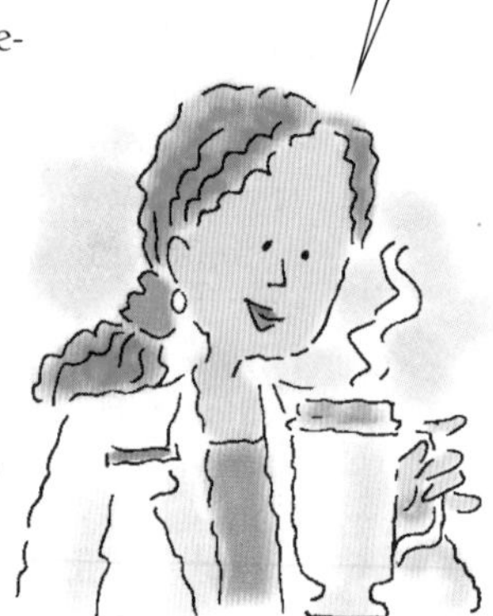
Don't give the patient access to liquids until he's fully alert.

Practice pointers

- Fear, pain, anxiety, hypothermia, confusion, and immobility can upset the patient and jeopardize his safety and postoperative status. Offer emotional support to the patient and his family. Keep in mind that the patient who has lost a body part or who has been diagnosed with an incurable disease will need ongoing emotional support. Refer him and his family for counseling as needed.

After general anesthesia

- As the patient recovers from general anesthesia, reflexes appear in reverse order to that in which they disappeared. Hearing recovers first, so avoid speaking inappropriately in his presence.
- The patient under general anesthesia can't protect his own airway because his muscles are relaxed. As he recovers, his cough and gag reflexes reappear. If he can lift his head without assistance, he should be able to breathe on his own.

After spinal anesthesia

- If the patient received spinal anesthesia, he'll need to remain in a supine position with the bed adjusted to between 0 and 20 degrees for at least 6 hours *to reduce the risk of spinal headache from leakage of cerebrospinal fluid.*
- The patient won't be able to move his legs, so reassure him that sensation and mobility will return.

After epidural anesthesia

- If the patient has had epidural anesthesia for postoperative pain control, monitor his respiratory status closely. *Respiratory arrest may result from paralysis of the diaphragm by the anesthetic.* He may also suffer nausea, vomiting, or itching.

For PCA

- If the patient will be using a patient-controlled anesthesia (PCA) unit, make sure he understands how to use it. Caution him to activate it only when he has pain and not when he feels sleepy.
- Review facility policy regarding PCA use. (See *Documenting postoperative care.*)

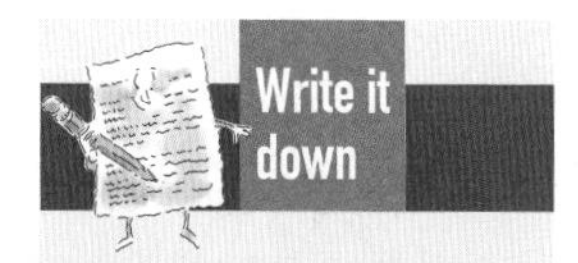

Documenting postoperative care

Document vital signs on the appropriate flowchart. In your notes, record:
- condition of dressings and drain
- characteristics of drainage
- interventions taken to alleviate pain and anxiety and the patient's responses to them
- complications and interventions taken.

Care of the dying patient

A patient needs intensive physical and emotional support as he approaches death. Signs and symptoms of impending death include reduced respiratory rate and depth, decreased or absent blood pressure, weak or erratic pulse rate, lowered skin temperature, decreased LOC, diminished sensorium and neuromuscular control, diaphoresis, pallor, cyanosis, and mottling.

Emotional support for the dying patient and his family usually involves reassuring them and being there *to help ease fear and loneliness.* More intense support is important at earlier stages, especially for a patient with a long-term progressive illness, who can work through the stages of dying. (See *Five stages of dying,* page 82.)

What you need

Clean bed linens * clean gowns * gloves * water-filled basin * soap * washcloth * towels * lotion * linen-saver pads * petroleum jelly * suction and resuscitation equipment, as necessary * optional: indwelling urinary catheter, pain medication.

How you do it

- Assemble equipment at the patient's bedside as needed.

Meeting physical needs

- Take vital signs often and observe the patient for pallor, diaphoresis, and decreased LOC.
- Reposition the patient in bed at least every 2 hours *because sensation, reflexes, and mobility diminish first in the legs and gradually in the arms.* Make sure the bed sheets cover him loosely *to reduce discomfort caused by pressure on arms and legs.*

Five stages of dying

According to Elisabeth Kübler-Ross, author of *On Death and Dying*, the dying patient may progress through five psychological stages in preparation for death. Although each patient experiences these stages differently, and not necessarily in this order, understanding the stages will help you meet your patient's needs.

Denial

When the patient first learns of his terminal illness, he'll refuse to accept the diagnosis. He may experience physical signs and symptoms similar to a stress reaction—shock, fainting, pallor, sweating, tachycardia, nausea, and GI disorders.

During this stage, be honest with the patient but not blunt or callous. Maintain communication with him so he can discuss his feelings when he accepts the reality of his impending death. Don't force him to confront this reality.

Anger

When the patient stops denying his impending death, he may show deep resentment toward anyone who will live on after he dies. Although you may instinctively draw back from the patient or even resent this behavior, remember that he's dying and that he has a right to be angry. After you accept his anger, you can help him find ways to express it and can help his family understand it.

Bargaining

Although the patient acknowledges his impending death, he attempts to bargain with God or fate for more time. He will probably strike this bargain secretly. If he does confide in you, don't urge him to keep his promises.

Depression

In this stage, the patient may first experience regrets about his past and then grieve about his condition. He may withdraw from his friends, family, doctor, and you. He may suffer from anorexia, increased fatigue, or self-neglect. You may find him sitting alone, in tears. Accept the patient's sorrow, and if he talks to you, listen. Provide comfort by touch, as appropriate. Resist the temptation to make optimistic remarks or cheerful small talk.

Acceptance

In this last stage, the patient accepts the inevitability and imminence of his death—without emotion. The patient may simply desire the quiet company of a family member or friend. If, for some reason, a family member or friend can't be present, stay with the patient to satisfy his final need. Remember, however, that many patients die before reaching this stage.

Watch what you say

- When the patient's vision and hearing start to fail, turn his head toward the light and speak to him from near the head of the bed. *Because hearing may be acute despite loss of consciousness,* avoid speaking inappropriately in his presence.
- Change the bed linens and the patient's gown as needed. Provide skin care during gown changes, and adjust the room temperature for patient comfort, if necessary.
- Observe the patient for incontinence or anuria, *which can result from diminished neuromuscular control or decreased renal function.* If necessary, obtain an order to catheterize the patient or place linen-saver pads beneath his buttocks. Put on gloves and wash the perineal area with soap and water. Dry thoroughly *to prevent irritation.*

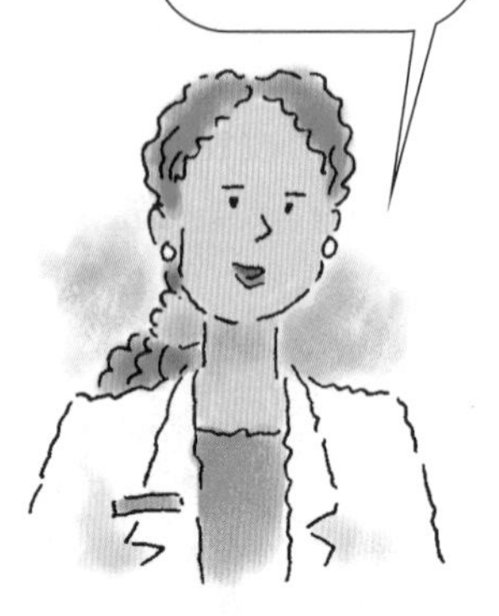
Make your patient's last days as comfortable as possible.

- With suction equipment, suction the patient's mouth and upper airway *to remove secretions*. Elevate the head of the bed *to decrease respiratory resistance*. As his condition deteriorates, he may breathe mostly through his mouth.
- Offer fluids frequently and lubricate the patient's lips and mouth with petroleum jelly *to counteract dryness*.
- If the comatose patient's eyes are open, provide appropriate eye care *to prevent corneal ulceration*, which can cause blindness.
- Provide ordered pain medication as needed. Keep in mind that, as circulation diminishes, medications given intramuscularly (I.M.) will be poorly absorbed. Medications should be given I.V., if possible, *for optimum results*.

Meeting emotional needs

- Fully explain all care and treatments to the patient even if he's unconscious *because he may still be able to hear*. Answer any questions as candidly as possible without sounding callous.
- Allow the patient to express his feelings, which may range from anger to loneliness. Take time to talk with him. Sit near the head of his bed and avoid looking rushed or unconcerned. Touch him often in neutral areas, such as on his arm or his hand, and allow him to hold your hand as desired.
- Notify family members, if absent, when the patient wishes to see them. Let the patient and family discuss death at their own pace.
- Offer to contact a member of the clergy or social services department, if appropriate.
- At an appropriate time, ask the family whether they've considered organ and tissue donation. Check the patient's records *to determine whether he completed an organ donor card*. (See *Understanding organ and tissue donation*.)

Understanding organ and tissue donation

A federal regulation enacted in 1998 requires facilities to report all deaths to the regional organ procurement organization. The regulation ensures that the family of every potential donor understands the option to donate. According to the American Medical Association, about 25 kinds of organs and tissues can be transplanted. Although donor organ requirements vary, the typical donor must be between the ages of newborn and 60 years and free from transmissible disease. Tissue donations are less restrictive, and some tissue banks will accept skin from donors up to age 75.

Collection of most organs—such as the heart, liver, kidney, or pancreas—requires that the patient be pronounced brain dead and kept physically alive until organ harvesting. Eyes, skin, bone, and heart valves may be taken after death.

Contact your regional organ procurement organization for specific organ donation criteria or to identify a potential donor. Or call the United Network for Organ Sharing at (804) 330-8500.

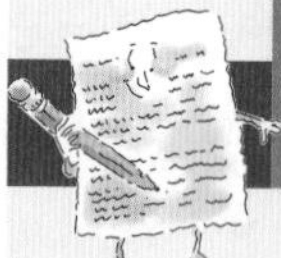

Write it down

Documenting care of the dying patient

Record changes in the patient's vital signs, intake and output, and LOC. Note the times of cardiac arrest and the end of respiration and notify the doctor when these occur.

Practice pointers

- If the patient has signed a living will, the doctor will write a "no code" order on his progress notes and order sheets. Know state policy regarding the living will.
- If it's legal, transfer the no code order to the patient's chart or Kardex and inform incoming staff of this order.

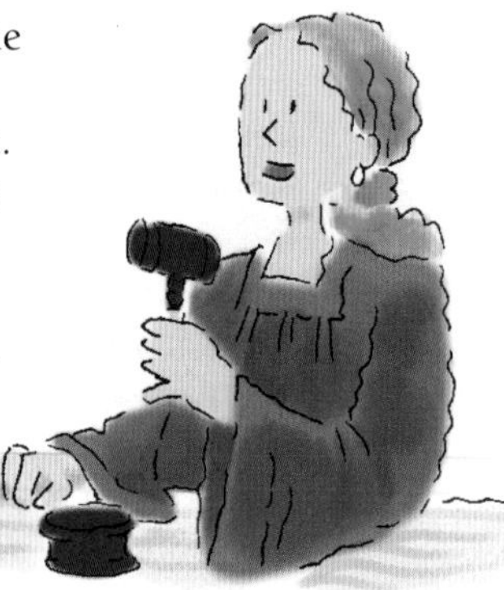
Know your state's policy regarding living wills.

Family matters

- If family members remain with the patient, show them where the bathrooms, lounges, and cafeterias are located.
- Explain the patient's needs, treatments, and plan of care to them.
- If appropriate, offer to teach them specific skills so they can take part in nursing care. Emphasize that their efforts are important and effective.
- As the patient's death approaches, give them emotional support. (See *Documenting care of the dying patient.*)

Postmortem care

After the patient dies, care includes preparing him for family viewing, arranging transportation to the morgue or funeral home, and determining the disposition of the patient's belongings. Postmortem care also entails comforting and supporting the patient's family and friends and providing for their privacy.

Postmortem care usually begins after a doctor certifies the patient's death. If the patient died violently or under suspicious circumstances, postmortem care may be postponed until the medical examiner completes an autopsy.

What you need

Gauze or soft string ties ✳ gloves ✳ chin straps ✳ ABD pads ✳ cotton balls ✳ plastic shroud or body wrap ✳ three identification tags ✳

adhesive bandages * plastic bag * tape * sheet * water-filled basin * soap * towels * washcloths * stretcher.

A commercial morgue pack usually contains gauze or string ties, chin straps, a shroud, and identification tags.

How you do it

- Document any auxiliary equipment, such as a mechanical ventilator, still present. Put on gloves.

Preparing for family viewing

- Place the body in the supine position, arms at sides and head on a pillow. Then elevate the head of the bed slightly *to prevent discoloration from blood settling in the face.*
- If the patient wore dentures and your facility's policy permits, gently insert them; then close his mouth. Close his eyes by gently pressing on his lids with your fingertips. If they don't stay closed, place moist cotton balls on the eyelids for a few minutes, and then try again to close them. Place a folded towel under his chin *to keep his jaw closed.*
- Remove indwelling urinary catheters, tubes, and tape and apply adhesive bandages to puncture sites. Replace soiled dressings.
- Collect all the patient's valuables *to prevent loss.* If you're unable to remove a ring, cover it with gauze, tape it in place, and tie the gauze to the wrist *to prevent slippage and subsequent loss.*
- Clean the body thoroughly using soap, a basin, and washcloths. Place one or more ABD pads between the buttocks *to absorb rectal discharge or drainage.*
- Cover the body up to the chin with a clean sheet.
- Offer comfort and emotional support to the family and intimate friends. If they wish to see the body, let them to do so in private. Ask if they would prefer to leave the patient's jewelry on the body.
- Support the family's needs for spiritual or religious rituals.
- After the family leaves, remove the towel from under the chin of the deceased patient. Pad the chin and wrap chin straps under the chin and tie them loosely on top of the head. Pad the wrists and ankles *to prevent bruises* and tie them together with gauze or soft string ties.

Preparing for transport

- Fill out the three identification tags. Each tag should include the deceased patient's name, room and bed numbers, date and time of death, and doctor's name. Tie one tag to the deceased patient's hand or foot, but don't remove his identification bracelet *to ensure correct identification.*

- Place the shroud or body wrap on the morgue stretcher and, after obtaining assistance, transfer the body to the stretcher. Wrap the body and tie the shroud or wrap with the string provided. Then attach another identification tag and cover the shroud or wrap with a clean sheet. If a shroud or wrap isn't available, dress the patient in a clean gown and cover the body with a sheet.
- If the patient died of an infectious disease, label the body according to facility policy.
- Close the doors of adjoining rooms if possible. Then take the body to the morgue. Use corridors that aren't crowded and, if possible, use a service elevator.

Handling personal belongings

- Place the deceased patient's personal belongings, including valuables, in a plastic bag and attach the third identification tag to it.

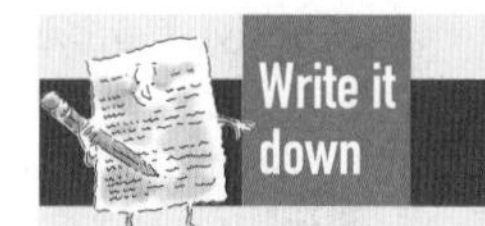

Documenting postmortem care

Although the extent of documentation varies among facilities, always record the disposition of the patient's possessions, especially jewelry and money. Also, note the date and time the patient was transported to the morgue.

Practice pointers

- Give the deceased patient's personal belongings to his family or bring them to the morgue. If you give the family jewelry or money, make sure a coworker is present as a witness. Obtain the signature of an adult family member *to verify receipt of valuables or to state their preference that jewelry remain on the patient.*
- Offer emotional support to the deceased patient's family and friends and to his facility roommate, if appropriate. (See *Documenting postmortem care.*)

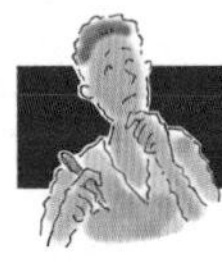

Quick quiz

1. Which heart rate in a neonate would be considered normal?
   A. 60 to 80 beats/minute
   B. 100 to 120 beats/minute
   C. 120 to 140 beats/minute
   D. 140 to 160 beats/minute

Answer: C. A heart rate of 120 to 140 beats/minute in a neonate is considered normal.

2. When giving a back massage, which stroke uses alternating kneading and stroking of the patient's back and upper arms?
   A. Pétrissage
   B. Massage
   C. Effleurage
   D. Palpation

Answer: A. Pétrissage involves using alternating kneading and stroking maneuvers on the patient's back and upper arms.

3. In which patient is digital removal of a fecal impaction contraindicated?

   A. Myasthenia gravis
   B. Diabetes mellitus
   C. Heart disease
   D. Stroke

Answer: C. Digital removal of a fecal impaction shouldn't be performed on a patient who has heart disease because stimulation of the vagus nerve can cause bradycardia or syncope.

Scoring

☆☆☆ If you answered all three items correctly, congratulations! You are a fundamentals phenom!

☆☆ If you answered two items correctly, great! You are fundamentally prepared for fundamentals!

☆ If you answered fewer than two correctly, don't despair. Just review the chapter and try again!

Selected References

Allbutt, H. (2014, May 18). Korotkoff sounds annotated video [Video file]. Retrieved from http://www.youtube.com/watch?v=VJrLHePNDQ4-

American Association of Nurse Anesthetists. (2014). *Latex allergy management (guidelines)*. Retrieved from http://www.aana.com/resources2/professionalpractice/Pages/Latex-Allergy-Protocol.aspx

American Society of Anesthesiologists Committee. (2011). Practice guidelines for preoperative fasting and the use of pharmacological agents to reduce the risk of pulmonary aspiration: Application to healthy patients undergoing elective procedures: An updated report by the American Society of Anesthesiologists Committee on Standards and Practice Parameters. *Anesthesiology, 114*(3), 495–511.

Atwood, D., Uttley, R., & Ortega, D. (2012). Organ donation considerations. *Nursing Management, 43*(6), 22–27.

Centers for Disease Control and Prevention. (2014). *Hand hygiene in healthcare settings.* Retrieved from http://www.cdc.gov/handhygiene

Centers for Medicare and Medicaid Services. (2014). *§482.13(e): Standard: Restraint or seclusion.* State Operations Manual Appendix A rev. CoP. Retrieved from http://www.cms.gov/Regulations-and-Guidance/Guidance/Manuals/downloads/som107ap_a_hospitals.pdf

Deans, B. (2013). Choosing and positioning a blood pressure cuff [Video file]. Retrieved from http://www.youtube.com/watch?v=II0ioJNLnyg

Drake, K. (2011). SCIP core measures: Deep impact. *Nursing Management, 42*(5), 24.

Lewis, S., Dirksen, S. R., Heitkemper, M. M., et al. (2011). *Medical-surgical nursing: Assessment and management of clinical problems* (8th ed.). St. Louis, MO: Mosby.

Nelson, A. (2008). *Safe patient handling and movement algorithms.* Retrieved from http://www.visn8.va.gov/patientsafetycenter/safepthandling/

Perry, A., & Potter, P. (2015). *Mosby's pocket guide to nursing skills and procedures* (8th ed.). St. Louis, MO: Elsevier.

Perry, A., Potter, P., & Ostendorf, W. (2014). *Clinical nursing skills & techniques.* St. Louis, MO: Elsevier.

Pickering, T. G., Hall, J. E., Appel, L. J., et al. (2005). Recommendations for blood pressure measurement in humans and experimental animals: Part 1: Blood pressure measurement in humans: A statement for professionals from the Subcommittee of Professional and Public Education of the American Heart Association Council on High Blood Pressure Research. *Hypertension, 45,* 142–161.

Siegel, J. D., Rhinehart, E., Jackson, M., et al. (2007). 2007 *Guideline for isolation precautions: Preventing transmission of infectious agents in healthcare settings.* Retrieved from http://www.cdc.gov/hicpac/pdf/isolation/isolation2007.pdf

Sumana, R. (1998). Latex allergy. *American Family Physician, 57*(1), 93–100.

The Joint Commission. (2009). *Provision of care, treatment and services: Restraint/seclusion for hospitals that use TJC for deemed status purposes.* Chicago, IL: Author.

Chapter 2

Specimen collection

Just the facts

In this chapter, you'll learn:

- about procedures for collecting specimens and how to perform them
- what patient care, complications, and patient teaching are associated with each procedure
- about essential documentation for each procedure.

Venipuncture

Venipuncture is the process of obtaining intravenous (I.V.) access for the purpose of venous blood sampling or for I.V. therapy. Nurses are often responsible for venipuncture, although many facilities employ phlebotomists for this function. The personnel who are able to draw blood specimens at your organization will be determined by state regulations and reflected in their policies.

Venipuncture is the most common method of obtaining blood specimens. It involves inserting a hollow-bore needle into the lumen of a vein to obtain a specimen using either a Vacutainer for multiple samples or a needle and syringe. The site may be used as a major site to obtain blood for laboratory testing and for infusion therapy. It is essential to maintain the integrity of the site and to follow safe practices when performing the procedure. You must be skilled in venipuncture to avoid injuries and complications that can occur with improper technique.

Anterior to and below the elbow—that's the usual spot for venipuncture.

What you need

Tourniquet (use latex-free tourniquets if patient has an allergy or is at high risk) ✳ clean gloves ✳ alcohol, chlorhexidine, or antiseptic pads ✳ color-coded collection tubes containing appropriate additives ✳ patient identification labels ✳ laboratory requisition ✳ 2″ × 2″ gauze pads ✳ adhesive bandage ✳ biohazard bag ✳ sharps container (OSHA approved) ✳ Warming devices or warm compresses

Guide to color-top collection tubes

Tube color	Draw volume	Additive	Purpose
Red (glass)	2 to 20 mL	None	Chemistry, serology, toxicology, and drug testing
Lavender	2 to 10 mL	K_2 EDTA	Whole-blood studies (ABO grouping, Rh typing, antibody screening)
Green	2 to 15 mL	Heparin (sodium, lithium, or ammonium)	Plasma studies
Light blue	2.7 or 4.5 mL	Sodium citrate and citric acid	Coagulation studies on plasma
Royal blue	2.7 or 4.5 mL	Sodium heparin, Na_2EDTA, or none	Trace elements, toxicology, nutritional chemistry
Gray	3 to 10 mL	Glycolytic inhibitor, such as sodium fluoride/ potassium oxalates or Na_2EDTA	Glucose determinations on serum or plasma
Yellow	12 mL	Acid-citrate-dextrose	Blood bank studies, human leukocyte antigen (HLA) phenotyping, DNA, paternity testing

Follow agency recommended order of tubes for drawing samples, such as yellow; red; light blue; speckled red, green, lavender; then gray. Blood cultures are always first if ordered.

may be used to dilate blood vessel and increase flow ✱ Ice or refrigerant should be available for specimens that require immediate chilling. (See *Guide to color-top collection tubes*.)

Venipuncture with syringe: sterile safety needles (20G to 21G for adults; 23G to 25G for children) ✱ sterile 10- to 20-mL luer-lock safety syringe ✱ needle-free blood transfer device.

Venipuncture with Vacutainer: Vacutainer and safety access device with luer-lock adapter ✱ sterile double-ended needles. (See "Venipuncture with syringe" for sizes.)

Getting ready

Universal precautions must be followed when obtaining blood specimens. Specimens from any patient could be infected with blood pathogens.

If you're using evacuated tubes, open the needle packet, attach the needle to its holder, and select the appropriate tubes. If you're using a syringe, choose one large enough to hold all the blood required for the test, and then attach the appropriate needle to it. Label all collection tubes clearly with the patient's name and room number, the doctor's name, and the date and time of collection.

Have your supplies laid out in order of use and in close proximity to the area you are accessing. The tubes should be in order of collection as specified by your organization's policies and procedures. This is important to avoid contamination of the specimens.

How you do it

- Determine if there are special circumstances that need to be met prior to drawing the specimen, such as NPO for a fasting level, a certain amount of time after a medication was given for peak and trough levels, or the specimen needing ice immediately after it is drawn.
- Assess for risks associated with venipuncture: (*You will need to hold the site for at least 5 minutes following the venipuncture to avoid a hematoma.*)
  - Anticoagulant therapy
  - Low platelet count
  - Bleeding disorders such as hemophilia
  - A medication history that includes drugs that increase risk of bleeding
- Identify the patient using two patient identifiers according to the facility's policies and procedures.
- Wash your hands thoroughly and put on gloves.
- Tell the patient that you're about to collect a blood sample and explain the procedure *to ease his anxiety and ensure his cooperation*. Ask him if he's ever felt faint, sweaty, or nauseated when having blood drawn. If he answers affirmatively, have the patient lie in a supine position during the venipuncture procedure.
- If the patient is on bed rest, ask him to lie in a supine position with his head slightly elevated and his arms at his sides; if he's ambulatory, ask him to sit in a chair and support his arm securely on an armrest or a table.

The best site

The median cubital and cephalic veins are most commonly used. Alternative sites are on the dorsum of the arm or dorsal hand veins. The basilic vein should only be used if there is no more prominent vein available. Because of its close proximity to the brachial nerve and artery, there is an increased risk of complications. The veins in the foot and ankle should only be used as a last resort because it limits the patient's mobility, can cause thrombophlebitis, and is a more painful site to access. Veins on the underside of the wrist should also be avoided because of the close proximity to nerves. (See *Contraindicated sites*, page 92.)

- Assess the patient's veins *to determine the best puncture site*. (See *Common venipuncture sites*, page 93.) Observe the skin for the vein's blue color. Use your index finger to palpate and trace the

Contraindicated sites

- Sites with extensive scarring from burns or surgery
- Arm on the side a mastectomy was performed because of increased risk for infection from decreased lymphatic drainage
- Hematoma at site from existing injury to blood vessel wall
- Site of I.V. therapy/blood transfusions—if there is a need to use that arm, go below the site of the infusion. If you must go above the site, the infusion needs to be turned off for at least 2 minutes before performing the venipuncture to reduce the risk of contamination. This should be noted on the specimen requisition and the lab will determine if it can be used.
- Extremity with a cannula, fistula, or vascular graft
- Edematous extremeties
- Sites with noticeable skin conditions such as eczema or infection because they can introduce pathogens into the venipuncture site
- Tattoos are similar to scars and can have impaired circulation and be more prone to infection. However, there is no conclusive evidence to date that the dye contaminates the sample.

path of the vein. Arteries pulsate more, have thicker walls than veins, and are more elastic. Thrombosed veins are cordlike, roll easily, and are not preferable. If you are using a tourniquet for vein selection, it should be released after 1 minute and left off for at least 2 minutes before reapplying for venipuncture.

- Tie a tourniquet 2″ (5.1 cm) proximal to the area chosen. *By impeding venous return to the heart while still allowing arterial flow, a tourniquet produces venous dilation.* It can be placed over a gown to protect the skin, especially in the elderly. If the veins are already dilated and prominent, you do not need to use a tourniquet.
  - Palpate the distal pulse below the tourniquet. If you cannot feel it, release the tourniquet, wait for 60 seconds, and reapply the tourniquet more loosely.
- WARNING: Do not leave the tourniquet on for more than a minute or it can cause hemodilution of the specimen, stasis, and localized acidemia.
- Have the patient open and close the fist several times and then leave it clenched. This will allow the blood to fill the vein and distend it.
- Palpate the vein you selected previously.

Don't cancel

- Clean the venipuncture site with antiseptic swabs. Take the first swab and move back and forth in a horizontal motion. Take the second swab and repeat, moving vertically this time. Finally, use a third

Common venipuncture sites

These illustrations show the most common sites for venipuncture. The best sites are the veins in the forearm, followed by those on the hand.

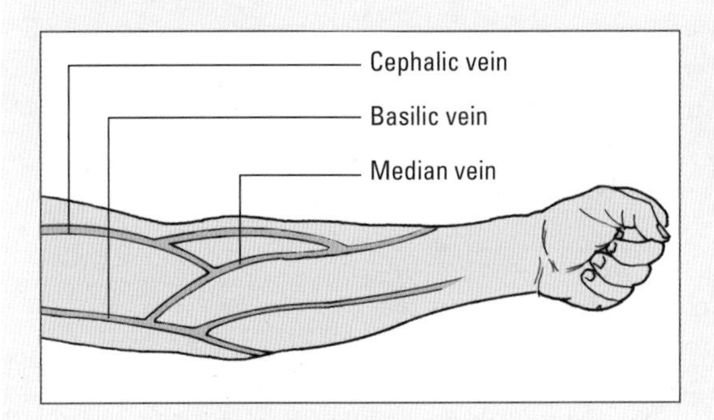

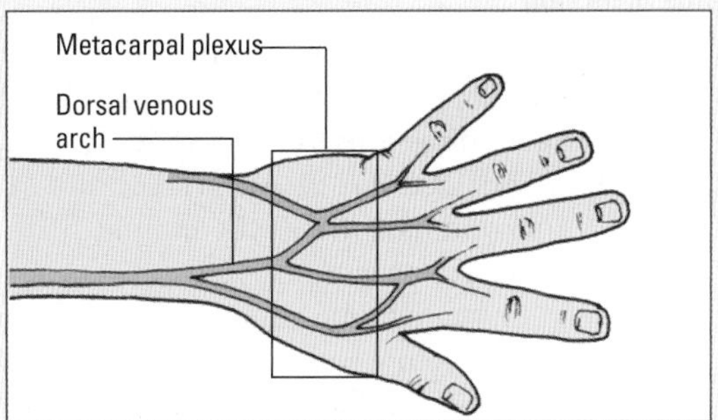

swab in a circular motion starting at the center and moving outward approximately 2″. Allow to dry so antimicrobial can work to the full extent and to reduce pain when inserting the needle. Alcohol swabs can be substituted; however, they should not be used for blood cultures or alcohol levels because they can alter the test results.

- Immobilize the vein by pressing just below the venipuncture site with your thumb and drawing the skin taut. DO NOT touch the cleaned site. If the site is touched, repeat the disinfection.

Hold that position

- Tell patients they will feel a sting or a pinch. To prepare them, ask them to count to three and tell them the sting will only last for that long. You can also ask them to count when you are inserting the needle to distract them.
- Remove the needle cover and inspect the needle for burrs or defects that can cause injury to the patient's veins and increase discomfort. Position the needle holder or syringe with the needle bevel up and the shaft parallel to the path of the vein and at a 30-degree angle to the arm. Insert the needle into the vein. If you're using a syringe, venous blood will appear in the hub. Withdraw the blood slowly, pulling the plunger of the syringe gently *to create steady suction* until you obtain the required sample. *Pulling the plunger too forcibly may collapse the vein.* If you're using a needle holder and an evacuated tube, grasp the holder securely to stabilize it in the vein and push down on the collection tube until the needle punctures the rubber stopper. Blood will flow into the tube automatically. Try not to move the needle between tubes because this will cause additional pain for the patient.

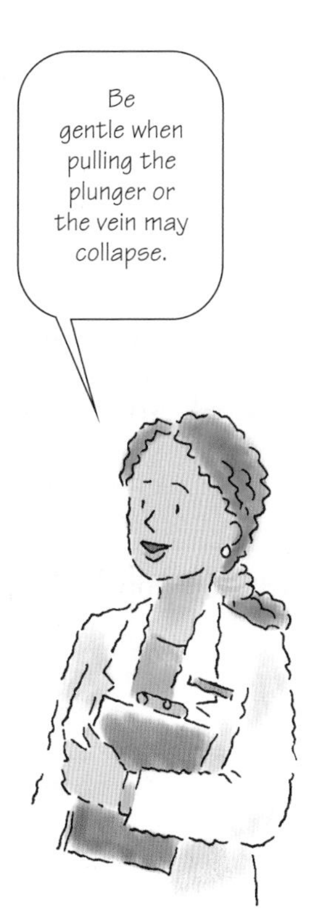
Be gentle when pulling the plunger or the vein may collapse.

- Remove the tourniquet as soon as blood flows adequately *to prevent stasis and hemoconcentration, which can impair test results.* If the flow is sluggish, leave the tourniquet in place longer, but always remove it before withdrawing the needle.

Gentle inversion

- Continue to fill the required tubes, removing one and inserting another. Gently invert each tube 8 to 10 times or per manufacturer's directions as you remove it *to help mix the additive with the sample.* DO NOT SHAKE THEM or it can hemolyze the specimen.
- After you have drawn the sample, place a gauze pad over the puncture site without putting pressure on the needle. When using an evacuated tube, remove it from the needle holder *to release the vacuum* before withdrawing the needle from the vein. Quickly but carefully withdraw the needle with the Vacutainer from the vein. If you used a syringe to draw the sample, activate the safety cover and immediately discard the needle in the appropriate container.

Gentle pressure

- Immediately apply gentle pressure to the puncture site for 2 to 3 minutes or until bleeding stops. *This prevents extravasation into the surrounding tissue, which can cause a hematoma.*
- After bleeding stops, apply an adhesive bandage or tape over the gauze pad.
- If you've used a syringe, a needle-free transfer device or double-ended needle for Vacutainer device will enable vacuum filling of blood tubes to the appropriate level. Gently invert each tube 8 to 10 times to disperse additives and prevent red blood cell hemolysis.
- Finally, check the venipuncture site *to see if a hematoma has developed.* If it has, apply warm soaks to the site.
- Discard syringes, needles, and used gloves in the appropriate containers.
- Verify that the requisition matches the patient identifiers on the label.
- Label the specimen and send it to the laboratory with the appropriate requisition.

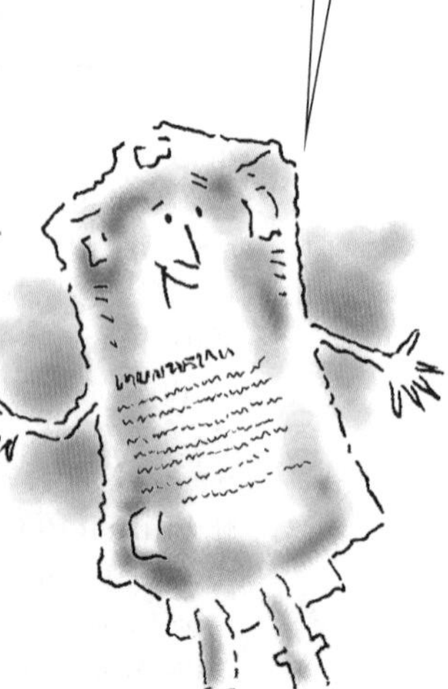
Don't collect a sample from a site that's already being used for I.V. therapy.

Practice pointers

- Consult with physician for prioritizing tests if venous access is poor and there is risk of not being able to obtain all required blood samples ordered.
- If signs and symptoms of infection occur at the venipuncture site, notify the physician and apply moist heat to the site.
- Prevent injury to a nerve, tendon, or muscle by carefully palpating the vein and using a 30-degree angle. Avoid excessive probing (moving the needle side to side).

- Prevent hemoconcentration by avoiding prolonged tourniquet application, massaging, flicking, squeezing, or probing the site. Other factors include long-term I.V. therapy and using sclerosed or occluded veins.
- Avoid hemolysis of the specimen when using a blood transfer device by allowing the vacuum to pull the blood into the tubes and not using the plunger to force the blood into the tubes.
- An individual should generally make only two venipuncture attempts before having someone else try.
- Blood minimization is used in some organizations to decrease the amount of blood drawn by using micro tubes that require less blood to run the test. Refer to your organization's policies and procedures for more information. (See *Documenting venipuncture.*)

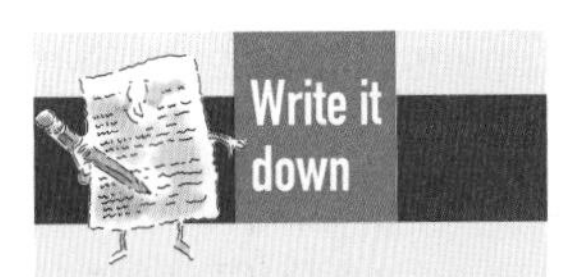

Documenting venipuncture

In your notes, record:

- date, time, and site of the venipuncture and/or method used to obtain blood specimen
- name of the test ordered
- time the sample was sent to the laboratory
- amount of blood collected
- patient's temperature
- description of venipuncture site and adverse reactions to the procedure.

Central or peripherally inserted central venous catheter

If the patient has a central venous catheter (CVC) or a peripherally inserted central catheter (PICC), draw venous blood sample using this special access per agency policy. Be sure to turn off all I.V. pumps and close all clamps and, when possible, clean the distal lumen with an alcohol wipe. Identify the type of cap on the device and follow the appropriate directions. Luer-lock caps impregnated with 70% isopropyl alcohol were recommended by the Infusion Nurses Society in 2011; if one is being used, remove it prior to wiping the lumen port.

After attaching only a 10-mL prefilled saline syringe, open clamp, aspirate gently, and flush with 5 to 10 mL of saline. Whether using a syringe or Vacutainer method, be prepared to waste the first 5 mL of blood obtained and flush the second line with 5 to 10 mL of saline using a push–pause method. Some caps have positive pressure, but if not, hold the syringe plunger down and close the slide clamp and then remove the syringe. Reattach an alcohol-impregnated cap if being used.

Blood culture

Blood cultures are performed to detect bacterial invasion (bacteremia) and the systemic spread of such an infection (septicemia) through the bloodstream. In this procedure, a laboratory technician, doctor, or nurse performs a venipuncture at the patient's bedside and then transfers the blood samples into two bottles: one containing an anaerobic (without oxygen) medium and the other an aerobic (with oxygen) medium. The bottles are incubated to encourage any organisms present in the sample to grow in the media. Blood cultures allow identification of about 67% of pathogens within 24 hours and up to 90% within 72 hours.

Timing may be everything

Although some authorities consider the timing of culture collections debatable and possibly irrelevant, others advocate two sets for those with multiple indicators of infective endocarditis, three sets with the third collected 4 to 6 hours later for suspected noncontaminant pathogens, and four sets when a common contaminant is suspected. The first of these should be collected at the earliest sign of suspected bacteremia or septicemia.

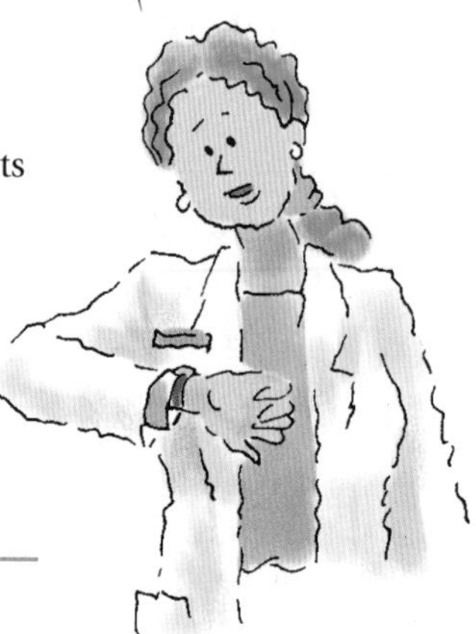
Many clinicians suggest drawing blood samples at least 1 hour apart.

What you need

Tourniquet ✳ gloves ✳ chlorhexidine skin prep ✳ 20-mL syringe for an adult or adequate syringe size for a child ✳ three or four 20G 1″ needles ✳ two or three blood culture bottles (50-mL bottles for adults or 20-mL bottles for infants and children) with sodium polyethanol sulfonate added (one aerobic bottle containing a suitable medium, such as trypticase soy broth with 10% carbon dioxide atmosphere; one anaerobic bottle with prereduced medium; and, possibly, one hyperosmotic bottle with 10% sucrose medium) ✳ laboratory requisition ✳ 2″ × 2″ gauze pads ✳ small adhesive bandages ✳ labels.

Getting ready

Check the expiration dates on the culture bottles and replace outdated bottles.

How you do it

- Tell the patient that you need to collect a series of blood samples to check for infection. Explain the procedure *to ease his anxiety and promote cooperation*. Explain that the procedure usually requires three blood samples collected at different times.
- Wash your hands and put on gloves.
- Tie a tourniquet 2″ (5.1 cm) proximal to the area chosen. (See "Venipuncture," page 89.)

Clean and dry

- Avoid contamination from skin flora for accurate testing. A recent literature review found cleansing the venipuncture site with 70% alcohol followed by 2% chlorhexidine and allowing the site to dry before puncture is effective. Start at the site and work outward in a circular motion. Wait 30 to 60 seconds for the skin to dry.
- After removing cap from culture bottles, cleanse the top with 70% alcohol and allow to dry.

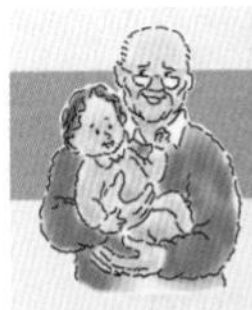

Ages and stages

Blood cultures from a child

When drawing blood for cultures from a child, follow weight-based quantity recommendations. A guideline is provided from a recent literature review:

- 1 mL for less than 8.6 kg
- 3 mL for 8.6 to 13.6 kg
- 5 mL for 13.6 to 27.3 kg
- 10 mL for 27.3 to 40.9 kg
- 15 mL for 40.9 to 54.4 kg.

Wipe the diaphragm tops of the culture bottles with 70% alcohol and change the needle on the syringe used to draw the blood. Next, inject half of the blood into each pediatric culture bottle.

- Perform a venipuncture, drawing 10 to 15 mL of blood from an adult from two different venipuncture sites to confirm culture growth. (See *Blood cultures from a child.*) With each specimen, activate the safety guard and discard the needle. Apply gentle pressure to the puncture site with a gauze pad for 2 to 3 minutes or until bleeding stops.
- After bleeding stops, apply an adhesive bandage.
- Wipe the diaphragm tops of the culture bottles with a povidone-iodine pad and change the needle on the syringe used to draw the blood.
- Inject 5 mL of blood into each 50-mL bottle. If both aerobic and anaerobic cultures are needed, fill the anaerobic bottle first because the organisms may take longer to grow. (Bottle size may vary according to facility protocol, but the sample dilution should always be 1:10.)

Culture ID

- Label the culture bottles with the patient's name and room number; doctor's name; and date, time, and site of collection. **Verify that the information on the label matches the requisition.** Indicate the suspected diagnosis and the patient's temperature, and note on the laboratory requisition any recent antibiotic therapy. Send the samples to the laboratory immediately.
- Discard syringes, needles, and gloves in the appropriate container.
- Check bottles for any signs of external contamination with blood. Decontaminate with 70% alcohol as needed.
- Remove gloves and perform hand hygiene after specimen is obtained and any spillage is cleaned.

Practice pointers

- Obtain each set of cultures from a different site.
- Avoid using existing I.V. lines for cultures or drawing them at time of I.V. catheter insertion to decrease false-positive rates from contamination and specimens from colonized devices. (See *Documenting blood culture collection.*)

Documenting blood culture collection

In your notes, record the:
- date, time, and site of blood sample collection
- name of the test
- amount of blood collected
- number of bottles used
- patient's temperature
- adverse reactions to the procedure.

Blood glucose tests

Reagent strip tests (such as Glucostix, Chemstrip bG, and Multistix), skin puncture equipment, and point-of-care monitors provide a quick, easy way to test a patient's blood glucose level. A drop of capillary blood—obtained by fingerstick, heelstick, or earlobe puncture—provides the blood sample.

These tests can detect or monitor blood glucose levels in patients with diabetes and improve tight control to slow progression of complications. They can also screen for diabetes mellitus and neonatal hypoglycemia and help distinguish diabetic coma from nondiabetic coma. What's more, they can be performed in the hospital, doctor's office, or patient's home.

Match the color to the chart

In blood glucose tests, a reagent patch on the tip of a handheld plastic strip changes color in response to the amount of glucose in the blood sample. Comparing the color change with a standardized color chart provides a semiquantitative measurement of blood glucose levels. More commonly today, inserting the reagent strip into a portable blood glucose meter (such as Glucometer II, Accu-Chek II, or OneTouch) provides quantitative measurements that are just as accurate as other laboratory tests. Some meters store successive test results electronically to help determine glucose patterns.

What you need

Reagent strips ✻ clean gloves ✻ portable blood glucose meter, if available ✻ alcohol pads ✻ gauze pads ✻ disposable lancets or mechanical blood-letting device ✻ small adhesive bandage ✻ watch or clock with a second hand.

How you do it

- Explain the procedure to the patient or the child's parents.
- Next, select the puncture site—usually the fingertip or earlobe for an adult or a child. (See *Not appropriate for all.*)
- Have the adult patient wash the hands to reduce the transmission of microorganisms at the puncture site.
- Wash your hands and put on gloves.
- If necessary, dilate the capillaries by applying warm, moist compresses to the area for about 10 minutes.
- Wipe the puncture site with an alcohol pad and dry it thoroughly with a gauze pad.

At the fingertip

- To collect a sample from the fingertip with a disposable lancet (smaller than 2 mm), position the lancet on the side of the patient's fingertip, perpendicular to the lines of the fingerprints. Pierce the skin sharply and quickly *to minimize the patient's anxiety and pain and to increase blood flow.* Alternatively, you can use a mechanical bloodletting device, such as an Autolet, which uses a spring-loaded lancet.
- After puncturing the fingertip, don't squeeze the puncture site: *Doing so can dilute the sample with tissue fluid.*
- Touch or wick a drop of blood to the reagent patch on the strip, following the manufacturer's direction and ensuring the patch is entirely covered for accurate results.

Under pressure

- After collecting the blood sample, briefly apply pressure to the puncture site *to prevent painful extravasation of blood into subcutaneous tissues.* Ask the adult patient to hold a gauze pad firmly over the puncture site until bleeding stops.
- Make sure you leave the blood on the strip for exactly 60 seconds on manually read reagent strips or according to manufacturer's directions. Blood glucose monitors can provide results in as little as 5 seconds. It allows blood glucose measurement between 20 and 800 mg/dl.

Color coordinated

- Compare the color change on the strip with the standardized color chart on the product container. If you're using a blood glucose meter, follow the manufacturer's instructions. Meter designs vary, but they all analyze a drop of blood placed on a reagent strip that comes with the unit and provide a digital display or audible message of the resulting glucose level.
- After bleeding has stopped, you may apply a small adhesive bandage to the puncture site.

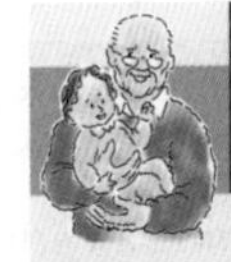

Ages and stages

Not appropriate for all

The fingertip or earlobe of an adult or a child is typically chosen as a venipuncture site for blood glucose testing. However, these sites are not appropriate for infants. The heel or great toe is commonly the preferred site for an infant.

Practice pointers

- Before using reagent strips, check the expiration date on the package and replace outdated strips. Check for special instructions related to the specific reagent. The reagent area of a fresh strip should match the color of the "0" block on the color chart. Protect the strips from light, heat, and moisture.
- There are more than 30 different glucose meters and many types of reagent strips; familiarity with the specific directions ensure accurate testing.
- Before using a blood glucose meter, calibrate it and run it with a control sample *to ensure accurate test results*. Follow the manufacturer's instructions for calibration. Routine competency demonstration is required in many facilities.
- Some patients may have an embedded continuous glucose monitor to provide instantaneous measures.

Stay away from the cold

- Avoid selecting cold, cyanotic, or swollen puncture sites *to ensure an adequate blood sample*. If you can't obtain a capillary sample, perform venipuncture and place a large drop of venous blood on the reagent strip. If you want to test blood from a refrigerated sample, allow the blood to return to room temperature before testing it. (See *Checking blood glucose*.)
- In order to help detect abnormal glucose metabolism and diagnose diabetes mellitus, the doctor may order other blood glucose tests. (See *Documenting blood glucose tests*.)

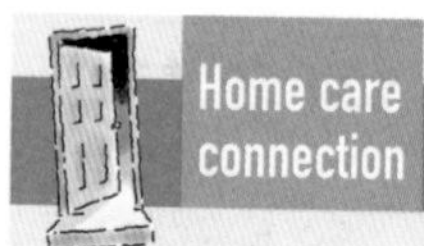
Home care connection

Checking blood glucose

If the patient will be using the reagent strip system at home, teach him the proper use of the lancet or Autolet, reagent strips and color chart, and portable blood glucose meter as necessary. Also, provide written guidelines to reinforce your teaching.

Arterial puncture for ABG analysis

Obtaining an arterial blood sample requires percutaneous puncture of the brachial, radial, or femoral artery or withdrawal of a sample from an arterial line. Low incidence of complications, ease of bedside testing, and quick results make arterial blood gas (ABG) analysis a valuable tool in assessing and directing patient treatment, especially when critically ill.

Breathing check

ABG analysis evaluates ventilation by measuring blood pH and the partial pressures of arterial oxygen ($Pa{O_2}$) and partial pressure of arterial carbon dioxide ($Pa{CO_2}$). Blood pH measurement reveals the blood's acid-base balance. $Pa{O_2}$ indicates the amount of oxygen that the lungs deliver to the blood, and $Pa{CO_2}$ indicates the lungs'

Write it down

Documenting blood glucose tests

Record the reading from the reagent strip (using a portable blood glucose meter or a color chart) in your notes or on a special flowchart, if available. Also record the time and date of the test. Note interventions you took.

capacity to eliminate carbon dioxide. ABG samples can also be analyzed for oxygen content and saturation and for bicarbonate values. Respiratory, metabolic, and mixed acid-base problems can be identified and treated.

Special training required

A doctor, however, usually performs collection from the femoral artery. Before attempting a radial puncture, Allen's test should be performed. (See *Performing a modified Allen's test.*)

Safety

Specific recommendations for arterial puncture:

- universal precautions including impervious gown or apron and face protection
- using extreme caution to avoid injury from needles
- cleansing hands and other skin immediately if blood exposure occurs and after gloves are removed.

Performing a modified Allen's test

Rest the patient's arm on the mattress or bedside stand, supporting the wrist with a rolled towel to perform this test. The patient is instructed to clench his fist. Then use your index and middle fingers to press on the radial and ulnar arteries, occluding them for a few seconds.

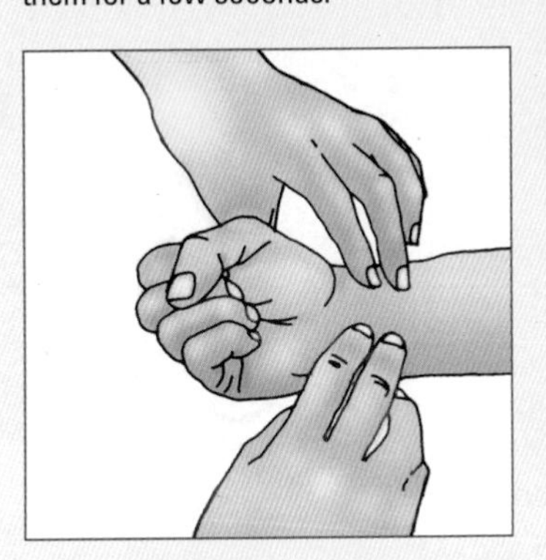

Without removing your fingers from the patient's arteries, ask him to unclench his fist and hold his hand in a relaxed position. The palm should be blanched because pressure from your fingers has impaired the normal blood flow.

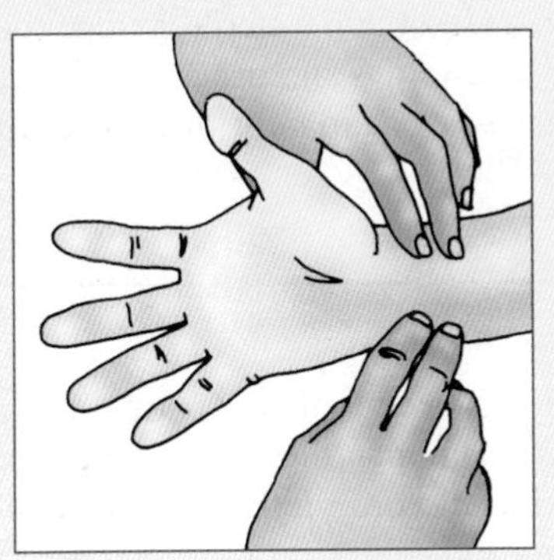

Release pressure on the patient's ulnar artery. If the hand becomes flushed within 5 to 15 seconds, which indicates blood filling the vessels, you can safely proceed with the radial artery puncture. If the hand doesn't flush, perform the test on the other arm.

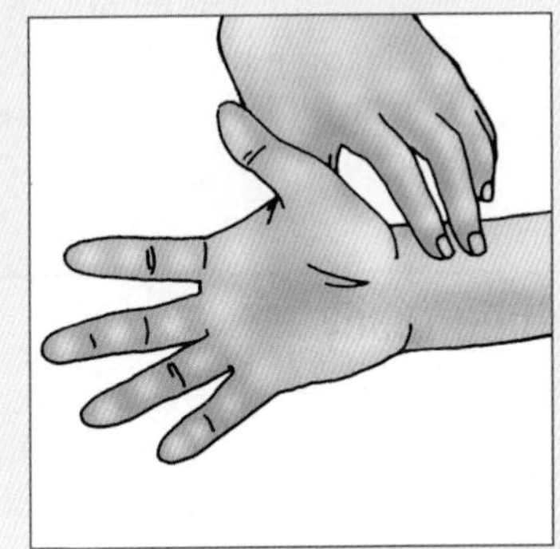

There is some controversy whether the modified Allen's test reliably screens adequate collateral circulation, and other tests may be employed such as a finger pulse plethysmography, Doppler flow measurements, or systolic pressure of the thumb.

Complications related to arterial sampling and how to prevent them

- Arteriospasm may be prevented by helping the patient to relax.
- A hematoma can be prevented by inserting the needle without puncturing the far side of the vessel and by applying pressure immediately after the needle is withdrawn. Pressure will need to be applied longer than when sampling from a vein and should be supervised closely to check for cessation of bleeding.
- Selecting an appropriate site and avoiding redirection of the needle can prevent nerve damage.
- Fainting or a vasovagal response can be prevented by placing the patient in a supine position.

What you need

ABG draw kit which typically contains biohazard bag ✳ 2″ × 2″ gauze ✳ standard syringe with 25G needle ✳ preheparinized 3-mL ABG syringe with needle, needle cap and protective sleeve, and chlorhexidine ✳ gloves ✳ towel ✳ filter cap ✳ ice-filled plastic bag ✳ label ✳ laboratory requisition ✳ adhesive bandage ✳ optional: 1% lidocaine solution without epinephrine.

A package deal

Many health care facilities use a commercial ABG kit, which contains everything you need to perform this procedure including preheparinized syringe and capillary design that minimizes air bubbles and does not need icing if the sample is tested within 30 minutes. Adhesive bandage, biohazard bag, and ice are not included in kits. If your facility doesn't use such a kit, obtain a sterile syringe specially made for drawing blood for ABG values and use a clean emesis basin filled with ice instead of the plastic bag to transport the sample to the laboratory.

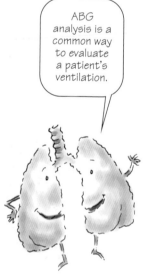

ABG analysis is a common way to evaluate a patient's ventilation.

Getting ready

Prepare everything you need before entering the patient's room. Wash your hands thoroughly, then open the ABG kit and remove the sample label and the plastic bag. Record on the label the patient's name and room number, date and collection time, and doctor's name. Fill the plastic bag with ice and set it aside.

The patient

- ABGs are corrected to patient temperature by adjusting the analyzer. The patient temperature must be obtained prior to performing ABGs.
- The patient should be in a comfortable position with stabilized breathing pattern for at least 5 minutes before a sample is drawn. Promote physical and mental comfort by quiet and reassuring talk.
- Patients receiving supplemental oxygen (FIO_2), positive end-expiratory pressure (PEEP), or continuous positive airway pressure (CPAP) should be maintained on the same settings for at least 20 minutes before sampling.

How you do it

- Absolute contraindications include an abnormal Allen's test, infection, distorted anatomy, peripheral vascular disease at puncture site, and the presence of arteriovenous fistulas or vascular grafts.
- Tell the patient you need to collect an arterial blood sample and explain the procedure *to help ease anxiety and promote cooperation.* Tell him that the needle stick will cause some discomfort but that he must remain still during the procedure.
- After washing your hands and putting on gloves, place a rolled towel under the patient's wrist *for support.* Locate the artery and palpate it for a strong pulse.

Site cleaning

- Clean the puncture site preferably with chlorhexidine pad. Don't wipe off the povidone-iodine with alcohol if used.
- Using a circular motion, clean the area, starting at the center of the site and spiralling outward. If you use alcohol, apply it with friction for 30 seconds or until the final pad comes away clean. Allow the skin to dry.
- Palpate the artery with the index and middle fingers of one hand while holding the syringe over the puncture site with the other hand.

What's the angle?

- Hold the needle bevel up at a 30- to 45-degree angle. When puncturing the brachial artery, hold the needle at a 60-degree angle. (See *Arterial puncture technique,* page 104.)
- Puncture the skin and arterial wall in one motion, following the path of the artery.
- Watch for blood backflow in the syringe. Don't pull back on the plunger *because arterial blood should enter the syringe automatically.* Fill the syringe to the 5-mL mark. (See *Consider the bone a no-touch zone,* page 104.)

5-minute pressure

- After collecting the sample, press a gauze pad firmly over the puncture site until the bleeding stops—at least 5 minutes. If the patient is receiving anticoagulant therapy or has a blood dyscrasia, apply pressure for 10 to 15 minutes; if necessary, ask a coworker to hold the gauze pad in place while you prepare the sample for transport to the laboratory, but don't ask the patient to hold the pad. *If sufficient pressure isn't applied, a large, painful hematoma may form, hindering future arterial punctures at that site.*

Tiny bubbles

- Activate the protective needle sleeve and dispose in sharps container.
- Check the syringe for air bubbles. If any appear, remove them by holding the syringe upright and slowly ejecting some of the blood onto a 2″ × 2″ gauze pad.
- Apply the enclosed needle cap directly on the needle hub. *This prevents the sample from leaking and keeps air out of the syringe.*

On the rocks

- Put the labeled sample in the ice-filled plastic bag. Attach a properly completed laboratory requisition and send the sample to the laboratory immediately.
- When the bleeding stops, apply a small adhesive bandage to the site.

Arterial puncture technique

The angle of needle penetration in ABG sampling depends on which artery is being sampled. For the radial artery, which is used most commonly, the needle should enter bevel up at a 30- to 45-degree angle over the radial artery, as shown below.

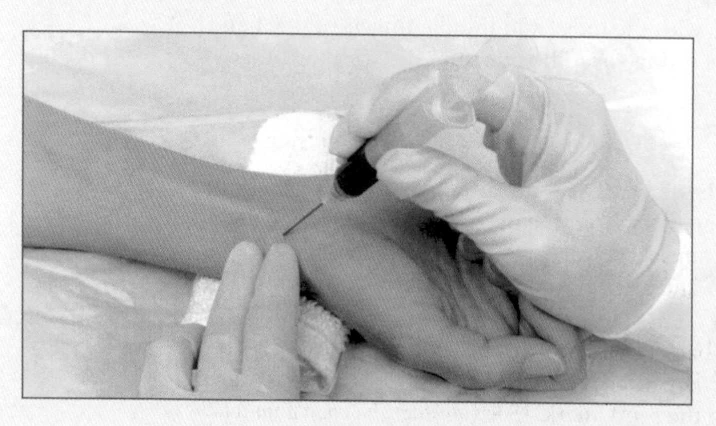

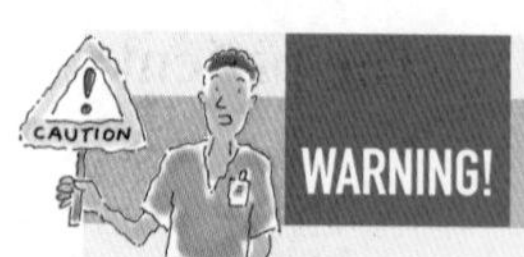

Consider the bone a no-touch zone

If you use too much force when attempting to puncture the artery, the needle may touch bone, causing the patient pain, or you may advance the needle through the opposite wall of the artery. If this happens, slowly pull the needle back a short distance and check to see if blood returns. If blood still fails to enter the syringe, withdraw the needle completely and start with a fresh needle.

Two is the limit
Don't make more than two attempts from the same site. Probing the artery may injure it and the radial nerve.

Get smaller
If arterial spasm occurs, blood won't flow into the syringe. Replace the needle with a smaller one and try the puncture again. A smaller bore needle is less likely to cause arterial spasm.

- Monitor the patient's vital signs and observe for signs and symptoms of circulatory impairment, such as swelling, discoloration, pain, numbness, or tingling in the bandaged arm or leg. Watch for bleeding at the puncture site.

Documenting arterial puncture

In your notes, record the:
- results of Allen's test
- time the sample was drawn
- patient's temperature
- arterial puncture site
- amount of time pressure was applied to the site to control bleeding
- type and amount of oxygen therapy the patient was receiving.

Practice pointers

- If the patient is receiving oxygen, make sure that his therapy has been underway for at least 20 minutes before collecting an arterial blood sample.
- Be sure to indicate on the laboratory request slip the amount and type of oxygen therapy the patient is receiving. Also note the patient's current temperature, most recent hemoglobin level, current respiratory rate, and, if he's on a ventilator, fraction of inspired oxygen and tidal volume. (See *Documenting arterial puncture*.)
- If the patient isn't receiving oxygen, indicate that he's breathing room air.
- If the patient has just received a nebulizer treatment, wait about 20 minutes before collecting the sample.
- Inappropriate collection and handling of ABGs can produce inaccurate results. Reasons for inaccurate blood result include:
  - presence of air in the sample
  - collection of venous rather than arterial blood
  - an improper quantity of heparin in the syringe or improper mixing after blood is drawn
  - a delay in specimen transportation.

Numbing effect

- If necessary, you can anesthetize the puncture site with 1% lidocaine solution. Consider such use of lidocaine carefully *because it can delay the procedure, the patient may prove allergic to the drug, or the resulting vasoconstriction may prevent successful puncture.*

Collecting a random urine specimen

A random urine specimen is collected as part of the physical examination or at various times during hospitalization. It permits laboratory screening for urinary and systemic disorders as well as for drug screening. Although there are no specific guidelines for how the specimen should be collected, avoiding the introduction of contaminants into the specimen is recommended. Instruct the patient not to touch the inside of the cup or lid. (See *Collecting urine*.)

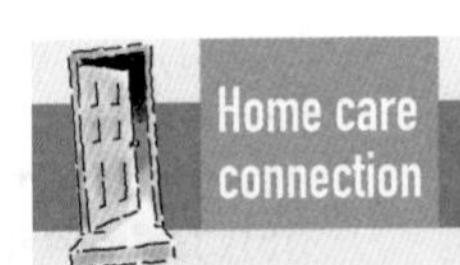

Collecting urine

If your patient will be collecting a random urine specimen at home, instruct him to collect the specimen in a clean container with a tight-fitting lid and to keep it on ice or in the refrigerator (separate from food items) for up to 24 hours.

What you need

Bedpan or urinal with cover, if necessary ✱ gloves ✱ graduated container ✱ specimen container with lid ✱ label ✱ laboratory requisition.

How you do it

- Tell the patient that you need a urine specimen for laboratory analysis. Explain the procedure to him and his family, if necessary, *to promote cooperation and prevent accidental disposal of specimens.*
- Provide privacy. Instruct the patient on bed rest to void into a clean bedpan or urinal or ask the ambulatory patient to void into either one in the bathroom.

Pour, record, discard

- Put on gloves. Then pour at least 120 mL of urine into the specimen container and cap it securely. If the patient's urine output must be measured and recorded, pour the remaining urine into the graduated container. Otherwise, discard the remaining urine. If you inadvertently spill urine on the outside of the container, clean and dry it *to prevent cross-contamination*. Remove and discard gloves. Wash your hands.
- After you label the specimen container with the patient's name and room number and the date and time of collection, attach the requisition and send it the laboratory immediately or refrigerate if there will be a delay. Clinical and Laboratory Standards Institute (CLSI) guidelines recommend testing the urine within 2 hours of collection, so it should be delivered within that time frame. If you are sending it in a pneumatic tube system, it must be in a compatible leakproof container/urine tube. **Verify that the information on the label matches the requisition before sending to the lab.** *Delayed transport of the specimen may alter test results.*

Clean and return

- Put on gloves. Clean the graduated container and urinal or bedpan and return them to their proper storage area. Discard disposable items.
- Wash your hands thoroughly *to prevent cross-contamination*. Offer the patient a washcloth and soap and water to wash his hands. (See *Documenting urine specimen collection.*)

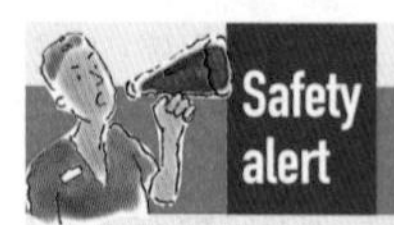

The label should always be placed on the container and not on the lid so it is always with the specimen. Always verify that the information on the requisition matches the label prior to sending to avoid a patient identification error that could lead to a diagnostic error.

Documenting urine specimen collection

Record the times of specimen collection and transport to the laboratory. Specify the test as well as the appearance, odor, color, and unusual characteristics of the specimen. If necessary, record the urine volume in the intake and output record.

Collecting a first morning specimen

This is the specimen of choice for urinalysis and microscopic analysis. The urine is generally more concentrated (because of the length of time the urine is in the bladder) and therefore will contain higher levels of cellular elements, such as protein, if present. The first morning specimen (FMS) is collected when the patient first wakes up in the morning, having emptied the bladder before going to sleep. Follow the collection practices in "Collecting a random urine specimen" and accurately record the collection time on the specimen label.

Collecting midstream clean-catch specimen

This is the preferred type of specimen for culture and sensitivity testing because of the reduced incidence of cellular and microbial contamination. This method can be conducted anytime day or night.

What you need

A kit is usually available with the required items for the collection ✱ gloves ✱ specimen container ✱ cleansing wipe ✱ label ✱ lab requisition.

How you do it

- The patient must follow a prescribed procedure of cleansing the urethral area where a cleansing wipe must be used to wipe from the front to back over the urethral area and discarded.
- Instruct the patient not to touch the inside of the cap or container.
- The patient should then void the first portion of the urine stream into the toilet. These first steps significantly reduce the opportunities for contaminants to enter into the urine stream.
- The urine midstream is then collected in the urine container and any excess is voided in the toilet. (See "Collecting a random urine specimen" for labelling and sending the specimen to the lab.)

Collecting from an indwelling catheter

Obtain an indwelling catheter specimen either by clamping the drainage tube and emptying the accumulated urine into a container or by aspirating a specimen with a syringe. Either way, it requires sterile collection technique to prevent catheter contamination and urinary tract infection. Clamping the drainage tube and emptying the urine into a container are contraindicated after genitourinary surgery.

What you need

Gloves ✳ alcohol pad ✳ 10-mL syringe ✳ 21G or 22G 1½″ needle ✳ tube clamp or rubber band ✳ sterile specimen container with lid ✳ label ✳ laboratory requisition.

How you do it

- About 30 minutes before collecting the specimen, bend the drainage tube and apply clamp or rubber band to allow urine to accumulate.
- Put on gloves. If the drainage tube has a built-in sampling port, wipe the port with an alcohol pad. Uncap the needle on the syringe and insert the needle into the sampling port at a 90-degree angle to the tubing. Aspirate the specimen into the syringe.

Rubber-made

- If the drainage tube doesn't have a sampling port and the catheter is made of rubber, obtain the specimen from the catheter. *Other types of catheters will leak after you withdraw the needle.* To withdraw the specimen from a rubber catheter, wipe it with an alcohol pad just above where it connects to the drainage tube. Insert the needle into the rubber catheter at a 45-degree angle and withdraw the specimen. Never insert the needle into the shaft of the catheter *because doing so may puncture the lumen leading to the catheter balloon.*
- Transfer the specimen to a sterile container, label it, and send it to the laboratory immediately or refrigerate if there will be a delay. CLSI guidelines recommend testing the urine within 2 hours of collection, so it should be delivered within that time frame. If you are sending it in a pneumatic tube system, it must be in a compatible leakproof container/urine tube. **Verify that the information on the requisition matches the label before sending to the lab.** If a urine culture is to be performed, list current antibiotic therapy on the laboratory requisition.

Not rubber-made

- If the catheter isn't made of rubber or has no sampling port, wipe the area where the catheter joins the drainage tube with an alcohol pad. Disconnect the catheter and allow urine to drain into the sterile specimen container. Avoid touching the inside of the sterile container with the catheter, and don't touch anything with the catheter drainage tube *to avoid contamination*. When you've collected the specimen, wipe both connection sites with an alcohol pad and join them. Cap the specimen container tightly, label it, and send it to the laboratory immediately or refrigerate if there will be a delay. CLSI guidelines recommend testing the urine within 2 hours of collection, so it should be delivered within that time frame. If you are sending it in a pneumatic tube system, it must be in a compatible leakproof container/urine tube. **Verify that the information on the label matches the requisition before sending to the lab.**
- Make sure you unclamp the drainage tube after collecting the specimen *to prevent urine backflow, which may cause bladder distention and infection*. (See *Documenting indwelling catheter specimen collection*.)

Documenting indwelling catheter specimen collection

In your notes, record:
- time of specimen collection and transport to the laboratory
- specific test
- appearance, odor, color, and unusual characteristics of the specimen
- fact that it came from an indwelling catheter.

If necessary, record the urine volume in the intake and output record.

Timed urine collection

Among the most commonly performed tests requiring timed specimens are those measuring creatinine, urine urea nitrogen, glucose, sodium, potassium, or catecholamines that are affected by diurnal variation.

A timed specimen is collected to measure the concentration of these substances in urine over a specific amount of time, usually 8 or 24 hours. This method requires the bladder to be emptied prior to the beginning of the timed specimen collection. During the designated timed period, all urine is collected and pooled into a collection container, with the final collection at the very end of the specified time period. The specimen should be refrigerated during the collection period, unless otherwise specified by the physician. The timing is critical to the calculations that are conducted to determine substance concentrations and ratios.

After the challenge

A timed urine specimen may also be collected after administering a challenge dose of a chemical—inulin, for example—to detect various renal disorders.

What you need

Large collection bottle with a cap or stopper or a commercial plastic container * preservative, if necessary * gloves * bedpan or urinal if patient doesn't have an indwelling catheter * graduated container if patient's intake and output must be measured * ice-filled container if a refrigerator isn't available * label * laboratory requisition * four patient care reminders.

Check with the laboratory to find out which preservatives may need to be added to the specimen or whether a dark collection bottle is required.

This test is sure to quench the patient's thirst.

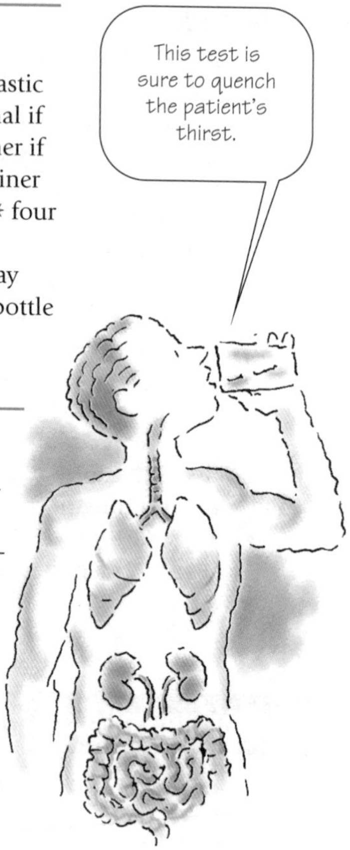

How you do it

- Explain the procedure to the patient and his family, as necessary, *to enlist their cooperation and prevent accidental disposal of urine during the collection period*. Emphasize that failure to collect even one specimen during the collection period invalidates the test and requires that it begin again.

Don't forget

- Place patient care reminders over the patient's bed, in his bathroom, on the bedpan hopper in the utility room if appropriate, and on the urinal or indwelling catheter collection bag. Include the patient's name and room number, the date, and the collection interval.
- Instruct the patient to save all urine during the collection period, to notify you after each voiding, and to avoid contaminating the urine with stool or toilet tissue. Explain any dietary or drug restrictions and make sure he understands and is willing to comply with them.

For 2-hour collection

- If possible, instruct the patient to drink two to four 8-oz (480 to 960 mL) glasses of water about 30 minutes before collection begins. After 30 minutes, tell him to void. Put on gloves and discard this specimen *so the patient starts the collection period with an empty bladder*.
- If ordered, administer a challenge dose of medication (such as glucose solution or corticotropin) and record the time.
- If possible, offer the patient a glass of water at least every hour during the collection period *to stimulate urine production*. After each voiding, put on gloves and add the specimen to the collection bottle.

15-minute warning

- Instruct the patient to void about 15 minutes before the end of the collection period, if possible, and add this specimen to the collection bottle. If you inadvertently spill urine on the outside of the container, clean and dry it *to prevent cross-contamination* before sending to the lab.
- At the end of the collection period, send the appropriately labeled collection bottle to the laboratory immediately, along with a properly completed laboratory requisition. **Verify that the information on the label matches the requisition before sending to the lab.**

For 12- and 24-hour collection

- Put on gloves and ask the patient to void. Then discard this urine *so the patient starts the collection period with an empty bladder.* Record the time.
- After putting on gloves and pouring the first urine specimen into the collection bottle, add the required preservative. Remove and discard your gloves. Then refrigerate the bottle or keep it on ice until the next voiding, as appropriate.

One more time

- After putting on gloves, collect all urine voided during the prescribed period. Just before the collection period ends, ask the patient to void again, if possible. Add this last specimen to the collection bottle and pack it in ice *to inhibit deterioration of the specimen.* If you inadvertently spill urine on the outside of the container, clean and dry it *to prevent cross-contamination.* Remove and discard your gloves. Label the collection bottle and send it to the laboratory with a properly completed laboratory requisition. **Verify that the information on the requisition matches the label before sending to the lab.**

Practice pointers

- Keep the patient well hydrated before and during the test *to ensure adequate urine flow.*
- Before collection of a timed specimen, make sure the laboratory will be open when the collection period ends *to help ensure prompt, accurate results.* Never store a specimen in a refrigerator that contains food or medication *to avoid contamination.* If the patient has an indwelling catheter in place, put the collection bag in an ice-filled container at his bedside.
- Tell the patient that exercise and ingestion of coffee, tea, or drugs can alter test results.

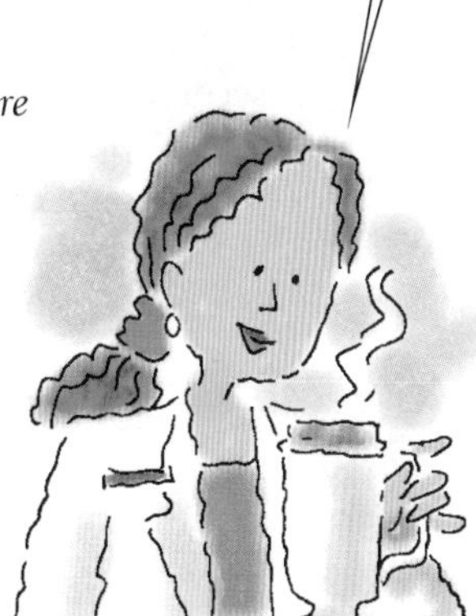
Be sure to tell your patient that exercise and ingestion of coffee, tea, or drugs can alter test results.

- If you accidentally discard a specimen during the collection period, you'll need to restart the collection. This may result in an additional day of hospitalization, which may cause the patient personal and financial hardship. Therefore, emphasize to everyone involved in his care as well as to family and other visitors the need to save all the patient's urine during the collection period. If you need to start over, you must get a new container. (See *Documenting timed urine collection.*)

Documenting timed urine collection

Record the date and intervals of specimen collection and when the collection bottle was sent to the laboratory.

Urine specific gravity

Urine specific gravity is determined by comparing the weight of a urine specimen with that of an equivalent volume of distilled water, which is 1.000. Because urine contains dissolved salts and other substances, it's heavier than 1.000. Urine specific gravity ranges from 1.003 (very dilute) to 1.035 (highly concentrated); normal values range from 1.010 to 1.025. Urine dipstick measurement can provide a rough estimate of specific gravity and can be performed easily in some health care settings following the strip manufacturer's directions for urine application, dwell time, and strip comparison. For more accurate results, a specimen is sent to the laboratory for analysis with urinometer or refractometer devices. (See *Documenting urine specific gravity collection.*)

Elevated specific gravity reflects an increased concentration of urine solutes, which occurs in conditions that cause renal hypoperfusion, and may indicate heart failure, dehydration, hepatic disorders, or nephrosis. Low specific gravity reflects failure to reabsorb water and concentrate urine; it may indicate hypercalcemia, hypokalemia, alkalosis, acute renal failure, pyelonephritis, glomerulonephritis, or diabetes insipidus.

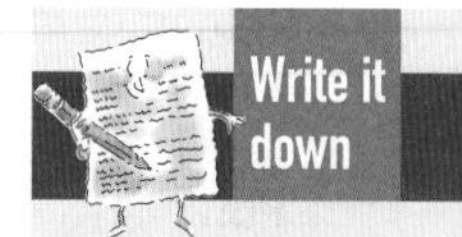

Documenting urine specific gravity collection

Record the specific gravity, volume, color, odor, and appearance of the collected urine specimen.

Measuring with a reagent strip

- Put on gloves and obtain a random or controlled urine specimen.
- Dip the reagent end of the test strip into the specimen for 2 seconds.
- Tap the strip on the rim of the specimen container to remove excess urine and compare the resultant color change with the color chart supplied with the kit.

Straining urine for calculi

Renal calculi, or kidney stones, may develop anywhere in the urinary tract. They may be excreted with the urine or become lodged in the urinary tract, causing hematuria, urine retention, renal colic, and, possibly, hydronephrosis.

Sizes vary

Ranging in size from microscopic to several centimeters, calculi form in the kidneys when mineral salts—principally calcium oxalate or calcium phosphate—collect around a nucleus of bacterial cells, blood clots, or other particles. Other substances involved in calculus formation include uric acid, xanthine, and ammonia.

Straining urine for stones is a team effort.

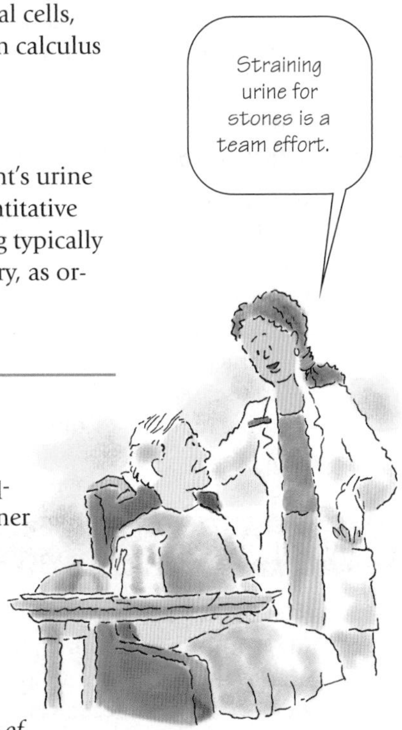

Strain carefully

Testing for calculi requires careful straining of all the patient's urine through a gauze pad or fine-mesh sieve and, at times, quantitative laboratory analysis of questionable specimens. Such testing typically continues until the patient passes the calculi or until surgery, as ordered.

What you need

Strainer or 4″ × 4″ gauze pad ✳ graduated container ✳ rubber band ✳ urinal or bedpan ✳ gloves ✳ laboratory requisition ✳ three patient care reminders ✳ specimen container (for use if calculi are found).

How you do it

- Explain the procedure to the patient and his family, if possible, *to ensure cooperation and to stress the importance of straining all the patient's urine.*
- Post a patient care reminder stating "STRAIN ALL URINE" over the patient's bed, in his bathroom, and on the collection container.
- Tell the patient to notify you after each voiding.

Improvise!

- If a commercial strainer isn't available, unfold a 4″ × 4″ gauze pad, place it over the top of a graduated measuring container, and secure it with a rubber band.

- Put on gloves. With the strainer secured over the mouth of the collection container, pour the specimen from the urinal or bedpan into the container. If the patient has an indwelling catheter in place, strain all urine from the collection bag before discarding it.

Detective work

- Examine the strainer for calculi. If you detect calculi or if the filter looks questionable, notify the doctor, place the filtrate in a specimen container, and send it to the laboratory with a laboratory requisition.
- If the strainer is intact, rinse it carefully and reuse it. If it has become damaged, discard it and replace it with a new strainer. Remove and discard your gloves.

Documenting straining urine for calculi

Chart the time of the specimen collection and transport to the laboratory, if necessary. Describe the filtrate passed and note whether pain or hematuria occurred during the voiding.

Practice pointers

- Save and send to the laboratory small or suspicious-looking residue in the specimen container *because even tiny calculi can cause hematuria and pain.*
- Be aware that calculi may appear in various colors, each of which has diagnostic value.
- If the patient will be straining his urine at home, teach him how to use a strainer and tell him how important it is to strain all his urine for the prescribed period. (See *Documenting straining urine for calculi.*)

Stool collection

Stool is collected to determine if blood, leukocytes, ova and parasites (protozoa or worms), bile, fat, pathogens, toxins, or substances such as ingested drugs are present. Multipathogen tests can evaluate 11 common infectious organisms at once. Visual examination of stool characteristics—such as color, consistency, and odor—can reveal such conditions as gastrointestinal (GI) bleeding and steatorrhea. Iatrogenic *Clostridium difficile* has become a huge focus recently. *C. difficile* toxin detection requires diarrheal stool specimens, but not all strains produce toxins.

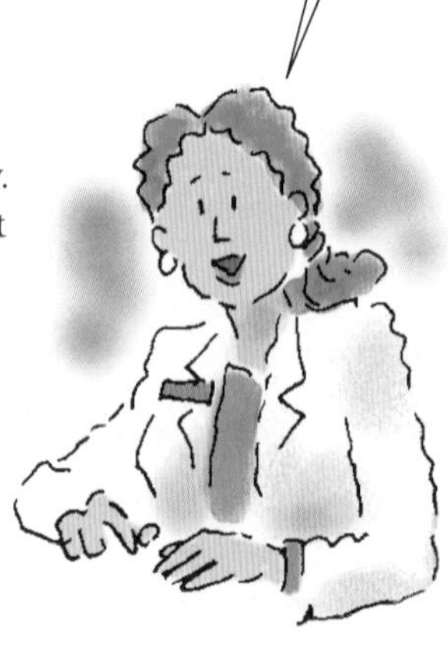
It's a fact—
stool specimens can't be obtained on demand. You'll have to work carefully with the patient to ensure proper collection.

Random or specific

Stool specimens are collected randomly or for specific periods, such as 72 hours. Because stool specimens can't be obtained on demand, proper collection requires careful instructions to the patient to ensure an uncontaminated specimen.

What you need

Specially designed stool specimen hat for toilet * specimen container with lid * gloves * tongue blade * paper towel or paper bag * bedpan or portable commode * three patient care reminders (for timed specimens) * laboratory requisition * patient identification labels.

How you do it

- Explain the procedure to the patient and to the family members, if possible, *to ensure their cooperation and prevent inadvertent disposal of timed stool specimens.*

Collecting a random specimen

- Tell the patient to notify you when he has the urge to defecate. Have him defecate into a clean, dry bedpan or portable commode. Instruct him not to contaminate the specimen with urine or toilet tissue *because urine inhibits fecal bacterial growth and toilet tissue contains bismuth, which interferes with test results.*
- Put on gloves.

Specimen representative

- Using a tongue blade, transfer the most representative stool specimen from the bedpan to the specimen container and cap the container. If the patient passes blood, mucus, or pus with the stool, be sure to include this with the specimen.
- Wrap the tongue blade in a paper towel or place it in a paper bag and discard it. Remove and discard your gloves and wash your hands thoroughly *to prevent cross-contamination.*

Collecting a timed specimen

- Place a patient care reminder stating "SAVE ALL STOOL" over the patient's bed, in his bathroom, and in the utility room.
- After putting on gloves, collect the first specimen and include this in the total specimen.

Complete transfer

- Obtain the timed specimen as you would a random specimen, but remember to transfer all stool to the specimen container.
- If stool must be obtained with an enema, use only tap water or normal saline solution.

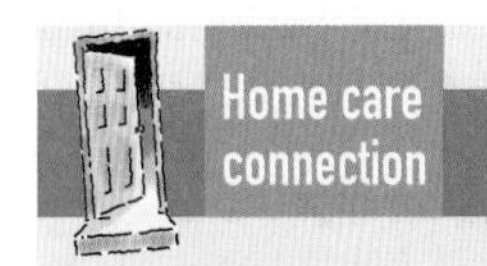

Collecting a stool specimen

If the patient is to collect a stool specimen at home, instruct him to collect it in a clean container with a tight-fitting lid, to wrap the container in a brown paper bag, and to keep it in the refrigerator (separate from food items) until it can be transported.

- Label the specimen with the patient name and other identifier, time, and date collected. **Verify that the information on the label matches the lab requisition.** Send each specimen to the laboratory immediately with a laboratory requisition or, if permitted, refrigerate the specimens collected during the test period and send them when collection is complete. Remove and discard gloves.
- Make sure the patient is comfortable after the procedure and that he has the opportunity to thoroughly clean his hands and perianal area. Perineal care may be necessary for some patients.

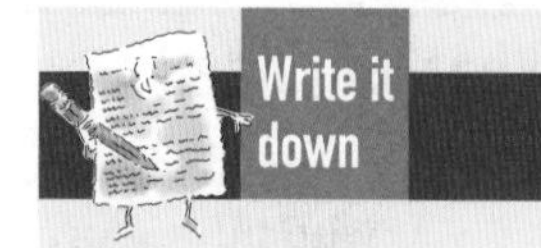

Documenting stool collection

In your notes, record:
- time of specimen collection and transport to the laboratory
- color, odor, and consistency of the stool
- unusual characteristics
- whether the patient had difficulty passing the stool.

Practice pointers

- Never place a stool specimen in a refrigerator that contains food or medication *to prevent contamination.* (See *Collecting a stool specimen,* page 115.)
- Notify the doctor if the stool specimen looks unusual. (See *Documenting stool collection.*)

Fecal occult blood test

Fecal occult blood tests are valuable for detecting occult blood (hidden GI bleeding), which may be present with colorectal cancer, and for distinguishing between true melena and melena-like stools. Certain medications, such as iron supplements and bismuth compounds, can darken stools so that they resemble melena.

Look for blue

Two common occult blood screening tests are Hematest (an orthotolidine reagent tablet) and the Hemoccult slide (filter paper impregnated with guaiac). Both tests produce a blue reaction in a fecal smear if occult blood loss exceeds 5 mL in 24 hours. A newer test, ColoCARE, requires no fecal smear and can be used at home for an initial screening.

Repeat three times

To confirm a positive result, the test must be repeated at least three times while the patient follows a meatless, high-residue diet. Even then, a confirmed positive result doesn't necessarily indicate colorectal cancer. It does indicate the need for further diagnostic studies because GI bleeding can result from many causes other than cancer, such as ulcers and diverticula. These tests are easily performed on collected specimens or smears from a digital rectal examination.

What you need

Test kit ✳ gloves ✳ stool specimen collection hat ✳ glass or porcelain plate ✳ tongue blade or other wooden applicator.

How you do it

- Put on gloves and collect a stool specimen.

Hematest reagent tablet test

- Use a tongue blade or other wooden applicator to smear a bit of the stool specimen on the filter paper supplied with the test kit. Or, after performing a digital rectal examination, wipe the finger you used for the examination on a square of the filter paper.
- Place the filter paper with the stool smear on a glass plate.
- Remove a reagent tablet from the bottle and immediately replace the cap tightly. Then place the tablet at the center of the stool smear on the filter paper.
- Add one drop of water to the tablet and allow it to soak in for 5 to 10 seconds. Add a second drop, letting it run from the tablet onto the specimen and filter paper. If necessary, tap the plate gently to dislodge water from the top of the tablet.

2-minute read

- After 2 minutes, the filter paper will turn blue if the test is positive. Don't read the color that appears on the tablet itself or that develops on the filter paper after the 2-minute period.
- Note the results and discard the filter paper.
- Remove and discard your gloves and wash your hands thoroughly.

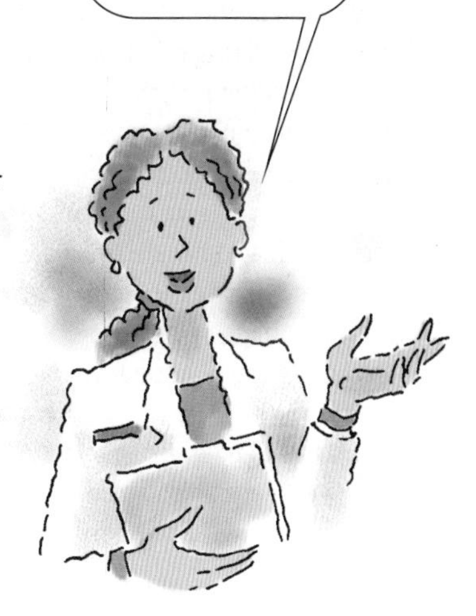
You'll get the best results if the patient maintains a high-fiber, meatless diet during the test period.

Hemoccult slide test

- Open the flap on the slide packet and use a tongue blade or other wooden applicator to apply a thin smear of the stool specimen to the guaiac-impregnated filter paper exposed in box A. Or, after performing a digital rectal examination, wipe the finger you used for the examination on a square of the filter paper.
- Apply a second smear from another part of the specimen to the filter paper exposed in box B *because some parts of the specimen may not contain blood.*
- Allow the specimens to dry for 3 to 5 minutes.

Positive result

- Open the flap on the reverse side of the slide package and place two drops of Hemoccult developer solution on the paper over each smear. A blue reaction will appear in 30 to 60 seconds if the test result is positive.
- Record the results and discard the slide package.
- Remove and discard your gloves and wash your hands thoroughly.

Practice pointers

- Make sure stool specimens aren't contaminated with urine, soap solution, or toilet tissue and test them as soon as possible after collection.
- Test samples from several portions of the same specimen *because occult blood from the upper GI tract isn't always evenly dispersed throughout the formed stool; likewise, blood from colorectal bleeding may occur mostly on the outer stool surface.*
- Discard outdated tablets. Protect Hematest tablets from moisture, heat, and light.

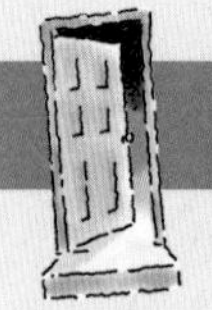

Home care connection

Home tests for fecal occult blood

Most fecal occult blood tests require the patient to collect a specimen of his stool and smear some of it on a slide. In contrast, some new tests don't require the patient to handle stool, making the procedure safer and simpler. One example is a test called ColoCARE. If your patient will be performing the ColoCARE test at home, include these instructions in your patient teaching:

- Tell him to avoid red meat and vitamin C supplements for 2 days before the test.
- Advise him to check with his doctor about the need for discontinuing medications before the test. Drugs that can interfere with test results include aspirin, indomethacin, corticosteroids, phenylbutazone, reserpine, dietary supplements, anticancer drugs, and anticoagulants.
- Tell him to flush the toilet twice just before performing the test to remove any toilet cleaning chemicals from the tank.
- Instruct him to defecate into the toilet—but to throw no toilet paper into the bowl—and, within 5 minutes, to remove the test pad from its pouch and float it printed side up on the surface of the water.
- Tell him to watch the pad for 15 to 30 seconds for evidence of blue or green color changes and have him record the result on the reply card.
- Emphasize that he should perform this test with three consecutive bowel movements and then send the completed card to his doctor. However, he should call his doctor immediately if he notes a positive color change in the first test.

Repeat if positive

- If repeat testing is necessary after a positive result, explain the test to the patient. Instruct him to maintain a high-fiber diet and to refrain from eating red meat, poultry, fish, turnips, and horseradish for 48 to 72 hours before the test as well as throughout the collection period *because these substances may alter test results.*
- As ordered, have the patient discontinue use of iron preparations, bromides, iodides, rauwolfia derivatives, indomethacin, colchicine, salicylates, potassium, phenylbutazone, oxyphenbutazone, bismuth compounds, steroids, and ascorbic acid for 48 to 72 hours before and during the test *to ensure accurate test results and avoid possible bleeding, which some of these compounds can cause.* (See *Home tests for fecal occult blood* and *Documenting a fecal occult blood test.*)

Write it down

Documenting a fecal occult blood test

Record the time and date of the test, the result, and unusual characteristics of the stool tested. Report positive results to the doctor.

Sputum collection

Sputum, which is secreted by mucous membranes lining the bronchioles, bronchi, and trachea, helps protect the respiratory tract from infection. When expelled from the respiratory tract, sputum carries saliva, nasal and sinus secretions, dead cells, and bacteria from the respiratory tract. Sputum specimens may be cultured to identify respiratory pathogens.

Three methods

Expectoration is the usual method of sputum specimen collection. It may require ultrasonic nebulization, hydration, or chest percussion and postural drainage. Less common methods for sputum specimen collection include tracheal suctioning and, rarely, bronchoscopy.

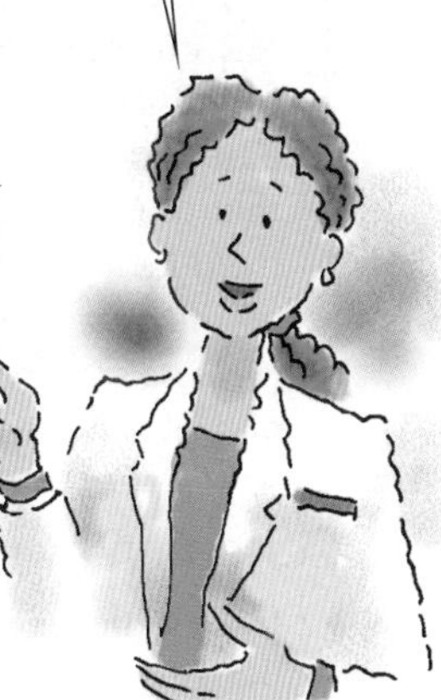
Expectoration is the most common method for collecting sputum.

What you need

Expectoration method

Sterile specimen container with tight-fitting cap ✳ gloves, if necessary ✳ label ✳ laboratory requisition.

For tracheal suctioning

#12 to #18 French sterile suction catheter (avoid trauma to nasal mucosa) ✳ laboratory requisition ✳ clean and sterile gloves ✳ mask ✳ protective eyewear ✳ sterile in-line specimen trap (Lukens trap) ✳ normal saline solution ✳ sterile water ✳ portable suction machine, if wall unit is unavailable ✳ oxygen therapy

* label * optional: nasal airway, to obtain a nasotracheal specimen with suctioning, if needed * biohazard transport bag.

Commercial suction kits contain all the equipment except the suction machine and an in-line specimen container.

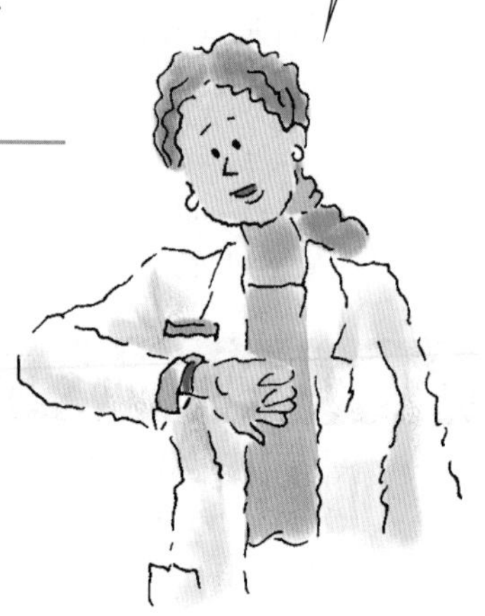
Sputum should be collected early in the morning.

Getting ready

Equipment and preparation depend on the method of collection. Gather the appropriate equipment for the task.

How you do it

- Tell the patient that you'll collect a specimen of sputum (not saliva) and explain the procedure *to promote cooperation.* If possible, collect the specimen early in the morning, before breakfast, *to obtain an overnight accumulation of secretions.* To minimize gagging and risk of aspiration, perform the suctioning 1 hour before a meal or 1 to 2 hours after.

Collection by expectoration

- Instruct the patient to sit in a chair or at the edge of the bed. If he can't sit up, place him in high Fowler's position.
- Ask the patient to rinse his mouth with water *to reduce specimen contamination.* (Avoid mouthwash or toothpaste *because they may affect the mobility of organisms in the sputum sample.*) Then tell him to cough deeply and expectorate directly into the specimen container. Ask him to produce at least 15 mL of sputum, if possible.
- Put on gloves.

Label and send

- Cap the container and, if necessary, clean its exterior. Remove and discard your gloves and wash your hands thoroughly. Label the container with the patient's name and room number, doctor's name, date and time of collection, and initial diagnosis. **Verify that the information on the label matches the requisition.** Also, include on the laboratory requisition whether the patient was febrile or taking antibiotics and whether sputum was induced (*because such specimens commonly appear watery and may resemble saliva*). Send the specimen to the laboratory immediately.

Collection by tracheal suctioning

- If the patient can't produce an adequate specimen by coughing, prepare to suction him to obtain the specimen. Explain the suctioning procedure to him and tell him that he may cough, gag, or feel short of breath during the procedure.

Testing . . . testing . . .

- Check the suction machine *to make sure it's functioning properly.* Then place the patient in high Fowler's or semi-Fowler's position.
- If the patient is on a ventilator, has a tracheostomy, or is already receiving oxygen, administer oxygen to the patient before beginning the procedure. (See *Suctioning can be dangerous.*)
- Wash your hands thoroughly.
- Put on sterile gloves. Consider one hand sterile and the other hand clean *to prevent cross-contamination.*
- Connect the suction tubing to the male adapter of the in-line specimen trap. Attach the sterile suction catheter to the rubber tubing of the trap. (See *Attaching a specimen trap to a suction catheter,* page 122.)
- Position a mask over your face. Tell the patient to tilt his head back slightly. Then lubricate the catheter with normal saline solution and gently pass it through the patient's nostril without suction.
- When the catheter reaches the larynx, the patient will cough. As he does, quickly advance the catheter into the trachea. Tell him to take several deep breaths through his mouth *to ease insertion.*
- To obtain the specimen, apply suction for 5 to 10 seconds but never longer than 15 seconds *because prolonged suction can cause*

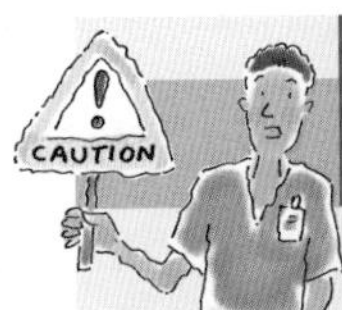

WARNING!

Suctioning can be dangerous

Tracheal suctioning can be dangerous because it deprives your patient of oxygen. If your patient becomes hypoxic or cyanotic during suctioning, remove the catheter immediately and administer oxygen.

If the patient has asthma or chronic bronchitis, watch for aggravated bronchospasms with the use of more than a 10% concentration of sodium chloride or acetylcysteine in an aerosol. If he's suspected of having tuberculosis, don't use more than 20% propylene glycol with water when inducing a sputum specimen *because a higher concentration inhibits growth of the pathogen and causes erroneous test results.* If propylene glycol isn't available, use 10% to 20% acetylcysteine with water or sodium chloride.

Patients with cardiac disease may develop arrhythmias during the procedure as a result of suctioning. Other potential complications include tracheal trauma or bleeding, vomiting, aspiration, and hypoxemia.

Attaching a specimen trap to a suction catheter

When collecting a sputum specimen using tracheal suctioning, you'll need to attach the specimen trap to the suctioning catheter. Follow the steps below for connecting and disconnecting the trap.

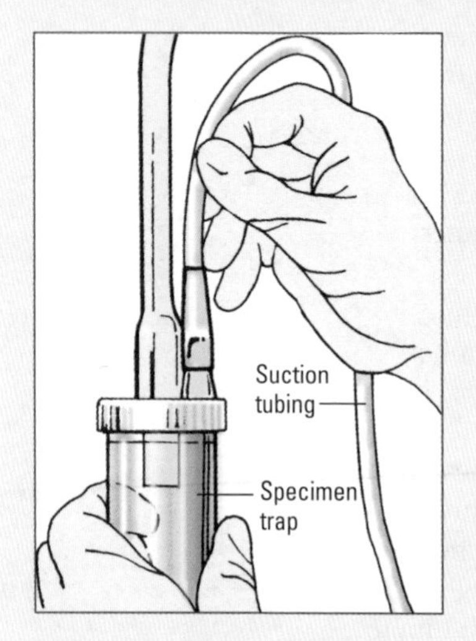

With gloves on, push the suction tubing onto the male adapter of the in-line trap.

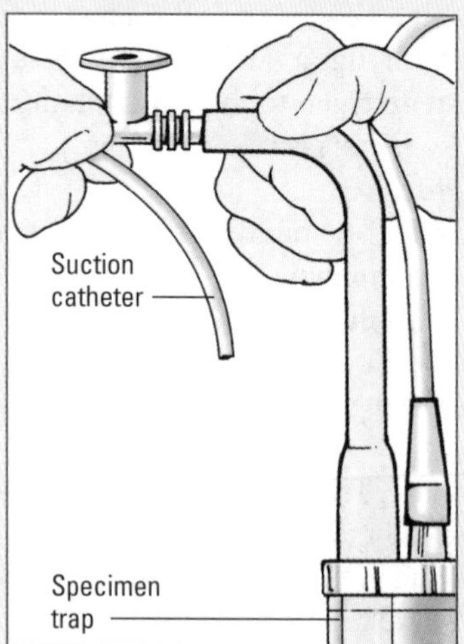

Insert the suction catheter into the rubber tubing of the trap.

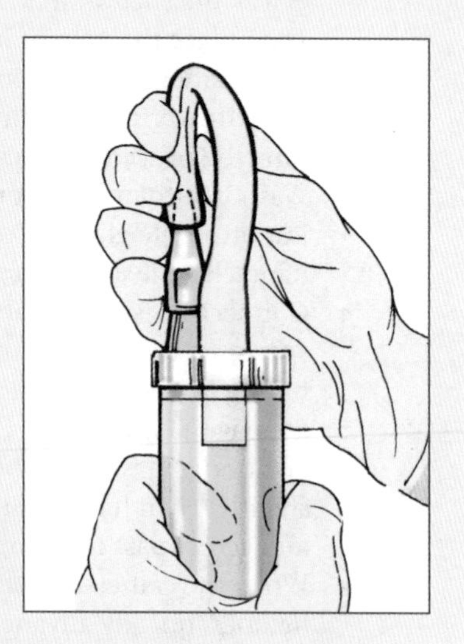

After suctioning, disconnect the in-line trap from the suction tubing and catheter. To seal the container, connect the rubber tubing to the male adapter of the trap.

hypoxia. If the procedure must be repeated, let the patient rest for four to six breaths. Collect 2 to 10 mL of sputum. When collection is completed, discontinue the suction, gently remove the catheter, and administer oxygen as indicated by patient's condition.

Careful clean-up

- Detach the catheter from the in-line trap, gather it up in your dominant hand, and pull the glove cuff inside out and down around the used catheter to enclose it for disposal. Remove and discard the other glove and your mask.
- Detach the trap from the tubing connected to the suction machine. Seal the trap tightly by connecting the rubber tubing to the male adapter of the trap. Examine the specimen *to make sure it's actually sputum, not saliva*. Label the trap's container as an expectorated specimen and send it to the laboratory immediately with a completed laboratory requisition. **Verify that the information on the requisition matches the label.**
- Offer the patient a glass of water or mouthwash.

Practice pointers

- If you can't obtain a sputum specimen through tracheal suctioning, perform chest percussion *to loosen and mobilize secretions* and position the patient for optimal drainage. After 20 to 30 minutes, repeat the tracheal suctioning procedure.
- Before sending the specimen to the laboratory, examine it to make sure it's actually sputum, not saliva, *because saliva will produce inaccurate test results.*
- Because expectorated sputum is contaminated by normal mouth flora, tracheal suctioning provides a more reliable specimen for diagnosis. (See *Documenting sputum collection.*)

Documenting sputum collection

In your notes, record:
- collection method used
- time and date of collection
- patient's response
- color and consistency of the specimen
- specimen's proper disposition.

Lumbar puncture

Lumbar puncture involves the insertion of a sterile needle into the subarachnoid space of the spinal canal, usually between the third and fourth lumbar vertebrae. This procedure is used to detect increased intracranial pressure (ICP) or the presence of blood in cerebrospinal fluid (CSF), to obtain CSF specimens for laboratory analysis, and to inject dyes or gases for contrast in radiologic studies. It's also used to administer drugs or anesthetics and to relieve ICP by removing CSF.

Proceed with caution

Performed by a doctor with a nurse assisting, lumbar puncture requires sterile technique and careful patient positioning. This procedure is contraindicated in patients with lumbar deformity or infection at the puncture site. It should be performed cautiously in patients with increased ICP because the rapid reduction in pressure that follows withdrawal of CSF can cause tonsillar herniation and medullary compression.

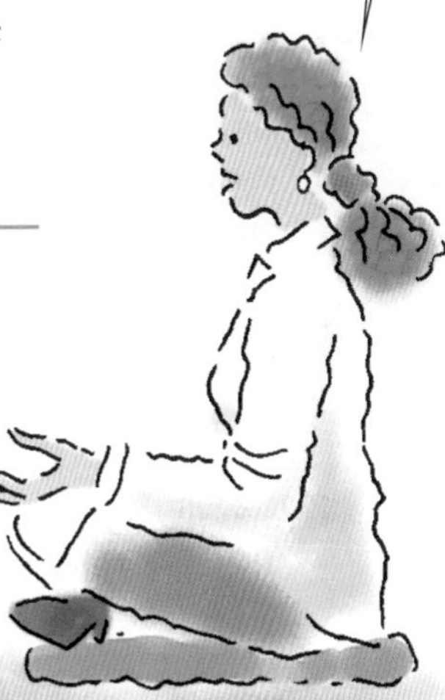
The nurse's role during lumbar puncture is to help the patient maintain the proper position.

What you need

Overbed table * one or two pairs of sterile gloves for the doctor * sterile gloves for the nurse * antiseptic solution * sterile gauze pads * alcohol pads * sterile fenestrated drape * 3-mL syringe for local anesthetic * 25G ¾" sterile needle for injecting anesthetic * local anesthetic (usually 1% lidocaine) * 18G or 20G 3½" spinal needle with stylet (22G needle for children) * three-way stopcock * manometer * small adhesive bandage * four sterile collection tubes with stoppers * laboratory requisitions ✱ labels ✱ light source such as a gooseneck lamp ✱ optional: patient care reminder.

Disposable lumbar puncture trays contain most of the needed sterile equipment.

Getting ready

Gather the equipment and take it to the patient's bedside. Allow the patient to empty his bladder and bowels. Ensure patients who take blood thinners have stopped according to recommendations by the health care provider.

How you do it

- Explain the procedure to the patient *to ease his anxiety and ensure his cooperation.* Make sure an informed consent form has been signed.
- Inform the patient that he may experience headache after lumbar puncture, but reassure him that his cooperation during the procedure minimizes such an effect. (See *Perils of lumbar puncture.*)
- Immediately before the procedure, provide privacy and instruct the patient to void.
- Wash your hands thoroughly.
- Open the equipment tray on an overbed table, being careful not to contaminate the sterile field when you open the wrapper.
- "Time out" to verify patient identifiers, procedure type, and site with patient and health care providers.

Model behavior

- Provide adequate lighting at the puncture site and adjust the height of the patient's bed *to allow the doctor to perform the procedure comfortably.*
- Position the patient and reemphasize the importance of remaining as still as possible *to minimize discomfort and trauma.* (See *Positioning for lumbar puncture.*)
- Assist the patient's relaxation efforts and facilitate comforting words or touch. Remind the patient not to strain, hold his breath, or talk; rather, he should breathe slowly and deeply.

Careful preparation

- The doctor cleans the puncture site with sterile gauze pads soaked in antiseptic solution, wiping in a circular motion away from the puncture site; he uses three different pads *to avoid contaminating spinal tissues with the body's normal skin flora.* Next, he drapes

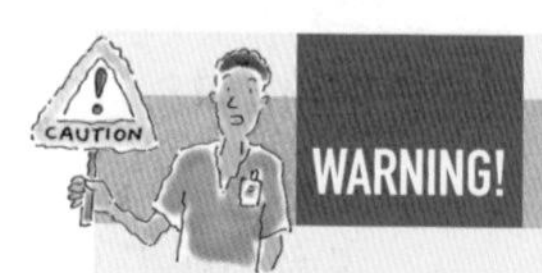

Perils of lumbar puncture

Headache is the most common adverse effect of lumbar puncture and may include blurred vision and tinnitus. Other adverse reactions include:

- a reaction to the anesthetic
- meningitis
- epidural or subdural abscess
- bleeding into the spinal canal
- CSF leakage through the dural defect remaining after needle withdrawal resulting in decreased level of consciousness, hearing loss, dilated pupils, and decreased ICP
- local pain caused by nerve root irritation
- edema or hematoma at the puncture site
- transient difficulty voiding and fever.

The most serious complications of lumbar puncture, although rare, are tonsillar herniation and medullary compression.

Positioning for lumbar puncture

Have the patient lie on his side at the edge of the bed, with his chin tucked to his chest and his knees drawn up to his abdomen (fetal position). Make sure the patient's spine is curved and his back is at the edge of the bed (as shown below). This position widens the spaces between the vertebrae, easing insertion of the needle.

To help the patient maintain this position, place one of your hands behind his neck and the other hand behind his knees and pull gently. Hold the patient firmly in this position throughout the procedure to prevent accidental needle displacement.

Needle insertion site

Typically, the doctor inserts the needle between the third and fourth lumbar vertebrae (as shown below).

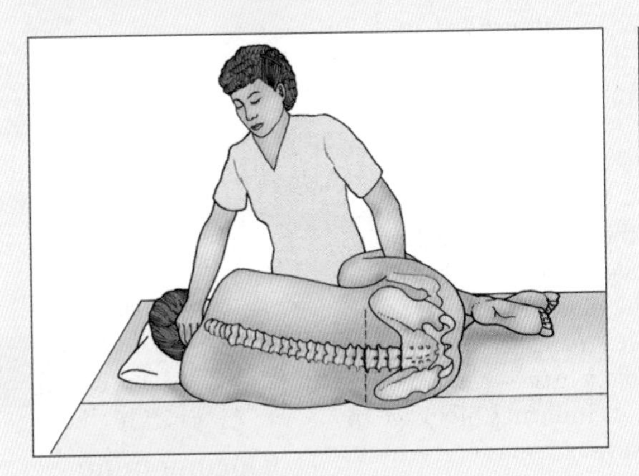

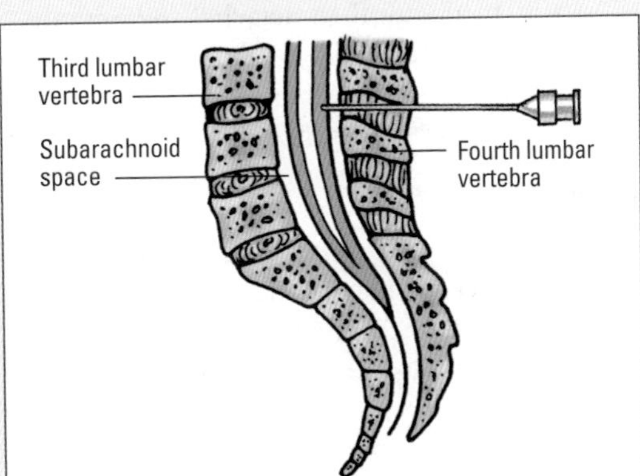

the area with the fenestrated drape *to provide a sterile field.* (If the doctor uses povidone-iodine pads instead of sterile gauze pads, he may remove his sterile gloves and put on another pair *to avoid introducing povidone-iodine into the subarachnoid space with the lumbar puncture needle.*)

- If no ampule of anesthetic is included on the equipment tray, clean the injection port of a multidose vial of anesthetic with an alcohol pad. Then invert the vial 45 degrees so that the doctor can insert a 25G needle and syringe and withdraw the anesthetic for injection.
- Before the doctor injects the anesthetic, tell the patient he'll experience a transient burning sensation and local pain. Ask him to report other persistent pain or sensations *because they may indicate irritation or puncture of a nerve root, requiring repositioning of the needle.*

Still and steady

- When the doctor inserts the sterile spinal needle into the subarachnoid space between the third and fourth lumbar vertebrae, instruct the patient to remain still and breathe normally. If necessary, hold the patient firmly in position *to prevent sudden movement that may displace the needle.*

- If the lumbar puncture is being performed to administer contrast media for radiologic studies or spinal anesthetic, the doctor injects the dye or anesthetic at this time.

Meter reader

- When the needle is in place, the doctor attaches a manometer with a three-way stopcock to the needle hub *to read CSF pressure.* If ordered, help the patient extend his legs *to provide a more accurate pressure reading.*
- The doctor then detaches the manometer and allows CSF to drain from the needle hub into the collection tubes. When he has collected 2 to 3 mL in each tube, mark the tubes in sequence, insert a stopper to secure them, and label them.

Stop sign

- If the doctor suspects an obstruction in the spinal subarachnoid space, he may check for Queckenstedt's sign. After he takes an initial CSF pressure reading, compress the patient's jugular vein for 10 seconds as ordered. *This increases ICP in 15 to 40 seconds of jugular occlusion and—if no subarachnoid block exists—causes CSF pressure to rise as well.* No rise in 10 seconds indicates blockage of spinal canal. The doctor then takes pressure readings every 10 seconds until the pressure stabilizes.

Finishing touches

- After the doctor collects the specimens and removes the spinal needle, put on sterile gloves, clean the puncture site with povidone-iodine, and apply a small adhesive bandage. Remove gloves and wash your hands.
- Send the CSF specimens to the laboratory immediately, with completed laboratory requisitions. **Verify that the labels match the information on the requisition.**

Practice pointers

- During lumbar puncture, watch closely for signs of adverse reaction: elevated pulse rate, pallor, and clammy skin. Alert the doctor immediately to significant changes.
- The patient may be ordered to lie flat for 8 to 12 hours after the procedure. If necessary, place a patient care reminder on his bed to this effect. (See *Documenting lumbar puncture.*)
- Educate the patient to report severe back pain, numbness or tingling in lower extremities, more than minor bleeding, headache lasting longer than 24 hours, and/or temperature above 101 ° F.

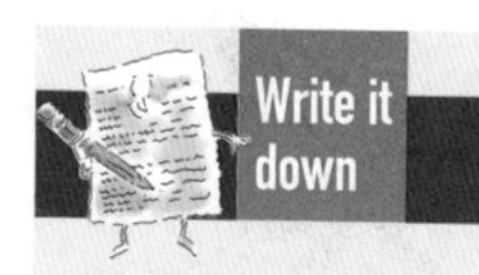

Documenting lumbar puncture

In your notes, record:

- initiation and completion times of the procedure
- patient's response including vitals every 15 minutes × 4, every 30 minutes × 4, and every 1 hour × 4 along with neuro status and puncture site assessment
- administration of drugs
- number of specimen tubes collected
- time of transport to the laboratory
- color, consistency, and other characteristics of the collected specimens.

Papanicolaou test

Also known as the Pap test or Pap smear, the Papanicolaou test developed in the 1920s by George N. Papanicolaou allows early detection of cervical cancer. The cytologic test involves scraping or aspirating secretions from the cervix, spreading them on a slide, and immediately coating the slide with fixative spray or solution to preserve specimen cells for nuclear staining. Cytologic evaluation then outlines cell maturity, morphology, and metabolic activity.

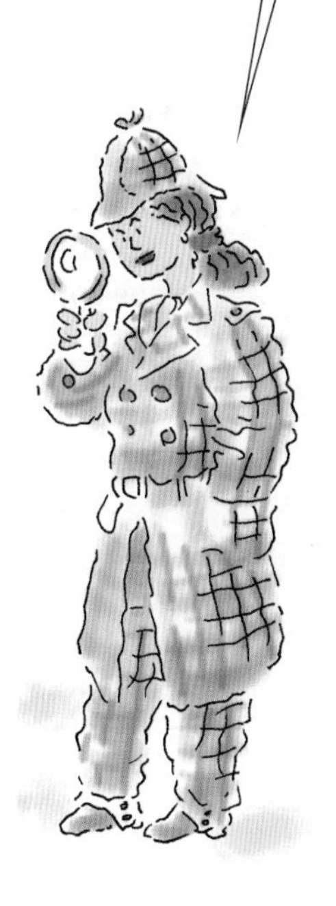
There's no speculation involved. You'll definitely need a speculum to perform a Pap test.

What you need

Bivalve vaginal speculum ✳ sterile gloves ✳ Pap stick (wooden spatula), cytobrush, or cervical brush ✳ pipette ✳ long cotton-tipped applicator ✳ three glass microscope slides ✳ thin prep Pap container (for liquid option) ✳ fixative (a commercial spray or 95% ethyl alcohol solution) ✳ adjustable lamp ✳ drape ✳ laboratory requisitions.

Getting ready

Select a speculum of the appropriate size and gather the equipment in the examining room. Label each glass slide with the patient's name and an "E," "C," or "V" *to differentiate endocervical, cervical, and vaginal specimens.* **Verify that the information on the labels matches the requisition.**

How you do it

- Explain the procedure to the patient and wash your hands.
- Instruct the patient to void *to relax the perineal muscles and facilitate bimanual examination of the uterus.*

Privacy, please!

- Provide privacy, allow patient to empty bladder as needed, and instruct the patient to undress below the waist. Then instruct her to sit on the examination table and to drape her genital region.
- Place the patient in the dorsal lithotomy position, with her feet in the stirrups and her buttocks extended slightly beyond the edge of the table. Adjust the drape to minimize exposure.
- Adjust the lamp so that it fully illuminates the genital area. Then fold back the corner of the drape to expose the perineum.
- If you're performing the procedure, first put on gloves. Then take the speculum in your dominant hand and moisten it with warm

water *to ease insertion*. Avoid using water-soluble lubricants, *which can interfere with accurate laboratory testing.*

- Warn the patient that you're about to touch her *to avoid startling her*. Then gently separate the labia with the thumb and forefinger of your nondominant hand.

Promote relaxation

- Instruct the patient to take several deep breaths and insert the speculum into the vagina. After it's in place, slowly open the blades to expose the cervix. Then lock the blades in place.

Fix immediately

- Insert a cotton-tipped applicator, cytobrush, or aspirator through the speculum ⅕″ (5 mm) into the cervical os. Rotate the applicator 360 degrees to obtain an endocervical specimen. Then remove the applicator and gently roll it in a circle across the slide marked "E." Refrain from rubbing the applicator on the slide *to prevent cell destruction*. Immediately place the slide in a fixative solution or spray it with a fixative *to prevent drying of the cells, which interferes with nuclear staining and cytologic interpretation*.
- Insert the small curved end of the Pap stick through the speculum and place it directly over the cervical os. Rotate the stick gently but firmly *to scrape cells loose of exocervix*. Remove the stick, spread the specimen across the slide marked "C," and fix it immediately, as before.
- The cervical broom obtains cells from the endocervix and exocervix and is the preferred method of Pap testing now. The broom's handle is removed and the sampling end is placed in a liquid medium.
- Insert the opposite end of the Pap stick or a cotton-tipped applicator through the speculum and scrape the posterior fornix or vaginal pool, an area that collects cells from the endometrium, vagina, and cervix. Remove the stick or applicator, spread the specimen across the slide marked "V," and fix it immediately.
- Unlock the speculum *to ease removal and avoid accidentally pinching the vaginal wall*. Then withdraw the speculum.

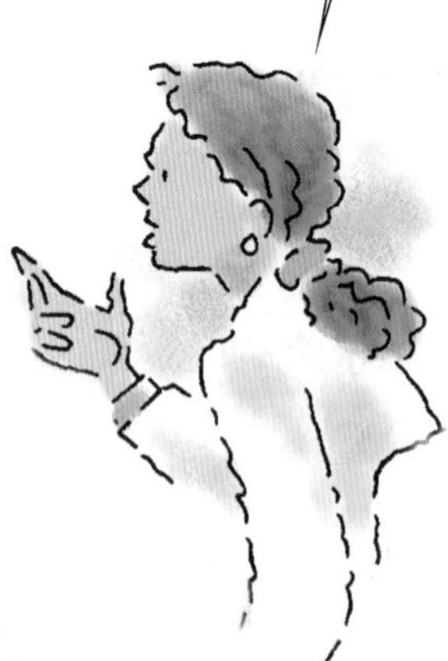
Rotate the Pap stick gently but firmly. That will scrape cells loose.

Finish up

- Remove the glove from your nondominant hand to perform the bimanual examination, which usually follows the Pap test. Then remove your other glove and discard both gloves.
- Gently remove the patient's feet from the stirrups and assist her to a sitting position. Provide privacy for her to dress.
- Fill out the appropriate laboratory requisitions, including the date of the patient's last menses.

Practice pointers

- Many preventable factors can interfere with the Pap test's accuracy, so provide appropriate patient teaching beforehand. For example, use of a vaginal douche in the 48-hour period (varying recommendation from 18 to 72 hours) before specimen collection washes away cellular deposits and prevents adequate sampling. Instillation of vaginal medications in the same period makes cytologic interpretation difficult. Collection of a specimen during menstruation prevents adequate sampling because menstrual flow washes away cells; ideally, such collection should take place 5 to 6 days before menses or 10 to 20 days after it. Application of topical antibiotics promotes rapid, heavy shedding of cells and requires postponement of the Pap test for at least 1 month.
- If the patient has had a complete hysterectomy, collect test specimens from the vaginal pool and cuff. (See *Documenting a Pap test.*)

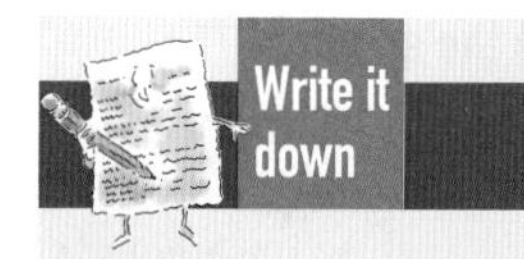

Documenting a Pap test

On the patient's chart, record the date and time of specimen collection, complications, and the nursing action taken.

Throat specimen collection

Correct collection and handling of a throat specimen helps the laboratory staff identify pathogens accurately with a minimum of contamination from normal bacterial flora. Collection normally involves using a swab to sample inflamed tissues and exudates from the throat.

What you need

Gloves ✻ tongue blade ✻ penlight ✻ sterile cotton-tipped swab ✻ sterile culture tube with transport medium (or commercial collection kit) ✻ label ✻ laboratory requisition.

How you do it

- Explain the procedure to the patient *to ease his anxiety and ensure cooperation.*
- Tell the patient that he may gag during the swabbing but that the procedure will probably take less than 1 minute.
- Instruct the patient to sit erect at the edge of the bed or in a chair, facing you. Then wash your hands and put on gloves.

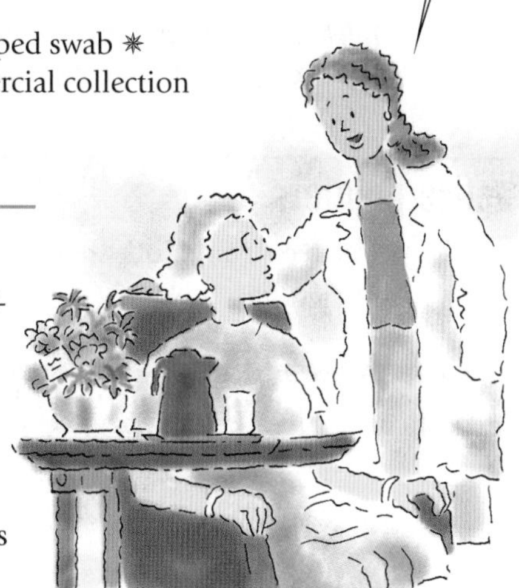
Collecting a throat specimen may cause you to gag, but the procedure will be over quickly.

In the spotlight

- Ask the patient to tilt his head back. Depress his tongue with the tongue blade and illuminate his throat with the penlight *to check for inflamed areas.*
- If the patient starts to gag, withdraw the tongue blade and tell him to breathe deeply. After he's relaxed, reinsert the tongue blade but not as deeply as before.

From side to shining side

- Using the cotton-tipped swab, wipe the tonsillar areas from side to side, including any inflamed or purulent sites. Make sure you don't touch the tongue, cheeks, lips, or teeth with the swab *to avoid contaminating it with oral bacteria.*
- Withdraw the swab and immediately place it in the culture tube. If you're using a commercial kit, crush the ampule of culture medium at the bottom of the tube and then push the swab into the medium *to keep the swab moist.*
- Remove and discard your gloves and wash your hands.
- Label the specimen with the patient's name and room number; the doctor's name; and the date, time, and site of collection.

Identify your suspect

- On the laboratory requisition, indicate whether any organism is strongly suspected, especially *Corynebacterium diphtheriae* (patchy gray pseudomembrane over lesion surrounded by red inflamed tissue, as this would require two swabs and special growth medium), *Bordetella pertussis* (requires a nasopharyngeal culture and special growth medium), and *Neisseria meningitidis* (requires enriched selective media).
- Send the specimen to the laboratory immediately *to prevent growth or deterioration of microbes* or refrigerate it. **Verify that the information on the label matches the requisition.**

Documenting throat specimen collection

In your notes, record:
- time, date, and site of specimen collection
- recent or current antibiotic therapy
- unusual appearance or odor of the specimen.

Practice pointers

- Note recent antibiotic therapy on the laboratory requisition. (See *Documenting throat specimen collection.*)

Nasopharyngeal specimen collection

Nasopharyngeal specimen collection involves using a sterile cotton-tipped swab to collect a specimen from the nasopharynx to help identify pathogens. After the specimen has been collected, the swab is immediately placed in a sterile tube containing a transport medium.

What you need

Gloves ✻ penlight ✻ sterile, flexible cotton-tipped swab ✻ tongue blade ✻ sterile culture tube with transport medium ✻ label ✻ laboratory requisition.

How you do it

- Tell the patient that he may gag or feel the urge to sneeze during the swabbing but that the procedure takes less than 1 minute.
- Have the patient sit erect at the edge of the bed or in a chair, facing you. Then wash your hands and put on gloves.

Clear passages

- Ask the patient to blow his nose to clear his nasal passages. Then check his nostrils for patency with a penlight.
- Tell the patient to occlude one nostril first and then the other as he exhales. Listen for the more patent nostril because *you'll insert the swab through it.*
- Ask the patient to cough *to bring organisms to the nasopharynx for a better specimen.*
- While the sterile swab is still in the package, bend it in a curve, and then open the package without contaminating the swab.
- Ask the patient to tilt his head back and gently pass the swab through the more patent nostril 3″ to 4″ (8 to 10 cm) into the nasopharynx, keeping the swab near the septum and floor of the nose. Rotate the swab quickly and remove it. (See *Obtaining a nasopharyngeal specimen,* page 132.)
- Alternatively, depress the patient's tongue with a tongue blade and pass the bent swab up behind the uvula. Rotate the swab and withdraw it, ensuring that other parts of the mouth are not touched with the swab.
- Remove the cap from the culture tube, insert the swab, and break off the contaminated end. Then close the tube tightly.
- Remove and discard your gloves and wash your hands.
- Label the specimen for culture, complete a laboratory requisition, and send the specimen to the laboratory immediately. **Verify that the information on the label matches the requisition.** If you're collecting a specimen to isolate a possible virus, check with the laboratory for the recommended collection technique. (See *Documenting nasopharyngeal specimen collection.*)

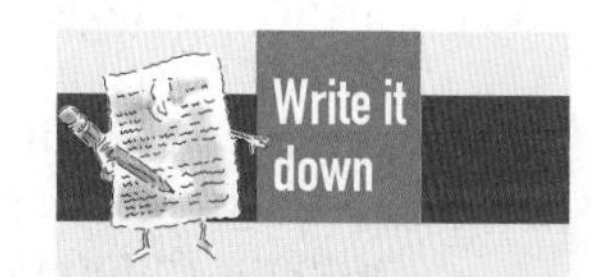

Documenting nasopharyngeal specimen collection

In your notes, record:
- time, date, and site of specimen collection
- recent or current antibiotic therapy
- unusual appearance or odor of the specimen.

Obtaining a nasopharyngeal specimen

After you've passed the swab into the nasopharynx, quickly but gently rotate the swab to collect the specimen twice, leave in place for 15 seconds, and remove slowly, taking care not to injure the nasal mucous membrane.

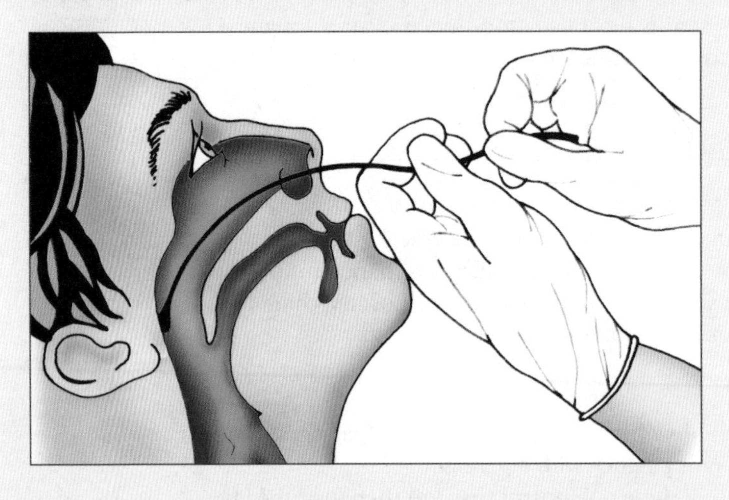

Wound specimen collection

Wound specimen collection involves using a sterile cotton-tipped swab to collect a specimen from inflamed tissues or exudate to help identify pathogens. After the specimen is collected, the swab is immediately placed in a sterile tube containing a transport medium and, in the case of sampling for anaerobes, an inert gas. Size up the wound to determine the proper method. Superficial wounds are swabbed with the cotton-tipped end of a culturette, whereas large wounds must have several different areas swabbed. Deep wounds may require aspiration of drainage with a needle, and if anaerobic pathogens are suspected, any extra air must be removed from the specimen.

What you need

Sterile gloves ✳ sterile forceps ✳ alcohol or povidone-iodine pads ✳ sterile swabs ✳ sterile 10-mL syringe ✳ sterile 21G needle ✳ sterile culture tube with transport medium (or commercial collection kit for aerobic culture) ✳ labels ✳ special anaerobic culture tube containing carbon dioxide or nitrogen ✳ fresh dressings for the wound ✳ laboratory requisition ✳ optional: rubber stopper for needle.

How you do it

- Determine patient's pain level and need for analgesic; premedicate as needed 30 minutes prior to the procedure.
- Wash your hands, prepare a sterile field, and put on sterile gloves. With sterile forceps, remove the dressing to expose the wound. Dispose of the soiled dressings properly.
- Clean the area around the wound with an alcohol, antiseptic pad, or a povidone-iodine pad *to reduce the risk of contaminating the specimen with skin bacteria.* Then allow the area to dry.

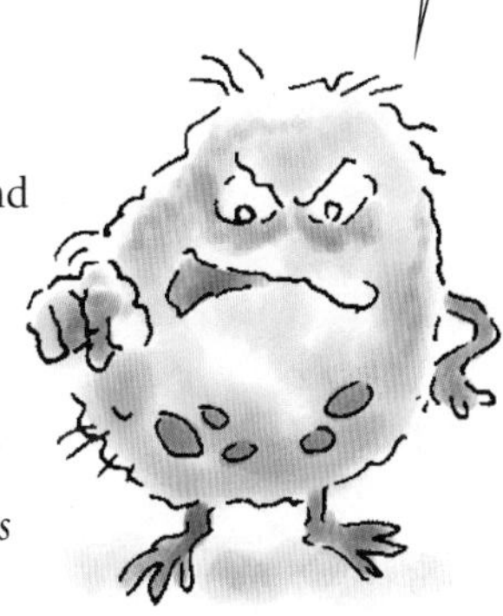
Avoiding contamination with skin bacteria is a key part of wound specimen collection.

Aerobic culture

- For an aerobic culture, use a sterile cotton-tipped swab to collect as much exudate as possible or insert the swab tip into the wound and gently rotate it. Remove the swab from the wound and immediately place it in the aerobic culture tube. Label the culture tube and send the tube to the laboratory immediately with a completed laboratory requisition. **Verify that the information on the requisition matches the labels.** Never collect exudate from the skin and then insert the same swab into the wound; *this could contaminate the wound with skin bacteria.*

Anaerobic culture

- For an anaerobic culture, insert the sterile cotton-tipped swab deeply into the wound, rotate it gently, remove it, and immediately place it in the anaerobic culture tube. (See *Anaerobic specimen collector*, page 134.) Alternatively, insert a sterile 10-mL syringe, without a needle, into the wound, and aspirate 1 to 5 mL of exudate into the syringe. Then attach the 21G needle to the syringe and immediately inject the aspirate into the anaerobic culture tube. If an anaerobic culture tube is unavailable, obtain a rubber stopper, attach the needle to the syringe, and gently push all the air out of the syringe by pressing on the plunger. Stick the needle tip into the rubber stopper, remove and discard your gloves, and send the syringe of aspirate to the laboratory immediately with a completed laboratory requisition. **Verify that the information on the requisition matches the label.**
- Put on sterile gloves.
- Apply a new dressing to the wound. (See chapter 3, Physical treatments.)

Practice pointers

- Note recent antibiotic therapy on the laboratory requisition.
- Although you would normally clean the area around a wound to prevent contamination by normal skin flora, don't clean a

Anaerobic specimen collector

Because most anaerobes die when exposed to oxygen, they must be transported in tubes filled with carbon dioxide or nitrogen. The anaerobic specimen collector shown here includes a tube filled with carbon dioxide, a small inner tube, and a swab attached to a plastic plunger.

Before specimen collection, the small inner tube containing the swab is held in place with the rubber stopper (as shown on the left). After collecting the specimen, quickly replace the swab in the inner tube and depress the plunger to separate the inner tube from the stopper (as shown on the right), forcing it into the larger tube and exposing the specimen to a carbon dioxide–rich environment.

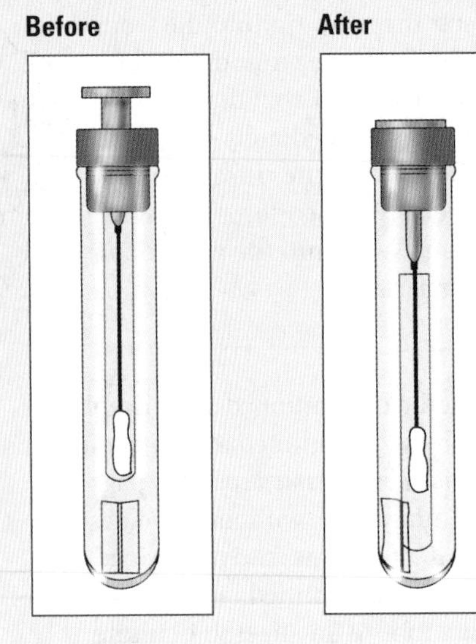
Before
After

Write it down

Documenting wound specimen collection

In your notes, record:
- time, date, and site of specimen collection
- recent or current antibiotic therapy
- unusual appearance or odor of the specimen.

perineal wound with alcohol *because this could irritate sensitive tissues*. Also, make sure that antiseptic doesn't enter the wound. (See *Documenting wound specimen collection*.)

- Remove old drainage and culture fresh exudate from center of wound.
- Assess for signs of fever, chills, excessive thirst, and pain.

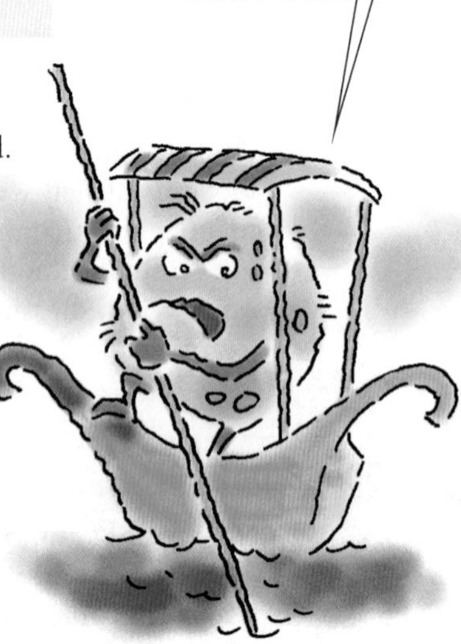
If I'm in the ear canal, ear specimen collection is the way to find out.

Ear specimen collection

Ear specimen collection involves using a sterile swab to collect a specimen from the ear canal to identify pathogens. After the specimen is collected, the swab is immediately placed in a sterile tube containing a transport medium.

What you need

Gloves ✳ normal saline solution ✳ two 2″ × 2″ gauze pads ✳ sterile swabs ✳ sterile culture tube with transport medium ✳ label ✳ 10-mL syringe and 22G 1″ needle (for tympanocentesis) ✳ laboratory requisition.

How you do it

- Wash your hands and put on gloves.
- Gently clean excess debris from the patient's ear with normal saline solution and gauze pads.
- Insert the sterile swab ⅛″ to ¼ ″ into the ear canal and rotate it gently along the walls of the canal *to avoid damaging the eardrum.*
- Withdraw the swab, being careful not to touch other surfaces *to avoid contaminating the specimen.*
- Place the swab in the sterile culture tube with transport medium.
- Remove and discard your gloves and wash your hands.
- Label the specimen for culture, complete a laboratory requisition, **verify the information on the label with the requisition**, and send the specimen to the laboratory immediately.

Collecting a middle ear specimen

- Put on gloves and clean the outer ear with normal saline solution and gauze pads.
- Remove and discard your gloves.
- After the doctor punctures the eardrum with a needle and aspirates fluid into the syringe, label the container, complete a laboratory requisition, **verify that the information on the label matches the requisition**, and send the specimen to the laboratory immediately.

Documenting ear specimen collection

In your notes, record:
- time, date, and site of specimen collection
- recent or current antibiotic therapy
- unusual appearance or odor of the specimen.

Practice pointers

- Note recent antibiotic therapy on the laboratory requisition. (See *Documenting ear specimen collection.*)

Eye specimen collection

Eye specimen collection involves using a sterile swab to collect specimen to identify pathogens. After the specimen is collected, the swab is immediately placed in a sterile tube containing a transport medium.

What you need

Sterile gloves * sterile normal saline solution * two 2″ × 2″ gauze pads * sterile swabs * sterile wire culture loop (for corneal scraping) * sterile culture tube with transport medium * label * laboratory requisition.

How you do it

- Wash your hands and put on sterile gloves.
- Gently clean excess debris from the outside of the eye with normal saline solution and gauze pads, wiping from the inner to the outer canthus.

Lowering the lower eyelid

- Retract the lower eyelid to expose the conjunctival sac. Gently rub the sterile swab over the conjunctiva, being careful not to touch other surfaces. Hold the swab parallel to the eye, rather than pointed directly at it, *to prevent corneal irritation or trauma from sudden movement.* (If corneal scraping is required, a doctor will perform the procedure using a wire culture loop.)
- Immediately place the swab or wire loop in the culture tube with transport medium.
- Remove and discard your gloves and wash your hands.
- Label the specimen for culture, complete a laboratory requisition, and send the specimen to the laboratory immediately.

Documenting eye specimen collection

In your notes, record:
- time, date, and site of specimen collection
- any recent or current antibiotic therapy
- unusual appearance or odor of the specimen.

Practice pointers

- Note recent antibiotic therapy on the laboratory requisition.
- Don't use an antiseptic before culturing *to avoid irritating the eye and inhibiting growth of organisms in the culture.* If the patient is a child or an uncooperative adult, ask a coworker to restrain the patient's head *to prevent eye trauma resulting from sudden movement.* (See *Documenting eye specimen collection.*)

Rectal specimen

Correct rectal specimen collection and handling of the swab specimen helps the laboratory staff identify pathogens accurately with a minimum of contamination from normal bacterial flora. Collection normally involves sampling inflamed tissues or exudate from the rectum with a sterile swab.

What you need

Gloves ✳ soap and water ✳ washcloth ✳ sterile swab ✳ normal saline solution ✳ sterile culture tube with transport medium ✳ label ✳ laboratory requisition.

How you do it

- Wash your hands and put on gloves.
- Clean the area around the patient's anus using a washcloth and soap and water.

Not far to go

- Insert the swab, moistened with normal saline solution or sterile broth medium, through the anus and advance it about 3⁄8″ (1 cm) for infants or 1½″ (4 cm) for adults. While withdrawing the swab, gently rotate it against the walls of the lower rectum to sample a large area of the rectal mucosa.
- Place the swab in a culture tube with transport medium.
- Remove and discard your gloves and wash your hands.
- Label the specimen for culture, complete a laboratory requisition, and send the specimen to the laboratory immediately.

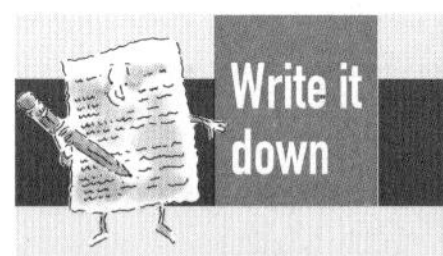

Documenting rectal specimen collection

In your notes, record:
- time, date, and site of specimen collection
- recent or current antibiotic therapy
- unusual appearance or odor of the specimen.

Practice pointers

Note recent antibiotic therapy on the laboratory requisition. (See *Documenting rectal specimen collection*.)

Bone marrow aspiration and biopsy

A specimen of bone marrow—the major site of blood cell formation—can be obtained by aspiration or needle biopsy. The procedure allows evaluation of overall blood composition, including blood elements such as red blood cells, white blood cells and platelets, precursor cells, iron stores, abnormal or malignant cells, and cultures for infectious agents.

Aspiration removes organic liquid through a needle inserted into the marrow cavity of the bone; a biopsy removes a small, solid core of marrow tissue through the needle. A doctor usually performs both procedures; however, some facilities authorize specially trained chemotherapy nurses or nurse clinicians to perform them with an assistant.

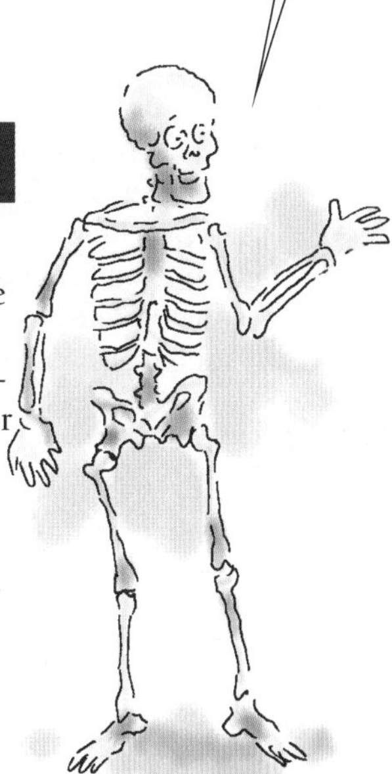

If you're specially trained, you can perform bone marrow aspiration and biopsy.

What you need

For aspiration

Prepackaged bone marrow set, which includes povidone-iodine pads ✱ two sterile drapes (one fenestrated, one plain) ✱ 4″ × 4″ gauze pads ✱ 2″ × 2″ gauze pads ✱ 12-mL syringe ✱ two bone marrow needles with inner stylet ✱ scalpel ✱ sedative ✱ sterile specimen containers or slides ✱ bone marrow needle ✱ 70% isopropyl alcohol ✱ 1% lidocaine (unopened bottle) ✱ 26G or 27G ½″ to ⅝″ needle ✱ 3-mL syringe ✱ adhesive tape ✱ sterile gloves ✱ mask ✱ goggles ✱ head cover ✱ labels.

For biopsy

All equipment listed earlier * Vim-Silverman, Jamshidi, Illinois sternal, or Westerman-Jensen needle * Zenker's fixative.

How you do it

- Ensure patient can maintain position required to perform the procedure and verify the patient's coagulation status.
- Time out—to verify the patient identification and also the procedure type and site with patient and health care team.
- Tell the patient that the doctor will collect a bone marrow specimen and explain the procedure *to ease his anxiety and ensure cooperation.*
- Make sure the patient or a responsible family member understands the procedure and signs a consent form obtained by the doctor.
- Alert the patient and his family that bleeding and infection are potentially life-threatening complications of aspiration or biopsy at any site.
- Inform the patient that the procedure normally takes 20 minutes, that test results usually are available in 1 day, and that more than one marrow specimen may be required.

Historically sensitive?

- Check the patient's history for hypersensitivity to the local anesthetic. Inform him that he'll receive a local anesthetic and feel heavy pressure from insertion of the biopsy or aspiration needle as well as a brief, pulling sensation. Tell him that the doctor may make a small incision to avoid tearing the skin.
- Tell him which bone—sternum or anterior iliac crest or proximal tibia—will be sampled.

- If the patient has osteoporosis, tell him that the needle pressure may be minimal. If he has osteopetrosis, inform him that a drill may be needed.
- Provide a sedative, as ordered, before the test.
- Position the patient according to the selected puncture site. (See *Common sites for bone marrow aspiration and biopsy*.)
- Using sterile technique, clean the puncture site with povidone-iodine pads and allow it to dry, then drape the area.

Numbing needed

- To anesthetize the site, the doctor infiltrates it with 1% lidocaine using a 26G or 27G ½″ to ⅝″ needle to inject a small amount intradermally and then a larger 22G 1″ to 2″ needle to anesthetize the tissue down to the bone.
- When the needle tip reaches the bone, the doctor anesthetizes the periosteum by injecting a small amount of lidocaine in a circular area about ¾″ (2 cm) in diameter. The needle should be withdrawn from the periosteum after each injection.
- After allowing about 1 minute for the lidocaine to take effect, a scalpel may be used to make a small stab incision in the patient's

Common sites for bone marrow aspiration and biopsy

The posterior superior iliac crest is the preferred site for bone marrow aspiration because no vital organs or vessels are nearby. The patient is placed either in the lateral position with one leg flexed or in the prone position.

For aspiration or biopsy from the anterior iliac crest, the patient is placed in the supine or side-lying position. This site is used with patients who can't lie in the prone position because of severe abdominal distention.

Aspiration from the sternum involves the greatest risk. However, it may be used because this site is near the surface, the cortical bone is thin, and the marrow cavity contains numerous cells and relatively little fat or supporting bone. This site is seldom used for biopsy.

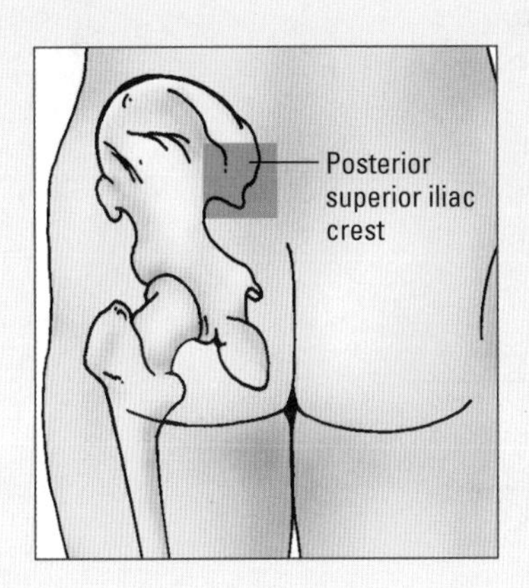

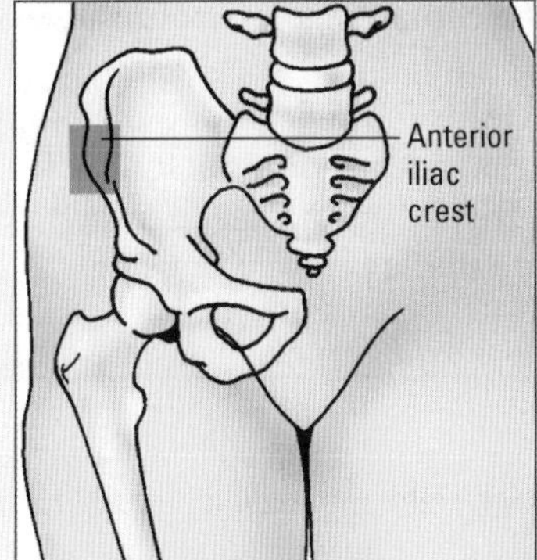

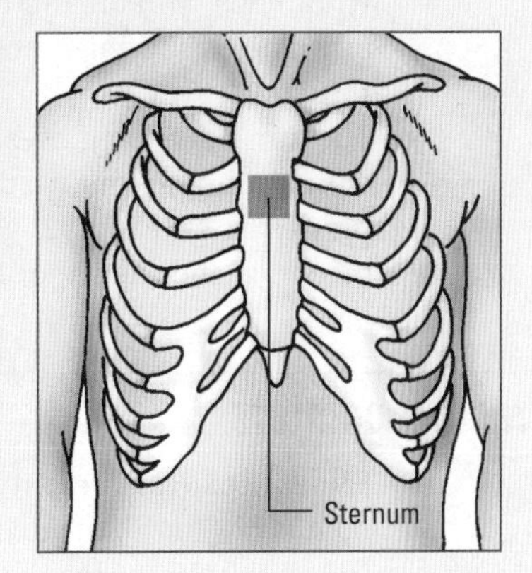

skin to accommodate the bone marrow needle. *This technique avoids pushing skin into the bone marrow and also helps avoid unnecessary skin tearing to help reduce the risk of infection.*

Bone marrow aspiration

- The doctor inserts the bone marrow needle and lodges it firmly in the bone cortex. If the patient feels sharp pain instead of pressure when the needle first touches bone, the needle was probably inserted outside the anesthetized area. If this happens, the needle should be withdrawn slightly and moved to the anesthetized area.
- The needle is advanced by applying an even, downward force with the heel of the hand or the palm while twisting it back and forth slightly. A crackling sensation means that the needle has entered the marrow cavity.
- Next, the doctor removes the inner cannula, attaches the syringe to the needle, aspirates the required specimen, and withdraws the needle.
- The nurse puts on gloves and applies pressure to the aspiration site with a gauze pad for 5 minutes to control bleeding while an assistant prepares the marrow slides. The area is then cleaned with alcohol to remove the povidone-iodine, the skin is dried thoroughly with a 4″ × 4″ gauze pad, and a sterile pressure dressing is applied.

Bone marrow biopsy

- The doctor inserts the biopsy needle into the periosteum and advances it steadily until the outer needle passes into the marrow cavity.
- The biopsy needle is directed into the marrow cavity by alternately rotating the inner needle clockwise and counterclockwise. Then a plug of tissue is removed, the needle assembly is withdrawn, and the marrow specimen is expelled into a properly labeled specimen bottle containing Zenker's fixative or formaldehyde.
- The nurse puts on gloves, cleans the area around the biopsy site with alcohol to remove the povidone-iodine solution, firmly presses a sterile 2″ × 2″ gauze pad against the incision to control bleeding, and then applies a sterile pressure dressing.

Practice pointers

- Faulty needle placement may yield too little aspirate. If no specimen is produced, the needle must be withdrawn from the bone (but not from the overlying soft tissue), the stylet replaced, and the needle inserted into a second site within the anesthetized field.

- Bone marrow specimens shouldn't be collected from irradiated areas *because radiation may have altered or destroyed the marrow.*
- Monitor for bleeding, pressure dressing performance, infection, drainage, redness, swelling, and pain.
- If a hematoma occurs around the puncture site, apply warm soaks. Give analgesics for site pain or tenderness. (See *Documenting bone marrow aspiration and biopsy.*)

Documenting bone marrow aspiration and biopsy

Chart the time, date, location, patient response, and the specimen obtained.

Skin biopsy

Skin biopsy is a diagnostic test in which a small piece of tissue is removed from a lesion that's suspected of being malignant, infected, or inflamed while the patient is under local anesthesia.

Pick one, any one. . .

One of four techniques may be used: shave biopsy, punch biopsy, and incisional or excisional biopsy. Shave biopsy cuts the lesion and a superficial layer of the skin (only used with benign lesions). Punch biopsy removes an oval core from the center of the lesion extending from the surface to the subcutaneous fat to assess inflammation. Incisional biopsy removes a cross-section piece through the center of a lesion too large to totally remove. Excisional biopsy removes the entire lesion plus adjacent tissue down to adipose layer and is indicated for rapidly expanding lesions; suspect melanoma; and sclerotic, bullous, or atrophic lesions.

What you need

Gloves ✳ #15 scalpel for shave or excisional biopsy ✳ local anesthetic ✳ specimen bottle containing 10% formaldehyde solution ✳ 4-0 sutures for punch or excisional biopsy ✳ adhesive bandage ✳ forceps.

How you do it

- Explain to the patient that the biopsy provides a skin specimen for microscopic study. Describe the procedure and tell him who will perform it. Typically, a doctor or an advanced practice nurse performs the biopsy. Answer questions he may have *to ease anxiety and ensure cooperation.*
- Inform the patient that he need not restrict food or fluids.
- Tell him that he'll receive a local anesthetic for pain.

- Inform him that the biopsy will take about 15 minutes and that the test results are usually available in 1 day.
- Have the patient or an appropriate family member sign a consent form after the physician has discussed the procedure, risks, benefits, and alternatives to the procedure with the patient.
- Check the patient's history for hypersensitivity to the local anesthetic.
- Position the patient comfortably. Wash your hands and put on gloves. The doctor cleans the biopsy site before the local anesthetic is administered.

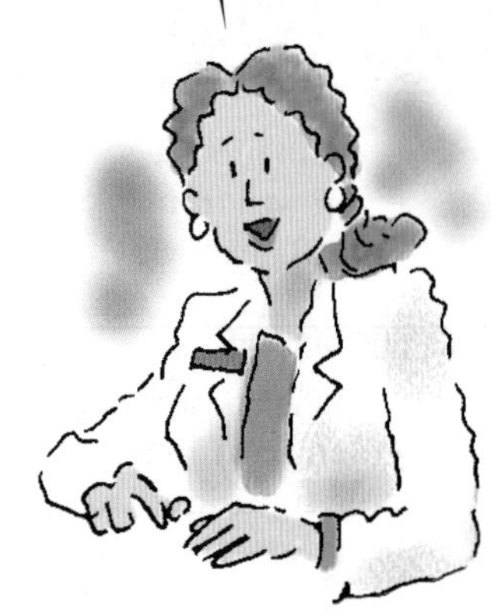
Bleeding is a possible complication associated with any biopsy.

Shave . . .

- For a shave biopsy, the protruding growth is cut off at the skin line with a #15 scalpel.
- The tissue is placed immediately in a properly labeled specimen bottle containing 10% formaldehyde solution.
- Apply pressure to the area *to stop the bleeding* as well as an adhesive bandage.

. . . punch . . .

- For a punch biopsy, the skin surrounding the lesion is pulled taut and the punch is firmly introduced into the lesion and rotated to obtain a tissue specimen. The plug is lifted with forceps or a needle and is severed as deeply into the fat layer as possible.
- The specimen is placed in a properly labeled specimen bottle containing 10% formaldehyde solution or in a sterile container if indicated.
- Closing the wound depends on the size of the punch: A 3-mm punch requires only an adhesive bandage, a 4-mm punch requires one suture, and a 6-mm punch requires two sutures.

. . . or incisional or excisional

- For an incisional or excisional biopsy, a #15 scalpel is used to excise part or the entire lesion, respectively; the incision is made as wide and as deep as necessary.
- The tissue specimen is removed and placed immediately in a properly labeled specimen bottle containing 10% formaldehyde solution.
- Apply pressure to the site *to stop the bleeding*.
- The wound is closed using a 4-0 suture. If the incision is large, a skin graft may be required.
- Check the biopsy site for bleeding.
- Remove and discard gloves; wash your hands.
- Send the specimen to the laboratory immediately.
- If the patient experiences pain, administer an analgesic.

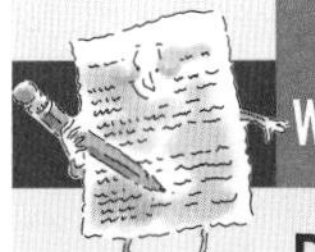

Write it down

Documenting skin biopsy

In your notes, record:

- time and location where the specimen was obtained
- appearance of the site and specimen
- whether bleeding occurred at the biopsy site.

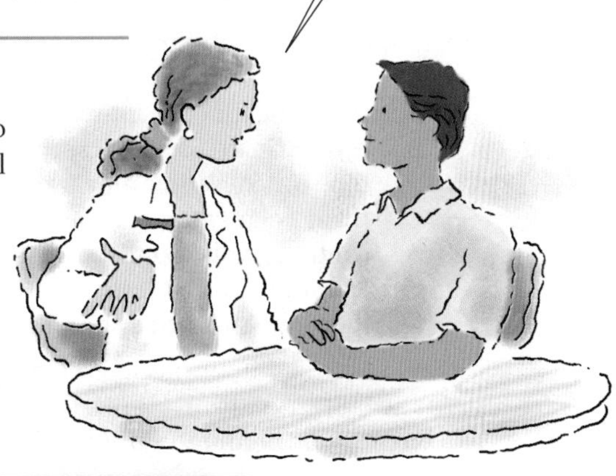
Keep your sutures dry and your strips in place.

Practice pointers

- Advise the patient going home with sutures to keep the area clean and as dry as possible. Tell him that facial sutures will be removed in 3 to 5 days and trunk sutures in 7 to 14 days.
- Instruct the patient with adhesive strips to leave them in place for 14 to 21 days. (See *Documenting skin biopsy*.)
- Educate the patient to report increased bleeding and signs of infection.

Quick quiz

1. Where should the tourniquet be applied before performing a venipuncture?

A. 1″ proximal to chosen site
B. 2″ distal to the chosen site
C. 2″ proximal to the chosen site
D. Directly at the chosen site

Answer: C. Before performing a venipuncture, apply a tourniquet 2″ proximal to the area chosen.

2. The patient suddenly develops a fever. The nurse notified the health care provider who orders blood cultures. Which statement describes appropriate procedure in drawing blood cultures?

A. Draw blood sample of 5 mL from right arm and 10 mL from left leg.
B. Add blood specimen to anaerobic culture bottle first.
C. Always first cleanse the diaphragm top with Betadine.
D. The blood may be drawn from any extremity.

Answer: B. When drawing both aerobic and anaerobic specimen, inoculate the anaerobic culture bottle first to minimize exposure of specimen to oxygen.

3. The patient suddenly develops respiratory distress, and the health care provider orders ABG levels. Which test should the nurse conduct before performing a radial puncture to obtain the arterial sample?

A. Allen's test
B. Queckenstedt's test
C. Schilling's test
D. Pulse oximeter

Answer: A. Before attempting a radial puncture, Allen's test should be performed.

4. The nurse is instructing a patient to collect a 24-hour urine specimen at home. Which statement made by the patient indicates the need for further teaching?

A. I will urinate, discard that specimen, but mark the time as start time for collection time frame.
B. I will urinate, save that specimen, and note time as start time for collection time frame.
C. If I accidently forget to save urine, mark down the time and continue collection.
D. Start the urine collection with the first void after midnight, then add each urine specimen until the container is filled.

Answer: A. A 24-hour specimen is accurately collected by having the patient discard the first urine, start collection, and save last voided specimen about 10 minutes prior to collection completion time.

5. Which food item should the patient avoid for 48 to 72 hours before fecal occult blood testing as well as throughout the collection period?

A. Horseradish
B. Tomatoes
C. Beets
D. Kale

Answer: A. The patient should maintain a high-fiber diet and refrain from eating red meat, poultry, fish, turnips, and horseradish for 48 to 72 hours before the test as well as throughout the collection period.

Scoring

☆☆☆ If you answered all five items correctly, Wowwee! You're quite a specimen!

☆☆ If you answered three or four items correctly, Yowzer! Your collection knowledge is impressive!

☆ If you answered fewer than three correctly, relax, review, and give it another go!

Selected References

Chernecky, C. C., & Berger, B. J. (2013). *Laboratory tests and diagnostic procedures* (6th ed.). St. Louis, MO: Elsevier Saunders.

Danckers, M., & Fried, E. D. (2013). *Arterial blood sampling*. Retrieved from http://emedicine.medscape.com/article/1902703-overview

Elkin, M. K., Perry, A. G., & Potter, P. A. (2000). *Nursing interventions and clinical skills* (2nd ed.). St. Louis, MO: Mosby.

Ellis, J. R., & Hartley, C. L. (2000). *Managing and coordinating nursing care* (3rd ed.). Philadelphia, PA: Lippincott Williams & Wilkins.

Fortunato, N. H. (2000). *Berry & Kohn's operating room technique* (9th ed.). St. Louis, MO: Mosby.

Goldman, L., & Schafer, A. I. (2012). *Goldman's Cecil medicine* (24th ed.). Philadelphia, PA: Elsevier Saunders.

Hadaway, L. C. (1999). I.V. infiltration. Not just a peripheral problem. *Nursing Management, 29*(9), 41–47.

Hess, C. T. (2002). *Clinical guide to wound care* (4th ed.). Spring House, PA: Springhouse.

Hinkle, J. L., & Cheever, K. H. (2014). *Brunner and Suddarth's textbook of medical-surgical nursing* (13th ed.). Philadelphia, PA: Lippincott Williams & Wilkins.

Hogan-Quigley, B., Palm, M. L., & Bickley, L. (2012). *Bates' nursing guide to physical examination and history taking*. Philadelphia, PA: Lippincott Williams & Wilkins.

Horne, C., & Derrico, D. (1999). Mastering ABGs. The art of arterial blood gas measurement. *The American Journal of Nursing, 99*(8), 26–32.

Ignatavicius, D. D., & Workman, M. L. (2001). *Medical-surgical nursing: Critical thinking for collaborative care* (4th ed.). Philadelphia, PA: W.B. Saunders.

Jagger, J., & Perry, J. (1999). Power in numbers: Reducing your risk of bloodborne exposures. *Nursing, 29*(1), 51–52.

Joint Commission on Accreditation of Healthcare Organizations. (2001). *Comprehensive accreditation manual for hospitals*. Oakbrook Terrace, IL: Author.

Lanken, P. N., Hanson, C. W., & Manaker, S. (2001). *The intensive care unit manual*. Philadelphia, PA: W.B. Saunders.

Lynn-McHale, D. J., & Carlson, K. K. (Eds.). (2001). *AACN procedure manual for critical care* (4th ed.). Philadelphia, PA: W.B. Saunders.

Maklebust, J., & Sieggreen, M. (2001). *Pressure ulcers: Guidelines for prevention and management* (3rd ed.). Spring House, PA: Springhouse.

Nicol, M., Bavin, C., Bedford-Turner, S., et al. (2000). *Essential nursing skills*. St. Louis, MO: Mosby.

Perry, A. G., & Potter, P. A. (2014). *Clinical nursing skills & techniques* (8th ed.). St. Louis, MO: Elsevier.

Phillips, L. D. (2001). *Manual of I.V. therapeutics* (3rd ed.). Philadelphia, PA: F.A. Davis.

Phippen, M. L., & Wells, M. P. (2000). *Patient care during operative and invasive procedures*. Philadelphia, PA: W.B. Saunders.

Pierson, F. M. (1999). *Principles and techniques of patient care* (2nd ed.). Philadelphia, PA: W.B. Saunders.

Shoemaker, W. C., Ayres, S. M., Grenvik, A., et al. (2000). *Textbook of critical care* (4th ed.). Philadelphia, PA: W.B. Saunders.

Springhouse. (2000). *Nursing procedures* (3rd ed.). Spring House, PA: Author.

Springhouse. (2001). *Diagnostic: An A-to-Z guide to laboratory tests & diagnostic procedures*. Spring House, PA: Author.

Chapter 3

Physical treatments

Just the facts

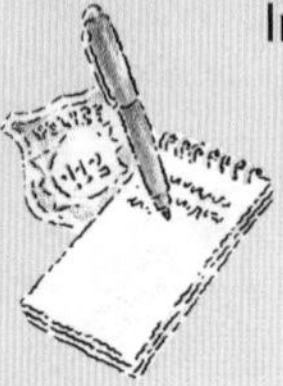

In this chapter, you'll learn:

- about physical treatments and how to perform them
- what patient care is associated with each treatment
- how to manage complications
- what patient teaching and documentation are associated with each treatment.

Antiembolism stocking application

Graduated compression stockings (GCS; also called gradient stockings, thromboembolic deterrent [TED] hose, and antiembolism hose) are knee-, thigh-, or waist-high garments worn to compress the leg veins. The application of pressure reduces venous stasis, edema, and the formation of venous leg ulcers and thrombi (i.e., blood clots) within the leg veins (i.e., deep vein thrombosis [DVT]). Prevention of DVT is crucial because, once formed, thrombi within the leg veins can enter the general circulation and cause pulmonary embolism and other ischemic events.

What you need

Tape measure ✳ antiembolism stockings of correct size and length.

Getting ready

Measure the patient for the correct size stocking according to the manufacturer's specifications. (See *Measuring for antiembolism stockings.*)

Measuring for antiembolism stockings

Measure the patient carefully to ensure that his antiembolism stockings provide enough compression for adequate venous return.

To choose the correct knee-length stocking, measure the circumference of the calf at its widest point (top left) and the leg length from the bottom of the heel to the back of the knee (bottom left).

To choose a thigh-length stocking, measure the calf as for a knee-length stocking and the thigh at its widest point (top right). Then measure the leg length from the bottom of the heel to the gluteal fold (bottom right).

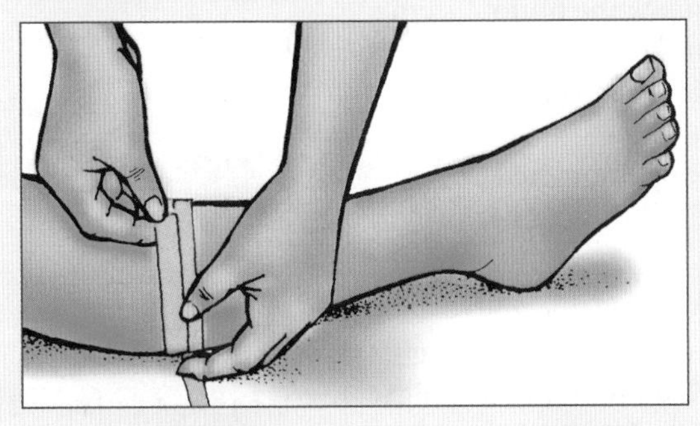

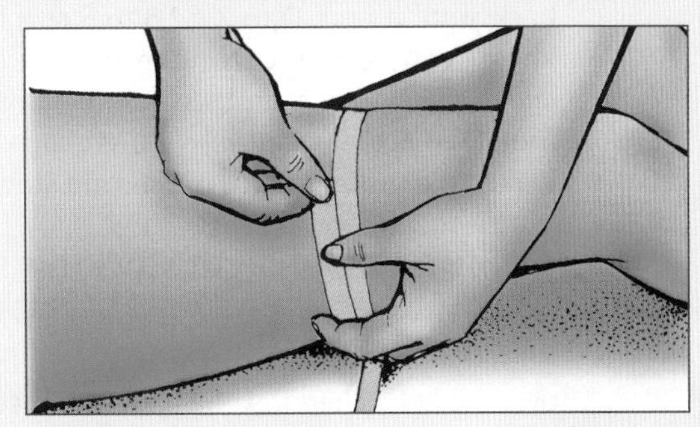

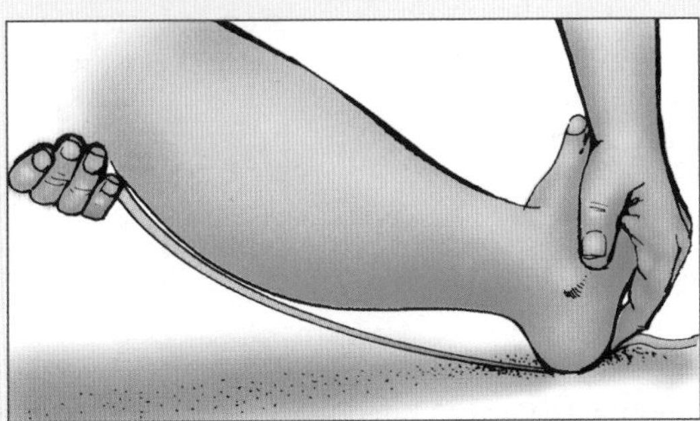

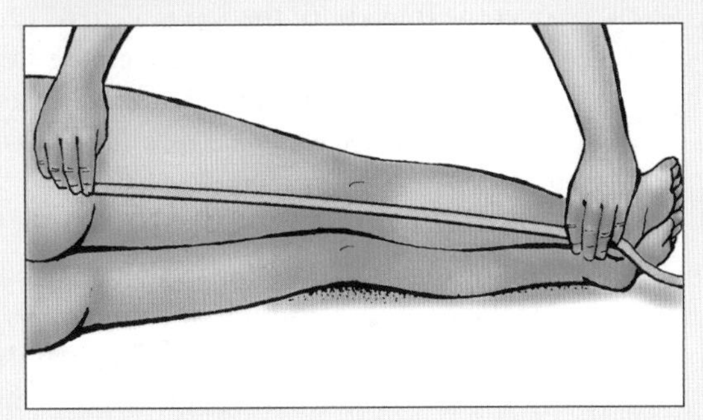

Ensure that patients who develop edema or postoperative swelling have their legs remeasured and antiembolism stockings refitted.

How you do it

- First, check the doctor's order, then identify the patient using two patient identifiers.
- Assess the patient's condition. If his legs are cold or cyanotic, notify the doctor before proceeding.
- After explaining the procedure to the patient, provide privacy and perform hand hygiene.
- Have the patient lie down.

Applying a knee-length stocking

- Begin by turning the stocking inside out until the foot part remains inside the stocking.
- Ease the turned-in foot section over the toes while supporting the ankle, and stretch it until the heel rests in the heel pocket. The toe should be visible through the toe window, if any.
- Gather the loose material at the ankle and slide the rest of the stocking up over the heel with short pulls, alternating front and back, until it rests 1″ to 2″ (2.5 to 5 cm) below the bottom of the knee. Gently snap the fabric around the ankle *to ensure a tight fit and to eliminate gaps* and see that the fabric is smooth over the foot. (See *Applying antiembolism stockings*.)
- Repeat the procedure for the second stocking, if ordered.

Applying a thigh-length stocking

- Follow the procedure for applying a knee-length stocking.
- With the patient's leg extended, stretch the rest of the stocking over the knee, then flex the patient's knee and pull the stocking over the thigh until the top is 1″ to 3″ (2.5 to 7.5 cm) below the gluteal fold. Remember to stretch the stocking from the top, front, and back *to distribute the fabric evenly*. Gently snap the fabric behind the knee *to eliminate gaps, which could reduce pressure*.

Applying a waist-length stocking

- Follow the procedure for applying knee-length and thigh-length stockings and extend the stocking top to the gluteal fold.
- Fit the patient with the adjustable belt that accompanies the stockings, making sure that the waistband and the fabric don't interfere with any incision, drainage tube, catheter, or other device.

Applying antiembolism stockings

Gather the loose part of the stocking at the toes and pull this portion toward the heel.

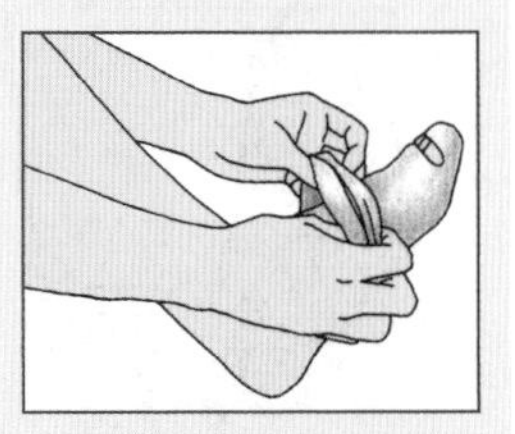

Then gather the loose part of the stocking and bring it over the heel with short, alternating front and back pulls.

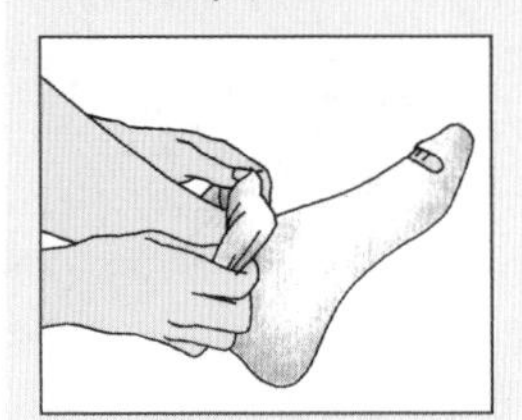

Insert the index and middle fingers into the gathered part of the stocking at the ankle and ease it upward by rocking it slightly up and down.

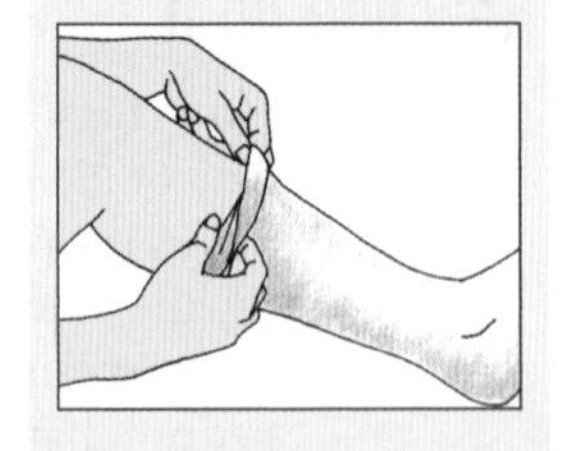

Practice pointers

- Antiembolism stockings usually aren't used on patients with skin lesions; fragile tissue; gangrene; poor circulation; peripheral neuropathy; or other sensory impairment, massive edema, major limb deformity, cardiac failure, recent vein ligation, unusual leg size or shape, or skin grafts.
- If you find the patient's measurements are outside the range indicated, ask the doctor if he wants to order custom-made stockings.
- Use caution and clinical judgment when applying antiembolism stockings over venous ulcers or wounds.
- Stockings should be applied in the morning, *before edema develops*. If the patient has been walking, have him lie down and elevate his legs for 15 to 30 minutes before applying the stockings *to facilitate venous return*.

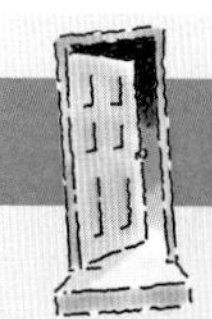

Home care connection

Reviewing antiembolism stocking care

If the patient requires antiembolism stockings after discharge, teach him or a family member how to apply them correctly and explain the benefits of wearing them.

Instruct the patient or family member to care for the stockings properly and to replace them when they lose elasticity. Tell the patient that he should wear the stockings at all times (except during bathing) to provide continuous protection against thrombosis. Ensure the patient and family know what to look for when checking the skin, such as skin marking and discoloration, particularly over bony prominences. Tell him to keep a second pair handy to wear while the first pair is being laundered. Ensure the family knows whom to call if there is a problem.

Write it down

Documenting antiembolism stocking application

In your notes, record:

- date and time of stocking application and removal
- patient education
- stocking length and size
- condition of the leg before and after treatment
- condition of the toes during treatment
- complications
- patient's tolerance of the treatment.

- Don't allow the stockings to roll or turn down at the top or toe *because this can cut off circulation.*
- Check the patient's toes at least once every 4 hours, noting skin color and temperature, sensation, swelling, and ability to move. If complications occur, remove the stockings and notify the doctor immediately. Remove the stockings once daily *to bathe the skin and to observe for irritation and breakdown.*
- Discontinue the use of antiembolism stockings if there is marking, blistering, or discoloration of the skin, especially over bony prominences. A mechanical compression device such as a sequential compression device (SCD) should be considered as an alternative.
- Review antiembolism stocking application with the patient, if necessary. (See *Reviewing antiembolism stocking care* and *Documenting antiembolism stocking application.*)

Sequential compression device therapy

SCD therapy mimics muscle activity during ambulation by massaging the legs in a wavelike, milking motion that promotes blood flow and deters thrombosis. It may be used with other measures to prevent DVT, such as antiembolism stockings and anticoagulant medications. Antiembolism stockings and sequential compression sleeves are commonly used preoperatively and postoperatively because blood clots tend to form during surgery. SCD therapy is effective for patients at moderately high risk for venous thromboembolism (VTE).

Sequential compression therapy uses a wavelike motion to massage the legs, which promotes blood flow.

It should begin upon admission and continue as long as the patient has limited mobility.

What you need

Measuring tape ✳ sizing chart for the brand of sleeves you're using ✳ pair of compression sleeves in correct size ✳ connecting tubing ✳ compression controller.

Getting ready

Identify the patient using two patient identifiers and verify the order. Perform hand hygiene. Explain the procedure to the patient. Have the patient rest in bed so that you can measure the circumference of the upper thigh at the gluteal fold. Find the patient's thigh measurement on the sizing chart and locate the corresponding size of the compression sleeve. Follow manufacturer directions to determine size correctly. Conduct a baseline skin and neurovascular assessment before placing the sleeves on the patient and again at least every 8 hours or immediately in the event of complications. (See *Skin and neurovascular assessment.*)

Remove the compression sleeves from the package and unfold them, laying them with the cotton lining facing up.

How you do it

- Place the patient's leg on the cotton sleeve lining, positioning the back of the knee over the popliteal opening and the back of the ankle over the ankle marking.

Skin and neurovascular assessment

Skin and neurovascular assessment should include:

- pain assessment
- color of skin
- palpable or Doppler pulses
- paresthesia ("pins and needles" sensation)
- paralysis
- skin abnormalities under the sleeve
- pain associated with movement or touch
- edema of the extremity
- swelling, redness, or pain *which could indicate a blood clot is present.*

Report any assessment abnormalities to the physician or licensed independent practitioner.

- Starting at the side opposite the clear plastic tubing, wrap the sleeve snugly around the patient's leg, beginning with the ankle and calf and then the thigh, and secure it with Velcro fasteners.
- Using the same procedure, apply the second sleeve.

Connect with a click

- Connect each sleeve to the tubing leading to the controller, making sure the tubing isn't kinked. Line up the arrows on the connectors and push the ends together firmly. Listen for a click, signaling a firm connection.
- Plug the compression controller into the wall outlet and turn on the power. The controller automatically sets the compression sleeve pressure at 45 mm Hg, which is the midpoint of the normal range (35 to 55 mm Hg). Stay with the patient to assess sleeve inflation and deflation through one full cycle.
- Check the AUDIBLE ALARM key. The green light should be lit, indicating that the alarm is working.
- The sleeve should be removed during bathing and when the patient ambulates. Instruct the patient to call for assistance to ambulate *to prevent falls.*
- If the patient complains of sweating or itching under the sleeves, initiate the cooling system on the SCD pump. To relieve itching, apply cornstarch.
- Caution patients to never remove the sleeves without consulting a nurse because *it increases their risk of VTE.*
- When discontinuing the therapy, dispose of the sleeves because they are one-time use but store the tubing and compression controller according to your facility's protocol.

Practice pointers

- Be sure that there are no contraindications to therapy. If there are, discuss the situation with the doctor. (See *Contraindications to sequential compression therapy.*)

Two-finger test

- The sleeve should fit snugly, but you should still be able to insert two fingers between the sleeve and the patient's leg at the knee opening. Loosen or tighten the sleeve by readjusting the Velcro fastener.
- If you're applying only one sleeve—for example, if the patient has a cast—leave the unused sleeve folded in the plastic bag. Cut a small hole in the bag's sealed bottom edge and pull the sleeve connector (the part that holds the connecting tubing) through the hole. Then you can join both sleeves to the compression controller.

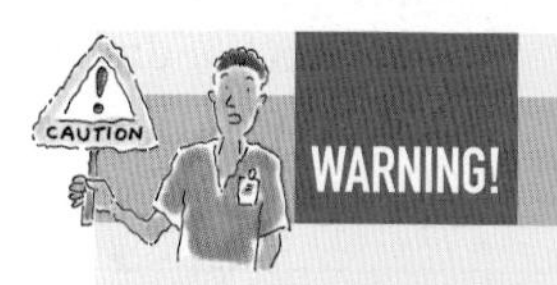

Contraindications to sequential compression therapy

Consult with the doctor before use if the patient has:

- acute DVT
- DVT diagnosed within the past 6 months
- severe arteriosclerosis or other ischemic vascular disease
- massive edema of the legs
- dermatitis
- vein ligation
- gangrene
- skin grafting.

A patient with a pronounced leg deformity also would be unlikely to benefit from compression sleeves.

- The compression sleeves should function continuously until the patient is fully ambulatory. Be sure to check the sleeves at least once each shift *to ensure proper fit and inflation.* (See *Documenting sequential compression therapy.*)

Write it down

Documenting sequential compression therapy

In your notes, record:
- procedure
- date and time it was initiated and discontinued
- patient education and understanding of the procedure
- patient's response and compliance
- status of the alarm and cooling settings.

Elastic bandage application

Elastic bandages exert gentle, even pressure on a body part. By supporting blood vessels, these rolled bandages promote venous return and prevent pooling of blood that can lead to thrombophlebitis and pulmonary embolism.

Elastic bandages are used postoperatively, on bedridden patients, to minimize joint swelling after trauma, to secure a splint, or to immobilize a fracture. They also can provide hemostatic pressure and anchor dressings after surgical procedures such as vein stripping.

What you need

Elastic bandage of appropriate width * tape or pins * gauze pads or absorbent cotton. Bandages usually come in 2″ to 6″ widths and 4′ and 6′ (1.2 and 1.8 m) lengths. The 3″ width is adaptable to most applications. An elastic bandage with self-closures is also available.

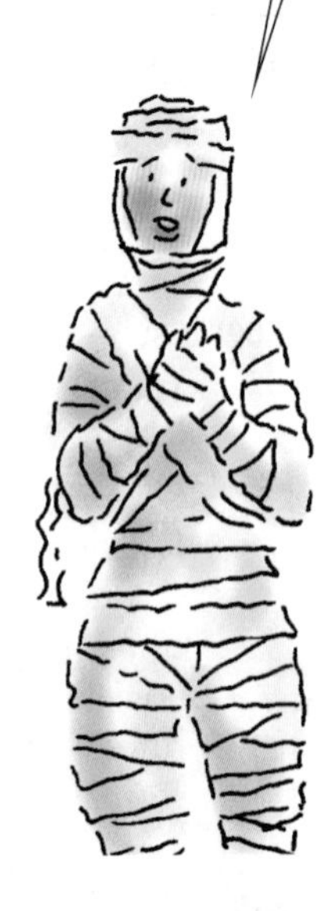
I think this bandage is too long!

Getting ready

Select a bandage that wraps the affected body part completely but isn't excessively long. In most cases, use a narrower bandage for wrapping the foot, lower leg, hand, or arm and a wider bandage for the thigh or trunk. The bandage should be clean and rolled before application.

How you do it

- Check the doctor's order and identify the patient using two patient identifiers. Examine the area to be wrapped for lesions or skin breakdown. If these conditions are present, consult the doctor before applying the elastic bandage.
- Explain the procedure to the patient, provide privacy, and perform hand hygiene. Explain the procedure to the patient and family if the bandage is to be used at home. Position him comfortably, with the body part to be bandaged in normal

functioning position *to promote circulation and prevent deformity and discomfort*. If the extremity has been dependent, elevate it for 15 to 30 minutes before application *to facilitate venous return*.

- Place gauze or absorbent cotton as needed between skin surfaces, such as toes or fingers, or under breasts and arms *to prevent skin irritation*.
- Hold the bandage close to the part being bandaged with the roll facing upward in one hand and the free end of the bandage in the other hand.

That special twist

- Unroll the bandage as you wrap the body part in a spiral or spiral-reverse method and overlap each layer of bandage by one-half to two-thirds the width of the strip. (For an explanation of these and other techniques, see *Bandaging techniques*, page 154.)
- Wrap firmly, applying even pressure.
- When wrapping an extremity, anchor the bandage initially by circling the body part twice. *To prevent the bandage from slipping out of place on the foot or to go around a joint*, wrap it in a figure eight around the foot and ankle before continuing. Remember to leave the toes (or fingers) exposed *to detect impaired circulation*.

Better than metal

- When you're finished wrapping, secure the end of the bandage with tape, pins, or self-closures. Avoid using metal clips *because they typically come loose and can injure the patient*.
- Check distal circulation after the bandage is on and be sure to elevate a wrapped extremity for 15 to 30 minutes *to facilitate venous return*. (See *Complications of elastic bandages*.)
- Remove the bandage every 8 hours, or as ordered, to inspect the skin for irritation or breakdown. It also should be changed at least once daily and the area bathed and dried thoroughly.

Practice pointers

- If the bandage becomes loose and wrinkled, unwrap it and roll it up as you unwrap *for reuse*. Observe the area and provide skin care before rewrapping the bandage.
- Wrap an elastic bandage from the distal area to the proximal area *to promote venous return*. Avoid leaving gaps in bandage layers or exposed skin surfaces *because this may result in uneven pressure on the body part*. (See *Documenting elastic bandage application*, page 155.)

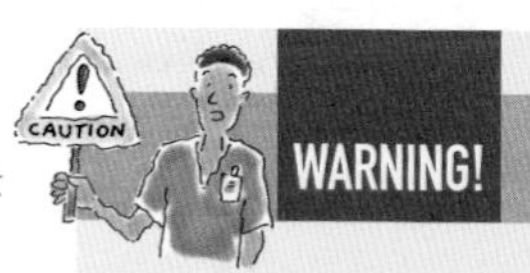

Complications of elastic bandages

Check distal circulation once or twice every 8 hours and assess the skin underneath.

Too tight

If the elastic bandage is too constricting, arterial obstruction can occur. This can cause a decreased or an absent distal pulse, blanching or bluish discoloration of the skin, dusky nail beds, numbness and tingling or pain and cramping, and cold skin. Edema is caused by obstruction of venous return. Less serious complications include allergic reaction and skin irritation.

Bandaging techniques

Here are several techniques for applying elastic bandages.

Circular
Each turn encircles the previous one, covering it completely. Use this technique to anchor a bandage.

Spiral
Each turn partially overlaps the previous one. Use this technique to wrap a long, straight body part or one of increasing circumference.

Spiral-reverse
Anchor the bandage and then reverse direction halfway through each spiral turn. Use this technique to accommodate the increasing circumference of a body part.

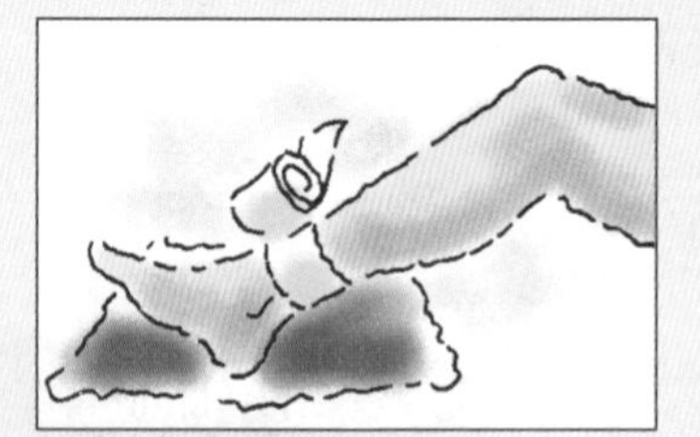

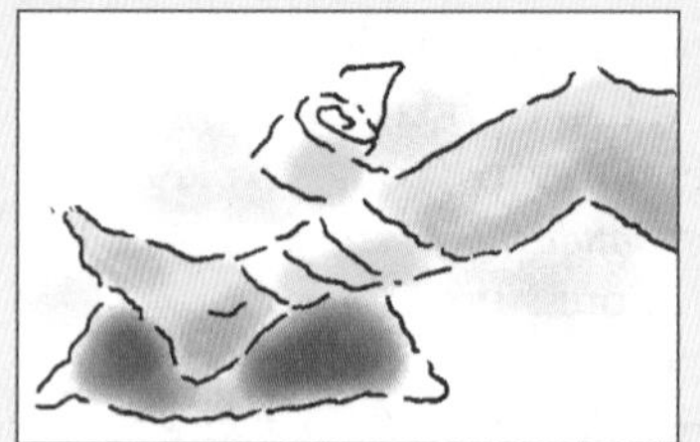

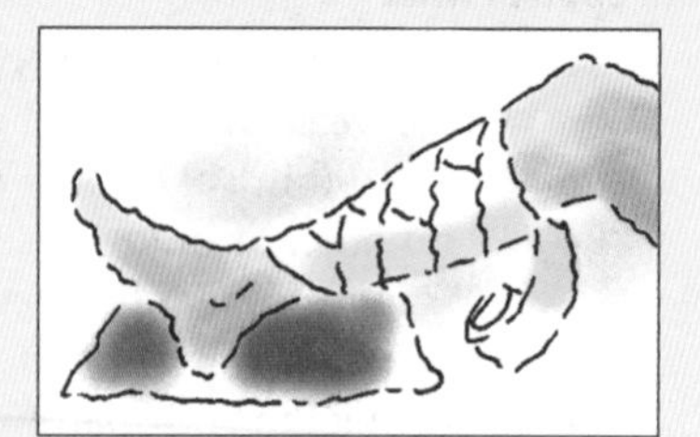

Figure eight
Anchor below the joint, and then use alternating ascending and descending turns to form a figure eight. Use this technique around joints.

Recurrent
This technique includes a combination of recurrent and circular turns. Hold the bandage as you make each recurrent turn and then use the circular turns as a final anchor. Use this technique for a stump, a hand, or the scalp.

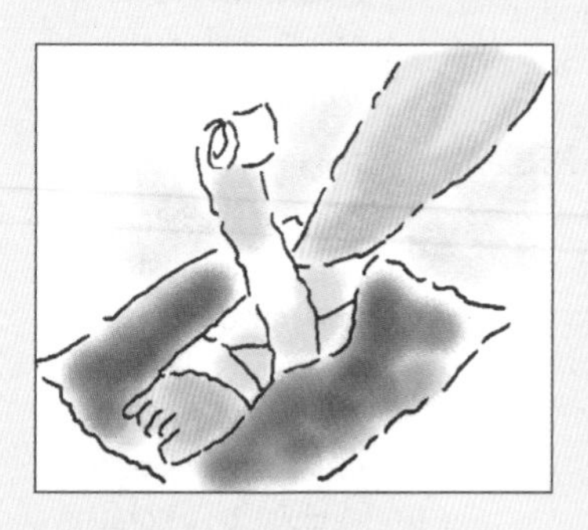

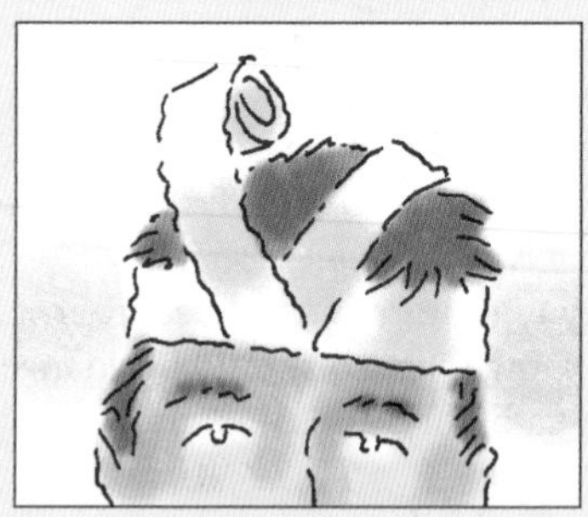

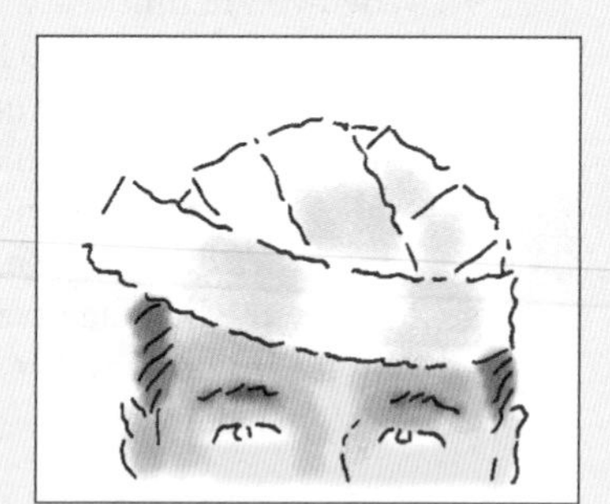

Pressure dressing application

Pressure dressing is a temporary treatment to control excessive, unexpected bleeding. It is essential to stop the flow of blood and promote clotting at the site until other measures can be taken to control the bleeding. In this procedure, a bulky dressing is held in place with a glove-protected hand and then bound into place with a pressure bandage or held under pressure by an inflated air splint or blood pressure cuff.

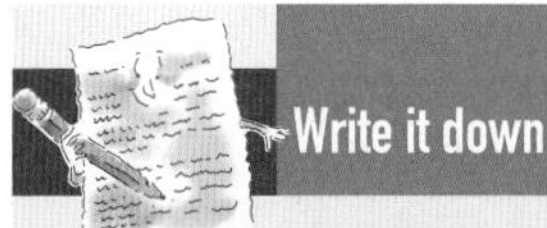

Write it down

Documenting elastic bandage application

In your notes, record:

- date and time of bandage application and removal
- application site and bandage size
- skin condition before application
- skin care provided after removal
- complications
- patient's tolerance of the treatment
- patient teaching provided.

Check, please!

A pressure dressing requires frequent checks for wound drainage to determine its effectiveness in controlling bleeding.

What you need

Two or more sterile gauze pads ✳ ABD pads ✳ hemostatic dressings ✳ roller gauze ✳ adhesive tape, hypoallergenic if necessary ✳ clean gloves ✳ metric ruler ✳ gown, goggles, and mask or face shield ✳ equipment for vital signs.

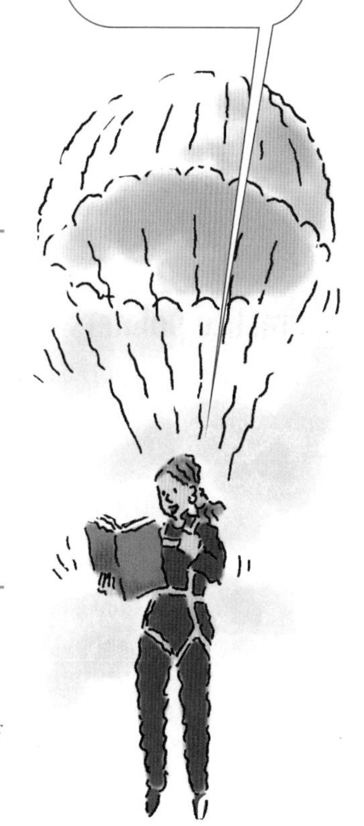
When applying the dressing, elevate the injured area to reduce bleeding.

Getting ready

Obtain the pressure dressing quickly to avoid excessive blood loss or have another staff member obtain the equipment while you apply manual pressure and monitor the patient. Use a clean cloth for the dressing if sterile gauze pads aren't available. Given the urgent nature of an acute bleeding episode, aseptic technique is secondary to stopping the bleeding. The wound can be cleaned and the dressing changed after the emergency situation is controlled.

How you do it

- Quickly explain the procedure to the patient *to help decrease his anxiety.*
- Identify the site and source of the external bleeding. (See *Source of bleeding,* page 156.) Look underneath large abdominal dressings

if present. Apply immediate manual pressure to the bleeding site. See assistance.

- The second nurse can elevate the injured body part *to help reduce bleeding.*
- First nurse will continue to apply pressure. The second nurse can prepare the roller gauze and cut strips of adhesive for the bandage and place in close proximity.

That's a wrap

- In a coordinated fashion, the second nurse will quickly cover the wound with the new gauze and the first nurse lifts the dressing off and continues to apply pressure after the new dressing is applied.
- Place adhesive strips 3″ to 4″ beyond the width of the dressing with continued pressure at the center of the dressing. Secure tape on the distal end over the center of the dressing to the proximal end.
- Remove the fingers quickly and apply another strip of tape firmly over the center of the dressing. Continue overlapping strips of tape to reinforce the dressing. Keep applying pressures.
- For an extremity or a trunk wound, hold the dressing firmly over the wound and wrap the roller gauze tightly across it by wrapping two circles around the outer sides of the wound and then the center *to provide pressure on the wound.* Continue with figure-eight turns. Secure the bandage with adhesive tape.
- Check pulse, temperature, and skin condition distal to the wound site *because excessive pressure can obstruct normal circulation.*
- Check the dressing frequently *to monitor wound drainage.*
- Obtain additional medical care as soon as possible.

Practice pointers

- To apply a dressing to the neck, shoulder, or another location that can't be tightly wrapped, apply tape directly over the dressing *to provide the necessary pressure at the wound site.*
- If the dressing becomes saturated, don't remove it *because this will interfere with the pressure.* Instead, reinforce the original dressing by applying an additional dressing over the saturated one and continue to monitor and record drainage. (See *Documenting pressure dressing application.*)
- Mark drainage on wound dressing.
- **Report immediately to the physician or licensed independent practitioner (LIP)** the present status of the bleeding control, when it was discovered, actions taken, estimated blood loss, vital signs, mental status changes, and the need for the physician or LIP to see the patient as soon as possible.

Source of bleeding

Arterial bleeding is bright red and flows in waves with the heart rate. Venous bleeding is dark red and flows slowly. Capillary bleeding oozes dark red blood; self-sealing controls this bleeding.

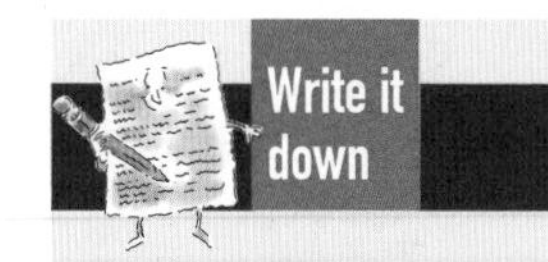

Documenting pressure dressing application

When the bleeding is controlled, record:

- date and time of dressing application
- whether reinforcement was necessary
- presence or absence of distal pulses
- integrity of distal skin
- amount of wound drainage
- complications.

Surgical wound management

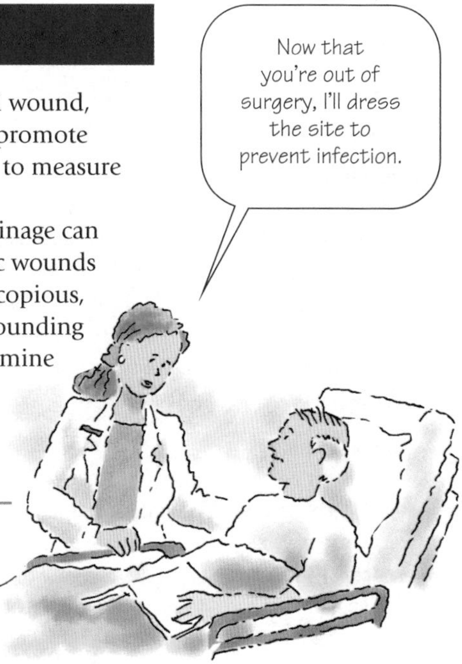

Two primary methods for managing a draining surgical wound, dressing and pouching can help prevent infection and promote patient comfort and healing. Pouching also allows you to measure wound drainage.

Lightly seeping wounds with drains or minimal drainage can be managed with packing and gauze dressings. Chronic wounds may require an occlusive dressing, whereas those with copious, excoriating drainage need pouching to protect the surrounding skin. You may use the color of the wound to help determine which type of dressing to apply. (See *Tailoring wound care to wound color,* page 158.) When handling wound drainage, always follow standard precautions.

Now that you're out of surgery, I'll dress the site to prevent infection.

What you need

Waterproof trash bag ✻ clean gloves ✻ sterile gloves ✻ gown and face shield or goggles and mask, if indicated ✻ sterile 4″ × 4″ gauze pads ✻ large absorbent dressings, if indicated ✻ sterile cotton-tipped applicators ✻ sterile dressing set ✻ povidone-iodine swabs ✻ topical medication, if ordered ✻ adhesive or other tape ✻ soap and water ✻ optional: forceps, skin protectant, nonadherent pads, collodion spray or acetone-free adhesive remover, sterile normal saline solution, graduated container, and Montgomery straps or a T-binder.

For a wound with a drain

Sterile scissors ✻ sterile 4″ × 4″ gauze pads without cotton lining ✻ sump drain ✻ sterile precut tracheostomy pads or drain dressings ✻ adhesive tape (paper or silk tape if the patient is hypersensitive) ✻ surgical mask.

For pouching a wound

Collection pouch with drainage port ✻ sterile gloves ✻ skin protectant ✻ sterile gauze pads.

Getting ready

Ask the patient about allergies to tapes, dressings, and solutions you'll be using such as povidone-iodine. Assemble all equipment in the patient's room; check the expiration date on each sterile package and inspect for tears.

Place a waterproof bag near the patient's bed, but avoid reaching across the sterile field or the wound when disposing of soiled articles.

Tailoring wound care to wound color

With any wound, promote healing by keeping it moist, clean, and free from debris. For open wounds, use wound color to guide the specific management approach and to assess how well the wound is healing.

Red wounds

Red, the color of healthy granulation tissue, indicates normal healing. Cover a red wound, keep it moist and clean, and protect it from trauma. Use a transparent dressing (such as Tegaderm or Opsite), a hydrocolloidal dressing (such as DuoDerm), or gauze dressing moistened with sterile normal saline solution or impregnated with petroleum jelly or an antibiotic.

Yellow wounds

Yellow is the color of exudate produced by microorganisms in an open wound. Exudate usually appears whitish yellow, creamy yellow, yellowish green, or beige. Dry exudate appears darker.

If your patient has a yellow wound, clean it and remove exudate using high-pressure irrigation; then cover it with a moist dressing. Use absorptive products (for example, Debrisan beads and paste) or a moist gauze dressing with or without an antibiotic ointment as per order. You may also use hydrotherapy with whirlpool or high-pressure irrigation.

Black wounds

Black, the least healthy color, signals necrosis. Notify physician immediately. Debridement is usually necessary. As ordered, use enzyme products (such as Elase or Travase), surgical debridement, hydrotherapy with a whirlpool or high-pressure irrigation, or a moist gauze dressing.

Multicolored wounds

You may note two or even all three colors in a wound. In this case, classify the wound according to the least healthy color present. For example, if your patient's wound is red and yellow, classify it as a yellow wound.

Form a cuff by turning down the top of the trash bag *to provide a wide opening and to prevent contamination of instruments or gloves by touching the bag's edge.*

How you do it

- Check the doctor's order for specific wound care and medication instructions. Note the location of surgical drains *to avoid dislodging them during the procedure.*
- Identify the patient using two patient identifiers.
- Explain the procedure to the patient *to allay his fears and ensure his cooperation.*
- Provide teaching to the patient as well as responsible family members if the dressing will be changed at home. (See *Caring for surgical wounds.*)

Removing the old dressing

- Assess the patient's condition, provide privacy, and position him as necessary, exposing only the wound site.
- Perform hand hygiene and put on a gown, face shield (if necessary), and gloves.

- Loosen the soiled dressing by holding the patient's skin and pulling the tape or dressing toward the wound *to prevent stress on the incision.*
- Slowly remove the soiled dressing. If the gauze adheres to the wound, loosen the gauze by moistening it with sterile normal saline solution.
- Observe the dressing for the amount, type, color, and odor of drainage, then discard the dressing and gloves in the waterproof trash bag.

Caring for the wound

- Identify the patient with two identifiers.
- Perform hand hygiene.
- Establish a sterile field with all the equipment and supplies you'll need for suture line care and the dressing change. Squeeze ointment (if ordered) onto the sterile field. If you're using an antiseptic from an unsterile bottle, pour the antiseptic cleaning agent into a sterile container *so you won't contaminate your gloves.* Then don sterile gloves. Also don moistureproof gown, mask, and goggles if at risk for spray from the wound.
- Saturate the sterile gauze pads with the prescribed cleaning agent.
- If ordered, obtain a wound culture (see chapter 2, Specimen collection), then proceed to clean the wound.
- Pick up the moistened gauze pad or swab and squeeze out the excess solution.

Start from the top

- Working from the top of the incision, wipe once to the bottom and then discard the gauze pad. With a second moistened pad, wipe from top to bottom next to the incision and then continue to work outward from the incision in lines running parallel to it.
- Use sterile, cotton-tipped applicators for efficient cleaning of tight-fitting wire sutures, deep and narrow wounds, and wounds with pockets. Remember to wipe only once with each applicator.
- If the patient has a surgical drain, clean the drain's surface last by wiping in half or full circles from the drain site outward.
- Clean to at least 1" (2.5 cm) beyond the end of the new dressing. If you aren't applying a new dressing, clean to at least 2" (5 cm) beyond the incision.

Infection detection

- Check to make sure that the edges of the incision are lined up properly, and check for signs of infection (heat, redness, swelling, induration, and odor) or separation. If you observe such signs or if the patient reports pain at the wound site, notify the doctor.
- Irrigate the wound, as ordered. (See "Wound irrigation," page 173.)

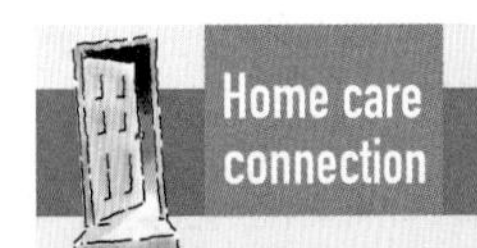

Caring for surgical wounds

If your patient needs wound care after discharge, provide appropriate teaching to the patient and support person who will be assisting the patient. If he's caring for the wound himself, stress the importance of using aseptic technique and teach him how to examine the wound for signs of infection and other complications.

Put on a show

Also show him and the support person how to change dressings. Give him written instructions with pictures for all procedures to be performed at home *to meet the needs of visual learners and those with low literacy.* Have the patient and support person practice the dressing change during their stay with guidance from the nurse. Consult with case management to determine if other services such as home health care are needed.

- Wash the skin surrounding the wound with soap and water and pat dry using a sterile 4″ × 4″ gauze pad. Avoid oil-based soap *because it may interfere with pouch adherence*. Apply any prescribed topical medication and skin protectant, if needed.
- If ordered, pack the wound with gauze pads or strips folded to fit using sterile forceps. Pack the wound, but not tightly, using the wet-to-damp method and make sure to wring out the pad so that it's slightly moist.

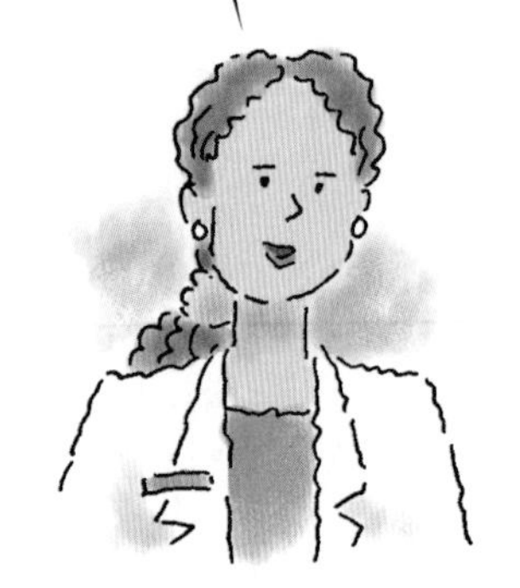
Oil alert! Using an oil-based soap may prevent the pouch from adhering.

Applying a fresh gauze dressing

- Gently place sterile 4″ × 4″ gauze pads at the center of the wound and move progressively outward to the edges of the wound site. Extend the gauze at least 1″ (2.5 cm) beyond the incision in each direction and cover the wound evenly with enough sterile dressings (usually two or three layers) to absorb all drainage until the next dressing change. Place additional dressings at the lower part of the wound to absorb drainage as it collects there. Use large absorbent dressings to form outer layers, if needed, *to provide greater absorbency*.
- Secure the dressing's edges to the patient's skin with strips of tape or with a T-binder or Montgomery straps *to prevent skin excoriation*, which may occur with repeated dressing changes. (See *How to make Montgomery straps*.)
- Label the dressing with the date and time of the dressing change with indelible ink or label the dressing according to your facility's policy.
- Properly dispose of the solutions and trash bag and clean or discard soiled equipment and supplies according to your facility's policy.

Dressing a wound with a drain

- Prepare a drain dressing by using sterile scissors to cut a slit in a sterile 4″ × 4″ gauze pad or use prepackaged dressings. Don't use a cotton-lined gauze pad *because cutting the gauze opens the lining and releases cotton fibers into the wound*.
- Gently press one pad close to the skin around the drain so that the tubing fits into the slit. Press the second pad around the drain from the opposite direction so that the two pads encircle the tubing.
- Layer as many uncut sterile 4″ × 4″ gauze pads or large absorbent dressings around the tubing as needed *to absorb expected drainage*. Tape the dressing in place or use a T-binder or Montgomery straps.

How to make Montgomery straps

An abdominal dressing requiring frequent changes can be secured with Montgomery straps to promote the patient's comfort. If ready-made straps aren't available, follow these steps to make your own:

- Cut four to six strips of 2″ or 3″ wide hypoallergenic tape of sufficient length to allow the tape to extend about 6″ (15 cm) beyond the wound on each side.
- Fold one of each strip 2″ to 3″ back on itself (sticky sides together) to form a nonadhesive tab. Then cut a small hole in the folded tab's center, close to its top edge. Make as many pairs of straps as you'll need to snugly secure the dressing.
- Clean the patient's skin to prevent irritation. After the skin dries, apply a skin protectant. Then apply the sticky side of each tape to a skin barrier sheet composed of opaque hydrocolloidal or nonhydrocolloidal materials and apply the sheet directly to the skin near the dressing. Next, thread a separate piece of twill tape (about 12″ [30.5 cm]) through each pair of holes in the straps and fasten each tie as you would a shoelace. Don't secure the ties too tightly.
- Repeat this procedure according to the number of Montgomery straps needed.
- Replace Montgomery straps whenever they become soiled (every 2 to 3 days). If skin maceration occurs, place new tapes about 1″ (2.5 cm) away from the irritation.

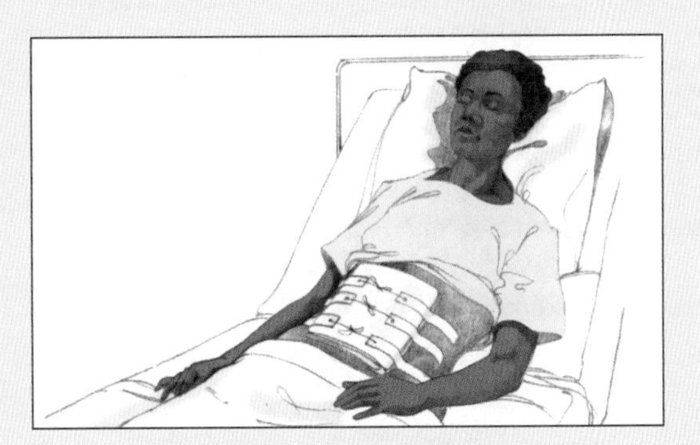

Pouching a wound

- If your patient's wound is draining heavily or if drainage may damage surrounding skin, you'll need to apply a pouch, as per doctor's orders, or wound care protocol. First, measure the wound and then cut an opening 3/8″ (0.9 cm) larger than the wound in the facing of the collection pouch.
- Apply a skin protectant as needed. Some protectants are incorporated within the collection pouch and also provide adhesion.
- Make sure that the drainage port at the bottom of the pouch is closed firmly *to prevent leaks*. Then gently press the contoured pouch opening around the wound, starting at its lower edge, *to catch any drainage*. The pouch drain may be directed toward the side if the patient is on bed rest and directed toward the patient's leg if he's ambulatory *to allow ease of emptying*.

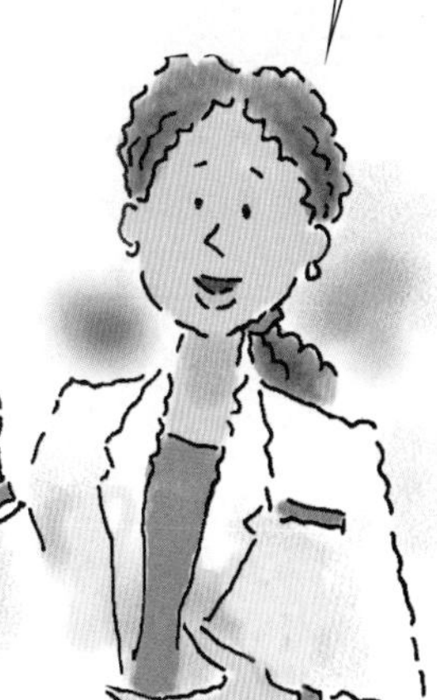
If the wound is draining heavily, you need to apply a pouch.

Gloves and goggles

- To empty the pouch, put on gloves and a face shield or mask and goggles to avoid any splashing. Then insert the pouch's bottom half into a graduated biohazard container and open the drainage port. Note the color, consistency, odor, and amount of fluid. If ordered, obtain a culture specimen and send it to the laboratory immediately. (See chapter 2, Specimen collection, for sputum culture.) Remember to follow standard precautions when handling infectious drainage.

- Wipe the bottom of the pouch and the drainage port with a gauze pad *to remove drainage* and reseal the port. Change the pouch only if it leaks or fails to adhere.
- Dispose of all materials, dressings, and personal protective equipment (PPE) in the appropriate container per facility policy.

Practice pointers

- If the patient has two wounds in the same area, cover each wound separately with layers of sterile 4″ × 4″ gauze pads. Then cover each site with a large absorbent dressing secured to the patient's skin with tape. Don't use a single large absorbent dressing to cover both sites *because drainage quickly saturates a pad, promoting cross-contamination.*
- When packing a wound, don't pack it too tightly *because this compresses adjacent capillaries and may prevent the wound edges from contracting.* Avoid overlapping damp packing onto surrounding skin *because it macerates the intact tissue.*

Be sensitive to sensitivity

- If your patient is sensitive to adhesive tape, use paper or silk tape *because it's less likely to cause a skin reaction and peels off more easily than adhesive tape.*
- If a sump drain isn't adequately collecting wound drainage, reinforce it with an ostomy pouch or another collection bag and connect the tubing to the suction pump. *This method frees the drainage port at the bottom of the pouch so you don't have to remove the tubing to empty the pouch.*

Do it yourself

- Because many doctors prefer to change the first postoperative dressing themselves to check the incision, don't change the first dressing unless you have specific instructions to do so. If you have no such order and drainage comes through the dressings, reinforce the dressing with fresh sterile gauze. Request an order to change the dressing or ask the doctor to change it as soon as possible. A reinforced dressing shouldn't remain in place longer than 24 hours *because it's an excellent medium for bacterial growth.*
- For the recent postoperative patient or a patient with complications, check the dressing every 15 to 30 minutes or as ordered. For the patient with a properly healing wound, check the dressing at least once every 8 hours or per facility policy/protocol. (See *Documenting surgical wound management.*)

Write it down

Documenting surgical wound management

In your notes, record:
- date, time, and type of wound management procedure
- pain assessment
- amount of soiled dressing and packing removed
- wound appearance (size, condition of margins, presence of necrotic tissue) and odor
- type, color, consistency, and amount of drainage
- presence and location of drains
- additional procedures such as irrigation
- topical medication application
- type and amount of new dressing or pouch applied
- patient's tolerance of the procedure.

Document special or detailed wound care instructions and pain management steps on the plan of care. Record drainage color and amount on the intake and output sheet.

Suture removal

The goal of suture removal is to remove skin sutures from a healed wound without damaging newly formed tissue. Usually, for a sufficiently healed wound, sutures are removed 7 to 10 days after insertion. Suture and staple removal are minimally invasive procedures that typically cause little or no pain unless infection is present or the sutures or staples are left in place too long and have become embedded in the skin. Techniques for removal depend on the method of suturing, but all require sterile procedure to prevent contamination. Although sutures usually are removed by a doctor, in many facilities, a nurse may remove them with a doctor's order.

What you need

Waterproof trash bag ✳ adjustable light ✳ clean gloves, if the wound is dressed ✳ sterile gloves ✳ sterile forceps or sterile hemostat ✳ normal saline solution ✳ sterile gauze pads ✳ antiseptic cleaning agent ✳ sterile curve-tipped suture scissors ✳ povidone-iodine pads ✳ optional: adhesive butterfly strips or Steri-Strips and compound benzoin tincture or other skin protectant.

Prepackaged, sterile suture removal trays are available.

Getting ready

Assemble all equipment in the patient's room. Check the expiration date on each sterile package and inspect for tears. Open the waterproof trash bag and place it near the patient's bed, but avoid reaching across the sterile field or the suture line when disposing of soiled articles. Form a cuff by turning down the top of the trash bag.

How you do it

- If your facility allows you to remove sutures, check the doctor's order *to confirm the details for this procedure.*
- Verify the order and identify the patient using two patient identifiers.
- Check for patient allergies, especially to adhesive tape and povidone-iodine or other topical solutions or medications.
- Explain the procedure to the patient, provide privacy, and position him so he's comfortable without placing undue tension on the suture line.
- Perform hand hygiene, don gloves, and carefully remove the dressing. Discard the dressing and gloves in the waterproof trash bag.

All healed up?

- Observe the patient's wound for possible gaping, drainage, inflammation, signs of infection, and embedded sutures. Notify the doctor if the wound has failed to heal properly.
- Establish a sterile work area with all the equipment and supplies you'll need for suture removal and wound care. Put on sterile gloves and open the sterile suture removal tray if you're using one.
- Clean the suture line. Soften them further, if needed, with normal saline solution.
- Then proceed according to the type of suture you're removing. (See *Methods for removing sutures.*) *Because the visible part of a suture is exposed to skin bacteria and considered contaminated,* be sure to cut sutures at the skin surface on one side of the visible part of the suture. Remove the suture by lifting and pulling the visible end off the skin *to avoid drawing this contaminated portion back through subcutaneous tissue.*

Consider the visible part of a suture contaminated. After all, I might be there.

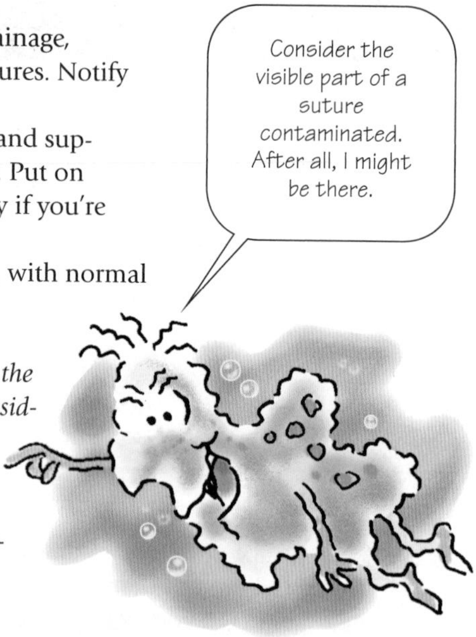

Skip over for support

- If ordered, remove every other suture *to maintain some support for the incision.* Then go back and remove the remaining sutures.

Methods for removing sutures

Removal techniques depend in large part on the type of sutures to be removed. The illustrations here show removal steps for four common suture types. Keep in mind that for all suture types, it's important to grasp and cut sutures in the correct place to avoid pulling the exposed (thus contaminated) suture material through subcutaneous tissue.

Plain interrupted sutures

Using sterile forceps, grasp the knot of the first suture and raise it off the skin. This will expose a small portion of the suture that was below skin level. Place the rounded tip of sterile curved-tip suture scissors against the skin and cut through the exposed portion of the suture. Then, still holding the knot with the forceps, pull the cut suture up and out of the skin in a smooth continuous motion to avoid causing the patient pain. Discard the suture. Repeat the process for every other suture, initially; if the wound doesn't gape, you can then remove the remaining sutures as ordered.

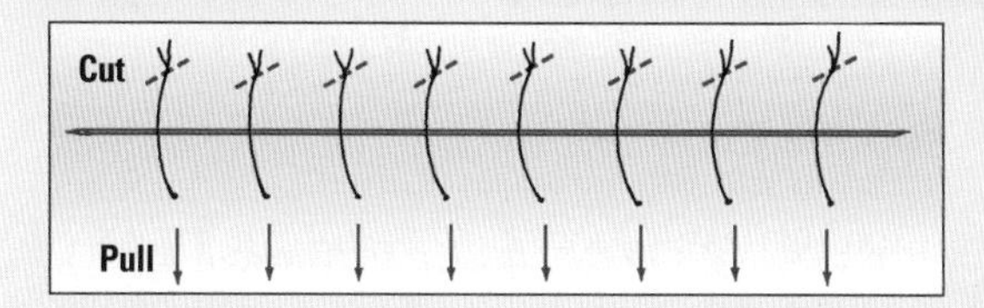

Plain continuous sutures

Cut the first suture on the side opposite the knot. Next, cut the same side of the next suture in line. Then lift the first suture out in the direction of the knot. Proceed along the suture line, grasping each suture where you grasped the knot on the first one.

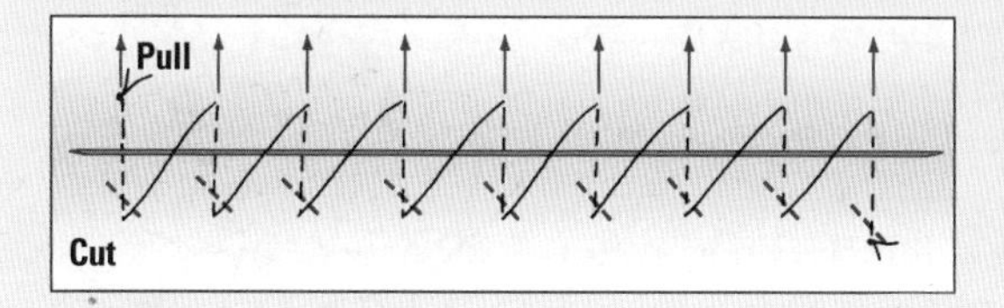

Mattress interrupted sutures

If possible, remove the small, visible portion of the suture opposite the knot by cutting it at each visible end and lifting the small piece away from the skin to prevent pulling it through and contaminating subcutaneous tissue. Then remove the rest of the suture by pulling it out in the direction of the knot. If the visible portion is too small to cut twice, cut it once and pull the entire suture out in the opposite direction. Repeat these steps for the remaining sutures and monitor the incision carefully for infection.

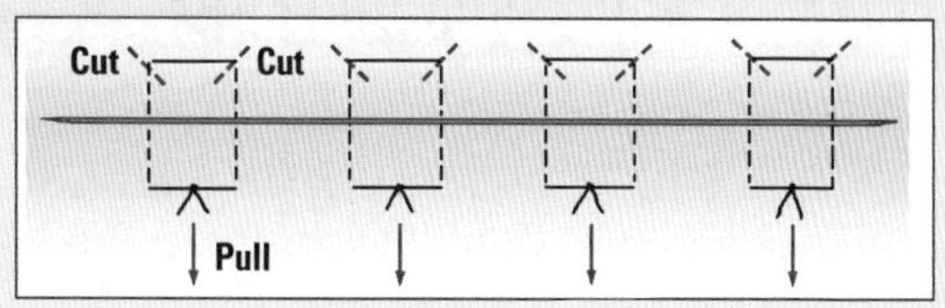

Mattress continuous sutures

Follow the procedure for removing mattress interrupted sutures, first removing the small visible portion of the suture, if possible, to prevent pulling it through and contaminating subcutaneous tissue. Then extract the rest of the suture in the direction of the knot.

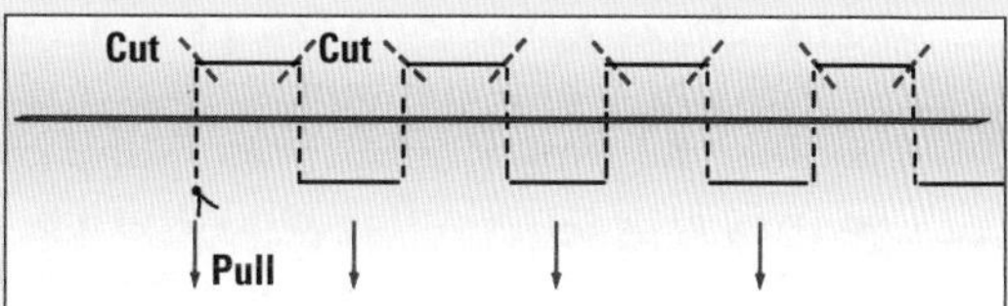

- After removing sutures, wipe the incision gently with gauze pads soaked in an antiseptic cleaning agent or with a povidone-iodine pad. Apply light sterile gauze dressing, if needed, then discard your gloves and soiled equipment and clean the equipment according to your facility's policy.

Practice pointers

- If the patient has interrupted sutures or an incompletely healed suture line, remove only those sutures specified by the doctor. He may want to leave some sutures in place for an additional day or two *to support the suture line.*
- If the patient has both retention and regular sutures in place, check the doctor's order for the sequence in which they are to be removed. *Because retention sutures link underlying fat and muscle tissue and give added support to the obese or slow-healing patient,* they usually remain in place for 14 to 21 days.
- If the wound dehisces during suture removal, apply butterfly adhesive strips or Steri-Strips to support and approximate the edges and call the doctor immediately to repair the wound. Leave the strips in place for 3 to 5 days, as ordered. (See *Documenting suture removal.*)

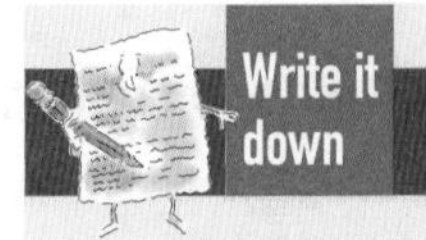

Write it down

Documenting suture removal

In your notes, record:
- date and time of suture removal
- type and number of sutures
- appearance of the suture line
- signs of wound complications
- dressings or butterfly strips applied
- patient's tolerance of the procedure.

Skin staple and clip removal

Skin staples or clips may be used instead of standard sutures to close lacerations or surgical wounds. When properly placed, staples and clips distribute tension evenly along the suture line with minimal tissue trauma and compression, facilitating healing and minimizing scarring. Usually, doctors remove skin staples and clips, but some facilities permit qualified nurses to perform this procedure.

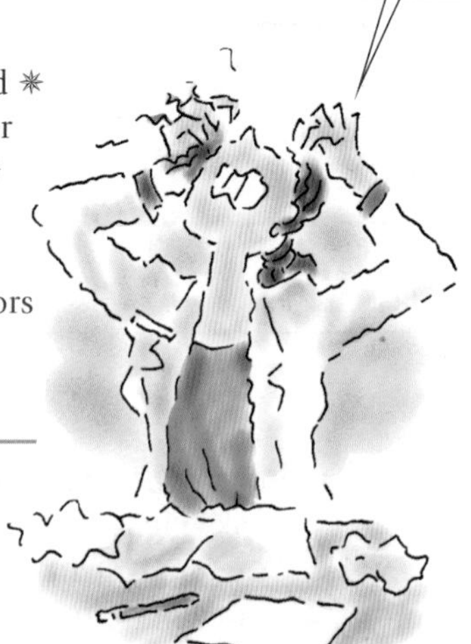
Staples and clips distribute tension evenly along the tissue line. If only I had something to distribute my tension!

What you need

Waterproof trash bag ✱ adjustable light ✱ clean gloves, if needed ✱ sterile gloves ✱ sterile gauze pads ✱ sterile staple or clip extractor ✱ povidone-iodine solution or other antiseptic cleaning agent ✱ sterile cotton-tipped applicators ✱ optional: butterfly adhesive strips or Steri-Strips, compound benzoin tincture or other skin protectant. Prepackaged, sterile, disposable staple or clip extractors are available.

Getting ready

Assemble all equipment in the patient's room. Check the expiration date on each sterile package and inspect for tears.

Open the waterproof trash bag and place it near the patient's bed, but avoid reaching across the sterile field or the wound. Form a cuff by turning down the top of the bag.

How you do it

- If your facility allows you to remove skin staples and clips, check the doctor's order *to confirm the exact timing and details for this procedure.*
- Identify the patient using two patient identifiers.
- Check for patient allergies, explain the procedure to the patient, provide privacy, and place him in a comfortable position that doesn't place undue tension on the incision. Adjust the light to shine directly on the incision.
- Perform hand hygiene, put on clean gloves, and carefully remove the dressing. Discard the dressing and the gloves in the waterproof trash bag.
- Assess the patient's incision and notify the doctor of gaping, drainage, inflammation, and other signs of infection.
- Establish a sterile work area with all the equipment and supplies you'll need for removing staples or clips and for cleaning and dressing the incision. Open the package containing the sterile staple or clip extractor, maintaining asepsis. Put on sterile gloves.
- Wipe the incision gently with sterile gauze pads soaked in an antiseptic cleaning agent or with sterile cotton-tipped applicators *to remove surface encrustations.*

#1: Extract. #2: Repeat step 1.

- Pick up the sterile staple or clip extractor. Then, starting at one end of the incision, remove the staple or clip. (See *Removing a staple,* page 168.) Hold the extractor over the trash bag and release the handle to discard the staple or clip. Repeat the procedure for each staple or clip until all are removed.
- Apply sterile gauze dressing, if needed, *to prevent infection and irritation from clothing.* Then discard your gloves and properly dispose of soiled equipment and supplies according to your facility's policy.

Practice pointers

- Carefully check the doctor's order for the time and extent of staple or clip removal. The doctor may want you to remove only alternate staples or clips initially and to leave the others in place for an additional day or two *to support the incision.*

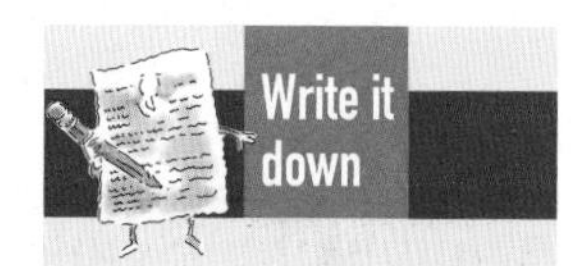

Documenting skin staple and clip removal

In your notes, record:
- date and time of staple or clip removal
- number of staples or clips removed
- appearance of the incision
- dressings or butterfly strips applied
- signs of wound complications
- patient's tolerance of the procedure.

Removing a staple

Follow these steps to remove a staple from a wound using an extractor.

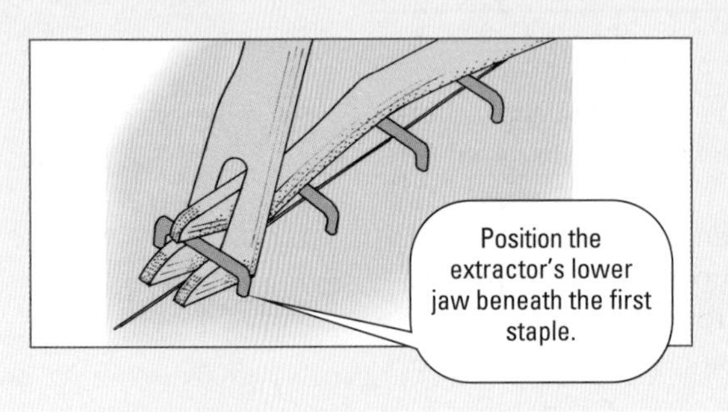

Position the
extractor's lower
jaw beneath the first
staple.

The extractor changes the shape of the staple and pulls the prongs out of the intradermal tissue.

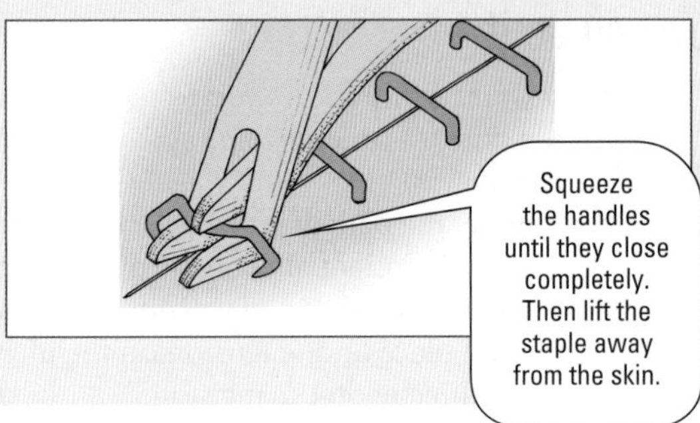

- If extraction is difficult, notify the doctor; *staples or clips placed too deeply within the skin or left in place too long may resist removal.*

If you need some support

- If the wound dehisces after staples or clips are removed, apply butterfly adhesive strips or Steri-Strips to approximate and support the edges and call the doctor immediately to repair the wound. Leave the strips in place for 3 to 5 days. (See *Documenting skin staple and clip removal*, page 167.)

Wound dehiscence and evisceration management

Occasionally, the edges of a wound may fail to join or may separate even after they seem to be healing normally. This development, called wound dehiscence, may lead to evisceration, in which a portion of the viscera (usually a bowel loop) protrudes through the incision. Evisceration, in turn, can lead to peritonitis and septic shock. **Notify the doctor immediately**. (See *Recognizing dehiscence and evisceration.*)

Dehiscence and evisceration are most likely to occur 6 to 7 days after surgery and may be caused by poor nutrition, chronic pulmonary or cardiac disease, localized wound infection, or stress on the incision (from coughing or vomiting).

What you need

Two sterile towels ✱ 1 L of sterile normal saline solution ✱ sterile irrigation set, including a basin, solution container, and 50-mL catheter-tip syringe ✳ several large abdominal dressings ✳ sterile, waterproof drape ✳ linen-saver pads ✳ sterile gloves.

If the patient will return to the operating room, gather the following equipment after the open wound is treated: intravenous (I.V.) administration set and I.V. fluids ✳ equipment for nasogastric (NG) intubation ✳ sedative, as ordered ✳ suction apparatus.

Getting ready

Provide reassurance and tell the patient to stay in bed. If possible, stay with him while someone else notifies the doctor and collects the necessary equipment.

Place a linen-saver pad under the patient *to keep the sheets dry when you moisten the exposed viscera.* Using sterile technique, unfold a sterile towel *to create a sterile field.* Open the package containing the irrigation set and place the basin, solution container, and 50-mL syringe on the sterile field.

Open the bottle of normal saline solution and pour 400 mL into the solution container and 200 mL into the sterile basin. Open several large abdominal dressings and place them on the sterile field.

How you do it

- Identify the patient using two patient identifiers.
- Perform hand hygiene.
- Put on the sterile gloves and place one or two of the large abdominal dressings into the basin *to saturate them with saline solution.*
- Place the moistened dressings over the exposed viscera, followed by a sterile, waterproof drape *to prevent the sheets from getting wet.*
- Moisten the dressings every hour by withdrawing saline solution from the container through the syringe and then gently squirting the solution on the dressings.

Darkness visible

- When you moisten the dressings, inspect the color of the viscera. **If it appears dusky or black, notify the doctor immediately.** *With its blood supply interrupted, a protruding organ may become ischemic and necrotic.*
- Keep the patient on absolute bed rest in low Fowler's position (no more than 20 degrees' elevation) with his knees flexed to *prevent injury and reduce stress on the incision.*
- Don't allow the patient to have anything by mouth and monitor the patient's pulse, respirations, blood pressure, and temperature every 15 minutes *to detect shock.*

Recognizing dehiscence and evisceration

Dehiscence or evisceration may occur as a surgical intervention.

Wound dehiscence

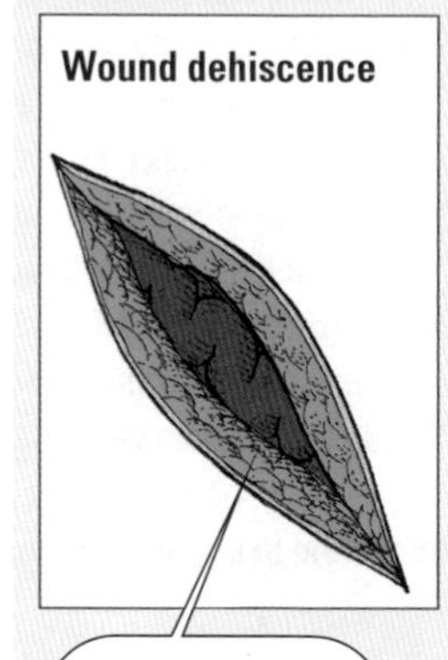

Surgical wound layers separate.

Evisceration of bowel loop

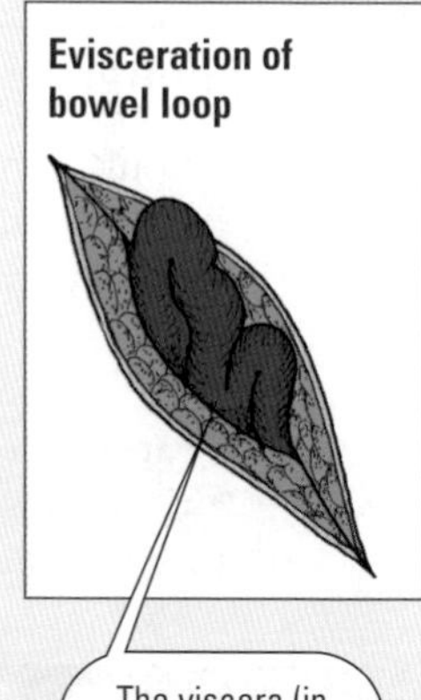

The viscera (in this case, the bowel loop) protrude through the incision.

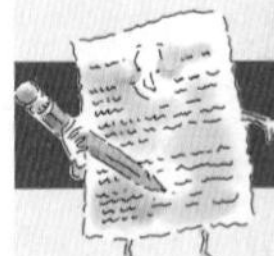

Write it down

Documenting dehiscence and evisceration management

In your notes, document:

- when the problem occurred
- patient's activity preceding the problem
- patient's condition
- time the doctor was notified
- appearance of the wound or eviscerated organ
- amount, color, consistency, and odor of drainage
- nursing actions taken
- patient's vital signs and response to the incident
- doctor's actions.

Finally, be sure to change the patient's plan of care to reflect nursing actions needed to promote proper healing.

- Continue to reassure the patient and, if necessary, prepare him to return to the operating room.

Practice pointers

- If you're caring for a postoperative patient who is at risk for poor healing, make sure he gets an adequate supply of protein, vitamins, and calories. Monitor his dietary deficiencies, and discuss any problems with the doctor and dietitian.
- Surgical intervention might be needed to close the wound; be aware of preoperative orders, such as nothing by mouth (NPO), NG tube insertion, and preoperative medication administration. (See *Documenting dehiscence and evisceration management.*)

Traumatic wound management

Traumatic wounds include abrasions, lacerations, puncture wounds, and amputations. In an abrasion, the skin is scraped, with partial loss of the skin surface. In a laceration, the skin is torn, causing jagged, irregular edges; the severity of a laceration depends on its size, depth, and location. A puncture wound occurs when a pointed object, such as a knife or glass fragment, penetrates the skin. Traumatic amputation refers to removal of part of the body, a limb, or part of a limb.

In cases of trauma, first stabilize the patient's airway, breathing, and circulation. Then treat the traumatic wound according to the type and cause.

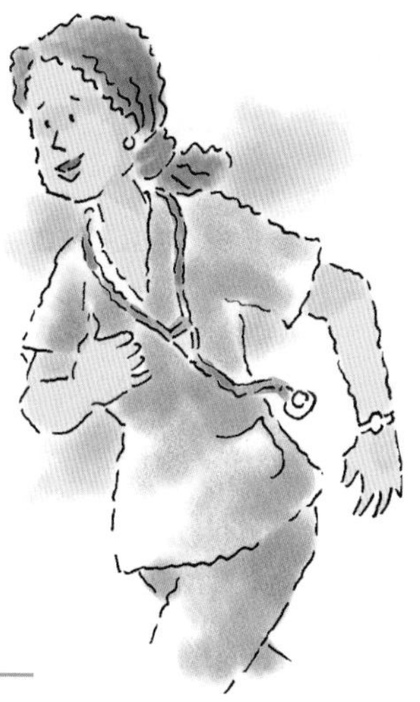
First focus on the ABCs. Then treat the traumatic wound.

What you need

Sterile basin ✱ normal saline solution ✱ sterile 4″ × 4″ gauze pads ✱ sterile gloves ✱ clean gloves ✱ sterile cotton-tipped applicators ✱ dry sterile dressing, nonadherent pad, or petroleum gauze ✱ linen-saver pad ✱ optional: scissors, towel, goggles, mask, gown, 50-mL catheter-tip syringe, surgical scrub brush, antibacterial ointment, porous tape, sterile forceps, sutures and suture set, hydrogen peroxide.

Getting ready

Place a linen-saver pad under the area to be cleaned. Remove any clothing covering the wound. If necessary, cut hair around the wound with scissors to promote cleaning and treatment.

Assemble needed equipment at the patient's bedside. Fill a sterile basin with normal saline solution. Make sure the treatment area has enough light to allow close observation of the wound.

How you do it

- Check the patient's medical history for previous tetanus immunization and, if needed and ordered, arrange for immunization as well as pain medication, if ordered.
- Perform hand hygiene and put on a gown, mask, gloves, and goggles if spraying or splashing of body fluids is possible. Depending on the type and location of the wound, wear sterile or clean gloves.

For an abrasion

- Flush the scraped skin with normal saline solution.
- Remove dirt or gravel with a sterile 4″ × 4″ gauze pad moistened with normal saline solution and rub in the opposite direction from which the dirt or gravel became embedded. If the wound is extremely dirty, you may use a surgical brush to scrub it.
- With a small wound, allow it to dry and form a scab. With a larger wound, you may need to cover it with a nonadherent pad or petroleum gauze and a light dressing. Apply antibacterial ointment if ordered.

For a laceration

- Moisten a sterile 4″ × 4″ gauze pad with normal saline solution. Clean the wound gently, working outward from its center to about 2″ (5 cm) beyond its edges. Discard the soiled gauze pad and use a fresh one as necessary. Continue until the wound appears clean.
- If the wound is dirty, you may irrigate it with a 50-mL catheter-tip syringe and normal saline solution.
- Assist the doctor in suturing the wound edges using the suture kit or apply sterile strips of porous tape.
- Apply the prescribed antibacterial ointment and a dry sterile dressing over the wound.

Write it down

Documenting traumatic wound management

In your notes, document:
- date and time of the procedure
- wound size and condition
- medication administration
- specific wound care measures
- patient teaching.

For a puncture wound

- If the wound is minor, allow it to bleed for a few minutes before cleaning it. For a larger puncture wound, you may need to irrigate it before applying a dry dressing.
- Stabilize any embedded foreign object until the doctor can remove it. After he removes the object and bleeding has stabilized, clean the wound as you would clean a laceration or deep puncture wound.

For an amputation

- Apply a gauze pad moistened with normal saline solution to the amputation site. Elevate the affected part and immobilize it for surgery.
- Recover the amputated part and prepare it for transport to a facility where microvascular surgery is performed.

Use hydrogen peroxide to clean traumatic wounds. The foaming action washes away debris.

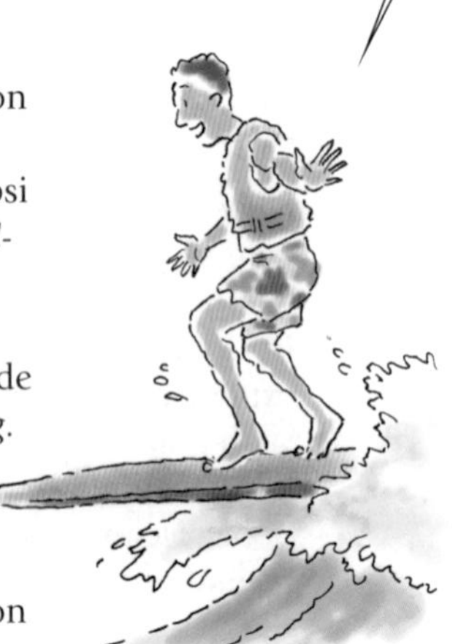

Practice pointers

- Before wound care, assess the patient's need for pain medication or an agent prescribed to promote comfort.
- When irrigating a traumatic wound, avoid using more than 8 psi of pressure *because higher pressure can seriously interfere with healing, kill cells, and allow bacteria to infiltrate the tissue.*
- *To clean the wound, use ordered solution.*
- After a wound has been cleaned, the doctor may want to debride it *to remove dead tissue and reduce the risk of infection and scarring.* If this is necessary, pack the wound lightly with gauze pads soaked in normal saline solution until debridement.
- Observe for signs and symptoms of infection, such as warm red skin at the site or purulent discharge. Be aware that infection

of a traumatic wound can delay healing, increase scar formation, and trigger systemic infection such as septicemia.

- Observe all dressings. If edema is present, loosen the dressing *to avoid impairing circulation (pulses, color, warmth) to the area.* (See *Documenting traumatic wound management.*)

Wound irrigation

Irrigation cleans tissues and flushes cell debris and drainage from an open surgical or chronic wound, such as a pressure ulcer. Irrigation with a commercial wound cleaner helps the wound heal properly from the inside tissue layers outward to the skin surface; it also helps prevent premature surface healing over an abscess pocket or infected tract.

The cleansing solution is instilled directly into the wound with a syringe, syringe with a soft catheter, or pulsed lavage device using strict sterile technique. If using a syringe, the tip is held 1″ above the wound. If it is a deep wound, use a syringe with a soft catheter to allow the solution to enter the wound. After irrigation, pack open wounds to absorb additional drainage. Always follow standard precautions.

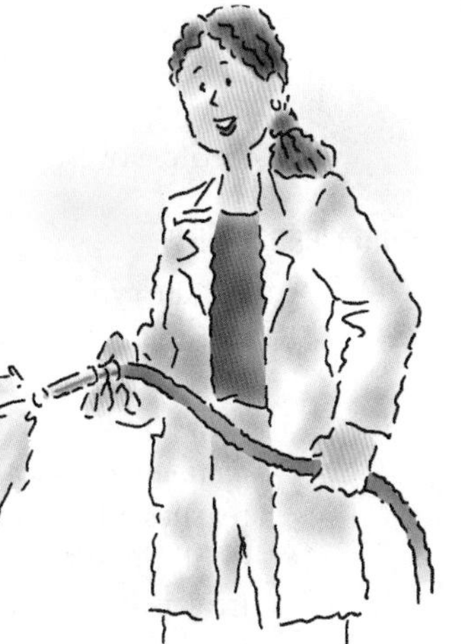
Hose it down! Irrigation cleans tissues and flushes away cell debris from an open wound.

What you need

Waterproof trash bag ✳ linen-saver pad ✳ emesis basin ✳ clean gloves ✳ sterile gloves ✳ goggles ✳ gown, if indicated ✳ prescribed irrigant such as sterile normal saline solution ✳ sterile water or normal saline solution ✳ soft rubber or plastic catheter ✳ sterile container ✳ materials as needed for wound care ✳ sterile irrigation and dressing set ✳ commercial wound cleaner ✳ 35-mL piston syringe with 19G needle or catheter ✳ skin protectant wipe ✳ wound assessment supplies.

Getting ready

Assemble all equipment in the patient's room. Check the expiration date on each sterile package and inspect for tears.

Use the prescribed irrigant. Don't use any solution that has been open longer than 24 hours.

Open the waterproof trash bag; place it near the patient's bed but avoid reaching across the sterile field or the wound when disposing of soiled articles. Form a cuff by turning down the top of the trash bag.

How you do it

- Check the doctor's order and identify the patient with two identifiers.
- Administer analgesia 30 to 45 minutes prior to wound irrigation as needed.
- Assess the patient's condition and identify allergies. Explain the procedure to the patient, provide privacy, and position him so that wound is vertical to collection basin. Place the linen-saver pad under the patient and place the emesis basin below the wound *so that the irrigating solution flows from the wound into the basin.*
- Warm the cleansing solution in a basin of hot water until it reaches body temperature. *Warmed solution increases comfort and reduces vascular constriction.*
- Perform hand hygiene and put on gloves.
- Remove the soiled dressing, then discard the dressing and gloves in the trash bag.
- Establish a sterile field with all the equipment and supplies you'll need for irrigation and wound care. Pour the prescribed amount of irrigating solution into a sterile container *so you won't contaminate your sterile gloves later by picking up unsterile containers.* Put on sterile gloves, gown, and goggles, if indicated.

From clean to dirty

- Fill the syringe with the irrigating solution and connect the catheter to the syringe. Gently instill a slow, steady stream of solution into the wound until the syringe empties. Make sure the solution flows from the clean to the dirty area of the wound *to prevent contamination of clean tissue by exudate.* Also make sure the solution reaches all areas of the wound.
- Refill the syringe, reconnect it to the catheter, and repeat the irrigation. Continue to irrigate the wound until you've administered the prescribed amount of solution or until the solution returns clear. Note the amount of solution administered. Then remove and discard the catheter and syringe in the waterproof trash bag.

Positioned for success

- Keep the patient positioned *to allow further wound drainage into the basin.*
- Clean the area around the wound with normal saline solution; wipe intact skin with a skin protectant wipe and allow it to dry.

Documenting wound irrigation

In your notes, record:

- patient education
- date and time of irrigation
- irrigation device used
- amount and type of irrigant
- wound appearance before and after irrigation
- sloughing tissue or exudate
- amount of solution returned
- skin care performed around the wound
- dressings applied
- patient's tolerance of the procedure.

- Apply appropriate dressing and label with time, date, and nurse's initials. Remove and discard your PPE in the appropriate container per facility policy.
- Make sure the patient is comfortable and dispose of drainage, solutions, trash bag, and soiled equipment and supplies according to facility policy and Centers for Disease Control and Prevention (CDC) guidelines.

Practice pointers

- Try to coordinate wound irrigation with the doctor's visit *so that he can inspect the wound.*
- Immediately report to physician or LIP any evidence of fresh bleeding, sharp increase in pain, retention of irrigant, or signs of shock.
- Do not force catheter into the wound because it can damage the tissue.
- Use a slow, continuous pressure to flush the wound *to loosen particulate matter on wound surface and promote healing.*
- Irrigate with a bulb syringe if the wound is small or not particularly deep or if a piston syringe is unavailable. However, use a bulb syringe cautiously *because this type of syringe doesn't deliver enough pressure to adequately clean the wound.* (See *Documenting wound irrigation.*)

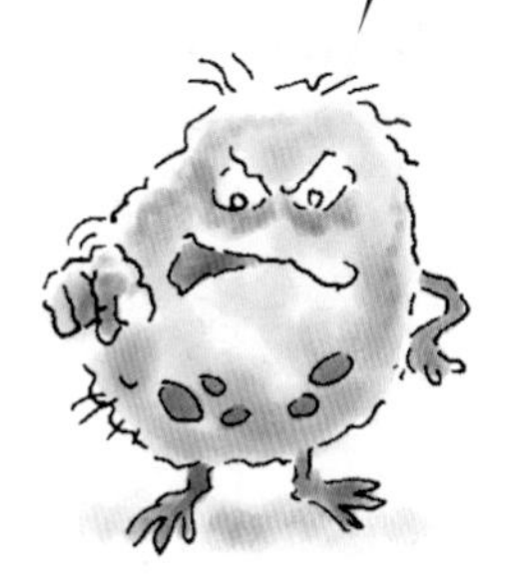
If you aren't careful during irrigation, my pathogenic friends and I will run rampant.

Vacuum-assisted closure therapy

Vacuum-assisted closure pressure therapy, also known as negative pressure wound therapy, is used to enhance delayed or impaired wound healing. The vacuum-assisted closure device applies localized subatmospheric pressure to draw the edges of the wound toward the center. A special dressing is placed in the wound or over a graft or flap, and vacuum-assisted closure therapy is applied. This wound packing removes fluids from the wound, reduces edema, and stimulates growth of healthy granulation tissue and perfusion.

Vacuum-assisted closure therapy is indicated for acute and traumatic wounds, pressure ulcers, and chronic open wounds, such as diabetic ulcers, meshed grafts, and skin flaps. It's contraindicated for fistulas that involve organs or body cavities, necrotic tissue with eschar, untreated osteomyelitis, and malignant wounds. This therapy should be used cautiously in patients with active bleeding, in those taking anticoagulants, and when achieving wound hemostasis has been difficult.

What you need

Waterproof trash bag ✱ goggles ✱ gown, if indicated ✱ emesis basin ✱ normal saline solution ✱ clean gloves ✱ sterile gloves ✱ sterile scissors ✱ linen-saver pad ✱ 35-mL piston syringe with 19G catheter ✱ reticulated foam ✱ fenestrated tubing ✱ evacuation tubing ✱ skin protectant wipe ✱ transparent occlusive air-permeable drape ✱ evacuation canister ✱ vacuum unit ✱ materials to assess the wound.

Getting ready

Assemble the vacuum-assisted closure device at the bedside according to the manufacturer's instructions. Set negative pressure according to the doctor's order (25 to 200 mm Hg).

How you do it

- Check the doctor's order and identify the patient using two patient identifiers.
- Assess the patient's condition.
- Explain the procedure to the patient, provide privacy, and perform hand hygiene. If necessary, put on a gown and goggles *to protect you from wound drainage and contamination.*
- Place a linen-saver pad under the patient *to catch any spills and avoid linen changes.* Position to allow maximum wound exposure. Place the emesis basin under the wound *to collect any drainage.*
- Put on clean gloves. Remove the soiled dressing and discard it in the waterproof trash bag. Attach the 19G catheter to the 35-mL piston syringe and irrigate the wound thoroughly using normal saline solution.
- Clean the area around the wound with normal saline solution; wipe intact skin with a skin protectant wipe and allow it to dry well. Assess the wound. Remove and discard your gloves.

Fun with foam

- Don sterile gloves. Using sterile scissors, cut the foam to the shape and measurement of the wound. More than one piece of foam may be necessary if the first piece is cut too small. Do not cut the foam over the wound *because particles may fall into the wound.*
- Carefully place the foam in the wound. Next, place the fenestrated tubing into the center of the foam. *The fenestrated tubing embedded into the foam delivers negative pressure to the wound.*
- Place the transparent occlusive air-permeable drape over the foam, enclosing the foam and the tubing together. Remove and

discard your gloves and PPE in the appropriate container per facility policy.
- Connect the free end of the fenestrated tubing to the tubing that's connected to the evacuation canister.

Flick the switch

- Turn on the vacuum unit.
- Make sure the patient is comfortable.
- Properly dispose of drainage, solution, linen-saver pad, and trash bag, and clean and dispose of soiled equipment and supplies according to facility policy and CDC guidelines.

Documenting vacuum-assisted closure therapy

In your notes, document:
- frequency and duration of therapy
- amount of negative pressure applied
- size and condition of the wound
- number of pieces of foam in the wound
- patient's response to the procedure.

Practice pointers

- Change the dressing every 48 hours. Try to coordinate the dressing change with the doctor's visit *so he can inspect the wound.*
- Do not place foam dressings in direct contact with exposed blood vessels, anastomotic sites, organs, or nerves.
- Measure the amount of drainage every shift.
- Audible and visual alarms alert you if the unit is tipped greater than 45 degrees, if the canister is full, if the dressing has an air leak, or if the canister becomes dislodged.
- Cleaning and care of wounds may temporarily increase the patient's pain and increases the risk for infection. (See *Documenting vacuum-assisted closure therapy.*)

Closed-wound drain management

A closed-wound drain, such as the Hemovac or Jackson-Pratt system, consists of perforated tubing connected to a portable vacuum unit. It's commonly inserted during surgery with the distal end of the tubing laying within the wound and leaving the body from another site.

A closed-wound drain helps reduce the risk of infection, skin breakdown, and the number of dressing changes. It also promotes healing. The drain is usually sutured to the skin, and the exit site is often treated as an additional surgical wound.

What you need

Graduated biohazard cylinder ✳ sterile laboratory container, if needed ✳ alcohol pads ✳ gloves ✳ trash bag ✳ sterile gauze pads ✳ antiseptic cleaning agent ✳ prepackaged povidone-iodine swabs.

Using a closed-wound drainage system

The portable closed-wound drainage system draws drainage from a wound site, such as the chest wall postmastectomy (as shown below left), by means of a Y tube.

To empty the drainage, remove the plug and empty it into a graduated cylinder. To reestablish suction, compress the drainage unit against a firm surface to expel air and, while holding it down, replace the plug with your other hand (as shown below center).

The same principle is used for the Jackson-Pratt bulb drain (as shown below right).

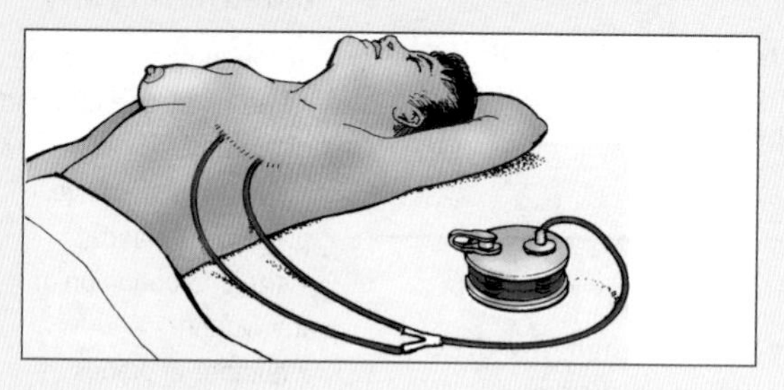

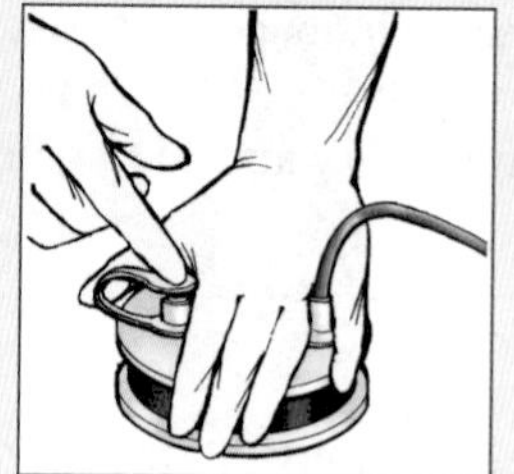

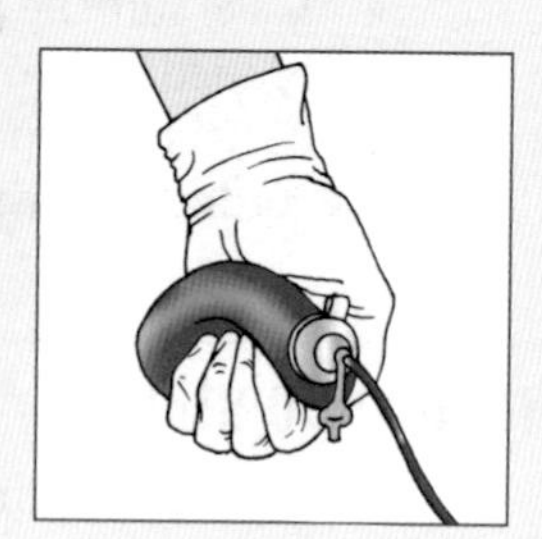

How you do it

- Identify the patient with two patient identifiers.
- Explain the procedure to the patient, provide privacy, and perform hand hygiene.
- Wearing gloves, unclip the vacuum unit from the patient's gown and release the vacuum by removing the spout plug on the collection chamber. The container will expand completely as it draws in air.
- Empty the unit's contents into a graduated cylinder and note the amount and appearance of the drainage. If diagnostic tests will be performed on the fluid specimen, pour the drainage directly into a sterile laboratory container.
- Use an alcohol pad to clean the unit's spout and plug, then reestablish the vacuum by fully compressing the vacuum unit with one hand and replacing the spout plug with your other hand. (See *Using a closed-wound drainage system.*)

(Un)do the twist

- Check the patency of the equipment, making sure the tubing is free from twists and kinks and working properly. (See *Complications of drains.*) If reinflation occurs, recompress the unit and make sure the spout plug is secure.
- Secure the vacuum unit to the patient's gown below the wound, making sure that there's no tension on the drainage tubing. Remove and discard your gloves and perform hand hygiene.

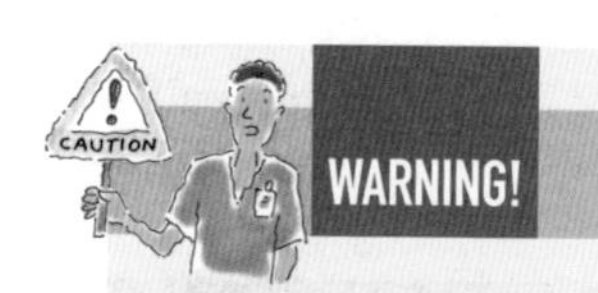

Complications of drains

With a closed-wound drain, monitor for occlusion of the tubing by fibrin, clots, or other particles that can reduce or obstruct drainage.

Bad mistake

Also, be careful not to mistake chest tubes for closed-wound drains. Unlike a closed-wound drain, the vacuum of a chest tube should never be released.

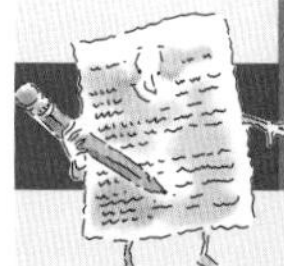

Write it down

Documenting closed-wound drain management

In your notes, record:

- date and time you empty the drain
- appearance of the drain site
- presence of swelling or other signs of infection
- equipment malfunction and nursing action taken
- patient's tolerance of the procedure.

On the intake and output sheet, record drainage color, consistency, type, and amount. If the patient has more than one closed-wound drain, number the drains and record the information above separately for each drainage site.

Suture surveillance

- Observe the sutures that secure the drain to the patient's skin; look for signs of pulling, tearing, swelling, or infection of surrounding skin. Gently clean the sutures per hospital protocol.
- Properly dispose of drainage, solutions, and the trash bag, and clean or dispose of soiled equipment and supplies according to facility policy.

Practice pointers

- Drainage must be emptied and measured frequently *to maintain maximum suction and prevent strain on the suture line.* Empty the drain and measure its contents once during each shift if drainage has accumulated and more often if drainage is excessive. If the patient is ambulatory, empty the device before ambulation *to remove excess drainage, maintain maximum suction, and avoid straining the drain's suture line.*
- If the patient has more than one closed drain, number the drains *so you can record drainage from each site.* (See *Documenting closed-wound drain management.*)

External radiation therapy

Also called radiotherapy, external radiation therapy delivers X-rays or gamma rays directly to the cancer site. Doses are given in increments, usually three to five times a week, until the total dose is reached.

Radiation therapy may be used to completely destroy the cancer, control its progress, or help relieve symptoms, such as bone pain, bleeding, and headache. Radiation therapy may be augmented by chemotherapy, brachytherapy (radiation implant therapy), or surgery, as needed.

Getting ready

Verify the order and identify the patient with two patient identifiers. Explain the treatment to the patient and his family and review its goals, adverse effects, complications, and treatment issues. Provide education on interventions to minimize adverse effects as well as available local cancer services.

Make sure the radiation oncology department has obtained informed consent and that it's alerted to any abnormalities in recent laboratory and imaging results. Transport the patient to the radiation oncology department.

How you do it

- Initially, the patient undergoes treatment planning in which the target area is mapped out and tattooed or marked in ink *to ensure*

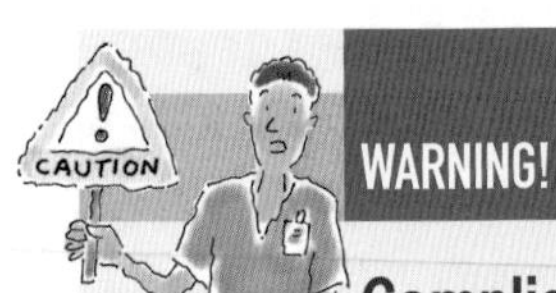

WARNING!

Complications of radiation therapy

Adverse reactions to radiation therapy arise gradually and diminish gradually after treatments. They may be acute, subacute (accumulating as treatment progresses), chronic (following treatment), or long term (arising months to years after treatment).

Adverse reactions are localized to the area of treatment, and their severity depends on the total radiation dose, underlying organ sensitivity, and the patient's overall condition.

Short but serious

Common acute and subacute adverse reactions can include altered skin integrity, altered gastrointestinal (GI) and genitourinary functions, altered fertility and sexual functions, altered bone marrow production, fatigue, and alopecia.

For the long haul

Long-term complications or adverse reactions may include radiation pneumonitis, neuropathy, skin and muscle atrophy, telangiectasia, fistulas, altered endocrine function, and secondary cancers. Other complications of treatment include headache, alopecia, xerostomia, dysphagia, stomatitis, altered skin integrity (wet or dry desquamation), nausea, vomiting, heartburn, diarrhea, cystitis, and fatigue.

accurate treatments. The doctor and radiation oncologist then determine the duration and frequency of treatments depending on the patient's body size, size of portal, extent and location of cancer, and treatment goals.
- The patient is positioned on the treatment table beneath the machine with treatments lasting from a few seconds to a few minutes. After treatment is complete, the patient may return home or to his room.

Documenting external radiation therapy

In your notes, record:
- radiation precautions taken during treatment
- adverse effects of therapy
- teaching given to the patient and his family and their responses
- patient's tolerance of isolation procedures and the family's compliance with them
- referrals to local cancer services.

Practice pointers

- Instruct the patient to report short- and long-term adverse effects. (See *Complications of radiation therapy*.)
- Reassure the patient that he won't feel anything and won't be radioactive. (See *Documenting external radiation therapy*.)

Radiation implant therapy

In this treatment, also called brachytherapy, the doctor uses implants of radioactive isotopes (encapsulated in seeds, needles, or sutures) to deliver ionizing radiation within a body cavity or interstitially to a tumor site. Implants may be permanent or temporary and deliver a continuous radiation dose over several hours or days to a specific site while minimizing exposure to adjacent tissues. Radiation implant therapy is commonly combined with external radiation therapy (teletherapy) for increased effectiveness.

What you need

Film badge or pocket dosimeter * RADIATION PRECAUTION sign for door * RADIATION PRECAUTION warning labels * masking tape * lead-lined container * long-handled forceps * optional: lead shield and lead strip.

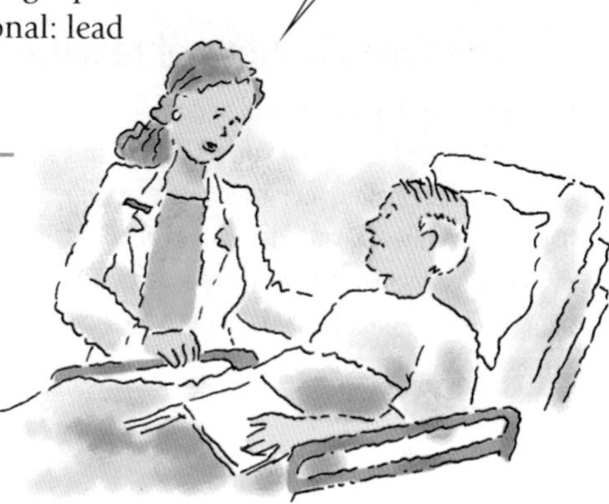
I won't be performing the radiation therapy, but I'll teach you what to expect.

Getting ready

The patient's room needs to be equipped with a lead-lined container, long-handled forceps, lead shield, and a "safe line" marked on the floor with masking tape 6′ (1.8 m) from the bed *to minimize radiation exposure*.

If an implant will be inserted in the oral cavity or neck, an emergency tracheotomy tray should also be placed in the room.

How you do it

- Explain the treatment, goals, long-term concerns, and home care issues to the patient. Review radiation safety procedures, visitation policies, potential adverse effects, and interventions for those effects. (See *Complications of radiation implant therapy.*)
- Place the RADIATION PRECAUTION sign on the door and affix warning labels to the patient's identification wristband, chart, and Kardex *to ensure staff awareness of radioactive status.*
- Check to see that informed consent has been obtained and laboratory tests have been performed before beginning treatment.

This badge means business

- Wear a film badge or dosimeter at waist level during the entire shift and turn in the badge monthly or according to your facility's policy.

Three important principles

- To minimize exposure to radiation, use the three principles of time, distance, and shielding. Give care in the shortest time possible to reduce your amount of exposure. Essential nursing care should only be provided. Distance your work as far away from the radiation source as possible, such as providing care from the side opposite the implant. Use a shield if needed and desired.
- Make sure that wipes, sanitary pads, and similar items are bagged correctly and monitored according to your facility's radiation policy. The patient's room must be monitored daily by the radiation oncology department, and disposables must be monitored and removed according to facility guidelines.

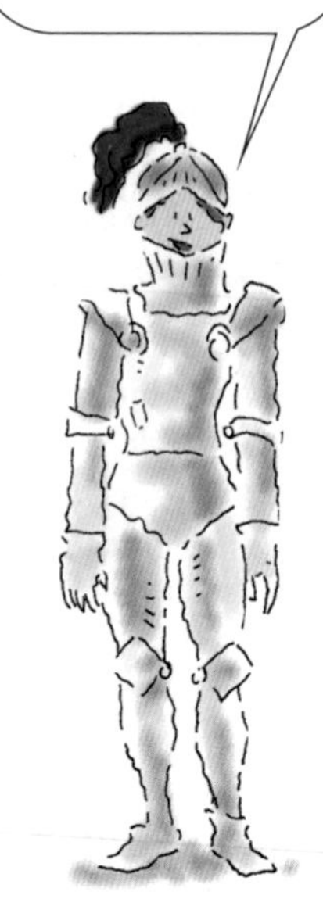
To minimize exposure to radiation, use the three principles of time, distance, and shielding.

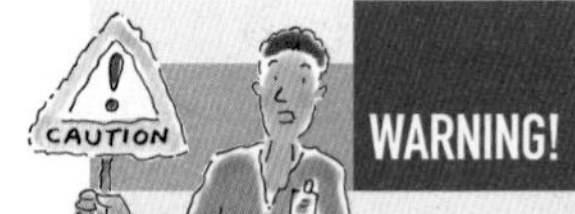
CAUTION

WARNING!

Complications of radiation implant therapy

Depending on the implant site and total radiation dose, complications of implant therapy may include dislodgment of the radiation source or applicator, tissue fibrosis, xerostomia, radiation pneumonitis, muscle atrophy, sterility, vaginal dryness or stenosis, fistulas, hypothyroidism, altered bowel habits, infection, airway obstruction, diarrhea, cystitis, myelosuppression, neurotoxicity, and secondary cancers. Encourage the patient and family members to contact the radiation oncology department if concerns or physical changes occur.

- Before discharge, a patient's temporary implant must be removed and properly stored by the radiation oncology department. A patient with a permanent implant may not be released until his radioactivity level is less than 5 millirems/hour at 1 m.

Practice pointers

- If laboratory work is required during treatment, it's the badged technician's responsibility to obtain the specimen, label the collection tube with a RADIOACTIVE PRECAUTION label, and alert laboratory personnel before bringing it.
- Dressing changes over an implanted area must be supervised by the radiation technician or another designated caregiver.

If there's a baby on the way

- Nurses and visitors who are pregnant or trying to conceive or father a child must not attend patients receiving radiation implant therapy.
- If the patient must be moved out of his room, notify the appropriate department and ensure that the route is clear of equipment and other people. Move the patient in a bed or wheelchair, accompanied by two badged caregivers.
- If a code is called on a patient with an implant, follow your facility's code procedures, alert the code team of the patient's radioactive status, and notify the radiation oncology department.

Don't touch

- If an implant becomes dislodged, notify the radiation oncology department staff and follow their instructions.
- If a patient with an implant dies on the unit, notify the radiation oncology department. (See *Documenting radiation implant therapy*.)

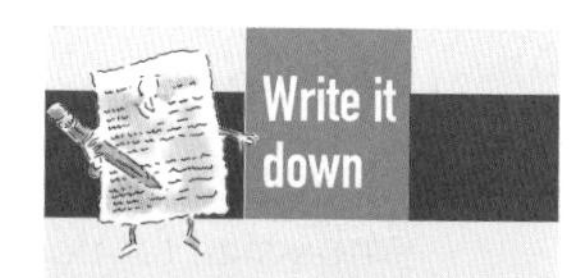
Write it down

Documenting radiation implant therapy

In your notes, record:
- radiation precautions
- adverse effects
- patient education
- patient's tolerance of isolation procedures and the family's compliance with them
- referrals to local cancer services.

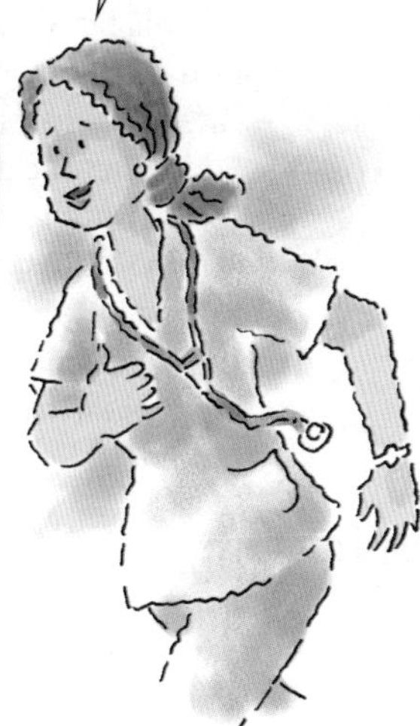
If a code is called, tell the code team that the patient is radioactive and place lead shielding over the implant site.

Radioactive iodine therapy

Radioactive iodine 131 (^{131}I) is an isotope used to treat primarily thyroid cancers as well as cancer that has spread. Because ^{131}I is absorbed systemically, all body secretions, especially urine, must be considered radioactive. For ^{131}I treatments, the patient usually is placed in a private room (with its own bathroom) located as far away from high-traffic areas as practical. Adjacent rooms and hallways may also need to be restricted. Consult your facility's radiation safety policy for specific guidelines. In lower doses, ^{131}I also may be used to treat hyperthyroidism on an outpatient basis with home care instructions.

What you need

Film badges, pocket dosimeters, or ring badges ✳ RADIATION PRECAUTION sign for door ✳ RADIATION PRECAUTION warning labels ✳ waterproof gowns ✳ clear and red plastic bags for contaminated articles ✳ plastic wrap ✳ absorbent plastic-lined pads ✳ masking tape ✳ radioresistant gloves ✳ trashcans ✳ optional: portable lead shield.

Getting ready

Assemble all necessary equipment in the patient's room. Keep an emergency tracheotomy tray just outside the room or in a handy place at the nurses' station. Place the RADIATION PRECAUTION sign on the door and affix warning labels to the patient's identification wristband, chart, and Kardex.

Place an absorbent plastic-lined pad on the bathroom floor, under the sink, over the bedside table, and over any carpeting. Secure plastic wrap over the telephone, television controls, bed controls, mattress, call button, and toilet with masking tape. *These measures prevent radioactive contamination of working surfaces.*

Keep large trashcans in the room lined with two clear bags inserted inside an outer red bag. Monitor all objects before they leave the room. Notify the dietitian to supply disposable containers and utensils.

How you do it

- Verify the order. Identify the patient using two patient identifiers.
- Explain the procedure and review treatment goals with the patient and his family as well as radiation safety procedures and visitation policies, potential adverse effects, interventions, and home care procedures. (See *What to do after treatment.*)
- Verify that the doctor has obtained informed consent.
- Check for allergies to iodine and review the medication history for thyroid-containing or thyroid-altering drugs and for lithium carbonate, *which may increase* ^{131}I *uptake.*
- If necessary, remove the patient's dentures *to avoid contaminating them and to reduce radioactive secretions.* Tell him that they'll be replaced 48 hours after treatment.

Tug three times

- Explain that the patient will need to use the toilet rather than a bedpan or urinal and to flush it three times after each use *to*

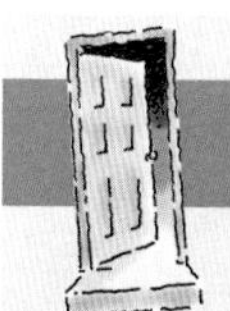

Home care connection

What to do after treatment

Instruct the patient to report adverse reactions. Review signs and symptoms of hypothyroidism and hyperthyroidism. Ask him to report signs and symptoms of thyroid cancer, such as enlarged lymph nodes, dyspnea, bone pain, nausea, vomiting, and abdominal discomfort.

Seeing less of you

Although the patient's radiation level at discharge will be safe, suggest that he take extra precautions during the 1st week, such as using separate eating utensils, sleeping in a separate bedroom, and avoiding body contact.

Avoid pregnancy

Sexual intercourse may be resumed 1 week after ^{131}I treatment. However, urge a female patient to avoid pregnancy for 6 months after treatment and tell a male patient to avoid impregnating his partner for 3 months after treatment.

reduce radiation levels. In addition, he'll need to remain in his room except for tests or procedures.
- Ensure that all laboratory tests are performed before beginning treatment.
- Wear a film badge or dosimeter at waist level during the entire shift. Turn in the radiation badge monthly or according to your facility's protocol and be sure to record your exposures accurately.
- Wear gloves to touch the patient or objects in his room and restrict visiting. (See *Visiting restrictions*, page 186.)

Only the essentials

- Give essential nursing care only and make sure that wipes, sanitary pads, and similar items are bagged correctly.
- If the patient vomits or urinates on the floor, notify the nuclear medicine department and use nondisposable radio-resistant gloves and waterproof gowns when cleaning the floor. After cleanup, wash your gloved hands, remove the gloves and leave them in the room, and perform hand hygiene.
- If the patient must be moved from his room, notify the appropriate department of his status *so that receiving personnel can make appropriate arrangements to receive him*. When moving the patient, ensure that the route is clear of equipment and other people. Move the patient in a bed or wheelchair, accompanied by two badged caregivers.

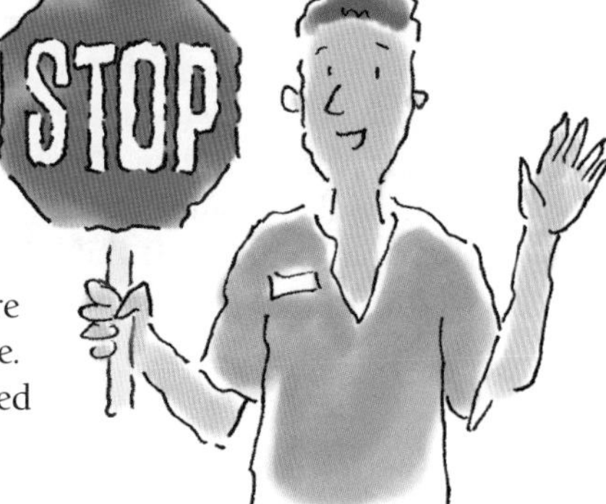
Keep a radioactive iodine patient away from high-traffic areas.
STOP

Who cleans up?

- The radiation oncology department, not housekeeping, must clean the patient's room. The room must be monitored daily, and disposables must be monitored and removed according to facility guidelines.
- At discharge, schedule the patient for a follow-up examination. Also arrange for a whole-body scan about 7 to 10 days after ^{131}I treatment.
- Inform the patient and his family of community support services for cancer patients.

Visiting restrictions

Allow visitors to patients undergoing radioactive iodine therapy to stay no longer than 30 minutes every 24 hours with the patient. Stress that no visitors who are pregnant or trying to conceive or father a child will be allowed. Visitors under age 18 are prohibited.

Practice pointers

- Unless contraindicated, instruct the patient to increase his fluid intake to 3 qt (3 L) daily. Encourage the patient to chew or suck on hard candy *to keep salivary glands stimulated and prevent them from becoming inflamed (which may develop in the first 24 hours).*

If you need labs

- If laboratory work is required, the badged laboratory technician obtains the specimen, labels the collection tube with a RADIATION PRECAUTION warning label, and alerts laboratory personnel before transporting it. If urine tests are needed, ask the radiation oncology department or laboratory technician how to transport the specimens safely.
- Nurses and visitors who are pregnant or trying to conceive or father a child must not attend or visit patients receiving ^{131}I therapy *because the gonads and developing embryo and fetus are highly susceptible to the damaging effects of ionizing radiation.*
- Restrict direct contact to no longer than 30 minutes or 20 millirems per day.
- If a code is called on a patient undergoing ^{131}I therapy, follow your facility's code procedures as well as notifying the radiation oncology department. Don't let anything leave the patient's room until it's monitored. The primary care nurse must remain in the room (as far as possible from the patient) *to act as a resource person and to provide film badges or dosimeters to code team members.*
- If the patient dies on the unit, notify the radiology safety officer who will determine which precautions to follow before postmortem care is provided and before the body can be removed to the morgue. (See *Documenting radioactive iodine therapy*.)

Documenting radioactive iodine therapy

In your notes, record:
- radiation precautions taken during treatment
- teaching given to the patient and his family
- patient's tolerance of isolation procedures and the family's compliance with them
- referrals to local cancer services.

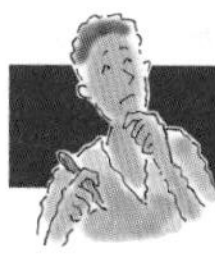

Quick quiz

1. The nurse is caring for a client who received radioactive iodine therapy and has vomited on the floor. What should be used to manage these secretions?
   A. Disposable gloves for cleanup
   B. Sterile gloves for cleanup
   C. Nondisposable radioresistant gloves for cleanup

Answer: C. Treat all secretions as radioactive and take appropriate precautions.

2. A patient with abdominal surgery states that he felt something "pop" when he was getting back into bed. The nurse examines his abdominal wound and found bowel protruding. What action should the nurse perform first?
   A. Place the patient in high Fowler's position.
   B. Place the patient in low Fowler's position.
   C. Place the patient flat in bed.
   D. Place the patient on his left side.

Answer: B. Place the patient in low Fowler's position to reduce tension on the wound.

3. When removing sutures, how should the nurse remove the sutures?
   A. Remove every other suture initially.
   B. Remove the middle sutures first.
   C. Remove the retention sutures last.
   D. Remove the ends first.

Answer: A. Remove every other suture initially to determine wound closure.

4. To irrigate a wound, which way should the nurse direct the flow of the irrigant?
   A. Toward the wound
   B. Away from the wound
   C. Toward the center of the wound
   D. Away from wound ends

Answer: B. Direct flow away from the wound to prevent contamination.

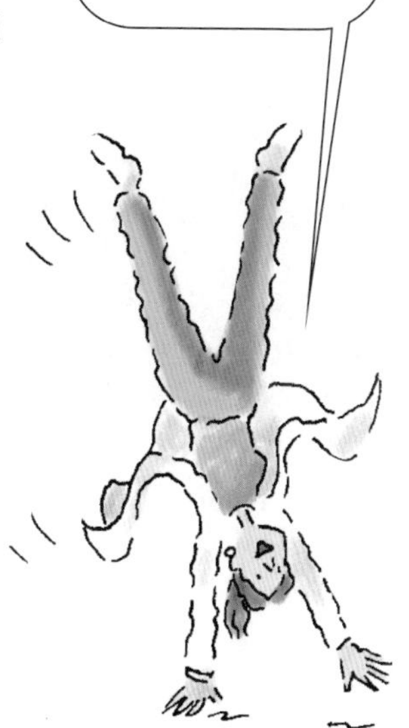
Time to flip from reviewing to testing. Try your hand at these quick quiz questions!

5. After applying antiembolism stockings, what is the next step the nurse should take?
   A. Check for circulation distally.
   B. Make sure the legs remain elevated for a short period.
   C. Remove the stockings periodically.
   D. Bend slightly at the knees bilaterally.

Answer: A. Circulation should be monitored to detect adequate perfusion.

6. Which technique is correct for obtaining a wound culture specimen from a surgical site?

A. Thoroughly irrigate the wound before collecting the specimen.
B. Use a sterile swab and wipe the crusty area around the outside of the wound.
C. Gently roll a sterile swab from the center of the wound outward to collect drainage.
D. Use a sterile swab to collect drainage from the dressing.

Answer: C. Rolling a swab from the center outward is the right way to obtain a culture specimen from a wound.

7. The nurse is caring for a client who is 4 days postoperative and is experiencing occasional vomiting. Which issue is the greatest concern?

A. Postsurgical hemorrhage and anemia
B. Wound dehiscence and evisceration
C. Decubitus skin integrity and decubitus ulcer
D. Loss of motility and paralytic ileus

Answer: C. Obesity and vomiting are high risk factors for dehiscence.

8. The nurse is changing a dressing and providing wound care. Which activity should she perform first?

A. Assess the drainage in the dressing.
B. Slowly remove the soiled dressing.
C. Wash hands thoroughly.
D. Put on latex gloves.

Answer: C. Wash hands before applying nonlatex gloves.

9. When bandaging a patient's foot, how should the nurse perform this technique?

A. Work from proximal to distal.
B. Work from anterior to posterior.
C. Cover the toes in a spiral.
D. Have the foot hyperextended.

Answer: B. Do not hyperextend, and toes should be visible to check circulation.

10. The nurse is teaching a female client with a leg ulcer about tissue repair and wound healing. Which statement by the client indicates effective teaching?

A. I will limit my intake of protein.
B. I will make sure that the bandage is wrapped tightly.
C. My foot should feel cold to touch.
D. I will eat plenty of fruits and vegetables and protein.

Answer: D. Healthy nutrition is important for wound healing.

Scoring

☆☆☆ If you answered all 10 items correctly, yippee! You're the Anti Em of antiembolism stocking application, you're De Bride of debridement, you're the . . . well, you get the picture—you're great!

☆☆ If you answered eight or nine items correctly, way to go! You're fit for physical treatments!

☆ If you answered fewer than seven items correctly, don't worry. Just review the chapter and try again!

Selected References

Baranoski, S., & Ayello, E. A. (2004). *Wound care essentials: Practice principles.* Philadelphia, PA: Lippincott Williams & Wilkins.

Elkin, M. K., Perry, A. G., & Potter, P. A. (2000). *Nursing interventions and clinical skills* (2nd ed.). St. Louis, MO: Mosby.

Ellis, J. R., & Hartley, C. L. (2000). *Managing and coordinating nursing care* (3rd ed.). Philadelphia, PA: Lippincott Williams & Wilkins.

Hess, C. T. (2005). *Clinical guide: Wound care* (5th ed.). Philadelphia, PA: Lippincott Williams & Wilkins.

KCI. (2013). *V.A.C® therapy indications and safety information.* Retrieved from http://www.kci-medical.ie/IE-ENG/indications

Lippincott. (2007). *Wound care made incredibly easy* (2nd ed.). Philadelphia, PA: Author.

Lippincott. (2012). Skin staple and clip removal. In *Lippincott's nursing procedures* (6th ed., pp. 658–660). Philadelphia, PA: Author.

Moore, C., Nichols-Willey, J., & Orlosky-Norvack, J. (2013). *Enhancing patient outcomes with sequential compression device therapy.* Retrieved from http://www.americannursetoday.com/enhancing-patient-outcomes-with-sequential-compression-device-therapy

National Institute for Health and Care Excellence. (2010). *NICE guidelines [CG92]: Venous thromboembolism: Reducing the risk of venous thromboembolism (deep vein thrombosis and pulmonary embolism) in patients admitted to hospital.* Retrieved from http://www.nice.org.uk/guidance/CG92

Perry, A. G., Potter, P. A., & Ostendorf, W. (2013). *Clinical nursing skills and techniques* (8th ed.). St. Louis, MO: Elsevier.

Chapter 4

Drug administration and I.V. therapy

Just the facts

In this chapter, you'll learn how to:

- safely administer drugs and I.V. fluids
- identify patient care associated with drug administration and I.V. therapy
- manage drug and I.V. complications
- complete patient education and proper documentation associated with drug therapy and I.V. administration.

New medication guidelines

- A review of the physician's order for accuracy and completeness is necessary.
- In order for medication administration to be error proof, follow the six rights of medication administration. These are the right patient, dose, medication, route, time, and documentation.
- One of The Joint Commission National Patient Safety Goals is to identify patients correctly using two patient identifiers. The most common patient identifiers are asking the patient to state his name and date of birth.
- Any verbal and telephone orders received by the nurse must be verified by "read back." The nurse reads back the order to the physician for accuracy.
- All facilities have been asked to develop a list to reduce medication errors of look-alike–soundalike drugs. The use of tall man lettering will help to reduce confusion and reduce medication errors.
- A "high-alert" medication list is part of each facility policy to reduce error and significant patient harm. The medications identified will need to have a "double check" by another health care professional at the time of administration, for example, insulin, chemotherapy.

- There are various medication scheduling terms used when administering medications. For instance, STAT, first time, loading doses, and one-time doses are to be given at the exact time. Medications such as antibiotics, insulins, anticonvulsants, and immunosuppressives can be given 30 minutes before and after the scheduled dose. Noncritical medications can be given 1 to 2 hours before or after a scheduled dose. Please check with the specific facility policy.
- Never administer medications from the same syringe to more than one patient, even if the needle is changed or you are injecting through an intervening length of intravenous (I.V.) tubing.
- Do not enter a medication vial, bag, or bottle with a used syringe or needle.
- Never use medications packaged as single-dose or single-use for more than one patient. This includes ampules, bags, and bottles of I.V. solutions.
- Always use aseptic technique when preparing and administering injections.

Skin medications

Topical drugs are applied directly to the skin surface and are absorbed through the epidermal layer into the dermis. They include lotions, pastes, ointments, creams, powders, shampoos, patches, and aerosol sprays.

Most topical medications are used for local effects, although some are used for systemic effects. Typically, topical medications should be applied two or three times a day to achieve their therapeutic effect.

What you need

Patient's medication record and chart ✳ prescribed medication ✳ gloves ✳ sterile tongue blades ✳ 4″ × 4″ sterile gauze pads ✳ transparent semipermeable dressing ✳ adhesive tape ✳ basin ✳ washcloths and towel.

Getting ready

Verify the order on the patient's medication record by checking it against the doctor's order on the chart and make sure the label on the medication agrees with the medication order. Read the label again before you open the container and as you remove the medication from the container. Check the expiration date. Check for allergies.

Confirm the patient's identity using two patient identifiers per facility policy.

How you do it

- Explain the procedure, perform hand hygiene, and don gloves.
- Help the patient assume a comfortable position that allows access to the area to be treated. Examine the skin or mucous membrane to be treated.
- If necessary, clean the skin of debris, including crusts, epidermal scales, and old medication. Change gloves if soiled.

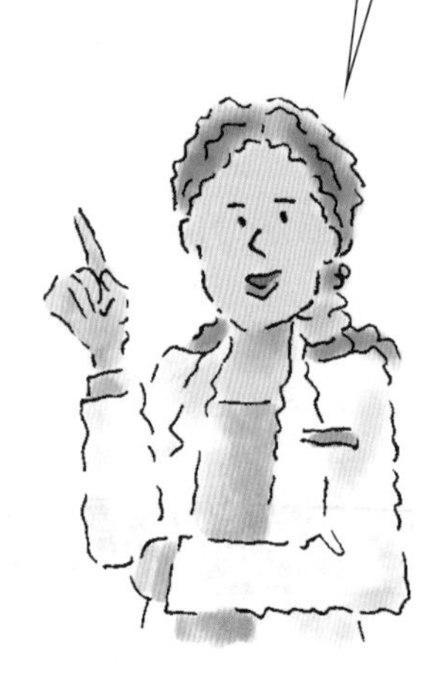
Help the patient into a comfortable position that allows access to the skin.

Applying paste, cream, or ointment

- Open the medication container and place the lid or cap upside down, remove a tongue blade from its sterile wrapper, and cover one end with medication from the tube or jar. Then transfer the medication from the tongue blade to your gloved hand.
- Apply the medication to the affected area with long, smooth strokes that follow the direction of hair growth; use a new tongue blade each time you remove medication from the container.

Removing ointment

- Perform hand hygiene and don gloves. Wash area with warm water and soap. Rinse and pat dry the affected area.

Applying other topical medications

- To apply shampoos, wet the patient's hair and wring out excess water, shake the bottle, and apply the proper amount as indicated by the label. Work the lather into the scalp, adding water as necessary. Leave the shampoo on the scalp as directed and then rinse thoroughly. A fine-tooth comb is used to remove nits, if necessary.
- To apply aerosol sprays, shake the container and hold it 6″ to 12″ (15 to 30.5 cm) from the skin or according to the manufacturer's recommendation. Spray a thin film of the medication evenly over the treatment area. Ask patient to turn head away from the spray.
- To apply powders, dry the skin surface, making sure to spread skin folds where moisture collects. Then apply a thin layer of powder over the treatment area. If ordered, a dressing may be used to cover the area.

They aren't fashionable anyway

- *To protect applied medications and prevent them from soiling the patient's clothes,* tape sterile gauze pads or a transparent semipermeable dressing over the treated area. In children, topical medications (such as steroids) should be covered only loosely with a diaper.
- Assess the patient's skin for signs of irritation, allergic reaction, or breakdown.

Practice pointers

- Never apply medication without removing previous applications *to prevent skin irritation from medication accumulation.*
- If the patient has an infectious skin condition or the area is open, use sterile gloves and dispose of old dressings according to your facility's policy.

Less is more

- Don't apply ointments to mucous membranes as liberally as you would to skin *because mucous membranes are usually moist and absorb ointment more quickly than skin does.*

The cover-up

- With certain medications (such as topical steroids), semipermeable dressings may be contraindicated. Check the medication's information and cautions. If you're applying a topical medication to the patient's hands or feet, cover the site with white cotton gloves for the hands or terry cloth scuffs for the feet.
- Inspect the treated area frequently for adverse effects such as signs of an allergic reaction. (See *Documenting use of skin medications.*)

Write it down

Documenting use of skin medications

In your notes, record:
- medication applied
- time, date, and site of application
- if patient refused
- if omitted or withheld and the reason
- patient education
- condition of the patient's skin at time of application.

Note subsequent effects of the medication, if any.

Transdermal medications

Through an adhesive patch or a measured dose of ointment applied to the skin, transdermal drugs deliver constant, controlled medication directly into the bloodstream for a prolonged systemic effect. Contraindications for transdermal drugs include skin allergies or skin reactions to the drug.

Transdermal drugs shouldn't be applied to broken or irritated skin *because they increase irritation* or to scarred or callused skin, *which might impair absorption.*

What you need

Patient's medication record and chart * gloves * prescribed medication (patch or ointment) * application strip or measuring paper (for nitroglycerin ointment) * adhesive tape * plastic wrap (optional for nitroglycerin ointment) or semipermeable dressing.

Getting ready

Verify the order on the patient's medication record by checking it against the doctor's order. Perform hand hygiene and, if necessary, don gloves.

How you do it

- Check the label on the medication and note the expiration date.
- Confirm the patient's identity using two patient identifiers.
- Explain the procedure to the patient and provide privacy.
- Remove any previously applied medication.

Applying transdermal ointment

- Place the prescribed amount of ointment on the application strip or measuring paper, taking care not to get any on your skin.
- Apply the strip to any dry, hairless area of the body but remember not to rub the ointment into the skin.
- Tape the strip and ointment to the skin.
- If desired, cover the application strip with the plastic wrap and tape the wrap in place.
- Instruct the patient to keep the area around the ointment as dry as possible.

Applying a transdermal patch

- Open the package and remove the patch.
- Without touching the adhesive surface, remove the clear plastic backing.
- Apply the patch to a dry, hairless area—behind the ear, for example, as with scopolamine. (See *Applying a transdermal medication patch.*)
- Write the date, time, and your initials on the dressing.

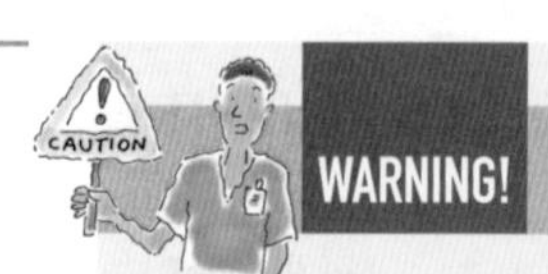

Transdermal drug pointers

Topical medications may cause skin irritation, such as pruritus and a rash. Watch for these symptoms and for adverse reactions to the specific medication.

A few examples

Transdermal nitroglycerin medications may cause headaches and, in elderly patients, orthostatic hypotension. Nitroglycerin ointment can be applied to chest area, abdomen, and front of thigh or back.

Know what the drug is that you are administering and be alert to its effects, implications, and adverse reactions.

Practice pointers

- Reapply daily transdermal medications at the same time every day *to ensure a continuous effect*, but alternate the application sites *to avoid skin irritation*. (See *Transdermal drug pointers.*)
- Review specific instructions with the patient regarding the type of medication, adverse effects, and interactions.
- Instruct the patient to keep the area around the patch as dry as possible. (See *Documenting transdermal medication use.*)

Eye medications

Eye medications typically include drops and ointments. Eyedrops can be used to anesthetize the eye, dilate the pupil for examination, and stain the cornea to identify corneal abrasions, scars, or anomalies. Eye medications can also be used to lubricate, treat certain eye conditions, and protect the vision of neonates.

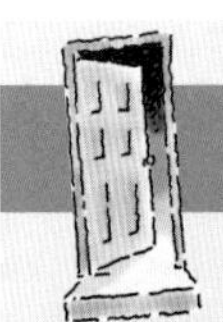

Home care connection

Applying a transdermal medication patch

If the patient receives medication by transdermal patch, instruct him in its proper use.

A layered affair

- Explain that the patch consists of several layers. The layer closest to his skin contains a small amount of the drug and allows prompt drug introduction into the bloodstream. The next layer controls drug release from the main portion of the patch. The third layer contains the main dose. The outermost layer consists of an aluminized polyester barrier.
- Teach the patient to apply the patch to the upper arm or chest and behind the ear. Warn him to avoid touching the gel or surrounding tape. Tell him to use a different site for each application to avoid skin irritation. If necessary, he can clip the hair at the site. Tell him to avoid any area that may cause uneven absorption, such as skin folds, scars, and calluses or any irritated or damaged skin areas. Also, tell him not to apply the patch below the elbow or knee.

More patch pointers

- Instruct the patient to wash his hands after application to remove any medication that may have rubbed off.
- Warn the patient not to get the patch wet. Tell him to discard it if it leaks or falls off and then to clean the site and apply a new patch at a different site.
- Instruct the patient to apply the patch at the same time at the prescribed interval. Bedtime application is ideal because body movement is reduced during the night. Finally, tell him to apply a new patch about 30 minutes before removing the old one.
- The patient must remove the old patch so he does not get a cumulative drug effect.

Write it down

Documenting transdermal medication use

In your notes, record:

- type of medication
- date, time, and site of application
- dose
- if patient refused the medication
- if omitted or withheld and the reason
- patient education
- adverse reactions
- patient's response to the medication
- removal of the old patch.

What you need

Prescribed eye medication ✳ patient's medication record and chart ✳ gloves ✳ warm water or normal saline solution ✳ sterile gauze pads ✳ facial tissues ✳ optional: ocular dressing.

Getting ready

Make sure the medication is labeled for ophthalmic use and check the expiration date. Remember to date the container the first time you use it and discard it in 2 weeks *to avoid contamination*.

Inspect ocular solutions for cloudiness, discoloration, and precipitation; don't use any solution that appears abnormal. If the tip of an eye ointment tube has crusted, turn the tip on a sterile gauze pad to remove the crust.

How you do it

- Verify the order on the patient's medication record by checking it against the doctor's order on his chart.
- Perform hand hygiene and check the medication label against the patient's medication record. Make sure you know which eye to treat because different medications or doses may be ordered for each eye.
- Confirm the patient's identity using two patient identifiers.
- Explain the procedure to the patient and provide privacy. Don gloves.
- If the patient is wearing an eye dressing, remove it by gently pulling it down and away from his forehead. Take care not to contaminate your hands.
- Remove any discharge by cleaning around the eye with sterile gauze pads moistened with warm water or normal saline solution, gently stroking from the inner to the outer canthus. Use a fresh sterile gauze pad for each stroke. Change gloves and remember to perform hand hygiene.
- Have the patient sit or lie in the supine position and tell him to tilt his head back and toward the side of the affected eye. Make sure the eyedrops are room temperature if they were refrigerated.

Instilling eye medications

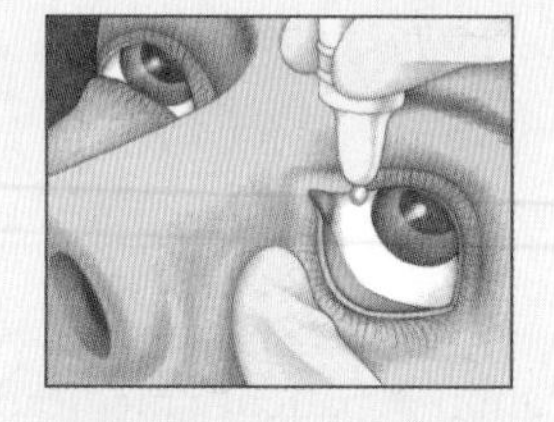

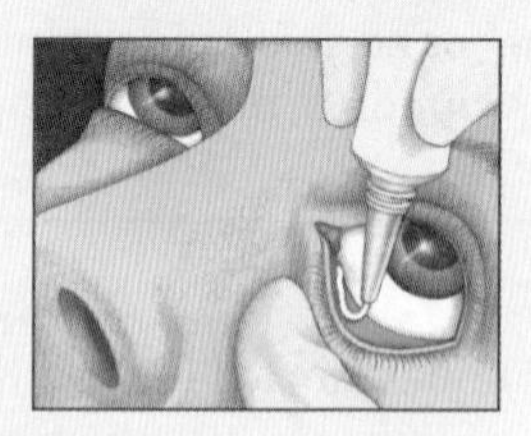

To instill eyedrops, pull the lower lid down to expose the conjunctival sac. Have the patient look up and away and then squeeze the prescribed number of drops into the sac. Release the patient's eyelid and have him blink to distribute the medication.

To apply an ointment, gently lay a thin strip of the medication along the conjunctival sac from the inner to the outer canthus. Avoid touching the tip of the tube to the patient's eye. Then release the eyelid and have the patient roll his eye behind closed lids to distribute the medication.

To apply an intraocular disc, perform hand hygiene and don gloves. Open package and press fingertip into the disc. Pull down on the patient's lower eyelid and place the disc between the iris and the conjunctival sac. Make sure the eyelid is pulled back up when finished. When removing the disc, pull down eyelid and pinch disc for removal.

Instilling eyedrops

- Remove the dropper cap from the medication container and draw the medication into it. Be careful to avoid contaminating the dropper tip or bottle top.
- Before instilling the eyedrops, instruct the patient to look up and away *to minimize the risk of touching the cornea with the dropper.*

Steady as she goes

- You can steady the hand holding the dropper by resting it against the patient's forehead. Then, with your other hand, gently pull down the lower lid and instill the drops in the conjunctival sac. (See *Instilling eye medications*.)
- Instruct the patient to blink to distribute the medicine.

Documenting use of eye medications

In your notes, record:

- medication instilled or applied
- eye or eyes treated
- date, time, and dose
- the patient refused the medication
- if it was omitted or withheld and the reason
- patient education
- adverse reactions
- patient's response.

Practice pointers

- After instilling eyedrops or ointment, do not wipe or blot the eye *because it will remove the medication.* If they eyes are tearing, only wipe under the eye with a clean tissue. Return the medication to the storage area, making sure you store it according to the label's instructions and then perform hand hygiene.

None in the duct

- When administering an eye medication that may be absorbed systemically (such as atropine), gently press your thumb on the inner canthus for 30 to 60 seconds after instilling drops while the patient closes his eyes. *This helps prevent medication from flowing into the tear duct.*
- To maintain the drug container's sterility, never touch the tip of the bottle or dropper to the patient's eyeball, lids, or lashes.
- Teach the patient to instill eye medications and to review the procedure, asking for a return demonstration. (See *Documenting use of eye medications*.)

Eardrops

Eardrops treat infection or inflammation, soften cerumen for removal, produce local anesthesia, or facilitate removal of an insect. Instillation of eardrops is usually contraindicated if the patient has a perforated eardrum, but it may be permitted with certain medications and adherence to sterile technique. Some conditions may prohibit instillation of certain medications into the ear such as hydrocortisone use in patients with viral or fungal infections.

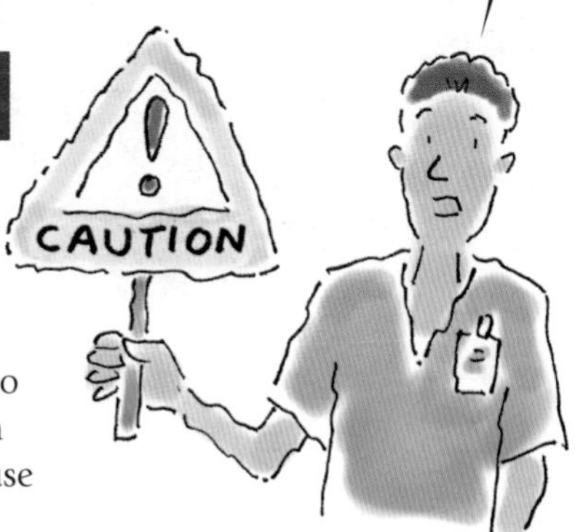
Yow! Test the medication's temperature by placing a drop on your wrist.
CAUTION

What you need

Prescribed eardrops * patient's medication record and chart * light source * facial tissue or cotton-tipped applicator * optional: cotton ball, bowl of warm water.

Getting ready

Verify the order on the patient's medication record by checking it against the doctor's order.

To avoid adverse reactions (such as vertigo, nausea, and pain), warm the medication to body temperature.

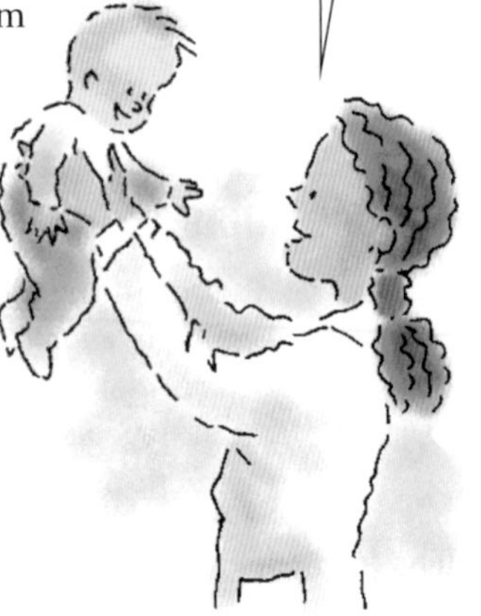
Be sure to pull the auricle down and back in a child under age 3.

How you do it

- Perform hand hygiene and confirm the patient's identity using two patient identifiers.
- Provide privacy, explain the procedure, and have the patient lie on the side opposite the affected ear.
- Straighten the patient's ear canal. For an adult, pull the auricle of the ear up and back. (See *Positioning the patient for eardrop instillation*.)

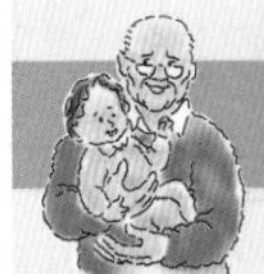

Ages and stages

Positioning the patient for eardrop instillation

Before instilling eardrops, have the patient lie on his side. Then straighten the patient's ear canal to help the medication reach the eardrum. For an adult, gently pull the auricle up and back. For an infant or a child under age 3, gently pull the auricle down and back because the ear canal is straighter at this age.

Adult

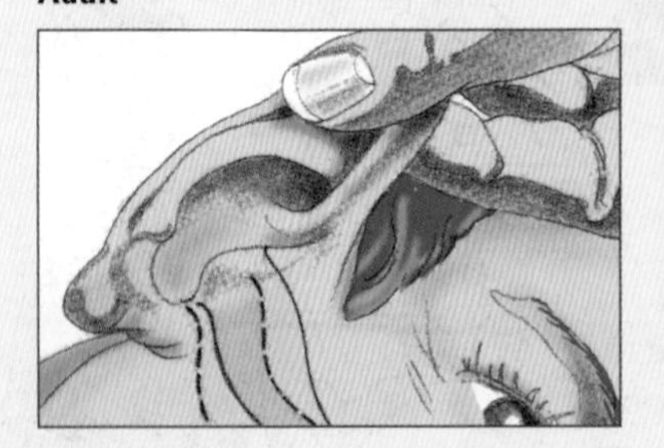

Child

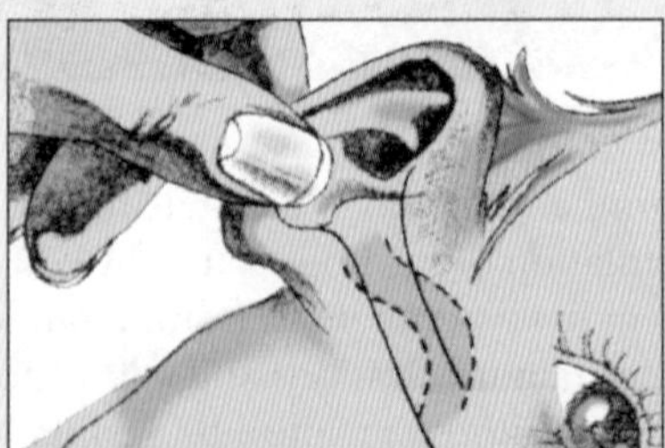

- Using a light source, examine the ear canal for drainage. If you find any, clean the canal with a tissue or cotton-tipped applicator *because drainage can reduce the medication's effectiveness.*
- Compare the label on the eardrops with the order on the patient's medication record. Check the label again while drawing the medication into the dropper. Check the label for the final time before returning the eardrops to the shelf or drawer.

Aim for the canal

- *To avoid damaging the ear canal with the dropper,* gently support the hand holding the dropper against the patient's head.
- Straighten the patient's ear canal once again and instill the ordered number of drops. *To avoid patient discomfort,* aim the dropper so that the drops fall against the sides of the ear canal, not on the eardrum.
- Hold the ear canal in position until you see the medication disappear down the canal, then release the ear.

Need a magazine?

- Instruct the patient to remain on his side for 5 to 10 minutes *to let the medication run down into the ear canal.*
- If ordered, tuck a cotton ball loosely into the opening of the ear canal *to prevent the medication from leaking out.* Be careful not to insert it too deeply into the canal *because this would prevent drainage of secretions and increase pressure on the eardrum. Cotton balls can be removed within 15 minutes.*
- Clean and dry the outer ear and, if ordered, repeat the procedure in the other ear after 5 to 10 minutes.
- Perform hand hygiene.

Documenting eardrop administration

In your notes, record:
- medication used
- ear treated
- date, time, and number of eardrops instilled
- patient refusal of the medication
- if the medication was omitted or withheld and the reason
- patient education
- signs or symptoms the patient experienced during the procedure, such as drainage, redness, vertigo, nausea, and pain.

Practice pointers

- *To prevent injury to the eardrum,* never insert a cotton-tipped applicator into the ear canal past the point where you can see the tip. After applying eardrops to soften the cerumen, irrigate the ear as ordered *to facilitate cerumen removal.*
- Teach the patient to instill the eardrops correctly so that he can continue treatment at home, if necessary. (See *Documenting eardrop administration*.)

Handheld oropharyngeal inhalers

Handheld inhalers include the metered-dose inhaler (or nebulizer), the turbo-inhaler, dry powder inhaler, and the nasal inhaler. These devices deliver topical medications to the respiratory tract, producing local and systemic effects. The mucosal lining of the respiratory tract absorbs the inhalant almost immediately.

Common inhalants are bronchodilators, used to improve airway patency and facilitate mucous drainage; mucolytics, which attain a high local concentration to liquefy tenacious bronchial secretions; and corticosteroids, used to decrease inflammation.

What you need

Patient's medication record and chart ✻ metered-dose inhaler, turbo-inhaler, or nasal inhaler ✻ prescribed medication ✻ normal saline solution (or another appropriate solution) for gargling ✻ optional: emesis basin. (See *Types of handheld inhalers*.)

How you do it

- Verify the order on the patient's medication record by checking it against the doctor's order.
- Perform hand hygiene.
- Check the label on the inhaler against the order on the medication record and verify the expiration date.
- Confirm the patient's identity using two patient identifiers.
- Explain the procedure to the patient.

Using a metered-dose inhaler

- Shake the inhaler bottle for 2 to 5 seconds and remove the mouthpiece and cap. Some metered-dose inhalers have a spacer built into the inhaler. Pull the spacer away from the section holding the medication canister until it clicks into place.
- Insert the metal stem on the bottle into the small hole on the flattened portion of the mouthpiece. Then turn the bottle upside down.
- Have the patient exhale, then place the mouthpiece in his mouth and close his lips around it.

Fill 'er up

- As you firmly push the bottle down against the mouthpiece, ask the patient to inhale slowly and to continue inhaling until his lungs feel full.
- Remove the mouthpiece from the patient's mouth, and tell him to hold his breath for 10 seconds and then exhale slowly through pursed lips.
- Rinse the mouthpiece with warm water *to prevent accumulation of residue.*

Types of handheld inhalers

Handheld inhalers use air under pressure to produce a mist containing medication. Drugs delivered in this form (such as mucolytics and bronchodilators) can travel deep into the lungs.

Inhalers with a spacer attachment provide greater therapeutic benefit for children and patients with poor coordination. A spacer attachment, an extension to the inhaler's mouthpiece, provides more dead air space for mixing medication.

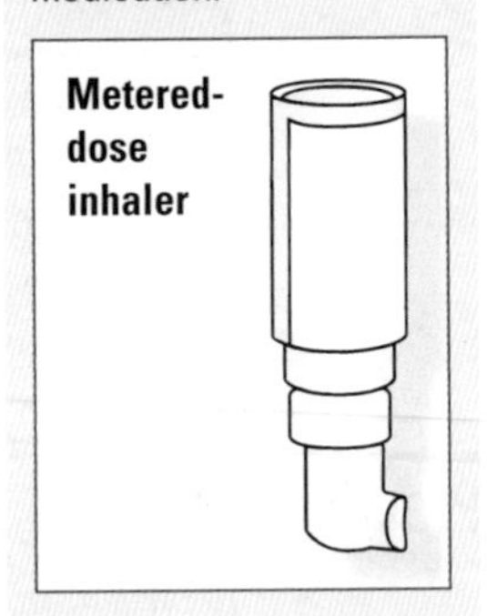

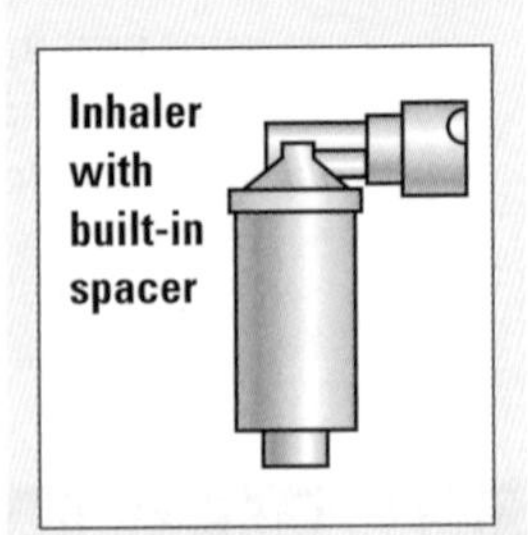

Using a turbo-inhaler

- Slide the sleeve away from the mouthpiece as far as possible and unscrew the tip of the mouthpiece by turning it counterclockwise.
- Firmly press the colored portion of the medication capsule into the propeller stem of the mouthpiece and screw the inhaler together again securely. Shake well.
- Holding the inhaler with the mouthpiece at the bottom, slide the sleeve all the way down and then up again *to puncture the capsule and release the medication*. Do this only once.
- Have the patient exhale and tilt his head back. Tell him to place the mouthpiece in his mouth, close his lips around it, and inhale once—quickly and deeply—through the mouthpiece.

Hold on there, pardner

- Tell the patient to hold his breath for 10 seconds, then remove the inhaler from the patient's mouth and have him exhale forcibly.
- Repeat the procedure until all the medication in the device is inhaled. Wait 20 to 30 seconds between inhalations.
- Discard the empty medication capsule, put the inhaler in its can, and secure the lid. Rinse the inhaler with warm water at least once a week. After 2 minutes, the patient may gargle.
- Teach the patient to initially use the inhaler in front of a mirror and watch for mist coming out of the inhaler. *If this happens, the medication is escaping into the air and not being inhaled.* The patient may need a spacer or further education.

Using dry powder inhaler

This inhaler comes in a disc shape. When ready to use, slide the side lever to load the medication into the mouthpiece. After placing lips on the mouth piece, instruct patient to take a deep breath and hold breath for 10 seconds.

Using a nasal inhaler

- Have the patient blow his nose *to clear his nostrils*.
- Shake the medication cartridge and then insert it in the adapter, removing the protective cap from the adapter tip.
- Hold the inhaler with your index finger on top of the cartridge and your thumb under the nasal adapter, pointing the adapter tip toward the patient.

Cover one, then go

- Have the patient tilt his head forward. Place the adapter tip into one nostril while occluding the other nostril with your finger.
- Instruct the patient to inhale gently as you press the adapter and the cartridge together firmly *to release a measured dose of medication*. Be sure to follow the manufacturer's instructions.

Documenting inhaler use

In your notes, record:
- inhalant administered
- dose
- time of inhaler use
- significant change in heart rate
- patient refusal of the medication
- omission or if the medication was withheld
- patient education
- other adverse reactions.

- Remove the inhaler and tell the patient to exhale through his mouth.
- Shake the inhaler and repeat the procedure in the other nostril.
- Remove the medication cartridge from the nasal inhaler and wash the nasal adapter in lukewarm water. Let the adapter dry thoroughly before reinserting the cartridge.

Practice pointers

- Teach the patient how to use the inhaler and explain that overdose can cause the medication to lose its effectiveness. Inform him of possible adverse reactions.
- If more than one inhalation is ordered, advise the patient to wait at least 2 minutes before repeating the procedure.

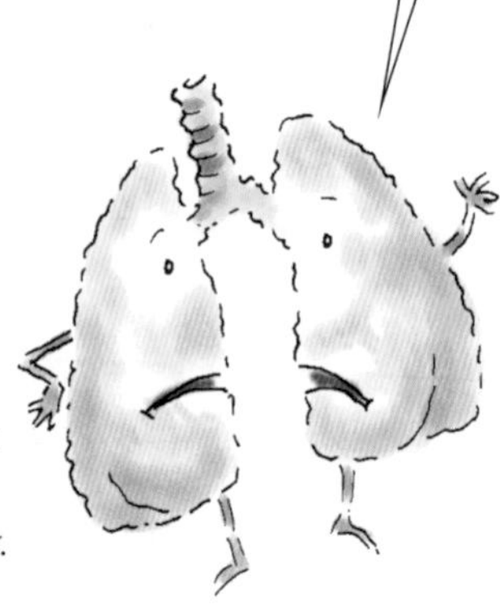

Steroid goes second

- If the patient is also using a steroid inhaler, instruct him to use the bronchodilator first and then wait 5 minutes before using the steroid. *This allows the bronchodilator to open the air passages for maximum effectiveness.* (See *Documenting inhaler use,* page 201.)
- Warn patients they can get hyperactive, anxious, and a rapid heart rate when using inhalers.
- Teach the patient the importance of using maintenance inhalers daily.
- Teach the patient to use the maintenance inhalers daily. The fast-acting inhaler (rescue inhaler) is used in addition if the patient is experiencing difficulty breathing.

Vaginal medications

Vaginal medications include suppositories, creams, gels, and ointments. These medications can be inserted as a topical treatment for infection or inflammation or as a contraceptive. Vaginal medications usually come with a disposable applicator and are most effective when the patient can lie down afterward to retain the medication.

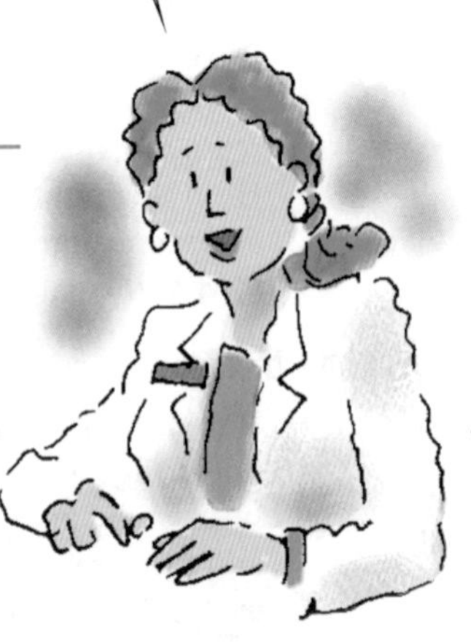
Give vaginal medications at bedtime, when the patient will be lying down.

What you need

Patient's medication record and chart ✳ prescribed medication and applicator, if necessary ✳ water-soluble lubricant ✳ gloves ✳ small sanitary pad.

Getting ready

If possible, plan to insert vaginal medications at bedtime, when the patient is recumbent.

Verify the order on the patient's medication record by checking it against the doctor's order. Confirm the patient's identity using two patient identifiers.

How you do it

- Perform hand hygiene, explain the procedure to the patient, and provide privacy.
- Ask the patient to void.
- Ask the patient if she would rather insert the medication herself. If so, provide appropriate instructions.
- Help her into the lithotomy position and expose only the perineum.

Inserting a suppository

- Remove the suppository from the wrapper and lubricate it with water-soluble lubricant.
- Put on gloves and expose the vagina.
- With an applicator or the forefinger of your free hand, insert the suppository about 3″ to 4″ (7.5 to 10 cm) into the vagina.

Inserting ointments, creams, gels, or foams

- Insert the plunger into the applicator. Then attach the applicator to the tube of medication.
- Gently squeeze the tube to fill the applicator with the prescribed amount of medication, detach the applicator from the tube, and lubricate the applicator.
- Put on gloves and expose the vagina.
- Insert the applicator 2″ to 3″ as you would a small suppository and administer the medication by depressing the plunger on the applicator.

When you're done

- Wash the applicator with soap and warm water and store it, unless it's disposable. If the applicator can be used again, label it *so that it will be used only for the same patient.*
- Remove and discard your gloves. Perform hand hygiene.

Practice pointers

- Refrigerate vaginal suppositories that melt at room temperature.
- *To prevent the medication from soiling the patient's clothing and bedding,* provide a sanitary pad.
- Help the patient return to a comfortable position and advise her to remain in bed as much as possible for the next several hours.

For the do-it-yourself type

- If possible, teach the patient how to insert the vaginal medication *because she may have to administer it herself after discharge*. Give her a patient teaching sheet if one is available.
- Instruct the patient not to wear a tampon after inserting vaginal medication and also to avoid sexual intercourse during treatment. (See *Documenting vaginal medications*.)

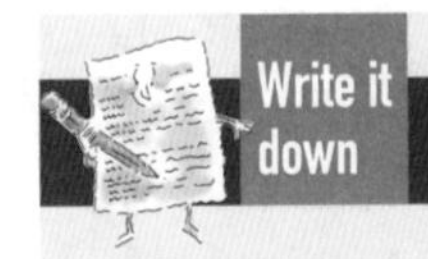

Documenting vaginal medications

In your notes, record:
- medication administered
- time and date
- adverse reactions
- vaginal drainage if present
- patient education
- other pertinent information.

Oral medications

Oral administration is usually the safest, most convenient, and least expensive method. For that reason, most drugs are administered orally in conscious patients who can swallow.

Drugs for oral administration are available in many forms: tablets, enteric-coated tablets, capsules, syrups, elixirs, oils, liquids, suspensions, powders, and granules. Some require special preparation before administration, such as mixing with juice to make them more palatable; oils, powders, and granules most often require such preparation.

What you need

Patient's medication record and chart * prescribed medication * medication cup * optional: appropriate vehicle, such as jelly or applesauce, for crushed pills commonly used with children or elderly patients, and juice, water, or milk for liquid medications; drinking straw; mortar and pestle for crushing pills.

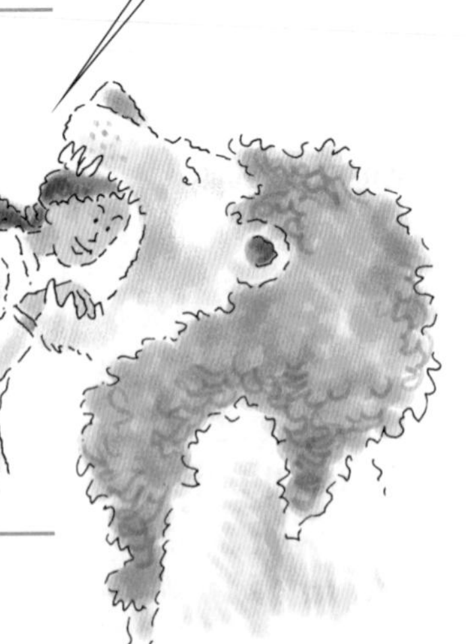
Oral administration is usually the safest, most convenient way to give drugs.

Getting ready

Verify the order on the patient's medication record by checking it against the doctor's order. Perform hand hygiene.

Check the label on the medication three times before administering it to the patient: when you take the container from the shelf, before you pour the medication into the cup, and again before returning the container to the shelf. If you're administering a unit-dose medication, check the label again at the bedside after pouring it and before discarding the wrapper.

How you do it

- Confirm the patient's identity using two patient identifiers.
- Assess the patient's condition, including level of consciousness and vital signs, as needed and indicated by the particular medication.

Need a drink?

- Give the patient his medication and liquid, as needed and indicated, *to aid swallowing, minimize adverse effects, or promote absorption*. If appropriate, some medications may be crushed *to facilitate swallowing*.

Close inspection

- Stay with the patient until he has swallowed the drug. If he seems confused or disoriented, check his mouth *to make sure he has swallowed it*. Return and reassess the patient's response within 1 hour after giving the medication.

Practice pointers

- Use care in measuring out the prescribed dose of liquid oral medication. (See *Measuring liquid medications*.)

Hey! Where did you get that?

- Never give a medication poured by someone else. Never return unwrapped or prepared medications to stock containers. Instead, dispose of them and notify the pharmacy. Keep in mind the

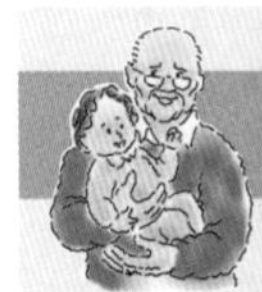

Ages and stages

Measuring liquid medications

Oral medications are relatively easy to give to infants because of their natural sucking instinct. Infants can take medications from the dropper or from pacifiers made to administer medications. For a liquid measured in drops, use only the dropper supplied with the medication.

Get an eyeful at eye level

To pour liquids, hold the medication cup at eye level. Use your thumb to mark off the correct level on the cup. Then set the cup down and read the bottom of the meniscus at eye level to ensure accuracy. If you've poured too much medication into the cup, discard the excess. Don't return it to the bottle.

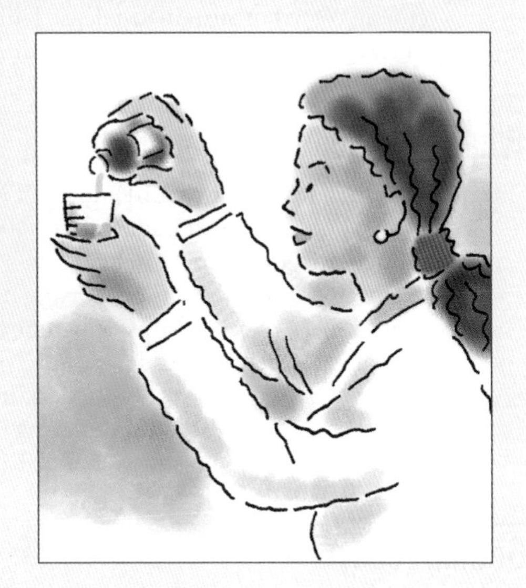

disposal of any narcotic drug must be cosigned by another nurse, as mandated by law.

- If the patient questions you about his medication or the dosage, check his medication record again. If the medication is correct, reassure him. Make sure you tell him about any changes in his medication or dosage and ask him to report anything he thinks may be an adverse effect.
    - Tell the patient what medication you are giving him and what it is for.
    - Teach the patient about any new medications and do a teach-back to verify understanding.

Plus, it's more fun

- If the patient can't swallow a whole tablet or capsule, ask the pharmacist if the drug is available in liquid form or if it can be administered by another route. If not, ask him if you can crush the tablet or open the capsule and mix it with food. Remember to contact the doctor for an order to change the administration route when necessary. (See *Documenting oral medications*.)

Documenting oral medications

In your notes, document:

- drug administration
- dose, date, and time
- patient education
- patient's reaction.

If the patient refuses a drug, document the refusal and notify the charge nurse and the patient's doctor, as needed. Also note if a drug was omitted or withheld for other reasons, such as radiology or laboratory tests, or if, in your judgment, the drug was contraindicated at the ordered time.

Sign out all narcotics given on the appropriate narcotics central record.

Nasogastric tubes

A nasogastric (NG) tube or gastrostomy tube allows direct instillation of medication into the gastrointestinal (GI) system of patients who can't ingest the drug orally. Before instilling the drug, you must check the patency and positioning of the tube. Oily medications and enteric-coated or sustained-release tablets (sublingual, chewable) or capsules are contraindicated for instillation through an NG tube.

What you need

Patient's medication record and chart ✻ prescribed medication ✻ towel or linen-saver pad ✻ 50- or 60-mL piston-type catheter-tip syringe ✻ feeding tubing ✻ two 4″ × 4″ gauze pads ✻ stethoscope ✻ gloves ✻ diluent ✻ cup for mixing medication and fluid ✻ spoon ✻ 50 mL of water ✻ gastrostomy tube and funnel, if needed ✻ optional: mortar and pestle, clamp.

For maximum control of suction, use a piston syringe instead of a bulb syringe. The liquid for diluting the medication can be juice, water, or a nutritional supplement.

Getting ready

Gather all necessary equipment at the bedside. Liquids should be at room temperature *so abdominal cramping doesn't occur.*

How you do it

- Verify the order on the patient's medication record by checking it against the doctor's order, perform hand hygiene, and don gloves. Check the label on the medication before preparing it for administration.

Liquid or crushed

- Request liquid forms of medications, if available. However, if the prescribed medication is in tablet form, crush the tablets *to dilute them with at least 30 mL of water unless otherwise specified* and bring the medication and equipment to the patient's bedside. All liquids should be at room temperature. *Cold liquids instilled in the enteral tube can cause abdominal cramping.*
- Explain the procedure to the patient, provide privacy, and confirm the patient's identity using two patient identifiers.
- Unpin the tube from the patient's gown and drape his chest with a towel or linen-saver pad.
- Elevate the head of the bed from 30 degrees to Fowler's position, as tolerated, to reduce the risk of aspiration.
- After unclamping the tube, confirm placement of the NG tube. (See "Nasogastric tube care," in chapter 8, page 389.)
- After you've established that the tube is patent and in the correct position, clamp the tube, detach the syringe, and lay the end of the tube on the 4″ × 4″ gauze pad.

Mix and stir

- Mix the crushed tablets or liquid medication with water unless otherwise specified. If the medication is in capsule form, open the capsules and empty their contents into the water. Pour liquid medications directly into the water. Stir well with the spoon. (If the medication was in tablet form, make sure the particles are small enough to pass through the eyes at the distal end of the tube.)
- Reattach the syringe, without the piston, to the end of the tube and open the clamp.
- Deliver the medication slowly and steadily. (See *Giving medications through an NG tube*, page 208.)

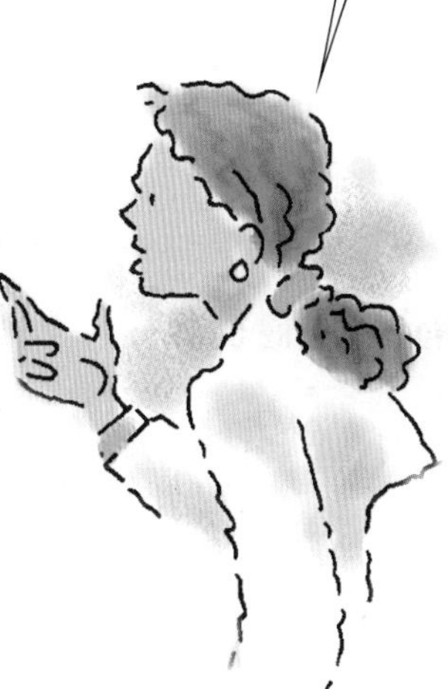
Slow and steady—that's the rule when delivering drugs through an NG tube.

How goes the flow?

- If the medication flows smoothly, slowly add more until the entire dose has been given. If the medication doesn't flow properly, don't force it. If it's too thick, dilute it with water. If you suspect that tube placement is inhibiting the flow, stop the procedure and reevaluate tube placement.

Giving medications through an NG tube

To give medication through an NG tube, hold the NG tube at a level above the patient's nose. Then pour up to 30 mL of diluted medication into the syringe barrel. For a child, irrigate the tube using only 15 to 30 mL of water.

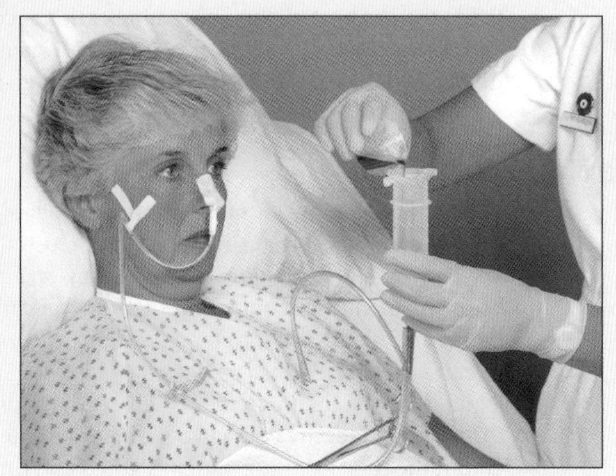

No air allowed

To prevent air from entering the patient's stomach, hold the tube at a slight angle, and add more medication before the syringe empties. If necessary, raise the tube slightly higher to increase the flow rate. After you have given the whole dose, position the patient on his right side, head slightly elevated, to minimize esophageal reflux.

- Watch the patient's reaction throughout the instillation. If he shows any sign of discomfort, stop the procedure immediately.
- As the last of the medication flows out of the syringe, start to irrigate the tube by adding 30 to 50 mL of water. *Irrigation clears medication from the sides of the tube and from the distal end, reducing the risk of clogging. If administering more than one medication, flush between each medication with 15 to 30 mL of water to maintain patency of the tube.*
- When the water stops flowing, quickly clamp the tube. Detach the syringe and dispose of it.
- Fasten the NG tube to the patient's gown, remove the towel or linen-saver pad, and replace linens as necessary.

No time to lie down

- Leave the patient in Fowler's position or have him lie on his right side with the head of the bed partially elevated for at least 30 minutes to 1 hour *to facilitate flow and prevent esophageal reflux.*
- If the patient has a gastrostomy feeding button, you may give a tablet or capsule dissolved in 30 to 50 mL of warm water (15 to 30 mL for children) and administer it if liquid form isn't available. Use the same procedure as for feeding the patient through the button. Draw up the dissolved medication into a syringe and inject it into the feeding tube. Withdraw the medication syringe, flush with 50 mL of warm water, replace the safety plug, and keep the patient at a 30-degree angle for 30 minutes to 1 hour.

Practice pointers

- The procedure is contraindicated if the tube is obstructed or improperly positioned, if the patient is vomiting around the tube, or if his bowel sounds are absent.
- Only warm water should be used as a diluent unless otherwise specified. *Cold liquid instilled in the enteral tube can cause abdominal cramping.*
- Dilute liquid medications that can cause local irritation such as potassium.
- Consult with a pharmacist if you are uncertain whether a medication can be crushed or given through an enteral tube.
- Only use enough diluent to dissolve the medication *to avoid fluid overload.*

Not on a full stomach

- *To prevent instillation of too much fluid* (for an adult, more than 400 mL of liquid at one time), don't schedule the drug instillation with the patient's regular tube feeding, if possible. If you must schedule a tube feeding and medication instillation simultaneously, give the medication first. Remember to avoid giving foods that interact adversely with the drug.
- If the patient receives continuous tube feedings, stop the feeding and check the quantity of residual stomach contents. If it's more than 50% of the previous hour's intake, withhold the medication and feeding and notify the doctor.
- If the NG tube is attached to suction, be sure to turn off the suction for 20 to 30 minutes after administering medication. (See *Documenting use of NG tube medications.*)

Write it down

Documenting use of NG tube medications

In your notes, record:

- instillation of medication
- date and time of instillation
- if the patient refuses the medication
- if omitted or if withheld and the reason
- patient education
- dose
- patient's tolerance of the procedure.

On the intake and output sheet, note the amount of fluid instilled.

Buccal, sublingual, and translingual medications

Certain drugs are given buccally, sublingually, or translingually to prevent their destruction or transformation in the stomach or small intestine. These drugs act quickly because the oral mucosa's thin epithelium and abundant vasculature allow direct absorption into the bloodstream.

What you need

Patient's medication record and chart ✳ prescribed medication ✳ medication cup.

Getting ready

Verify the order on the patient's medication record by checking it against the doctor's order on his chart. Perform hand hygiene and explain the procedure to the patient.

Check the label on the medication and the expiration date.

How you do it

- Confirm the patient's identity using two patient identifiers.

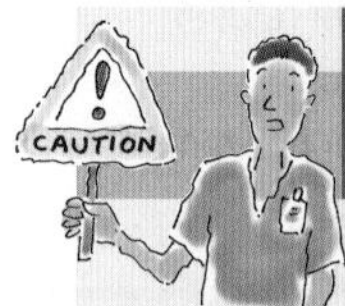

WARNING!

Placing drugs in the oral mucosa

Buccal and sublingual administration routes allow some drugs, such as nitroglycerin and methyltestosterone, to enter the bloodstream rapidly without being degraded in the GI tract.

What to do

To give a drug buccally, insert it between the patient's cheek and gum (as shown below left). Ask him to close his mouth and hold the tablet against his cheek until the tablet is absorbed.

To give a drug sublingually, place it under the patient's tongue (as shown below right) and ask him to leave it there until it's dissolved.

Problem solving

Some buccal medications may irritate the mucosa. Alternate sides of the mouth for repeat doses to prevent continuous irritation of the same site. Sublingual medications—such as nitroglycerin—may cause a tingling sensation under the tongue. If the patient finds this annoying, try placing the drug in the buccal pouch instead.

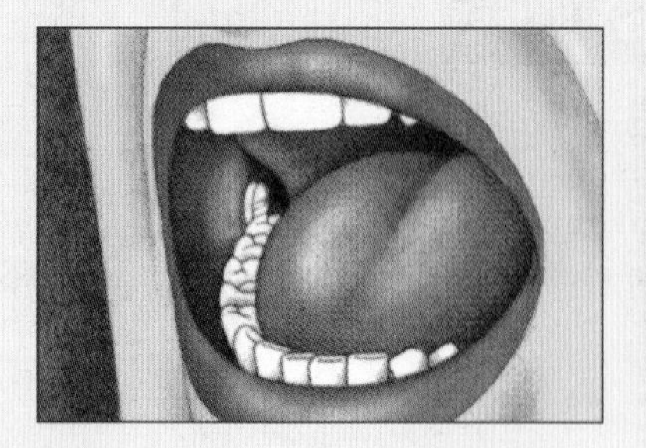

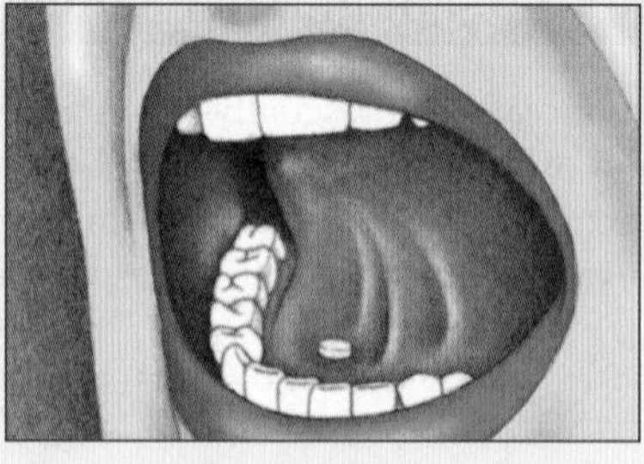

Write it down

Documenting use of buccal, sublingual, and translingual medications

In your notes, record:

- medication administered
- dose
- date and time
- if patient refuses
- if omitted or withheld and the reason
- patient education
- patient's reaction.

Buccal and sublingual administration

- For buccal administration, place the tablet in the buccal pouch, between the cheek and gum. For sublingual administration, place the tablet under the patient's tongue. The cheek and the area under the tongue have many small blood vessels and capillaries. The medication can be absorbed directly into the bloodstream without going through the digestive system. (See *Placing drugs in the oral mucosa.*)
- Instruct the patient to keep the medication in place until it dissolves and not to chew or touch it with his tongue *to prevent accidental swallowing.*

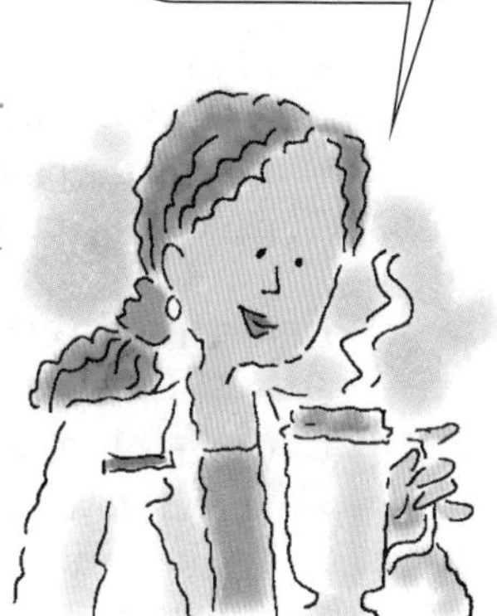
Don't drink liquids for 1 hour after taking buccal medication. Some drugs take up to an hour to be absorbed after buccal administration.

Practice pointers

- Tell the angina patient to wet the nitroglycerin tablet with saliva and to keep it under his tongue until it has been fully absorbed. (See *Documenting use of buccal, sublingual, and translingual medications.*)
  - Open sores in the mouth can be further irritated by the medication.
  - Eating, drinking, and smoking can have an effect on how much medication is absorbed and its effectiveness.

Rectal suppositories and ointments

A rectal suppository is a small, solid, medicated mass that may be inserted to stimulate peristalsis or defecation; relieve pain, vomiting, or local irritation; reduce fever; or induce relaxation. Rectal suppositories melt at body temperature and are absorbed slowly. They may be used when the medication interacts poorly with digestive enzymes or have a taste too offensive for oral use.

An ointment is a semisolid medication used to produce local effects. It may be applied externally to the anus or internally to the rectum. Rectal ointments commonly contain drugs that reduce inflammation or relieve pain and itching.

What you need

Rectal suppository or tube of ointment and applicator ✱ patient's medication record and chart ✱ gloves ✱ water-soluble lubricant ✱ 4″ × 4″ gauze pads ✱ optional: bedpan.

Getting ready

Store rectal suppositories in the refrigerator until needed *to prevent softening and decreased effectiveness.* A softened suppository is also difficult to handle and insert. To harden it again, hold the suppository (in its wrapper) under cold running water.

How you do it

- Verify the order on the patient's medication record by checking it against the doctor's order.
- Make sure the label on the medication package agrees with the medication order. Read the label again before you open the wrapper and again as you remove the medication. Check the expiration date.
- Perform hand hygiene and confirm the patient's identity using two patient identifiers.
- Explain the procedure and the purpose of the medication to the patient and provide privacy.

Inserting a rectal suppository

- Place the patient on his left side in Sims' position. Drape him with the bedcovers to expose only the buttocks.
- Put on gloves, remove the suppository from its wrapper, and lubricate it with water-soluble lubricant.
- Lift the patient's upper buttock with your nondominant hand and have him take slow deep breaths.

Here's the tough part

- Using your index finger, insert the suppository—tapered end first—about 4″ (8.6 cm), until you feel it pass the internal anal sphincter. Try to direct the tapered end toward the side of the rectum *so that it contacts the membranes.*
- Encourage him to retain the suppository for the appropriate length of time to be effective.
- Remove and discard your gloves. Perform hand hygiene.

Applying rectal ointment

- Put on gloves and squeeze the directed amount of ointment slowly onto a gauze pad or your gloved hand and *apply externally* over the anal area.
- *To apply internally,* attach the applicator to the tube of ointment and coat the applicator with water-soluble lubricant.
- Lift the patient's upper buttock with your nondominant hand *to expose the anus* and have him take several deep breaths through his mouth *to relax the anal sphincters and reduce anxiety or discomfort during insertion.*
- Gently insert the applicator, directing it toward the umbilicus, and slowly squeeze the tube to inject about 1″ (2.5 cm) of the medication.

- Remove the applicator and place a folded 4″ × 4″ gauze pad between the patient's buttocks *to absorb excess ointment.*
- Detach the applicator from the tube and recap it. Then clean the applicator thoroughly with soap and warm water.

Practice pointers

- Because insertion of a rectal suppository may stimulate the vagus nerve, this procedure is contraindicated in patients with potential cardiac arrhythmias. It may have to be avoided in patients with recent rectal or prostate surgery, rectal bleeding, rectal prolapse, or very low platelet counts *because of the risk of local trauma or discomfort during insertion.*

Mind the blinking light

- Make sure the patient's call button is handy and watch for his signal *because he may be unable to suppress the urge to defecate.*
- Be sure to inform the patient that the suppository may discolor his next bowel movement. (See *Documenting use of rectal medications.*)

Documenting use of rectal medications

In your notes, record:
- administration time
- dose
- if patient refuses
- if omitted or withheld and the reason
- patient education
- patient's response.

Intradermal injection

Intradermal injections are administered in small volumes (usually 0.5 mL or less) into the outer layers of the skin to produce a local effect, as in allergy or tuberculin testing.

The ventral forearm is the most commonly used site for intradermal injection because of its easy accessibility and lack of hair. In extensive allergy testing, the outer aspect of the upper arms may be used as well as the area of the back located between the scapulae. (See *Intradermal injection sites,* page 214.)

What you need

Patient's medication record and chart * tuberculin syringe with a 25G × 5/8″; 26G × 3/8″; 27G × 1/2″ needle * prescribed medication * gloves * alcohol pads.

Getting ready

Verify the order on the patient's medication record by checking it against the doctor's orders. Inspect the medication to make sure it isn't abnormally discolored or cloudy and doesn't contain precipitates.

Intradermal injection sites

The most common intradermal injection site is the ventral forearm. Other sites (indicated by dotted areas) include the upper chest, upper arm, and shoulder blades. Skin in these areas is usually lightly pigmented, thinly keratinized, and relatively hairless, facilitating detection of adverse reactions.

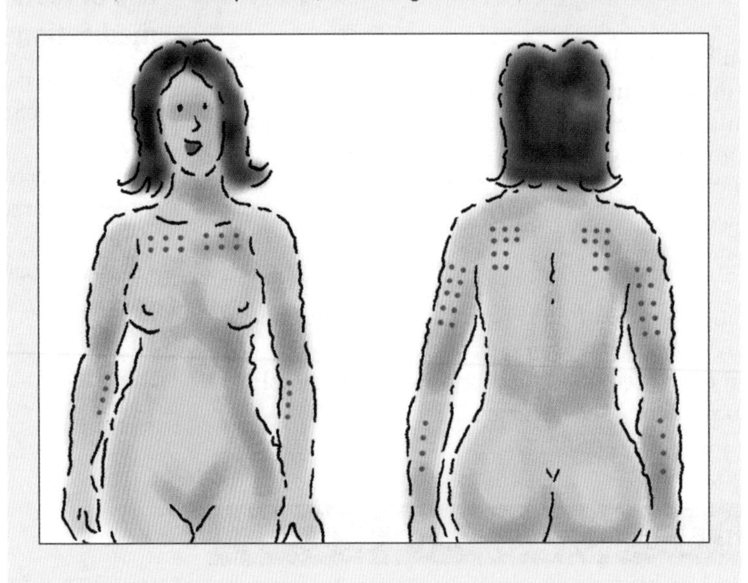

Perform hand hygiene. Choose equipment appropriate to the prescribed medication and injection site and make sure it works properly. Check the medication label against the patient's medication record. Read the label again as you draw up the medication for injection.

How you do it

- Verify the patient's identity using two patient identifiers.
- Check for allergies.
- Tell him where you'll be giving the injection.
- Instruct the patient to sit up and to extend his arm and support it on a flat surface, with the ventral forearm exposed.
- Don gloves.

Cleanliness first

- With an alcohol pad, clean the surface of the ventral forearm about two or three fingerbreadths distal to the antecubital space.

Be sure the test site you've chosen is free from hair or blemishes. Allow the skin to dry completely before administering the injection.

- While holding the patient's forearm in your hand, stretch the skin taut with your thumb.
- With your free hand, hold the needle at a 10- to 15-degree angle to the patient's arm, with its bevel up.

Mark of success

- Insert the needle about 1/8″ (0.3 cm) below the epidermis at sites 2″ (5 cm) apart. Stop when the needle's bevel tip is under the skin and inject the antigen slowly. You should feel some resistance as you do this, and a wheal should form as you inject the antigen. (See *Giving an intradermal injection.*) If no wheal forms, you have injected the antigen too deeply; withdraw the needle and administer another test dose at least 2″ from the first site.
- Withdraw the needle at the same angle at which it was inserted. Don't rub the site *because this could irritate the underlying tissue, affecting test results. Place a gauze dressing on the area.*

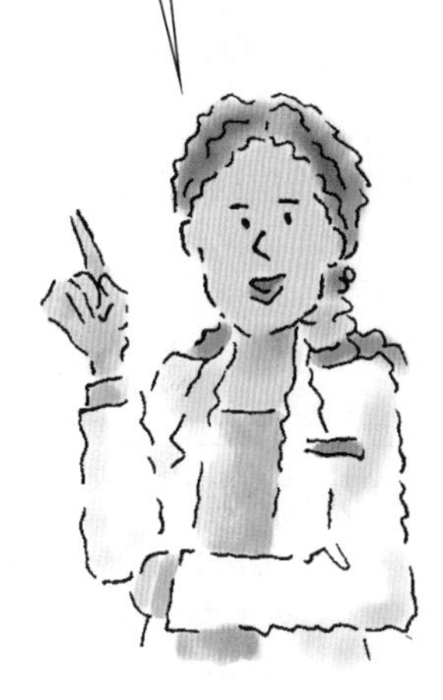
Watch for a wheal to form after giving an intradermal injection.

Circle marks the spot

- Circle each test site with a marking pen and label each site according to the recall antigen given. Instruct the patient to refrain from washing off the circles until the test is completed.
- Dispose of needles and syringes according to your facility's policy and discard your gloves.
- Assess the patient's response to the skin testing in 24 to 48 hours.
- If the injection is given for tuberculosis screening, the injection area is to be read within 48 to 72 hours by a nurse or physician.

Giving an intradermal injection

To give an intradermal injection, first secure the forearm. Then insert the needle at a 10- to 15-degree angle so that it just punctures the skin's surface. The antigen should raise a small wheal as it's injected.

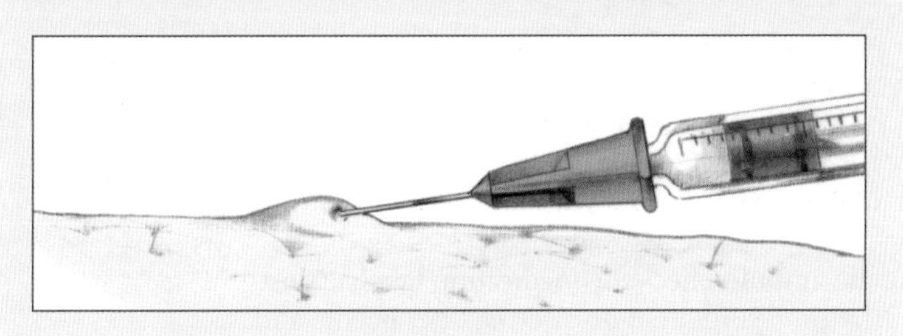

Practice pointers

- In patients who are hypersensitive to the test antigens, a severe anaphylactic response can result. This requires immediate epinephrine injection and other emergency resuscitation procedures. Be especially alert after giving a test dose of penicillin or tetanus antitoxin. (See *Documenting intradermal injection.*)

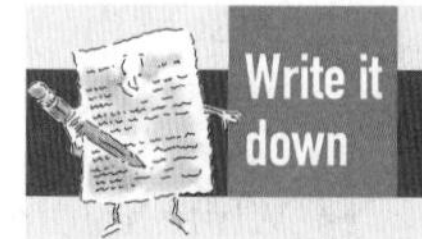

Documenting intradermal injection

On the patient's medication record, document:
- type and amount of medication given
- time it was given
- injection site
- patient education
- skin reactions and other adverse reactions.

Subcutaneous injection

Subcutaneous (S.C.) injections are delivered into the adipose (fatty) tissues beneath the skin. The result is a slower and more sustained drug administration than intramuscular injections. Small doses of medication less than 2 mL are given by this route. There's also less trauma to tissue and less risk of striking large blood vessels and nerves. Drugs and solutions are injected through short needles; common sites are the upper arms, anterior thigh, abdomen, upper hips, buttocks, and upper back. (See *Subcutaneous injection sites.*)

What you need

Patient's medication record and chart ✻ prescribed medication ✻ 25G to 27G 5/8″ to ½″ needle ✻ gloves ✻ 1- or 3-mL syringe ✻ alcohol pads.

Getting ready

Verify the order on the patient's medication record by checking it against the doctor's order. Also note whether the patient has any allergies, especially before the first dose.

Check the prescribed medication for color, clarity, and the expiration date. Choose equipment appropriate to the prescribed medication and injection site and make sure it works properly. Check for allergies to the medication.

If you use ampules . . .

- Perform hand hygiene.
- Wrap an alcohol pad around the ampule's neck and snap off the top, directing the force away from your body.
- Attach a filter needle to the needle and withdraw the medication.
- Tap the syringe *to clear air from it.*
- Before discarding the ampule, check the medication label against the patient's medication record, then discard the filter needle and the ampule.
- Attach the appropriate needle to the syringe.

Subcutaneous injection sites

Potential S.C. injection sites (indicated by the dotted areas) include the fat pads on the abdomen, upper hips, upper back, and lateral upper arms and anterior thighs.

Preferred injection sites for insulin are the arms, abdomen, thighs, and buttocks. For heparin, the preferred injection site is the lower abdominal fat pad, just below the umbilicus.

If repeated, rotate

For S.C. injections administered repeatedly, such as insulin, rotate sites. Choose one injection site in one area, move to a corresponding injection site in the next area, and so on. When returning to an area, choose a new site in that area.

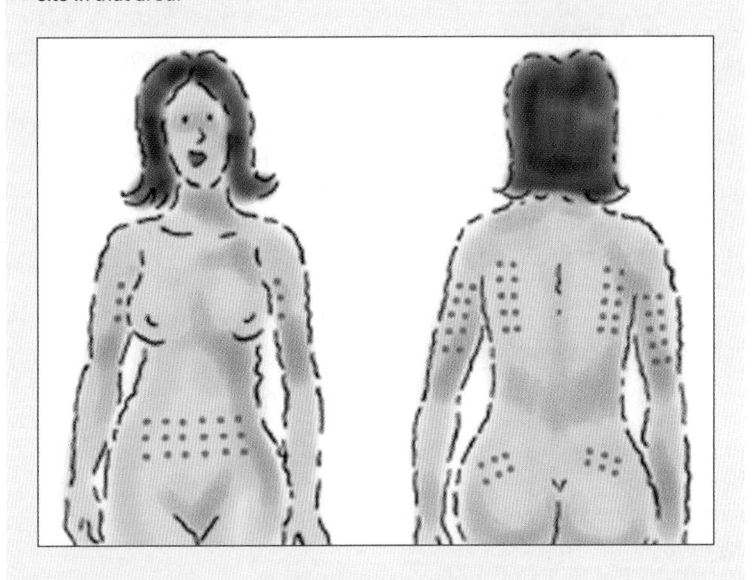

But for vials . . .

- Perform hand hygiene
- Reconstitute powdered drugs according to instructions, making sure all crystals have dissolved in the solution.
- Warm the vial by rolling it between your palms *to help the drug dissolve faster.*
- Wipe the stopper with an alcohol pad and draw up the prescribed amount of medication.
- Read the medication label as you select the medication, as you draw it up, and after you've drawn it up *to verify the correct dosage.*

How you do it

- Confirm the patient's identity using two patient identifiers.
- Provide privacy, explain the procedure to the patient, and perform hand hygiene.
- Select an appropriate injection site and rotate sites for repeated injections using different areas of the body unless contraindicated.
- Don gloves; position and drape the patient.
- Clean the injection site with an alcohol sponge, beginning at the center of the site and moving outward in a circular motion. Allow the skin to dry.

Grasp and lift

- Loosen the protective needle sheath. With your nondominant hand, grasp the skin around the injection site firmly to elevate the subcutaneous tissue.
- Holding the syringe in your dominant hand, insert the loosened needle sheath between the fourth and fifth fingers of your other hand while still pinching the skin around the injection site. Pull back the syringe with your dominant hand to uncover the needle.
- Position the needle with its bevel up and tell the patient he'll feel a needle prick.
- Insert the needle quickly in one motion at a 45- or 90-degree angle. (See *Technique for subcutaneous injections*.)

Check and inject

- Pull back the plunger slightly to check for blood return; if none appears, inject the drug slowly.
- After injection, remove the needle gently but quickly at the same angle used for insertion.
- Cover the site with an alcohol pad and apply a gauze dressing (delete massage gently); check the site for bleeding and bruising.
- Dispose of equipment according to your facility's policy.

Technique for subcutaneous injections

Before giving the injection, elevate subcutaneous tissue at the site by grasping it firmly. Insert the needle at a 45- or 90-degree angle to the skin surface, depending on needle length and the amount of subcutaneous tissue at the site. Some medications, such as heparin, should always be injected at a 90-degree angle.

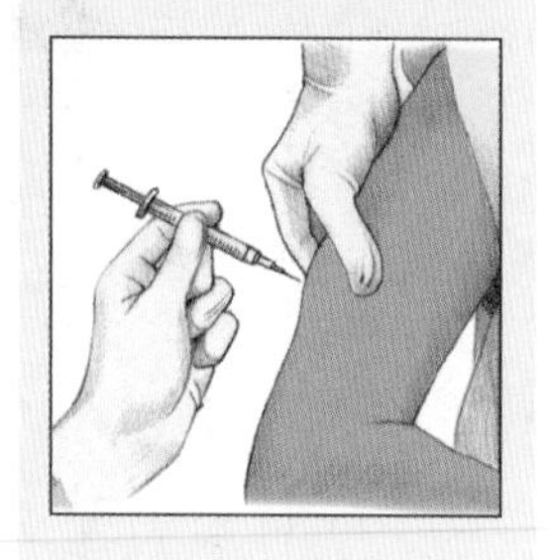

Practice pointers

- Never use medication that's cloudy or discolored or contains a precipitate unless the manufacturer's instructions allow it. If in doubt, check with the pharmacist.
- If blood appears on aspiration, withdraw the needle, prepare another syringe, and repeat the procedure.
- Don't aspirate for blood return when giving insulin or heparin. It isn't necessary with insulin and may cause a hematoma with heparin.
- To avoid needlestick injuries, don't resheath the needle.

Adjust for length

- When using prefilled syringes, adjust the angle and depth of insertion according to needle length.
- When combining insulins in a syringe, follow the facility's policy regarding which insulin to draw first. Remember to roll and invert the bottle gently when administering insulin.

Heparin hints

- The preferred site for heparin injection is the lower abdominal fat pad, 2″ (5 cm) beneath the umbilicus, between the right and left iliac crests.
- When injecting heparin, leave the needle in place for 10 seconds and then withdraw it; apply ice for 5 minutes if the patient bruises easily. Also, to prevent hemorrhages and bruising, don't rub or massage the site after the injection. (See *Documenting subcutaneous injection*.)
- If giving heparin in a prefilled syringe, do not expel the air bubble.

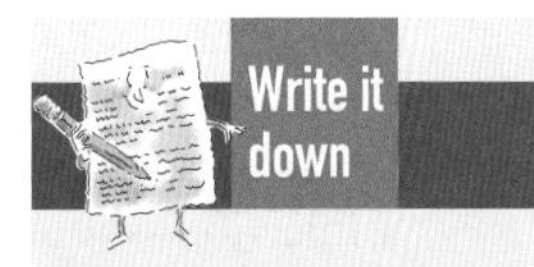
Write it down

Documenting subcutaneous injection

In your notes, record:
- time and date of the injection
- medication and dose administered
- injection site
- patient education
- if the patient refuses
- if omitted or withheld and the reason
- patient's reaction.

I.M. injection

Intramuscular (I.M.) injections deposit medication deep into muscle tissue. This route of administration provides rapid systemic action and absorption of relatively large doses (up to 5 mL in appropriate sites). Because there is a risk for injecting the medication into the blood vessels, the proper anatomic location of the injection site is important.

I.M. injections are recommended for patients who are uncooperative or can't take medication orally and for drugs that are altered by digestive juices. Because muscle tissue has few sensory nerves, I.M. injection allows less painful administration of irritating drugs.

What you need

Patient's medication record and chart ✳ prescribed medication ✳ diluent or filter needle, if needed ✳ 3- or 5-mL syringe ✳ 18G to 25G 1″ to 3″ needle ✳ gloves ✳ alcohol pads.

The prescribed medication must be sterile and the needle may be packaged separately or already attached to the syringe. Needles used for I.M. injections are longer than subcutaneous needles *because they must reach deep into the muscle.* Needle length also depends on the injection site, patient's size, and

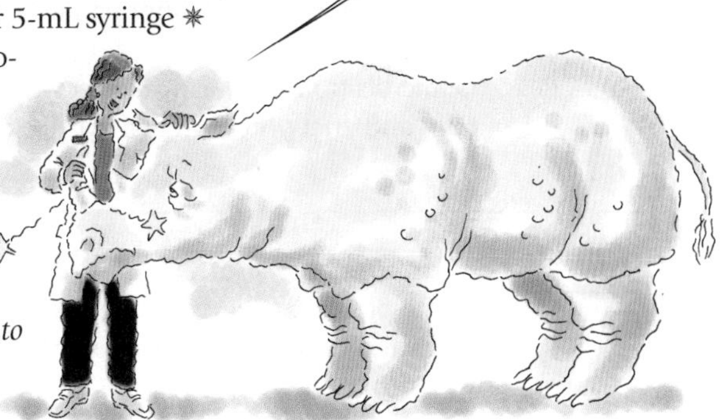
I told you that injection might hurt a little bit.

amount of subcutaneous fat covering the muscle. For example, a thin patient may need a needle length of 5/8″ to 1″, whereas an overweight person may need a 11/4 to 11/2 length. The needle gauge for I.M. injections should be larger to accommodate viscous solutions and suspensions.

Getting ready

Verify the order on the patient's medication record by checking it against the doctor's order. Also note whether the patient has any allergies, especially before the first dose.

Check the prescribed medication for color, clarity, and the expiration date.

Choose equipment appropriate to the prescribed medication and injection site and make sure it works properly.

For single-dose ampules

- Perform hand hygiene.
- Wrap an alcohol pad around the ampule's neck and snap off the top, directing the force away from your body.
- Attach a filter needle to the syringe and withdraw the medication.
- Tap the syringe *to clear air from it.*
- Before discarding the ampule, check the medication label against the patient's medication record, then discard the filter needle and the ampule.
- Attach the appropriate needle to the syringe.

For single-dose or multidose vials

- Perform hand hygiene.
- Reconstitute powdered drugs according to instructions, making sure all crystals have dissolved in the solution.
- Warm the vial by rolling it between your palms *to help the drug dissolve faster.*
- Wipe the stopper with an alcohol pad and draw up the prescribed amount of medication.
- Read the medication label as you select the medication, as you draw it up, and after you've drawn it up *to verify the correct dosage.*

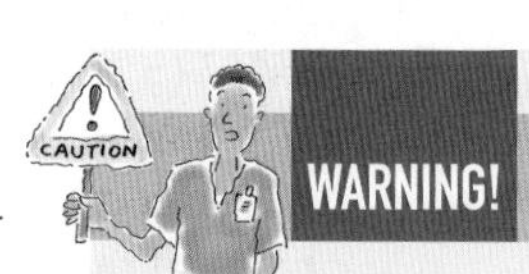

I.M. injection complications

If blood appears in the syringe on aspiration, the needle is in a blood vessel. Stop the injection, withdraw the needle, prepare another injection with new equipment, and inject another site. Don't inject the bloody solution.

If you miss

Accidentally injecting concentrated or irritating medications into subcutaneous tissue, or other areas where they can't be fully absorbed, can cause sterile abscesses. Failing to rotate sites in patients who require repeated injections may lead to deposits of unabsorbed medications. Such deposits can reduce the desired pharmacologic effect and cause abscess formation or tissue fibrosis.

How you do it

- Confirm the patient's identity using two patient identifiers.
- Provide privacy, explain the procedure to the patient, and perform hand hygiene.

- Select an appropriate injection site. The ventrogluteal and the vastus lateralis are the most common and safest I.M. site to use. The deltoid muscle may be used for a small-volume injection (2 mL or less). The dorsogluteal is not a common injection site because of the location of the sciatic nerve. If the injection is not in the proper area, damage to this nerve can cause partial or permanent paralysis. Remember to rotate injection sites for patients who require repeated injections. (See *Locating I.M. injection sites*, page 222.)
- Position and drape the patient appropriately, making sure the site is well exposed and that lighting is adequate.
- Loosen the protective needle sheath, but don't remove it.

Knock before entering

- Clean the skin at the site with an alcohol pad in a circular motion to a circumference of about 2″ (5 cm) from the injection site and allow the skin to dry. Keep the alcohol pad for later use.
- Don gloves. With the thumb and index finger of your nondominant hand, gently stretch the skin of the injection site taut.
- While you hold the syringe in your dominant hand, remove the needle sheath by slipping it between the free fingers of your nondominant hand.

Go deep

- Position the syringe at a 90-degree angle to the skin surface, with the needle a few inches from the skin. Tell the patient that he'll feel a prick as you insert the needle. Then quickly and firmly thrust the needle (use a darting motion) through the skin and subcutaneous tissue, deep into the muscle.
- Support the syringe with your nondominant hand, if desired. Pull back slightly on the plunger with your dominant hand to aspirate for blood. (See *I.M. injection complications*.) If no blood appears, *slowly* inject the medication into the muscle. *A slow, steady injection rate allows the muscle to distend gradually and accept the medication under minimal pressure.* You should feel little or no resistance against the force of the injection.
- After the injection, gently but quickly remove the needle at a 90-degree angle.

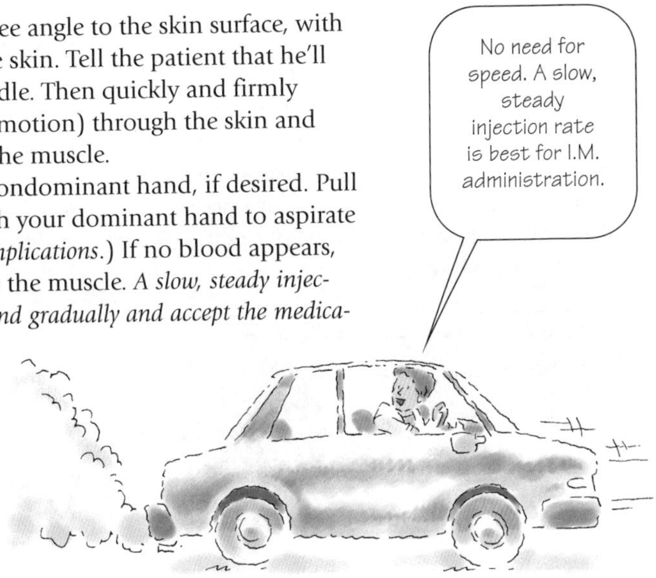

No need for speed. A slow, steady injection rate is best for I.M. administration.

Postaction rubdown

- Using a gloved hand, cover the injection site immediately with the used alcohol pad and apply gentle pressure.

Locating I.M. injection sites

The most common I.M. injection sites are discussed here. For infants and children, the vastus lateralis muscle of the thigh is used most often because it's usually the best developed and contains no large nerves or blood vessels, minimizing the risk of serious injury. The rectus femoris muscle may also be used in infants but is usually contraindicated in adults. The gluteal muscles can be used as the injection site only after a toddler has been walking for about 1 year.

Deltoid

Find the lower edge of the acromial process and the point on the lateral arm in line with the axilla. Insert the needle 1″ to 2″ (2.5 to 5 cm) below the acromial process, usually two or three fingerbreadths, at a 90-degree angle or angled slightly toward the process. Typical injection: 0.5 mL (range: 0.5 to 2.0 mL).

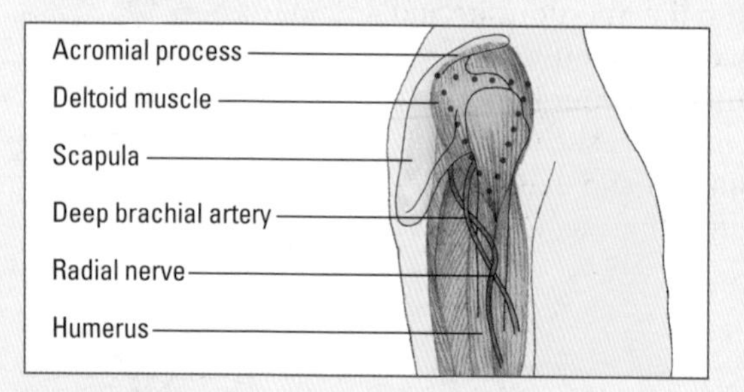

Dorsogluteal

Inject above and outside a line drawn from the posterior superior iliac spine to the greater trochanter of the femur. Or, divide the buttock into quadrants and inject in the upper outer quadrant, about 2″ to 3″ (5 to 7.6 cm) below the iliac crest. Insert the needle at a 90-degree angle. Typical injection: 1 to 4 mL (range: 1 to 5 mL).

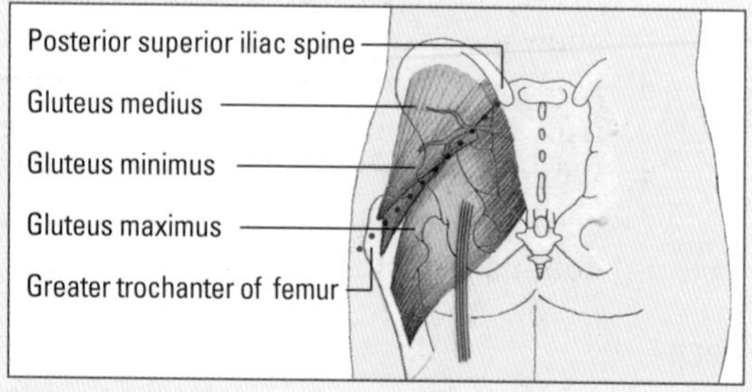

Ventrogluteal

Locate the greater trochanter of the femur with the heel of your hand. Then, spread your index and middle fingers from the anterior superior iliac spine to as far along the iliac crest as you can reach. Insert the needle between the two fingers at a 90-degree angle to the muscle. (Remove your fingers before inserting the needle.) Typical injection: 1 to 4 mL (range: 1 to 5 mL).

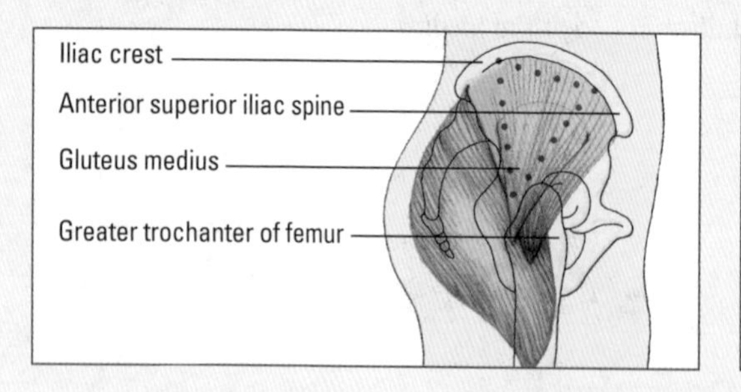

Vastus lateralis

Use the lateral muscle of the quadriceps group, from a handbreadth below the greater trochanter to a handbreadth above the knee. Insert the needle into the middle third of the muscle parallel to the surface on which the patient is lying. You may have to bunch the muscle before insertion. Typical injection: 1 to 4 mL (range: 1 to 5 mL; 1 to 3 mL for infants).

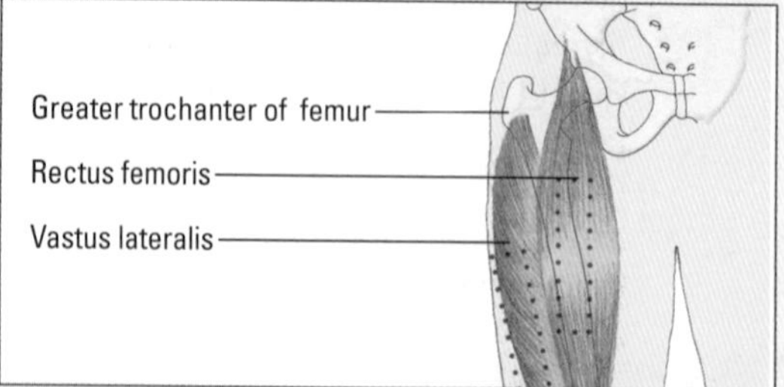

- Remove the alcohol pad and inspect the injection site for signs of active bleeding or bruising. If bleeding continues, apply pressure to the site; if bruising occurs, you may apply ice.
- Return to the patient's room in 15 to 30 minutes and ask the patient if he has any active pain, burning, numbness, or tingling at the injection site. *This may indicate injury to the underlying bone or nerves.*
- Discard all equipment according to standard precautions and your facility's policy. *Most syringes have a safety mechanism that encloses the needle after injection.* Don't recap needles; dispose of them in an appropriate sharps container *to avoid needlestick injuries.*

It's a low-tech solution, but ice works well for numbing sore injection sites.

Practice pointers

- Never use medication that's cloudy or discolored or contains a precipitate unless the manufacturer's instructions allow it. If in doubt, check with the pharmacist.
- I.M. injections shouldn't be administered at inflamed, edematous, sensitive, or irritated sites or at sites that contain moles, birthmarks, scar tissue, or other lesions and areas that twitch.

Stop the music

- I.M. injections may be contraindicated in patients with impaired coagulation mechanisms, occlusive peripheral vascular disease, edema, and shock; after thrombolytic therapy; and during an acute myocardial infarction.

Heavy rotation

- Keep a rotation record that lists all available injection sites divided into various body areas. Rotate from a site in the first area to a site in each of the other areas. Then return to a site in the first area that's at least 1″ (2.5 cm) away from the previous injection site in that area.
- If you must inject more than 5 mL of solution, divide the solution and inject it at two separate sites.
- I.M. injections can cause elevated serum enzyme levels. If measuring enzyme levels is important, suggest that the doctor switch to I.V. administration and adjust dosages accordingly.
- Dosage adjustments are usually necessary when changing from the I.M. route to the oral route. (See *Documenting I.M. injection*.)

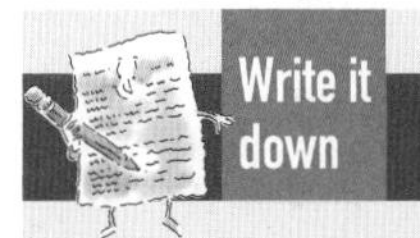

Documenting I.M. injection

In your notes, record:
- drug administered
- dose
- date and time
- injection site
- patient's tolerance of the injection
- patient education
- if patient refuses
- if omitted or withheld and the reason
- drug effects, including adverse reactions.

If the patient has any undesirable, effects notify the physician.

Z-track injection

The Z-track method of I.M. injection prevents leakage of irritating and discoloring medications (such as iron dextran) into the subcutaneous tissue. It may also be used in elderly patients who have decreased muscle mass. Lateral displacement of the skin during the injection helps to seal the drug in the muscle. The ventrogluteal site is the most common location for a Z-track injection.

What you need

Patient's medication record and chart ✳ two 20G 1¼″ to 2″ needles ✳ prescribed medication ✳ gloves ✳ 3- or 5-mL syringe ✳ two alcohol pads.

Getting ready

Verify the order on the patient's medication record by checking it against the doctor's order and perform hand hygiene. Check for allergies to the medication.

Measure up

Make sure the needle you're using is long enough to reach the muscle. As a rule of thumb, a 200-lb (91 kg) patient requires a 2″ needle; a 100-lb (45 kg) patient, a 1¼″ to 1½″ needle.

Attach one needle to the syringe and draw up the prescribed medication. Then draw 0.2 to 0.5 cc of air (depending on your facility's policy) into the syringe. Remove the first needle and attach the second *to prevent tracking the medication through the subcutaneous tissue as the needle is inserted.*

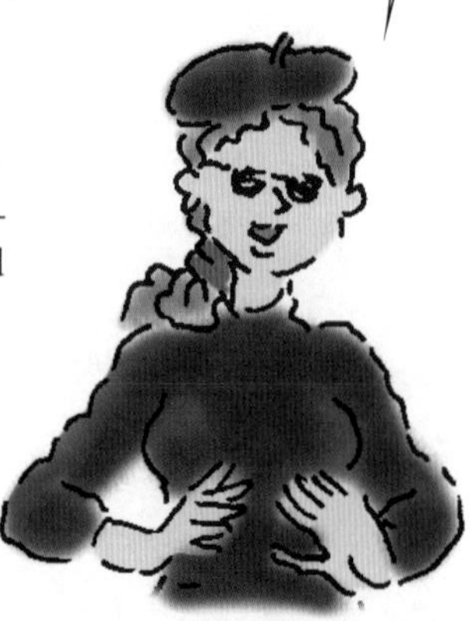
Dig this: The Z-track method is a cool way to prevent leakage into subcutaneous tissue.

How you do it

- Confirm the patient's identity using two patient identifiers, explain the procedure, and provide privacy.
- Place the patient in the lateral position, exposing the gluteal muscle to be used as the injection site. The patient may also be placed in the prone position.
- Clean an area on the upper outer quadrant of the patient's buttock with an alcohol pad.
- Put on gloves and displace the skin laterally by pulling it away from the injection site. (See *Displacing the skin for Z-track injection.*)

Displacing the skin for Z-track injection

Discomfort and tissue irritation may result from drug leakage into subcutaneous tissue. Displacing the skin helps prevent these problems.

Why to do it

By blocking the needle pathway after an injection, the Z-track technique allows I.M. injection while minimizing the risk of subcutaneous irritation and staining from drugs such as iron dextran. The illustrations below show how to perform a Z-track injection.

How to do it

To begin, place your finger on the skin surface and pull the skin and subcutaneous layers out of alignment with the underlying muscle. You should move the skin about 1" to 2" (2.5 to 3.5 cm).

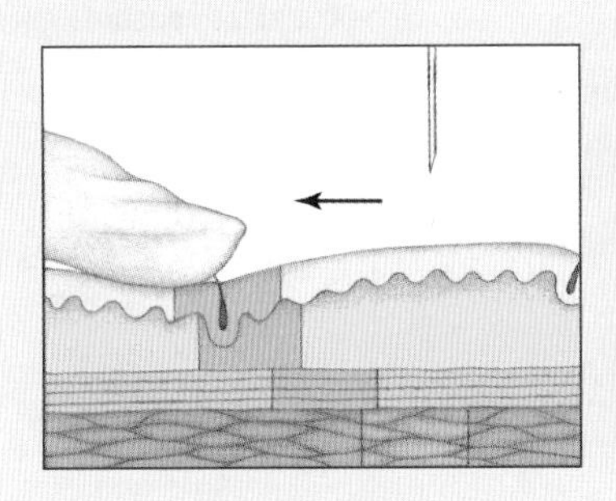

Insert the needle at a 90-degree angle at the site where you initially placed your finger. Inject the drug and withdraw the needle.

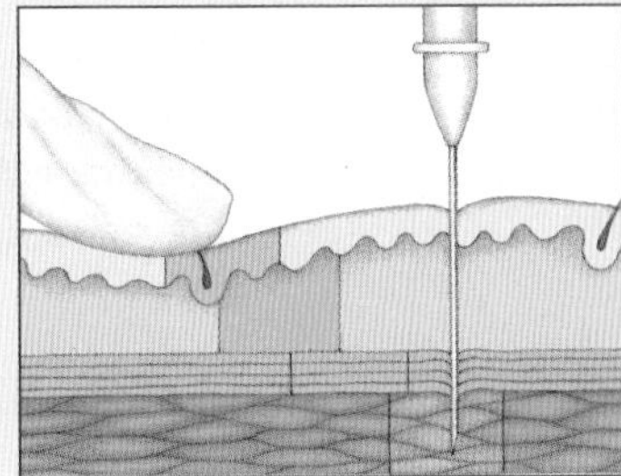

Finally, remove your finger from the skin surface, letting the layers return to normal. The needle track (shown by the dotted line) is now broken at the junction of each tissue layer, trapping the drug in the muscle.

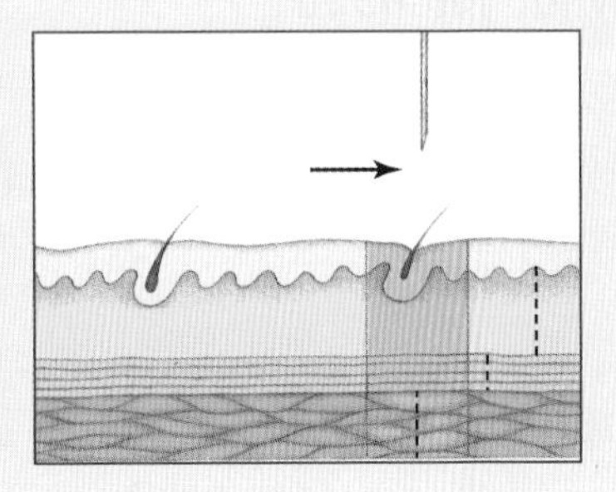

Follow with air

- Insert the needle into the muscle at a 90-degree angle and aspirate for blood return. If none appears, inject the drug slowly.
- Wait 10 seconds, withdraw the needle slowly, and release the displaced skin and subcutaneous tissue *to seal the needle track*. Don't massage or allow the patient to wear a tight-fitting garment over the site *because it could force the medication into subcutaneous tissue*. Encourage the patient to walk or move about in bed *to facilitate absorption of the drug from the injection site*.
- Discard the needles and syringe in an appropriate sharps container. Don't recap needles *to avoid needlestick injuries*.
- Remove and discard your gloves. Perform hand hygiene.

Practice pointers

- Never inject more than 5 mL of solution into a single site using the Z-track method. Alternate gluteal sites for repeat injections.

- I.M. injections can cause elevated serum enzyme levels. If measuring enzyme levels is important, suggest that the doctor switch to I.V. administration and adjust dosages accordingly. (See *Documenting Z-track injection*.)

Documenting Z-track injection

Record the medication, dosage, date, time, site of injection, and patient education on the patient's medication record. Include the patient's response to the injected drug. Note if the patient refuses the medication or if it is omitted or withheld and the reason.

Intraosseous infusion

When rapid venous infusion is difficult or impossible, intraosseous infusion allows delivery of fluids, medications, or whole blood into the bone marrow. It's typically performed on infants and children and is used in emergencies when I.V. access can't be obtained.

The site used most often is the anterior surface of the tibia, below the growth plate. Alternative sites include the iliac crest and spinous process. Only personnel trained in this procedure should perform it. Usually, a nurse assists. (See *Understanding intraosseous infusion*.)

What you need

Bone marrow biopsy needle or specially designed intraosseous infusion needle (cannula and obturator) ✳ povidone-iodine pads or alcohol ✳ sterile gauze pads ✳ sterile gloves ✳ sterile drape ✳ bone marrow set ✳ flush solution ✳ I.V. fluids and tubing ✳ 1% lidocaine ✳ 3- or 5-mL syringe ✳ tape.

Getting ready

Prepare I.V. fluids and high-pressure tubing as ordered.

How you do it

- Ensure that a responsible family member understands the procedure and consent form was signed. The physician is responsible for obtaining informed consent. Check the patient's history for hypersensitivity to the local anesthetic.
- Perform hand hygiene; consider and provide sedation, if appropriate; and position the patient based on the selected puncture site.
- Using sterile technique, the doctor cleans the puncture site with a povidone-iodine pad, allows it to dry, and covers the area with a sterile drape.

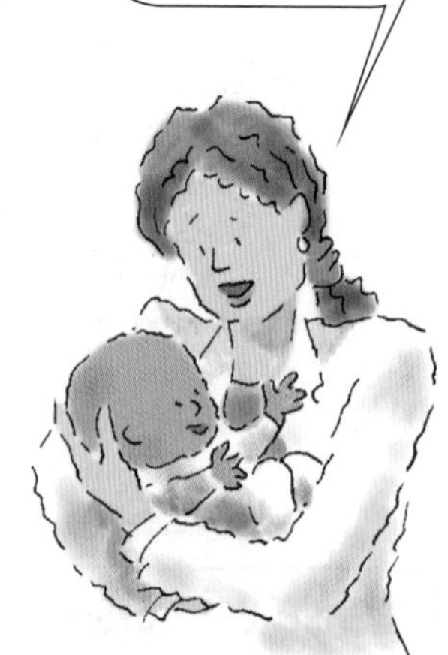
Intraosseous infusion is used only in emergencies. It's typically performed on infants and children when I.V. access can't be obtained.

Watch for the "give"

- Using sterile technique, the doctor inserts the intraosseous needle firmly through the skin and into the bone at a 90-degree angle, ¾″ to 1⅛″ (2 to 3 cm) below the anterior tibial growth plate. The needle should "give" suddenly as it enters the marrow and stand erect when released.

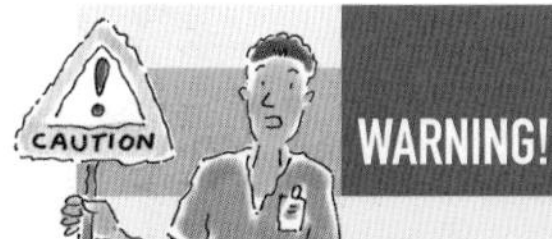

WARNING!

Understanding intraosseous infusion

During intraosseous infusion, the bone marrow serves as a noncollapsible vein. Thus, fluid infused into the marrow cavity rapidly enters the circulation by way of an extensive network of venous sinusoids. Here, the needle is shown positioned in the patient's tibia.

Common complications include extravasation of fluid into subcutaneous tissue, resulting from incorrect needle placement; subperiosteal effusion, resulting from failure of fluid to enter the marrow space; and clotting in the needle, resulting from delayed infusion or failure to flush the needle after placement. Other complications include subcutaneous abscess, osteomyelitis, and epiphyseal injury.

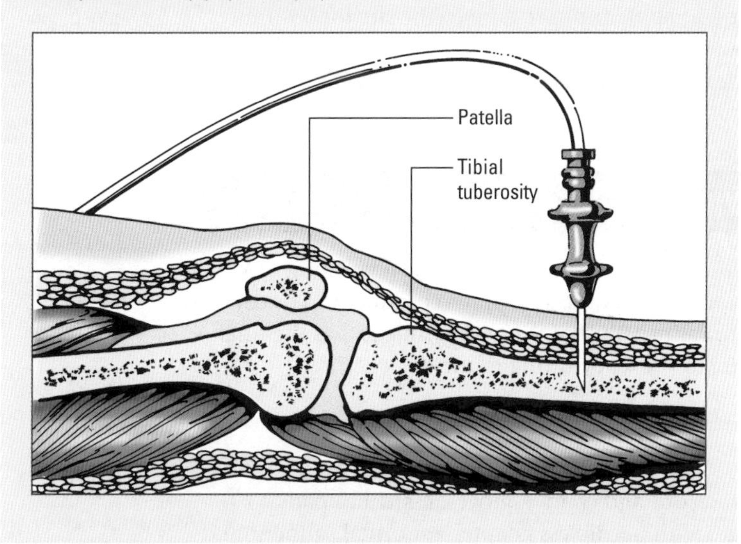

- Next, the doctor removes the obturator from the needle, attaches a 5-mL syringe, and aspirates bone marrow *to confirm needle placement.*
- The doctor replaces this syringe with a syringe containing 5 mL of saline and flushes the cannula.
- Next, the doctor removes the syringe and attaches pressurized I.V. tubing.

Now step in

- Don sterile gloves, clean the infusion site with povidone-iodine pads, and apply tape and sterile gauze dressing. Immobilize the site *to prevent dislodgment.*

- Monitor vital signs and check the infusion site for bleeding and extravasation.

Practice pointers

- This procedure is contraindicated in patients with osteogenesis imperfecta, osteopetrosis, and ipsilateral fracture *because of the potential for subcutaneous extravasation*. Infusion through an area with cellulitis or an infected burn *increases the risk of infection*.

Temporary measure

- Intraosseous infusion should be discontinued within 2 to 4 hours, if possible. *Prolonged infusion significantly increases the risk of infection.*
- After the needle has been removed, place a sterile dressing over the injection site and apply firm pressure to the site for 5 minutes.
- Intraosseous flow rates are determined by needle size and flow through the bone marrow. Fluids should flow freely if needle placement is correct. (See *Documenting intraosseous infusion*.)

Write it down

Documenting intraosseous infusion

In your notes, record:
- time, date, location of the infusion
- patient's tolerance of the procedure
- patient education.

Document the amount of fluid infused on the intake and output record.

Vascular access devices

An intermittent infusion injection device, or saline lock, allows I.V. administration without the need for multiple venipunctures or continuous I.V. infusion. Saline solution is typically injected as the final step in this procedure to prevent clotting in the device.

What you need

Patient's medication record and chart ✳ gloves ✳ alcohol pads ✳ three 3-mL syringes with needleless adapter ✳ normal saline solution ✳ extra intermittent infusion device ✳ prescribed medication in an I.V. container with administration set and needle (for infusion) or in a syringe with needle (for I.V. bolus or push) ✳ tourniquet ✳ tape ✳ optional: T-connector, sterile bacteriostatic water.

Getting ready

Verify the order on the patient's medication record by checking it against the doctor's order. Perform hand hygiene and then wipe the tops of the normal saline solution and medication containers with alcohol pads.

Fill two of the 3-mL syringes (bearing 22G needles) with normal saline solution.

Pump it up

If you'll be infusing medication, insert the administration set spike into the I.V. container, attach the needleless adapter, and prime the line. If you'll be giving an I.V. injection, fill a syringe with the prescribed medication.

Documenting intermittent infusion devices

Record the type and amount of drug administered and times of administration. On the intake record, include all I.V. solutions used to dilute the medication and flush the line.

How you do it

- Confirm the patient's identity using two patient identifiers. Explain the procedure.
- Don gloves and wipe the injection port of the intermittent infusion device with an alcohol pad. Then insert the needleless adapter of a saline-filled syringe.
- Aspirate the syringe and observe for blood *to verify the device's patency*.

Puffiness or pain?

- If you feel no resistance, watch for signs of infiltration (puffiness or pain at the site) as you slowly inject the saline solution. If these signs occur, insert a new intermittent infusion device.
- If blood is aspirated, slowly inject the saline solution and observe for signs of infiltration.
- Withdraw the saline syringe and needleless adapter.

Administering I.V. bolus or push injections

- Insert the needleless adapter and syringe, inject the medication at the required rate, and remove the needleless adapter and syringe.
- Insert the needleless adapter of the remaining saline-filled syringe into the injection port and slowly inject the saline solution *to flush all medication through the device*.
- Remove the needleless adapter and syringe.

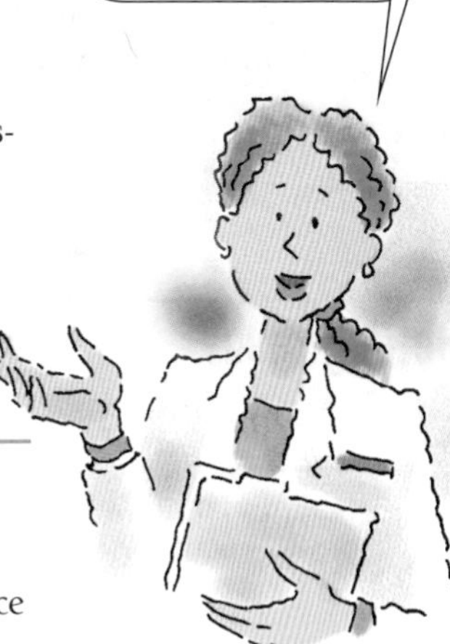
In some cases, you can flush the device with bacteriostatic water instead of saline solution.

Administering an infusion

- Insert and secure the needleless adapter attached to the administration set.
- Open the infusion line and adjust the flow rate as necessary.
- Infuse medication for the prescribed length of time, then flush the device with normal saline solution, as you would after a bolus or push injection, according to your facility's policy.

Practice pointers

- If you're giving a bolus injection of a drug that's incompatible with saline solution, such as diazepam (Valium), flush the device with bacteriostatic water.

- Intermittent infusion devices should be changed regularly (usually every 48 to 72 hours) according to standard precautions guidelines and your facility's policy.
- If you can't rotate injection sites because the patient has fragile veins, document this fact and discuss it with the patient's doctor. (See *Documenting intermittent infusion devices,* page 229.)

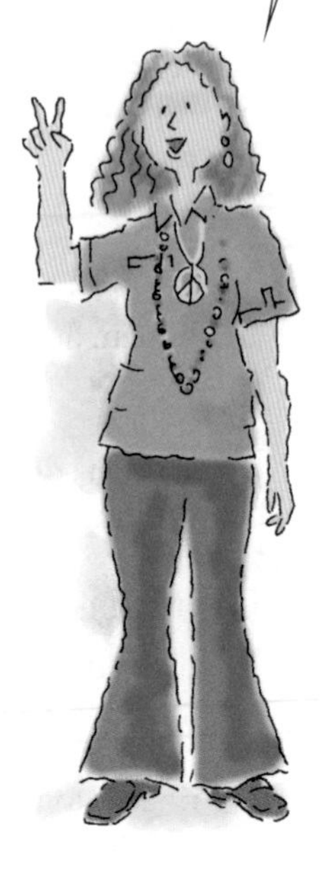
Like me, intermittent infusion devices become outdated. Change yours every 48 to 72 hours.

I.V. bolus injection

The I.V. bolus injection method allows rapid drug administration. It's used in an emergency, to administer drugs that can't be given intramuscularly, to achieve peak drug levels in the bloodstream, and to deliver drugs that can't be diluted.

The term *bolus* usually refers to the concentration or amount of a drug. Bolus doses of medication may be injected directly into a vein or through an existing I.V. line. Some facilities permit only specially trained nurses (such as emergency department, critical care, and chemotherapy nurses) to give bolus injections.

What you need

Patient's medication record and chart ✱ gloves ✱ prescribed medication ✱ 20G needle and syringe ✱ diluent, if needed ✱ tourniquet ✱ povidone-iodine or alcohol pad ✱ sterile 2″ × 2″ gauze pad ✱ adhesive bandage ✱ tape ✱ optional: winged-tip needle with catheter and second syringe (and needle) filled with normal saline solution, noncoring needle if used with a vascular access port (VAP), heparin flush solution.

When a wing-tip isn't a shoe

Winged-tip needles are commonly used for I.V. bolus injection because they can be quickly and easily inserted. They're ideal for repeated drug administration, as in weekly or monthly chemotherapy. Another useful dosage form is the ready injectable, which is a syringe already loaded with the medication (such as epinephrine).

Getting ready

Verify the order on the patient's medication record by checking it against the doctor's order. Know the actions, adverse reactions, and administration rate of the medication to be injected. Draw up the prescribed medication in the syringe and dilute it if necessary.

How you do it

- Confirm the patient's identity, perform hand hygiene, put on gloves, and explain the procedure.

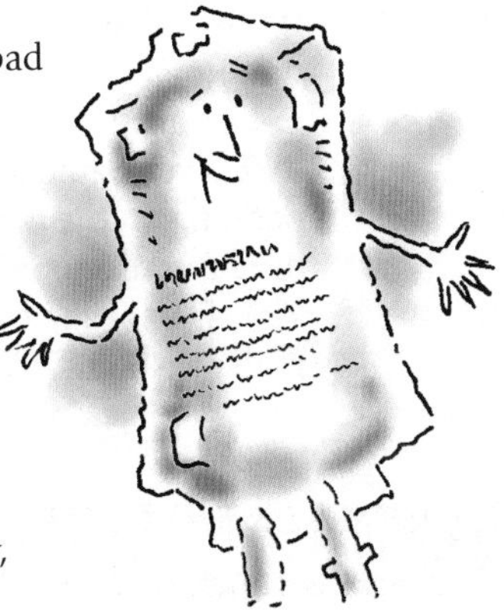
I need the largest vein suitable for an injection.

Giving direct injections

- Select the largest vein suitable for an injection, depending on the drug specified, and apply a tourniquet above the injection site *to distend the vein.*
- Clean the injection site with an alcohol or a povidone-iodine pad in a circular motion.
- If you're using the drug syringe's needle, insert it into the vein at a 30-degree angle with the bevel up. The bevel should reach ¼″ (0.6 cm) into the vein. If you're using a winged-tip needle, insert the needle (bevel up), tape the butterfly wings in place when you see blood return in the tubing, and attach the syringe containing the medication.

Backflow means go forward

- Pull back on the syringe plunger and check for blood backflow, *indicating that the needle is in the vein.*
- Remove the tourniquet and inject the medication at the appropriate rate.
- Pull back slightly on the syringe plunger and check for blood backflow again. Then flush the line with the normal saline solution from the second syringe *to ensure delivery of all the medication.*
- Withdraw the needle and apply pressure to the injection site with a sterile gauze pad for at least 3 minutes *to prevent hematoma formation.*
- Apply the adhesive bandage to the site after bleeding has stopped.

Giving injections through an existing I.V. line

- Check the compatibility of the medication with the I.V. solution.
- Close the flow clamp, wipe the injection port on the I.V. tubing (such as a T-connector or use a needleless adapter) with an alcohol pad, and inject the medication as you would a direct injection. Then open the flow clamp and readjust the flow rate.
- If the drug isn't compatible with the I.V. solution, flush the line with normal saline solution before and after the injection.

Practice pointers

- *Because drugs administered by I.V. bolus or push injections are delivered directly into the circulatory system and can produce an immediate effect,* an acute allergic reaction or anaphylaxis can develop rapidly. If signs of anaphylaxis (dyspnea, cyanosis, seizures, and increasing respiratory distress) occur, notify the doctor immediately and begin emergency procedures, as necessary. Also watch for signs of extravasation (redness and swelling). If extravasation occurs, stop the injection, estimate the amount of infiltration, and notify the doctor.

Sub for saline

- If you're giving diazepam or chlordiazepoxide through a winged-tip needle or an I.V. line, flush with bacteriostatic water instead of normal saline solution *to prevent drug precipitation resulting from incompatibility*.
- Excessively rapid administration may cause adverse reactions depending on the medication administered. You need to know the drug you're administering and the rate at which to inject the drug. You also need to be aware of the intended effects and monitor the patient as indicated by the medication given. (See *Documenting I.V. bolus injections*.)

Documenting I.V. bolus injections

In your notes, record:
- amount and type of drug administered
- time of injection
- appearance of the site
- duration of administration
- patient's tolerance of the procedure
- drug's effect and adverse reactions.

Epidural analgesics

Epidural analgesia helps manage acute and chronic pain, including moderate to severe postoperative pain. The epidural catheter, inserted near the spinal cord, eliminates the risks of multiple I.M. injections, minimizes adverse cerebral and systemic effects, and eliminates the analgesic peaks and valleys that usually occur with intermittent I.M. injections.

In this procedure, the anesthesiologist injects or infuses medication into the epidural space. The drug diffuses slowly into the subarachnoid space of the spinal canal and then into the cerebrospinal fluid (CSF), which carries it directly into the spinal area, bypassing the blood-brain barrier. In some cases, the doctor injects medication directly into the subarachnoid space. (See *Placement of a permanent epidural catheter*.)

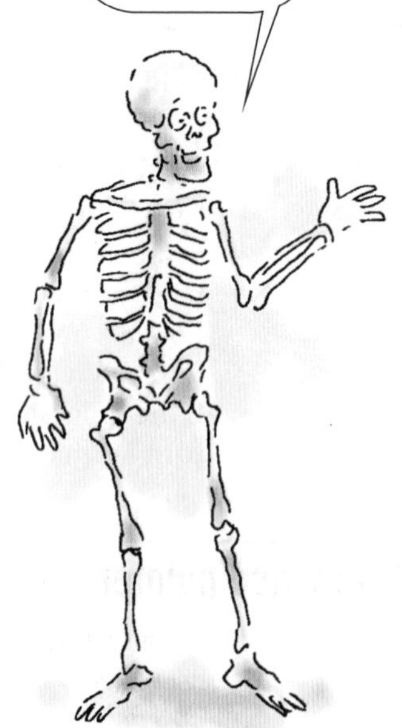

Delivering an analgesic near my spinal canal has impressive results.

What you need

Volume infusion device and epidural infusion tubing (depending on your facility's policy) ✻ patient's medication record and chart ✻ prescribed epidural solutions ✻ transparent dressing or sterile gauze pads ✻ epidural tray ✻ labels for epidural infusion line ✻ silk tape ✻ optional: monitoring equipment for blood pressure and pulse, apnea monitor.

Placement of a permanent epidural catheter

An epidural catheter is implanted beneath the patient's skin and inserted near the spinal cord at the first lumbar (L1) interspace. For temporary analgesic therapy (less than 1 week), the catheter may exit directly over the spine and be taped up the patient's back to the shoulder. For prolonged therapy, it may be tunneled subcutaneously to an exit site on the patient's side or abdomen or over his shoulder.

Dial down the dose

The most common complications of epidural infusions are numbness and leg weakness, which may occur after the first 24 hours and are drug- and concentration-dependent. The doctor must titrate the dosage to identify the dose that provides adequate pain control without causing excessive numbness and weakness. Other possible complications include respiratory depression during the first 24 hours, pruritus, nausea, and vomiting.

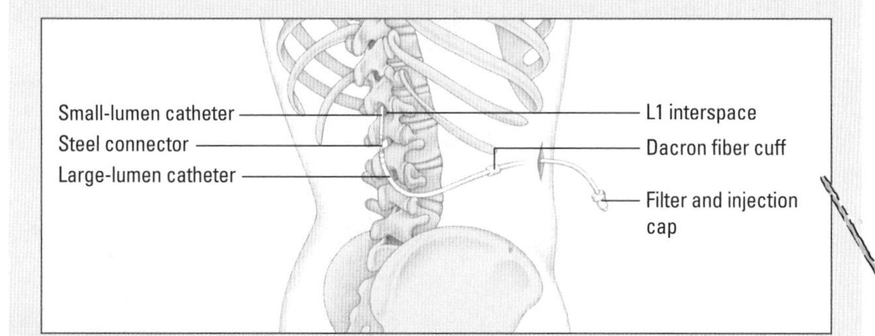

Have on hand the following drugs and equipment for emergency use: naloxone, 0.4 mg I.V.; ephedrine, 50 mg I.V. ✳ oxygen ✳ intubation set ✳ handheld resuscitation bag.

Getting ready

Prepare the infusion device according to the manufacturer's instructions and your facility's policy. Obtain an epidural tray. Check the medication concentration and infusion rate against the doctor's order.

How you do it

- Explain the procedure and possible complications to the patient. Tell him that he'll feel some pain as the catheter is inserted. Make sure that a consent form has been properly signed and witnessed. Perform hand hygiene.

- Position the patient on his side in the knee-chest position or have him sit on the edge of the bed and lean over a bedside table.
- After the catheter is in place, prime the infusion device, confirm the appropriate medication and infusion rate, and then adjust the device for the correct rate.
- Help the anesthesiologist connect the infusion tubing to the epidural catheter. Then connect the tubing to the infusion pump.
- Bridge-tape all connection sites and apply an EPIDURAL INFUSION label to the catheter, infusion tubing, and infusion pump *to prevent accidental infusion of other drugs*. Then start the infusion.

What's the score?

- Tell the patient to report any pain (according to facility policy, such as a scale of 1 to 10). If the patient reports a higher pain score, the infusion rate may need to be increased. Call the doctor or change the rate within the prescribed limits.
- The dressing is changed by the anesthesiologist or a specially trained nurse. The dressing is usually transparent *to allow inspection of drainage* and commonly appears moist or slightly blood-tinged.
- Change the infusion tubing every 48 hours or as specified by your facility's policy.

Removing an epidural catheter

- Typically, the anesthesiologist orders analgesics and removes the catheter. However, your facility's policy may allow a specially trained nurse to remove the catheter.

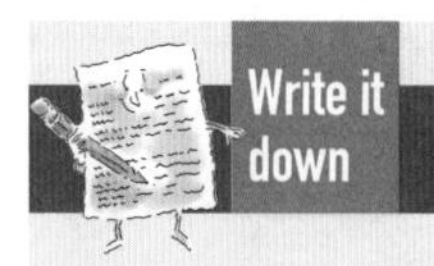

Documenting epidural analgesics

In your notes, record:
- catheter patency
- condition of dressing and insertion site
- patient's vital signs and assessment results
- labeling of the epidural catheter
- changing of infusion bags
- ordered analgesics, if any
- patient's response.

Practice pointers

- Epidural analgesia is contraindicated in patients who have local or systemic infection, neurologic disease, coagulopathy, spinal arthritis or a spinal deformity, hypotension, marked hypertension, or an allergy to the prescribed medication and in those who are undergoing anticoagulant therapy.

Regular check-in

- Assess the patient's vital signs, pain level, sedation, and motor and neurovascular status every 1 to 2 hours for 12 to 24 hours then every 4 hours as per facility policy; notify the doctor if the patient's respiratory rate is less than 10 breaths/minute or if his systolic blood pressure is less than 90 mm Hg.

- Notify the doctor if the patient appears drowsy; experiences nausea and vomiting, refractory itching, or an inability to void, *which are adverse reactions to certain narcotic analgesics;* or complains of unrelieved pain.

Push and pull

- Keep in mind that drugs given epidurally diffuse slowly and may cause adverse reactions, including excessive sedation, up to 12 hours after the infusion has been discontinued.
  - Monitor patients for respiratory depression.
- The patient should always have a peripheral I.V. line (either continuous infusion or saline lock) open *to allow immediate administration of emergency drugs.* (See *Documenting epidural analgesics.*)

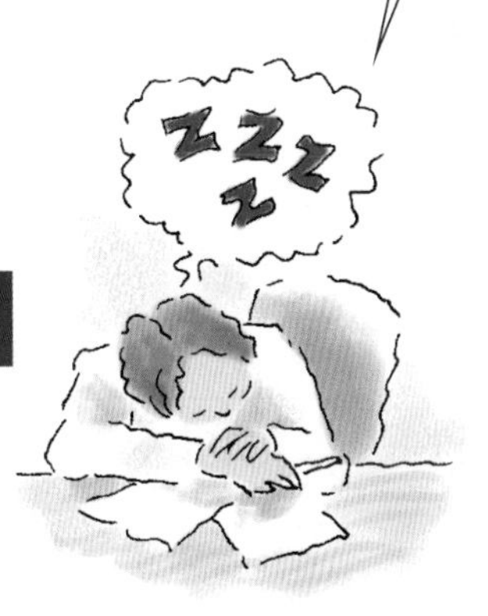
Epidurals can cause excessive sedation up to 12 hours after the infusion is discontinued.

Endotracheal medications

When an I.V. line isn't readily available, certain drugs (naloxone, atropine, diazepam, epinephrine, and lidocaine) can be administered into the respiratory system through an endotracheal (ET) tube in an emergency.

Drugs given endotracheally usually have a longer duration of action than drugs given I.V. because they are absorbed in the alveoli. A doctor, an emergency medical technician, or a critical care nurse usually administers ET drugs.

What you need

ET tube ✱ gloves ✱ stethoscope ✱ handheld resuscitation bag ✱ prescribed drug ✱ syringe or adapter ✱ sterile water or normal saline solution.

Getting ready

Verify the order on the patient's medication record by checking it against the doctor's order and perform hand hygiene.

Confirm ET tube placement by auscultation over the lungs with a stethoscope or via an exhaled carbon dioxide detector. Calculate the drug dose. Adult advanced cardiac life support guidelines recommend that drugs be administered at 2 to 2½ times the recommended I.V. dose.

Next, draw the drug up into a syringe and dilute it in 10 mL of sterile water or normal saline solution *to increase drug volume and contact with lung tissue.*

How you do it

- Verify it is the correct patient using two patient identifiers.
- Don gloves.
- Ventilate the patient three to five times with the resuscitation bag. Then remove the bag.
- Remove the needle from the syringe, insert the syringe tip into the ET tube, and inject the drug deep into the tube.

Jet propulsion

- Reattach the resuscitation bag and ventilate the patient briskly *to propel the drug into the lungs, oxygenate the patient*, and *clear the tube*.
- Discard the syringe in an appropriate sharps container and discard gloves.

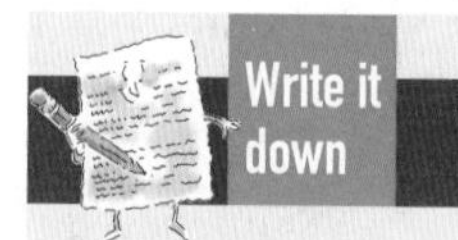

Documenting endotracheal medications

In your notes, record:
- date and time of drug administration
- drug administered
- patient's response.

Practice pointers

- Be aware that the drug's onset of action may be quicker than it would be by I.V. administration. If the patient doesn't respond quickly, the doctor may order a repeat dose. (See *Documenting endotracheal medications*.)

Peripheral I.V. catheter insertion

A peripheral line allows administration of fluids, medication, blood, and blood components. It also maintains I.V. access to the patient.

Peripheral I.V. line insertion involves selection of a venipuncture device and an insertion site, application of a tourniquet, preparation of the site, and venipuncture. Selection of a venipuncture device and site depends on the type of solution to be used; frequency and duration of infusion; patency and location of accessible veins; the patient's age, size, and condition; and, when possible, the patient's preference.

What you need

Alcohol pads or other approved antimicrobial solution, such as tincture of iodine 2% or 10% povidone-iodine ✳ gloves ✳ tourniquet (rubber tubing or a blood pressure cuff) ✳ I.V. access devices ✳ I.V. solution with attached and primed administration set ✳ I.V. pole ✳ sharps container ✳ sterile 2″ × 2″ gauze pads or a transparent semipermeable dressing ✳ 1″ hypoallergenic tape ✳ optional: arm board, roller gauze, tube gauze, warm packs, scissors.

Commercial venipuncture kits come with or without an I.V. access device. In many facilities, venipuncture equipment is kept on a tray or cart, allowing a choice of correct access devices and easy replacement of contaminated items.

Getting ready

Check the information on the label of the I.V. solution container, including the patient's name, room number, type of solution, time and date of its preparation, preparer's name, and ordered infusion rate and compare the doctor's orders. Then select the smallest-gauge device that's appropriate for the infusion.

If you're using a winged infusion set, connect the adapter to the administration set and unclamp the line until fluid flows from the open end of the needle cover. Then close the clamp and place the needle on a sterile surface such as the inside of its packaging. If you're using a catheter device, open its package to allow easy access.

How you do it

- Position the I.V. pole close to the patient and hang the I.V. solution with attached primed administration set on the I.V. pole.
- Verify the patient's identity by using two patient identifiers.
- Perform hand hygiene thoroughly and explain the procedure to the patient.

Selecting the site

- Select the puncture site. If long-term therapy is anticipated, start with a vein at the most distal site *so that you can move proximally as needed for subsequent I.V. insertion sites.*
- Place the patient in a comfortable, reclining position, leaving the arm in a dependent position *to increase capillary fill of the lower arms and hands.* If the patient's skin is cold, warm it by rubbing and stroking the arm or cover the entire arm with warm packs for 5 to 10 minutes.

Applying the tourniquet

- Apply a tourniquet about 6" (15 cm) above the intended puncture site *to dilate the vein.* Check for a radial pulse. If it isn't present, release the tourniquet and reapply it with less tension *to prevent arterial occlusion.*
- Lightly palpate the vein with the index and middle fingers of your nondominant hand. Stretch the skin *to anchor the vein.* If the vein feels hard or ropelike, select another.

Open sesame

- If the vein is easily palpable but not sufficiently dilated, one or more of the following techniques may help raise the vein. Place the extremity in a dependent position for several seconds, gently tap your finger over the vein, rub or stroke the skin upward toward the tourniquet, or have the patient open and close his fist several times.
- Leave the tourniquet in place for no longer than 3 minutes. If you can't find a suitable vein and prepare the site in that time, release the tourniquet for a few minutes. Then reapply it and continue the procedure.

Leave the tourniquet in place for no longer than 3 minutes.

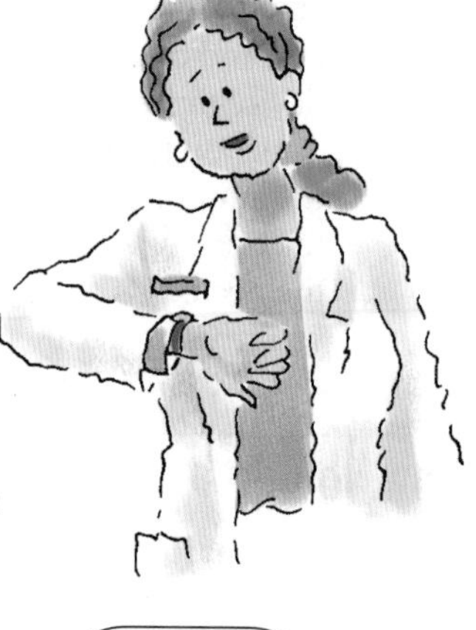

Preparing the site

- Perform hand hygiene and don gloves. Clip the hair around the insertion site if needed. Clean the site with alcohol pads or another approved antimicrobial solution according to your facility's policy. Don't apply alcohol after applying 10% povidone-iodine *because the alcohol negates the beneficial effect of the povidone-iodine*. Work in a circular motion outward from the site to a diameter of 2″ to 4″ (5 to 10 cm) and allow the solution to dry.
- Check your facility's policy for guidelines on how to use a local anesthetic before the venipuncture. Make sure the patient isn't sensitive to lidocaine.

Will this procedure ever end?

Round, firm, and resilient

- Lightly press the vein with the thumb of your nondominant hand about 1½″ (4 cm) from the intended insertion site. The vein should feel round, firm, fully engorged, and resilient.
- Grasp the access cannula. If you're using a winged infusion set, hold the short edges of the wings (with the needle's bevel facing upward) between the thumb and forefinger of your dominant hand. Then squeeze the wings together. If you're using an over-the-needle cannula, grasp the plastic hub with your dominant hand, remove the cover, and examine the cannula tip. If the edge isn't smooth, discard and replace the device.

Operation stabilization

- Using the thumb of your nondominant hand, stretch the skin taut below the puncture site *to stabilize the vein* and tell the patient that you're about to insert the device.
- Hold the needle bevel up and enter the skin parallel to the vein (a 10- to 30-degree angle) and push the needle directly through the skin and into the vein in one motion.

Check the flashback chamber behind the hub for blood return, signifying that the vein has been properly accessed. (You may not see a blood return in a small vein.)

- If using a winged-tip device, advance the needle, hold it in place, and release the tourniquet. Open the administration set clamp slightly and check for free flow or infiltration.
- For an over-the-needle catheter, advance the device to ensure that the cannula itself—not just the introducer needle—has entered the vein.
- Grasp the cannula hub to hold it in the vein and withdraw the needle. As you withdraw it, advance the cannula up to the hub or until you meet resistance.

Advance study

- To advance the cannula while infusing I.V. solution, release the tourniquet and remove the inner needle. Using aseptic technique, attach the I.V. tubing and begin the infusion. While stabilizing the vein with one hand, use the other to advance the catheter into the vein. When the catheter is advanced, decrease the I.V. flow rate. *This method reduces the risk of puncturing the vein's opposite wall because the catheter is advanced without the steel needle and because the rapid flow dilates the vein.*
- To advance the cannula before starting the infusion, first release the tourniquet. While stabilizing the vein with one hand, use the other to advance the catheter up to the hub. Next, remove the inner needle and, using aseptic technique, quickly attach the I.V. tubing. *This method often results in less blood being spilled.*

Dressing the site

- After the venous access device has been inserted, clean the skin completely. Dispose of the stylet in a sharps container. Then regulate the flow rate.
- You may use a transparent semipermeable dressing *to secure the device.* (See *How to apply a transparent semipermeable dressing.*)
- If you don't use a transparent dressing, cover the site with a sterile gauze pad or small adhesive bandage.

Loopy approach

- Loop the I.V. tubing on the patient's limb and secure the tubing with tape. *The loop allows some slack to prevent dislodgment of the cannula from tension on the line.* (See *Taping a venous access site,* page 240.)
- Label the last piece of tape with the type, gauge of needle, and length of cannula; date and time of insertion; and your initials. Adjust the flow rate as ordered.

How to apply a transparent semipermeable dressing

To secure the I.V. insertion site, you can apply a transparent semipermeable dressing as follows:

- Make sure the insertion site is clean and dry.
- Remove the dressing from the package. Using aseptic technique, remove the protective seal.
- Place the dressing directly over the insertion site and the hub, as shown. Don't cover the tubing or stretch the dressing.
- Tuck the dressing around and under the cannula hub to bar microorganisms.
- To remove the dressing, grasp one corner and then lift and stretch it. If removal is difficult, try loosening the edges with alcohol or water.

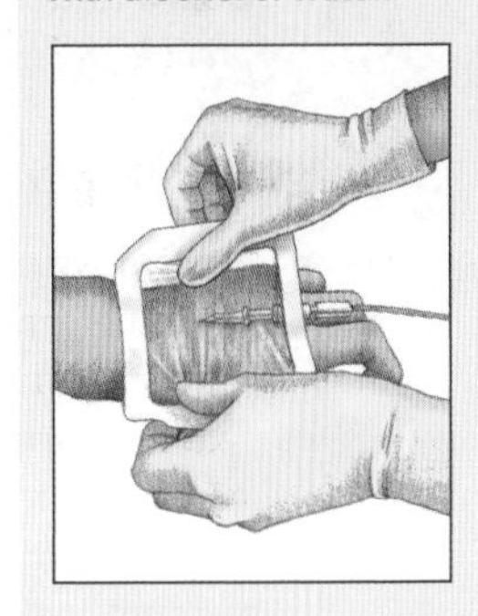

Taping a venous access site

You can use one of the methods shown below to tape a venous access site.

Chevron method

- Cut a long strip of ½″ tape and place it sticky side up under the cannula and parallel to the short strip of tape.
- Cross the ends of the tape over the cannula so that the tape sticks to the patient's skin (as shown).
- Apply a piece of 1″ tape across the two wings of the chevron.
- Loop the tubing and secure it with another piece of 1″ tape. When the dressing is secured, apply a label. On the label, write the insertion date, time, needle type, and gauge and your initials.

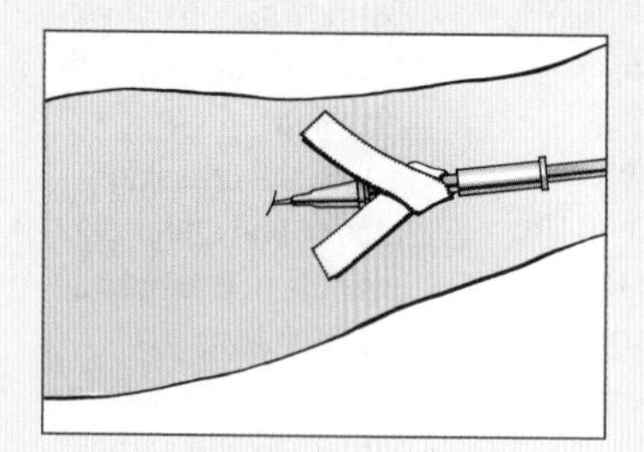

U method

- Cut a 2″ (5 cm) strip of ½″ tape. With the sticky side up, place it under the hub of the cannula.
- Bring each side of the tape up, folding it over the wings of the cannula in a U shape (as shown). Press it down parallel to the hub.
- Apply tape to stabilize the catheter.
- When a dressing is secured, apply a label. On the label, write the date and time of insertion, type and gauge of the needle or cannula, and your initials.

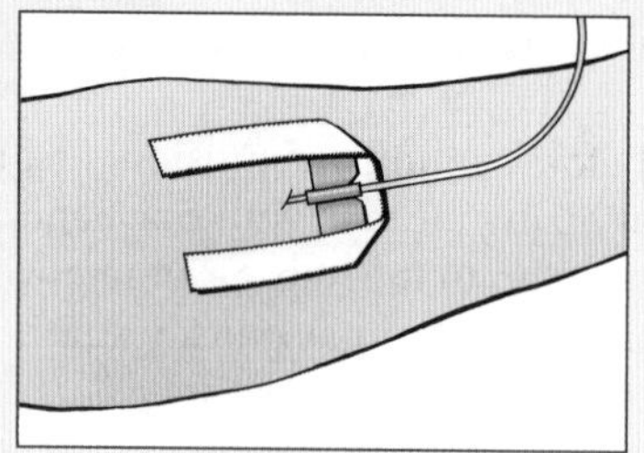

H method

- Cut three strips of 1″ tape.
- Place one strip of tape over each wing, keeping the tape parallel to the cannula (as shown).
- Now place the other strip of tape perpendicular to the first two. Put it either directly on top of the wings or just below the wings, directly on top of the tubing.
- Make sure the cannula is secure; then apply a dressing and a label. On the label, write the date and time of insertion, type and gauge of needle or cannula, and your initials.

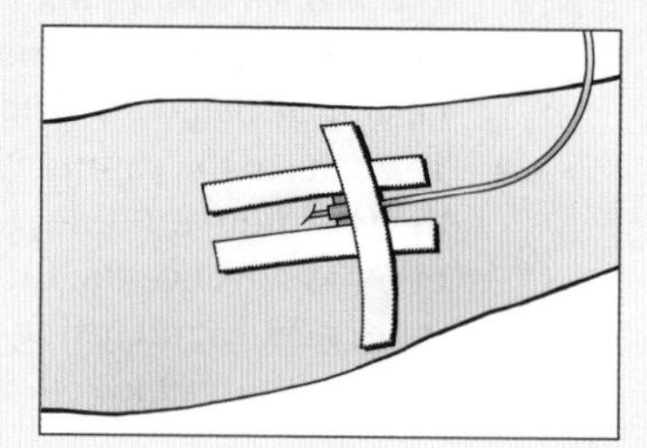

- If the puncture site is near a movable joint, place a padded arm board under the joint and secure it with roller gauze or tape *to provide stability*.

Removing a peripheral I.V. line

- To remove the I.V. line, clamp the I.V. tubing and gently remove the transparent dressing and all tape from the skin.
- Open a gauze pad and adhesive bandage and place them within reach. Perform hand hygiene. Don gloves. Hold the sterile gauze pad over the puncture site with one hand and use your other hand to withdraw the cannula slowly and smoothly, keeping it parallel to the skin. (Inspect the cannula tip; if it isn't smooth, assess the patient immediately and notify the doctor.)
- Using the gauze pad, apply firm pressure over the puncture site for 1 to 2 minutes after removal or until bleeding has stopped.

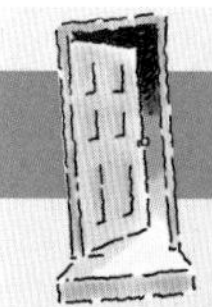

Home care connection

I.V. therapy in the home

Most patients who receive I.V. therapy at home have a central venous line. But if you're caring for a patient going home with a peripheral line, teach him how to care for the I.V. site and identify certain complications. If he must observe movement restrictions, make sure he understands them. Because the patient may have special drug delivery equipment that differs from the type used in the facility, be sure to demonstrate the equipment and have him give a return demonstration.

What's on the syllabus

Teach the patient and family member how to examine the site and instruct him to notify the doctor or home care nurse if redness, swelling, or discomfort develops; if the dressing becomes moist; or if blood appears in the tubing. Also tell the patient to report any problems with the I.V. line, for instance, if the solution stops infusing or an alarm goes off on an infusion pump. Explain that a home care nurse will change the I.V. site at established intervals.

If the patient is using an intermittent infusion device, teach him how and when to flush it. Finally, teach the patient to document daily whether the I.V. site is free from pain, swelling, and redness. Peripheral line complications can result from the needle or catheter (infection, phlebitis, and embolism) or from the solution (circulatory overload, infiltration, sepsis, and allergic reaction).

- Clean the site and apply the adhesive bandage or, if blood oozes, apply a pressure bandage and instruct the patient to restrict activity for about 10 minutes and to leave the dressing in place for at least 1 hour. If the patient experiences lingering tenderness at the site, apply warm packs and notify the doctor.

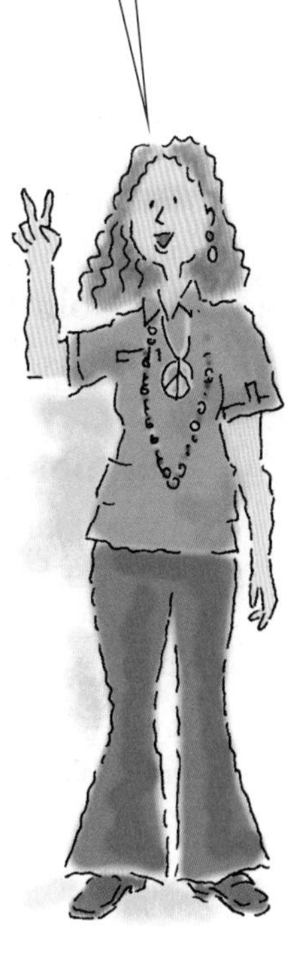
Flashback? I know just what you mean!

Practice pointers

- Insertion is contraindicated in a sclerotic vein, an edematous or impaired arm or hand, or a postmastectomy arm and in patients with a mastectomy, burns, or an arteriovenous fistula. Subsequent venipunctures should be performed proximal to a previously used or injured vein.
- If the patient is allergic to iodine-containing compounds, clean the skin with alcohol.
- If you fail to see blood flashback after the needle enters the vein, pull back slightly and rotate the device. If you still fail to see flashback, remove the cannula and try again with a new device or proceed according to your facility's policy.

- Change a gauze or transparent dressing whenever you change the administration set (every 48 to 72 hours or according to your facility's policy).
- If drainage appears at the puncture site when discontinuing the I.V., notify the physician. Then clean the area, apply a sterile dressing, and notify the doctor.
- Be sure to rotate the I.V. site, usually every 48 to 72 hours or according to your facility's policy.
- If the patient is to receive peripheral I.V. therapy at home, review teaching with him. (See *I.V. therapy in the home,* page 241 and *Documenting peripheral I.V. catheter insertion.*)

Documenting peripheral I.V. catheter insertion

In your notes or on the appropriate I.V. flowchart, record:
- date and time of the venipuncture
- needle type and gauge
- cannula length
- anatomic location of the insertion site
- reason the site was changed
- number of attempts at venipuncture (if you made more than one)
- type and flow rate of the I.V. solution
- name and amount of medication in the solution (if any)
- adverse reactions and nursing actions
- patient teaching and evidence of patient understanding.

Peripheral I.V. catheter maintenance

Routine maintenance of I.V. sites and systems includes regular assessment and rotation of the site. It also includes periodic changes of the dressing, tubing, and solution. These measures help prevent complications, such as thrombophlebitis and infection. They should be performed according to your facility's policy.

What you need

For dressing changes

Sterile gloves ✳ povidone-iodine or alcohol pads ✳ povidone-iodine or other antimicrobial ointment, according to your facility's policy ✳ adhesive bandage, sterile 2″ × 2″ gauze pad, or transparent semipermeable dressing ✳ 1″ adhesive tape.

For solution changes

Solution container ✳ alcohol pad.

For tubing changes

I.V. administration set ✳ sterile gloves ✳ sterile 2″ × 2″ gauze pad ✳ adhesive tape for labeling ✳ optional: hemostats.

For I.V. site change

Commercial kits containing the equipment for dressing changes are available.

Getting ready

- If you're changing the solution and the tubing, attach and prime the I.V. administration set before entering the patient's room.

How you do it

- Perform hand hygiene and explain the procedure to the patient.

Changing the dressing

- Remove the old dressing, open all supply packages, and put on sterile gloves.
- Hold the cannula in place with your nondominant hand and assess the venipuncture site for signs of infection (redness and pain at the puncture site), infiltration (coolness, blanching, and edema at the site), and thrombophlebitis (redness, firmness, pain along the path of the vein, and edema). If any such signs are present, cover the area with a sterile 2" × 2" gauze pad and remove the catheter or needle. Apply pressure to the area until the bleeding stops and apply an adhesive bandage. Then, using fresh equipment and solution, start the I.V. in another appropriate site, preferably on the opposite extremity.
- If the venipuncture site is intact, stabilize the cannula and carefully clean around the puncture site with a povidone-iodine or an alcohol pad, working in a circular motion. Allow the area to dry completely.
- Apply povidone-iodine and cover the site with a transparent semipermeable dressing to halfway up the cannula.

Changing the solution

- Perform hand hygiene and inspect the new solution container for cracks, leaks, and other damage. Check the solution for discoloration, turbidity, and particulates. Note the date and time the solution was mixed and its expiration date. Always verify that the solution is the same as the order in the chart.
- Clamp the tubing when inverting it *to prevent air from entering the tubing,* keeping the drip chamber half full.

Brand new bag

- If you're replacing a bag, remove the seal or tab from the new bag and remove the old bag from the pole. Remove the spike, insert it into the new bag, and adjust the flow rate.

- If you're replacing a bottle, remove the cap and seal from the new bottle and wipe the rubber port with an alcohol pad. Clamp the line, remove the spike from the old bottle, and insert the spike into the new bottle. Then hang the new bottle and adjust the flow rate.

Changing the tubing

- Reduce the I.V. flow rate, remove the old spike from the container, and hang it on the I.V. pole. Place the cover of the new spike loosely over the old one.
- Keeping the old spike in an upright position above the patient's heart level, insert the new spike into the I.V. container and prime the system. Hang the new I.V. container and primed set on the pole and grasp the new adapter in one hand. Then stop the flow rate in the old tubing.

Sterile steps

- Perform hand hygiene. Put on sterile gloves.
- Place a sterile gauze pad under the needle or cannula hub *to create a sterile field*. Press one of your fingers over the cannula to prevent bleeding.

You can use a hemostat or two to help disconnect the tubing.

Disconnect, but don't dislodge

- Gently disconnect the old tubing, being careful not to dislodge the I.V. device. A hemostat can be used to stabilize the hub. Or use one hemostat on the venipuncture device and another on the hard plastic end of the tubing and then twist the hemostats in opposite directions to loosen the connection.
- Remove the protective cap from the new tubing and connect the new adapter to the cannula while holding the hub securely.
- Observe for blood backflow into the new tubing *to verify that the needle or cannula is still in place.*
- Adjust the clamp to maintain the appropriate flow rate.
- Retape the cannula hub and I.V. tubing, recheck the I.V. flow rate, and be sure to label the new tubing and container with the date and time. Label the solution container with a time strip according to your facility's policy.

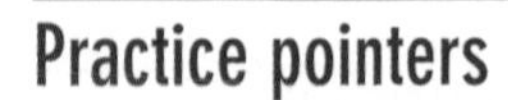

Practice pointers

- Check the prescribed I.V. flow rate before each solution change *to prevent errors*. If you crack the adapter or hub (or if you accidentally dislodge the cannula from the vein), remove the cannula.

Apply pressure and an adhesive bandage to stop any bleeding. Perform a venipuncture at another site and restart the I.V.

- Always verify that the pump is connected to the correct solution before changing the rate. Often, more than one solution may be hanging on a single pump and interchanged for intermittent infusions. (See *Documenting peripheral I.V. catheter maintenance*.)

Documenting peripheral I.V. catheter maintenance

Record the time, date, and rate and type of solution (and any additives) on the I.V. flowchart. Also record this information, dressing or tubing changes, and site appearance in your notes.

PICC insertion and removal

For a patient who needs central venous therapy for 1 to 6 months or who requires repeated venous access, a peripherally inserted central catheter (PICC) may be the best option. They're available in single- and double-lumen versions, with or without guide wires, and of varying diameters and lengths.

PICCs are being used increasingly for patients receiving home care. The device is easier to insert than other central venous devices and provides safe, reliable access for drug administration and blood sampling. A single catheter may be used for the entire course of therapy with greater convenience and at reduced cost. If your state nurse practice act permits, you may insert a PICC once you have obtained certification to do so.

What you need

Catheter insertion kit * three alcohol swabs or other approved antimicrobial solution, such as 10% povidone-iodine or tincture of iodine 2% * povidone-iodine ointment * 3-mL vial of heparin (100 U/mL) * injection port with short extension tubing * sterile and nonsterile measuring tape * vial of normal saline solution * sterile gauze pads * tape * linen-saver pad * sterile drapes * tourniquet * sterile transparent semipermeable dressing * two pairs of sterile gloves * sterile gown * mask * goggles * clean gloves.

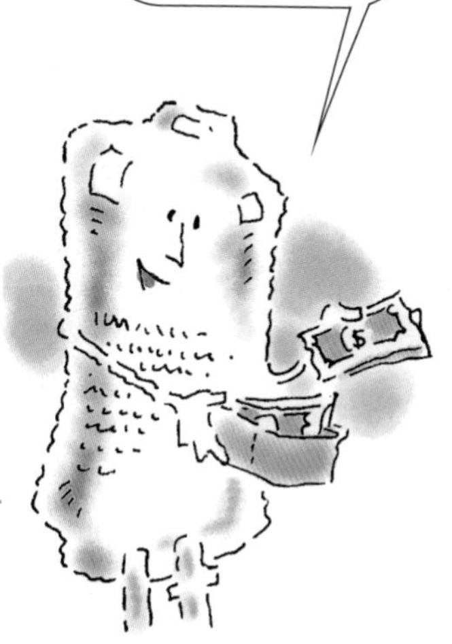
Because you only need one catheter for the entire theraphy, a PICC increases convenience and reduces costs.

Getting ready

Gather the necessary supplies. If you're administering PICC therapy in the patient's home, bring everything with you.

How you do it

- Describe the procedure to the patient and perform hand hygiene.
- Check the patient's chart to verify the order. Identify the patient using two patient identifiers.

Inserting a PICC

- Select the insertion site, place the tourniquet on the patient's arm, and assess the antecubital fossa.
- Remove the tourniquet and determine the spot at which the catheter tip will rest after insertion. For placement in the superior vena cava, measure the distance from the insertion site to the shoulder and from the shoulder to the sternal notch, then add 3″ (7.6 cm) to the measurement.
- Have the patient lie in a supine position with her arm at a 90-degree angle to her body and place a linen-saver pad under her arm.
- Open the PICC tray and drop the rest of the sterile items onto the sterile field. Put on the sterile gown, mask, goggles, and gloves.
- Using the sterile measuring tape, cut the distal end of the catheter according to specific manufacturer's recommendations and guidelines using the equipment provided.
- Using sterile technique, withdraw 5 mL of the normal saline solution and flush the extension tubing and the cap and then remove the needle from the syringe. Attach the syringe to the hub of the catheter and flush.

Rub down

- Prepare the insertion site by rubbing it with an alcohol swab or other approved antimicrobial solution using a circular motion and working outward about 6″ (15 cm). Allow the area to dry but be sure not to touch the intended insertion site.
- Remove gloves and apply the tourniquet about 4″ (10 cm) above the antecubital fossa.
- Don a new pair of sterile gloves and place a sterile drape under the patient's arm and another on top of the arm. Drop a sterile 4″ × 4″ gauze pad over the tourniquet.
- Stabilize the patient's vein and insert the catheter introducer at a 10-degree angle directly into the vein.
- After successful vein entry, you should see a blood return in the flashback chamber. Without changing the needle's position, gently advance the plastic introducer sheath until you're sure the tip is well within the vein. Remove the tourniquet using a sterile 4″ × 4″ gauze pad *to maintain sterile technique.*

Pressure point

- Carefully withdraw the needle while holding the introducer still. *To minimize blood loss,* try applying finger pressure on the vein just beyond the distal end of the introducer sheath.
- Using sterile forceps, insert the catheter into the introducer sheath and advance it into the vein 2″ to 4″ (5 to 10 cm).
- Remove the tourniquet using the 4″ × 4″ gauze pad.

- When you have advanced the catheter to the shoulder, ask the patient to turn her head toward the affected arm and place her chin on her chest. *This will occlude the jugular vein and ease the catheter's advancement into the subclavian vein.*
- Advance the catheter until about 4" (10 cm) remain. Then pull the introducer sheath out of the vein and away from the venipuncture.
- Grasp the tabs of the introducer sheath and flex them toward its distal end *to split the sheath,* then pull the tabs apart and away from the catheter until the sheath is completely split. Discard the sheath.
- Continue to advance the catheter until it's completely inserted. Flush with normal saline solution followed by heparin according to your facility's policy. A chest X-ray will need to be completed to confirm catheter placement.

Simon says: Hands down

- With the patient's arm below heart level, remove the syringe and connect the capped extension set to the hub of the catheter.
- Apply a sterile 2" × 2" gauze pad directly over the site and a sterile transparent semipermeable dressing over that. Leave this dressing in place for 24 hours.
- After the initial 24 hours, apply a new sterile transparent semipermeable dressing. The gauze pad is no longer necessary. You can place Steri-Strips over the catheter wings. Flush with heparin according to your facility's policy.

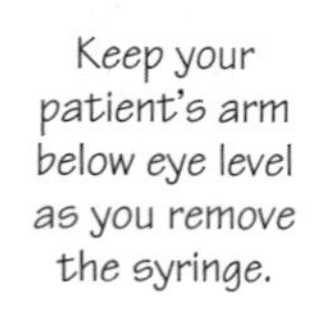

Keep your patient's arm below eye level as you remove the syringe.

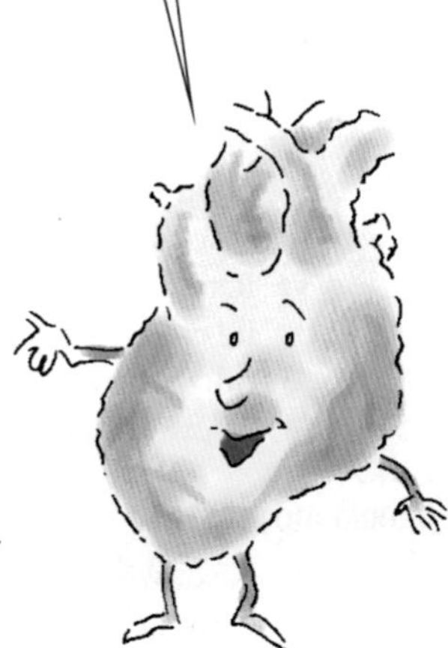

Administering drugs

- Check for blood return and flush with normal saline solution before administering a drug through a PICC line.
- Clamp the 7" (17.8 cm) extension tubing and connect the empty syringe to the tubing. Release the clamp and aspirate slowly *to verify blood return.* Flush with 3 mL of normal saline solution and then administer the drug. Be sure to check your hospital policy for guidelines.
- After giving the drug, flush again with 3 mL of normal saline solution in a 10-mL syringe. You should also flush the line between infusions of incompatible drugs or fluids.

Changing the dressing

- Change the dressing as per facility policy and more frequently if the integrity of the dressing becomes compromised. If possible, choose a transparent semipermeable dressing, *which has a high moisture vapor transmission rate.*

- Perform hand hygiene and assemble the necessary supplies. Position the patient with her arm extended away from her body at a 45- to 90-degree angle so that the insertion site is below heart level *to reduce the risk of air embolism*. Put on a sterile mask.

Today's star: The thumb

- Open a package of sterile gloves and use the inside of the package as a sterile field. Then open the transparent semipermeable dressing and drop it onto the field. Put on clean gloves and remove the old dressing by holding your left thumb on the catheter and stretching the dressing parallel to the skin. Repeat the last step with your right thumb holding the catheter. Free the remaining section of the dressing from the catheter by peeling toward the insertion site from the distal end to the proximal end *to prevent catheter dislodgment*. Remove the clean gloves.
- Don sterile gloves. Clean the area with an alcohol swab, starting at the insertion site and working outward.
- Apply the dressing carefully. Secure the tubing to the edge of the dressing over the tape with ¼″ adhesive tape.

Removing a PICC

- Done by a specially trained nurse. Check the patient's chart to verify the order. Identify the patient using two patient identifiers.
- Assemble the necessary equipment at the patient's bedside, explain the procedure to the patient, perform hand hygiene, and place a linen-saver pad under the patient's arm.
- Remove the tape holding the extension tubing and open two sterile gauze pads on a clean, flat surface. After putting on gloves, stabilize the catheter at the hub and remove the dressing by pulling it toward the insertion site.

Smooth move

- Next, withdraw the catheter with smooth, gentle pressure in small increments. If you feel resistance, stop and apply slight tension to the line by taping it down. Try to remove it again in a few minutes. If you still feel resistance, notify the doctor for further instructions. (See *PICC removal complications*.)
- After removing the catheter, apply pressure to the site with a sterile gauze pad for 1 minute.
- Measure and inspect the catheter. If any part has broken off during removal, notify the doctor immediately and monitor the patient for signs of distress.
- Cover the site with povidone-iodine ointment and tape a new folded gauze pad in place. Dispose of used items properly and perform hand hygiene.

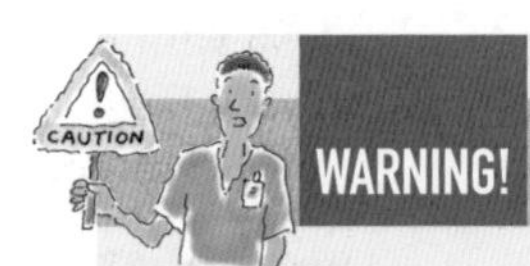

PICC removal complications

If a portion of the PICC breaks during removal, immediately apply a tourniquet to the upper arm, close to the axilla, to prevent advancement of the catheter piece into the right atrium. Then check the patient's radial pulse. If you don't detect the radial pulse, the tourniquet is too tight. Keep the tourniquet in place until an X-ray can be obtained, the doctor is notified, and surgical retrieval is attempted.

What else can happen? Catheter occlusion is also relatively common. Air embolism, always a potential risk of venipuncture, poses less danger in PICC therapy. Catheter tip migration may occur with vigorous flushing.

Practice pointers

- For a patient receiving intermittent PICC therapy, the catheter will need to be flushed with 10 mL of normal saline solution and 3 mL of heparin (100 U/mL) after each use or according to your facility's policy. For catheters that aren't being used routinely, flushing every 12 hours with 3 mL (100 U/mL) of heparin will maintain patency.
- If a patient will be receiving blood or blood products through the PICC, use at least an 18G cannula.
- Assess the catheter insertion site through the transparent semi-permeable dressing every 24 hours. Although oozing is common for the first 24 hours after insertion, excessive bleeding after that should be evaluated. (See *Documenting PICC insertion and removal.*)

Documenting PICC insertion and removal

In your notes, document:
- entire procedure, including problems with catheter placement
- patient education
- size, length, and type of catheter
- condition of the insertion site
- catheter insertion location.

Flow rate calculation and control

Calculated from a doctor's orders, flow rate is usually expressed as the total volume of I.V. solution infused over a prescribed interval or as the total volume given in milliliters per hour.

Same flow, different measure

When regulated by a clamp, flow rate is usually measured in drops per minute; by a volumetric pump, in milliliters per hour. The flow regulator can be set to deliver the desired amount of solution, also in milliliters per hour. Flow regulators are less accurate than infusion pumps and are most reliable when used with inactive adult patients.

With any device, flow rate can be easily monitored by using a time tape, which indicates the prescribed solution level at hourly intervals.

What you need

I.V. administration set with clamp ✱ 1″ paper or adhesive tape (or premarked time tape) ✱ infusion pump and controller (if infusing medication) ✱ watch with second hand ✱ drip rate chart, as necessary ✱ pen.

Standard macrodrip sets deliver from 10 to 20 drops/mL, depending on the manufacturer; microdrip sets, 60 drops/mL; and blood transfusion sets, 10 drops/mL. A commercially available adapter can convert a macrodrip set to a microdrip system.

Getting ready

Verify the doctor's orders before calculating the rate.

How you do it

- Flow rate requires close monitoring and correction *because factors, such as venous spasm, venous pressure changes, patient movement or manipulation of the clamp, and bent or kinked tubing, can cause the rate to vary markedly.*

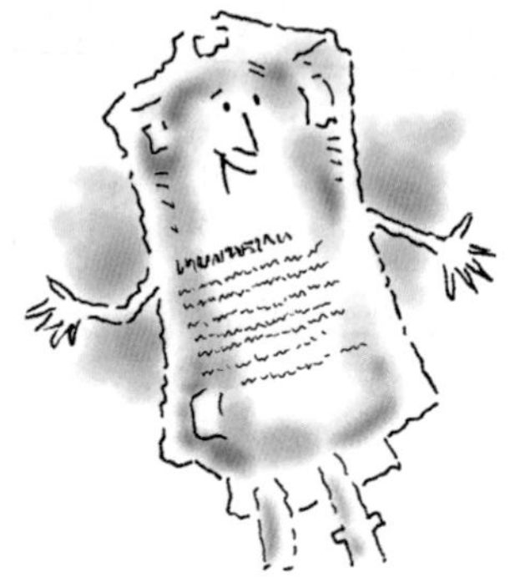
Keep a close watch on my flow rate—especially at the start of an infusion.

Calculating and setting the drip rate

- To determine the proper drip rate, divide the volume of the infusion (in milliliters) by the time of infusion (in minutes) and then multiply this by the drip factor (in drops per milliliter) or use your unit's drip rate chart.
- After calculating the desired drip rate, remove your watch and hold it next to the drip chamber *so that you can observe the watch and drops simultaneously.*
- Release the clamp to the approximate drip rate. Then count drops for 1 minute *to account for flow irregularities.*
- Adjust the clamp, as necessary, and count drops for 1 minute. Continue to adjust the clamp and count drops until the correct rate is achieved.

Making a time tape

- Calculate the number of milliliters to be infused per hour. Place a piece of tape vertically on the container alongside the volume-increment markers.
- Starting at the current solution level, move down the number of milliliters to be infused in 1 hour and mark the appropriate time and a horizontal line on the tape at this level. Then continue to mark 1-hour intervals until you reach the bottom of the container.
- Check the flow rate every 15 minutes until stable, then every hour or according to facility policy; adjust as needed.
- With each check, inspect the I.V. site for complications and assess the patient's response to therapy.

Practice pointers

- If the infusion rate slows significantly, a slight rate increase may be necessary. If the rate must be increased by more than 30%, consult the doctor. When infusing drugs, use an I.V. pump, if possible, *to avoid flow rate inaccuracies*. Always use a pump when infusing solutions through a central line.

- Large-volume solution containers have about 10% more fluid than the amount indicated on the bag *to allow for tubing purges*. Thus, a 1,000-mL bag or bottle contains an additional 100 mL. (See *Documenting flow rate control*.)

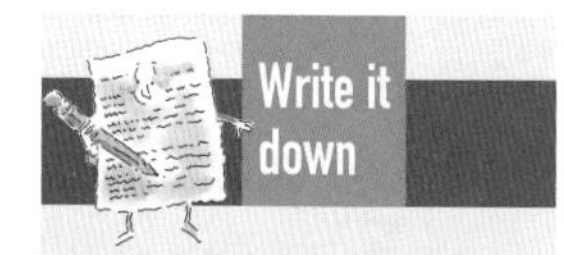

Documenting flow rate control

Record the original flow rate when setting up a peripheral line. If you adjust the rate, record the change, date, and time.

I.V. infusion pump use

Various types of pumps electronically regulate the flow of I.V. solutions or drugs with great accuracy.

Volumetric pumps, used for high-pressure infusion of drugs or for highly accurate delivery of fluids or drugs, have mechanisms to propel the solution at the desired rate under pressure. (Pressure is brought to bear only when gravity flow rates are insufficient to maintain preset infusion rates.) The peristaltic pump applies pressure to the I.V. tubing to force the solution through it. (Not all peristaltic pumps are volumetric; some count drops.) The piston-cylinder pump pushes the solution through special disposable cassettes. Most of these pumps operate at high pressures (up to 45 psi), delivering from 1 to 999 mL/hour with about 98% accuracy. (Some pumps operate at 10 to 25 psi.)

Specialty items

The portable syringe pump, another type of volumetric pump, delivers small amounts of fluid over a long period. It's used to administer fluids to infants and to deliver drugs such as antibiotics.

What you need

Peristaltic pump ✳ I.V. pole ✳ I.V. solution ✳ sterile administration set ✳ sterile peristaltic tubing or cassette, if needed ✳ alcohol pads ✳ adhesive tape. Tubing and cassettes vary among manufacturers.

Getting ready

To set up a volumetric pump

Attach the pump to the I.V. pole. Then swab the port on the I.V. container with alcohol, insert the administration set spike, and fill the drip chamber completely *to prevent air bubbles from entering the tubing*. Next, prime the tubing and close the clamp. Follow the manufacturer's instructions for tubing placement.

How you do it

- Position the pump on the same side of the bed as the I.V. or anticipated venipuncture site. If necessary, perform the venipuncture.
- Plug in the machine and attach its tubing to the needle or catheter hub.
- Turn it on and press the START button. Set the appropriate dials on the front panel to the desired infusion rate and volume. Set the volume dial at 50 mL less than the prescribed volume or 50 mL less than the volume in the container *so that you can hang a new container before the old one empties.*
- Check the patency of the I.V. line and watch for infiltration.
- Tape all connections and recheck the controller's drip rate *because taping may alter it.* Turn on the alarm switches and explain the alarm system to the patient. If the patient is to go home using an I.V. pump, review teaching with him. (See *Using an I.V. pump in the home.*)

Practice pointers

- Monitor the pump and the patient frequently to ensure the device's correct operation and flow rate and to detect infiltration and complications, such as infection and air embolism.
- Check the manufacturer's recommendations before administering opaque fluids, such as blood, *because some pumps fail to detect opaque fluids and others may cause hemolysis of infused blood.* (See *Documenting I.V. pump use.*)

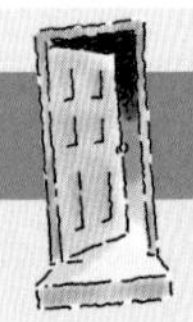

Home care connection

Using an I.V. pump in the home

Make sure the patient and his family understand the purpose of using the pump. Demonstrate how the device works and how to maintain the system (tubing, solution, and site assessment and care) until you're confident they can proceed safely. Have the patient and/or family do a repeat demonstration to verify technique, safety, and understanding. It is also helpful to give the patient a DVD of the procedure if available.

Discuss which complications to watch for, such as infiltration, and review measures to take if complications occur. Schedule a teaching session with the patient or family so you can answer questions they may have about the procedure before discharge.

Write it down

Documenting I.V. pump use

In addition to routine documentation of the I.V. infusion, record the use of a pump on the I.V. record and in your notes.

Total parenteral nutrition

When a patient can't meet his nutritional needs by oral or enteral feedings, he may require I.V. nutritional support, also known as parenteral nutrition.

Total parenteral nutrition (TPN) refers to any nutrient solution, including lipids, given through a central venous line. The most common delivery route for TPN is through a central venous line into the superior vena cava. Depending on the solution, it may be used to boost the patient's caloric intake, to supply full caloric needs, or to surpass the patient's caloric requirements.

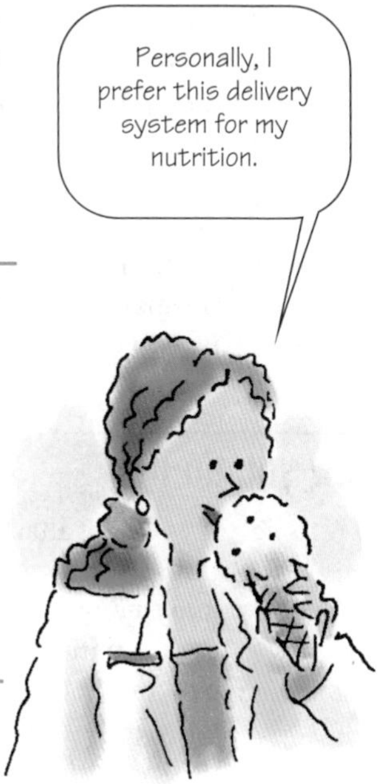

Personally, I prefer this delivery system for my nutrition.

What you need

Bag or bottle of prescribed parenteral nutrition solution ✳ sterile I.V. tubing with attached extension tubing ✳ 0.22-micron filter (or 1.2-micron filter if solution contains lipids or albumin) ✳ reflux valve ✳ time tape ✳ tape ✳ alcohol pads ✳ electronic infusion pump ✳ scale ✳ intake and output record ✳ sterile gloves ✳ syringes filled with normal saline solution for flush.

Getting ready

Make sure the solution, the patient, and the equipment are ready. Remove the solution from the refrigerator at least 1 hour before use. Check the solution against the doctor's order for correct patient name, expiration date, and formula components. Observe the container for cracks and the solution for cloudiness, turbidity, and particles. If any of these is present, return the solution to the pharmacy.

When you're ready to administer the solution, explain the procedure to the patient. Check the name on the solution container against the name on the patient's wristband and use two patient identifiers. Perform hand hygiene. Don gloves and, if specified by facility policy, a mask.

There's an order to it

- In sequence, connect the pump tubing, the micron filter with attached extension tubing (if the tubing doesn't contain an in-line filter), and the reflux valve.
- Insert the filter as close to the catheter site as possible. If the tubing doesn't have luer-lock connections, tape all connections *to prevent accidental separation, which could lead to air embolism, exsanguination,* or *sepsis.*

- Squeeze the I.V. drip chamber and, holding it upright, insert the tubing spike into the I.V. bag or bottle. Then release the drip chamber. Next, prime the tubing.
- Invert the filter at the distal end of the tubing and open the roller clamp. Let the solution fill the tubing and the filter. Gently tap it to dislodge air bubbles trapped in the Y-ports.
- If indicated, attach a time tape to the parenteral nutrition container for accurate measurement of fluid intake.
- Record the date and time you hung the fluid and initial the parenteral nutrition solution container.
- Attach the setup to the infusion pump and prepare it according to the manufacturer's instructions. Remove and discard your gloves. Perform hand hygiene.
- With the patient in the supine position, flush the catheter with normal saline solution and put on gloves. Clean the catheter injection cap with an alcohol pad.

How you do it

- If you'll be attaching the container of parenteral nutrition solution to a central line, clamp the central line before disconnecting it *to prevent air from entering the catheter*. If a clamp isn't available, ask the patient to perform Valsalva's maneuver or instruct the patient to take and deep breath and hold just as you change the tubing. Or, if the patient is being mechanically ventilated, change the I.V. tubing immediately after the machine delivers a breath at peak inspiration. *Both of these measures increase intrathoracic pressure and prevent air embolism.*
- Using aseptic technique, attach the tubing to the designated luer-locking port and remove the clamp, if applicable.
- Set the infusion pump at the ordered flow rate and start the infusion. Make sure the catheter junction is secure.
- Tag the tubing with the date and time of change.

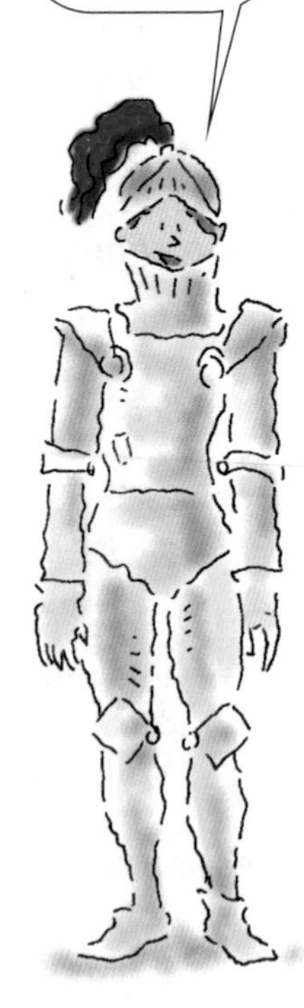
You don't need armor — just gloves and a mask.

Starting the infusion

- Depending on the patient's tolerance, parenteral nutrition is usually initiated at a rate of 40 to 50 mL/hour and then advanced by 25 mL/hour every 6 hours (as tolerated) until the desired infusion rate is achieved. However, when the glucose concentration is low, as occurs in most formulas, you can initiate the rate necessary to infuse the complete 24-hour volume and discontinue the solution without tapering.

Changing solutions

- Prepare the new solution and I.V. tubing as described earlier and put on gloves. Remove the protective caps from the solution containers and wipe the tops with alcohol pads.
- Turn off the infusion pump, close the flow clamps, remove the spike from the solution container that's hanging, and insert it into the new container.

Matching sets

- Hang the new container and tubing alongside the old. Turn on the infusion pump, set the flow rate, and open the flow clamp completely.
- If you'll be attaching the solution to a peripheral line, examine the skin above the insertion site for redness and warmth and assess for pain. If you suspect phlebitis or if the I.V. has been in place for 72 hours, remove the existing I.V. line and start a line in a different vein.
- Next, turn off the infusion pump and close the flow clamp on the old tubing. Disconnect the tubing from the catheter hub and connect the new tubing. Open the flow clamp on the new container to a moderately slow rate.
- Remove the old tubing from the infusion pump and insert the new tubing according to the manufacturer's instructions. Then turn on the infusion pump, set it to the desired flow rate, and open the flow clamp completely. Remove the old equipment and dispose of it properly.

Practice pointers

- Always infuse a parenteral nutrition solution at a constant rate without interruption *to avoid blood glucose fluctuations*. If the infusion slows, consult the doctor before changing the infusion rate.

Check points

- Monitor the patient's vital signs every 4 hours or more often if necessary. Watch for an increased temperature, *an early sign of catheter-related sepsis*.
- Check the patient's blood glucose every 6 hours. Some patients may require supplementary insulin, which the pharmacist may add directly to the solution. The patient may also require additional subcutaneous doses.
- Change the dressing over the catheter according to your facility's policy or whenever the dressing becomes wet, soiled, or nonocclusive.

- Weigh the patient at the same time every morning. Maintain accurate intake and output records.
- Change the tubing and filters every 24 hours or according to facility policy. (See *Documenting total parenteral nutrition.*)

Documenting total parenteral nutrition

In your notes, document:
- times of the dressing, filter, and solution changes
- condition of the catheter insertion site
- your observations of the patient's condition
- patient education
- complications and interventions taken.

Lipid emulsion administration

Lipid emulsions may be given alone or in conjunction with parenteral nutrition to provide a source of calories and essential fatty acids. They can be administered through either a peripheral or a central venous line.

What you need

Lipid emulsion ✳ I.V. administration set with vented spike (a separate adapter may be used if an administration set with a vented spike isn't available) ✳ access pin with reflux valve ✳ gloves ✳ tape ✳ time tape ✳ alcohol pads.

If administering the lipid emulsion as part of a 3-in-1 solution, also obtain a filter that's 1.2 microns or greater *because lipids will clog a smaller filter.*

Getting ready

Inspect the lipid emulsion for opacity and consistency of color and texture; if you think its stability or sterility is questionable, return the bottle to the pharmacy.

Make sure you have the correct lipid emulsion and verify with the doctor's order and patient name.

Documenting lipid emulsion administration

In your notes, record:
- times of all dressing changes and solution changes
- condition of the catheter insertion site
- your observations of the patient's condition
- patient education
- complications and nursing actions taken.

How you do it

- Identify the patient with two patient identifiers.
- Explain the procedure to the patient.

Connecting the tubing

- First, connect the I.V. tubing to the access pin. Access pins with reflux valves take the place of needles when connecting piggyback tubing to primary tubing.
- Close the flow clamp on the I.V. tubing. If the tubing doesn't contain luer-lock connections, tape all connections securely.
- Perform hand hygiene. Don gloves and remove the protective cap from the lipid emulsion bottle; wipe the rubber stopper with an alcohol pad.

Hold, invert, squeeze

- Hold the bottle upright and insert the vented spike through the inner circle of the rubber stopper, then invert the bottle and squeeze the drip chamber until it fills to the level indicated in the tubing package instructions.
- Open the flow clamp and prime the tubing. Gently tap the tubing *to dislodge air bubbles trapped in the Y-ports*. If necessary, attach a time tape to the lipid emulsion container *to allow accurate measurement of fluid intake.*
- Label the tubing, noting the date and time the tubing was hung.

Starting the infusion

- If this is the patient's first lipid infusion, administer a test dose at the rate of 1 mL/minute for 30 minutes; monitor the patient's vital signs and watch for signs and symptoms of an adverse reaction or allergy.
- If the patient has no adverse reactions to the test dose, begin the infusion at the prescribed rate. Use an infusion pump if you'll be infusing the lipids at less than 20 mL/hour. The maximum infusion rate is 125 mL/hour for a 10% lipid emulsion and 60 mL/hour for a 20% lipid emulsion.

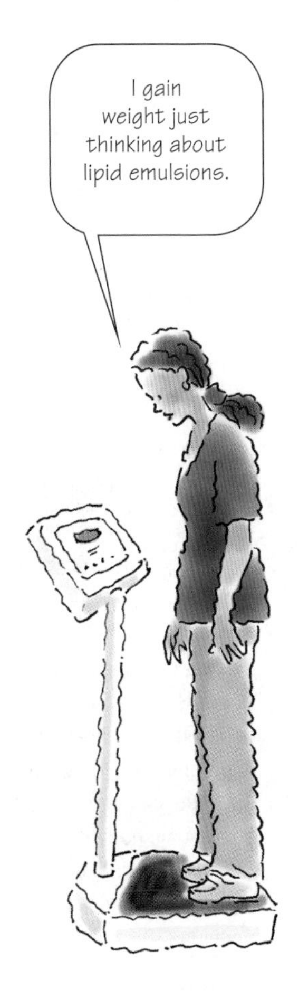
I gain weight just thinking about lipid emulsions.

Practice pointers

- Lipid emulsions are contraindicated in patients who have a condition that disrupts normal fat metabolism, such as pathologic hyperlipidemia, lipid nephrosis, or acute pancreatitis. They must be used cautiously in patients who have liver disease, pulmonary disease, anemia, or coagulation disorders and in those who are at risk for developing a fat embolism.
- Change the I.V. tubing and the lipid emulsion container every 24 hours.
- Whenever possible, draw blood for triglyceride levels at least 6 hours after the completion of the lipid emulsion infusion *to avoid falsely elevated results*. (See *Documenting lipid emulsion administration*.)

Blood transfusion

Whole blood transfusion replenishes both the volume and the oxygen-carrying capacity of the circulatory system. You may also transfuse packed red blood cells (RBCs) from which 80% of the plasma has been removed; this, however, restores only the oxygen-carrying capacity. Both types of transfusions treat decreased hemoglobin levels and hematocrit.

Two nurses must identify the patient and blood products before administering a transfusion to prevent errors and a potentially fatal reaction. It is essential that the right blood be given to the right patient at the right time. (See *Transfusion complications*.) If the patient is a Jehovah's Witness, a transfusion requires special written permission.

What you need

Blood recipient set (filter and tubing with drip chamber for blood or combined set) ✻ I.V. pole ✻ gloves ✻ gown ✻ face shield ✻ multiple-lead tubing ✻ whole blood or packed RBCs ✻ 250 mL of normal saline solution ✻ venipuncture equipment, if necessary (should include 20G or larger catheter) ✻ optional: ice bag, warm compresses.

Getting ready

Avoid obtaining either whole blood or packed RBCs until you're ready to begin the transfusion. Prepare the equipment when you're ready to start the infusion.

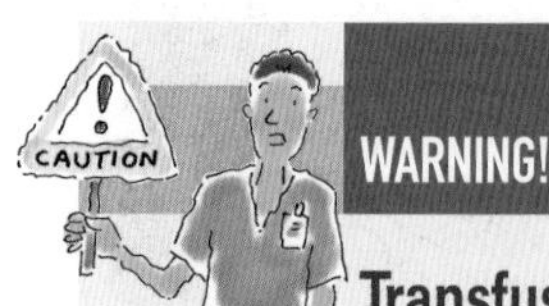

WARNING!

Transfusion complications

Despite improvements in crossmatching precautions, transfusion reactions can still occur. Unlike a transfusion reaction, an infectious disease transmitted during a transfusion may go undetected until days, weeks, or even months later when it produces signs and symptoms. Hepatitis C accounts for most posttransfusion hepatitis cases. The tests that detect hepatitis B and C can produce false-negative results and may allow some hepatitis cases to go undetected.

When testing for antibodies to human immunodeficiency virus (HIV), keep in mind that antibodies don't appear until 6 to 12 weeks after exposure. The estimated risk of acquiring HIV from blood products varies from 1 in 40,000 to 1 in 153,000.

What else can go wrong?

Circulatory overload and hemolytic, allergic, febrile, and pyogenic reactions can result from any transfusion. Coagulation disturbances, citrate intoxication, hyperkalemia, acid-base imbalance, ammonia intoxication, and hypothermia can result from massive transfusion.

How you do it

- Explain the procedure to the patient, make sure he has signed an informed consent form, and record baseline vital signs.
- Obtain whole blood or packed RBCs from the blood bank within 30 minutes of the transfusion start time. Check the expiration date on the blood bag and observe for abnormal color, RBC clumping, gas bubbles, and extraneous material. Return outdated or abnormal blood to the blood bank.

ID issues

- Compare the name and number on the patient's wristband with those on the blood bag label. Check the blood bag identification number, ABO blood group, and Rh compatibility. Also, compare the patient's blood bank identification number, if present, with the number on the blood bag. Identification of blood and blood products is performed at the patient's bedside by two licensed professionals according to the facility's policy.
- Don gloves, a gown, and a face shield. Using a Y-type set, close all the clamps on the set. Then insert the spike of the line you're using for the normal saline solution into the bag of saline solution. Next, open the port on the blood bag and insert the other spike. Hang the bags on the I.V. pole, open the clamp on the line of saline solution, and squeeze the drip chamber until it's half full.
- If the patient doesn't have an I.V. line in place, perform a venipuncture using a 20G or larger diameter catheter. Avoid using an existing line if the needle or catheter lumen is smaller than 20G. Central venous access devices also may be used for transfusion therapy.

Shaken, not stirred

- If you're administering whole blood, gently invert the bag several times *to mix the cells.*
- Attach the prepared blood administration set to the venipuncture device and flush it with normal saline solution. Then close the clamp to the saline solution and open the clamp between the blood bag and the patient. Adjust the flow clamp closest to the patient to deliver the blood at the calculated drip rate.
- Remain with the patient and watch for signs of a transfusion reaction, such as fever, chills, and wheezing. If such signs develop, record vital signs and stop the transfusion. Infuse saline solution at a moderately slow infusion rate and notify the doctor at once. If no signs of a reaction appear within 15 minutes, you'll need to adjust the flow clamp to the ordered infusion rate. A unit of RBCs may be given over 1 to 4 hours as ordered. Review the facility policy on blood transfusion for specific information. This is a high-risk procedure that requires strict adherence to the policy guidelines.

- After completing the transfusion, you'll need to put on gloves and remove and discard the used infusion equipment. Then remember to reconnect the original I.V. fluid, if necessary, or discontinue the I.V. infusion.

Sorry, you can't use the ATM

- Return the empty blood bag to the blood bank and discard the tubing and filter in the appropriate container per facility policy.
- Record the patient's vital signs.

Practice pointers

- Although some microaggregate filters can be used for up to 10 units of blood, always replace the filter and tubing if more than 1 hour elapses between transfusions. Blood transfusion sets should be changed after a maximum of 6 hours.
- After an RBC or plasma transfusion, a new blood administration set should be used to infuse platelets.
- Once a unit of blood has been removed from controlled storage, the transfusion should be commenced immediately on delivery to the clinical area. If the transfusion cannot be initiated promptly, the blood should be returned to the hospital transfusion laboratory for storage, unless the transfusion to the intended recipient can be completed within 4 hours. Blood should be returned to the hospital transfusion laboratory for documented disposal if out of controlled storage for more than 30 minutes.
- Routine warming of blood is not indicated. Patients who would benefit from warmed blood are adults and children receiving massive infusion and infants requiring an exchange transfusion.
- For rapid blood replacement, a pressure bag may be needed.
- If you're administering packed RBCs with a Y-type set, you can add saline solution to the bag *to dilute the cells* by closing the clamp between the patient and the drip chamber and opening the clamp from the blood. Then lower the blood bag below the saline solution container and let 30 to 50 mL of saline solution flow into the packed cells. Finally, close the clamp to the blood bag, rehang the bag, rotate it gently *to mix the cells and saline solution*, and close the clamp to the saline container.
- There are over 70 steps in the blood administration process. It is essential to adhere to all steps to prevent errors that could be fatal. The most frequently occurring errors are involving:
  - patient identification
  - sampling/labeling of the crossmatch sample
  - removal of blood from the fridge before transfusion
  - checking the identification of both the patient and the blood component at the bedside. (See *Documenting blood transfusions*.)

Documenting blood transfusions

In your notes, record:
- date and time of the transfusion
- type and amount of transfusion product
- patient's vital signs
- your check of all identification data
- patient's response
- patient education
- transfusion reaction and nursing actions taken.

Transfusion reaction management

A transfusion reaction typically stems from a major antigen-antibody reaction and can result from a single or massive transfusion of blood or blood products.

Although many reactions occur during the transfusion or within 96 hours afterward, infectious diseases transmitted during a transfusion may go undetected until days, weeks, or months later when signs and symptoms appear. A transfusion reaction requires immediate recognition and prompt nursing action to prevent further complications and, possibly, death.

Two nurses must identify the patient and blood products before a transfusion.

What you need

Normal saline solution ✱ I.V. administration set ✱ sterile urine specimen container ✱ needle, syringe, and tubes for blood samples ✱ transfusion reaction report form ✱ optional: oxygen, epinephrine, hypothermia blanket, leukocyte removal filter.

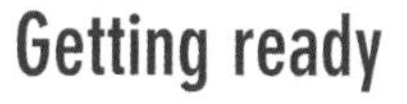

Getting ready

As soon as you suspect an adverse reaction, stop the transfusion and start the saline infusion at a keep-vein-open rate and notify the doctor. Monitor vital signs every 15 minutes or as indicated by the severity and type of reaction.

How you do it

- Compare the labels on all blood containers with corresponding patient identification forms *to verify that the transfusion was the correct blood or blood product.*
- Notify the blood bank of a possible transfusion reaction and collect blood samples, as ordered. Immediately send the samples, all transfusion containers (even if empty), and the administration set to the blood bank. *The blood bank will test these materials to further evaluate the reaction.*
- Collect the first posttransfusion urine specimen, mark the collection slip, "Possible transfusion reaction," and send it to the laboratory immediately. *The laboratory tests this urine specimen for the presence of hemoglobin (Hb), which indicates a hemolytic reaction.*
- Closely monitor intake and output. Note evidence of oliguria or anuria *because Hb deposition in the renal tubules can cause renal damage.*

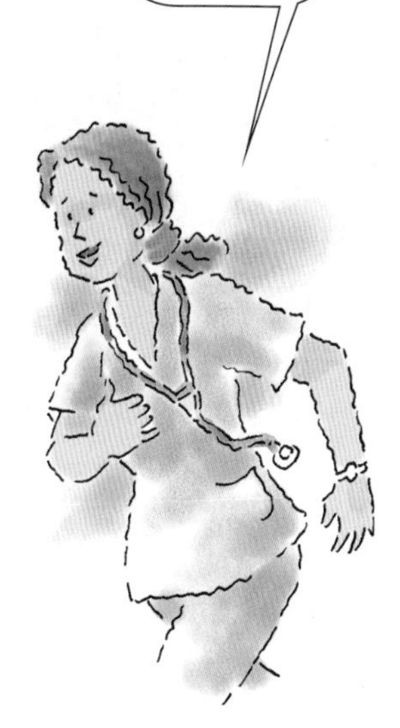
Every moment counts if your patient has a transfusion reaction.

- If prescribed, administer oxygen, epinephrine, or other drugs, and apply a hypothermia blanket *to reduce fever*.

Practice pointers

- Treat all transfusion reactions as serious until proven otherwise. If the doctor anticipates a transfusion reaction, such as one that may occur in a leukemia patient, he may order prophylactic treatment with antihistamines or antipyretics to precede blood administration. (See *Documenting transfusion reaction management*.)

Documenting transfusion reaction management

In your notes, record:
- time and date of the transfusion reaction
- type and amount of infused blood or blood products
- clinical signs of the transfusion reaction in order of occurrence
- patient's vital signs
- specimens sent to the laboratory for analysis
- treatment given and patient's response.

If required by your facility's policy, complete the transfusion reaction form.

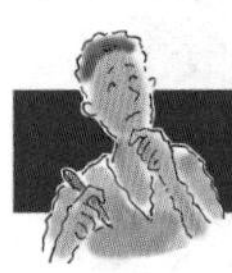

Quick quiz

1. The nurse is instilling eyedrops for her patient. Which instruction should the nurse provide?
   A. Look up and away.
   B. Look down and away.
   C. Look straight ahead.
   D. Look to the side.

Answer: A. Before instilling eyedrops, instruct the patient to look up and away to minimize the risk of touching the cornea with the dropper.

2. Before instilling eardrops, the nurse must straighten the patient's ear canal. How will the nurse accomplish this in an adult patient?
   A. Pull the auricle of the ear up and back.
   B. Pull the auricle of the ear down and back.
   C. Pull the auricle of the ear up and forward.
   D. Pull the auricle down and forward.

Answer: A. To straighten the ear canal of an adult, pull the auricle up and back; for an infant or young child, gently pull down and back.

3. After administering the patient his medication through an NG tube, how long should the nurse leave the head of his bed elevated?
   A. 15 minutes
   B. 30 minutes
   C. 60 minutes
   D. 90 minutes

Answer: B. After administering medication through an NG tube, leave the head of his bed elevated for at least 30 minutes.

4. The nurse is administering a rectal suppository to his patient. How should the patient be positioned?
   A. Supine
   B. On his left side in Sims' position
   C. In slight Trendelenburg's position
   D. Lithotomy

Answer: B. Before inserting a rectal suppository, place the patient on his left side in Sims' position.

5. In assessing the patient's I.V. site, which, findings indicate the patient is experiencing an I.V. infiltration?
   A. Redness, firmness, pain along the path of the vein, and edema
   B. Redness and pain at the puncture site
   C. Coolness, blanching, and edema at the site
   D. Red, warm with yellow drainage at the I.V. site

Answer: C. Signs of infiltration include coolness, blanching, and edema at the site.

Scoring

☆☆☆ If you answered all five items correctly, outstanding! You're the doyenne of drug administration.

☆☆ If you answered three or four items correctly, congratulations! You're on the track to exactness.

☆ If you answered fewer than three items correctly, give it another shot! Review this chapter and you'll be infusing more knowledge in no time.

Selected References

Kinman, T. (2013). *Sublingual and buccal medication administration*. Retrieved from http://www.healthline.com/health/sublingual-and-buccal-medication-administration#Definition1

National Blood Users Group. (2004). *Guidelines for the administration of blood and blood components*. Retrieved from https://www.giveblood.ie/Clinical_Services/Haemovigilance/Publications/Guidelines_for_the_Administration_of_Blood_and_Blood_Components.pdf

Perry, A., Potter, P., & Desmarais, P. (2015). *Mosby's pocket guide to nursing skills & procedures* (8th ed.). St. Louis, MO: Elsevier.

Weinstein, R. (2012). *2012 Clinical practice guide on red blood cell transfusion: Quick reference*. Retrieved from http://www.hematology.org/Clinicians/Guidelines-Quality/Quick-Ref/527.aspx

Chapter 5

Cardiovascular care

Just the facts

In this chapter, you'll learn:

- about cardiovascular procedures
- what patient care and patient teaching are associated with each procedure
- how to manage complications associated with each procedure
- about essential documentation for each procedure.

Electrocardiography

Electrocardiography (ECG), which measures the heart's electrical activity as waveforms, is one of the most valuable and commonly used diagnostic tools. An ECG uses electrodes attached to the skin to detect electric currents moving through the heart. It then transmits these signals to an instrument that produces a record (the electrocardiogram) of cardiac activity.

The ECG detects cumulative electrical signals generated by pacemaker cells of the heart. This electrical stimulus is what triggers a cardiac contraction. ECG can be used to identify myocardial ischemia and infarction, conduction abnormalities and abnormal heart rhythms, chamber enlargement (hypertrophy), electrolyte imbalances, and drug toxicity.

It's like 12 cameras

The standard 12-lead ECG uses a series of electrodes placed on the extremities and the chest wall to assess the heart from 12 different views (leads). The 12 leads consist of three standard bipolar limb leads (designated I, II, III), three unipolar augmented leads (aV_R, aV_L, aV_F), and six unipolar precordial leads (V_1 to V_6). The limb leads and augmented leads show the heart from the frontal plane. The precordial leads show the heart from the horizontal plane.

Using these leads, the ECG device measures and averages the differences between the electrical potential of the electrode sites for each lead and graphs them over time. This creates the standard ECG complex, called P-QRS-T. The P wave represents atrial depolarization; the QRS complex, ventricular depolarization; and the T wave, ventricular repolarization. The U wave, sometimes present, represents the recovery period of ventricular conduction fibers. (See *Reviewing ECG components*.)

ECGs are performed as a resting ECG, exercise ECG, and/or an ambulatory (Holter monitor) ECG. The intended population can be adult, pediatric, and neonatal and can be done in the hospital, clinic, ambulance, or ambulatory (Holter monitor) settings.

Where's the remote?

ECG is typically accomplished using a multichannel method. All electrodes are attached to the patient at once, and the machine prints a simultaneous view of all leads.

Reviewing ECG components

This strip shows the components of a normal ECG waveform.

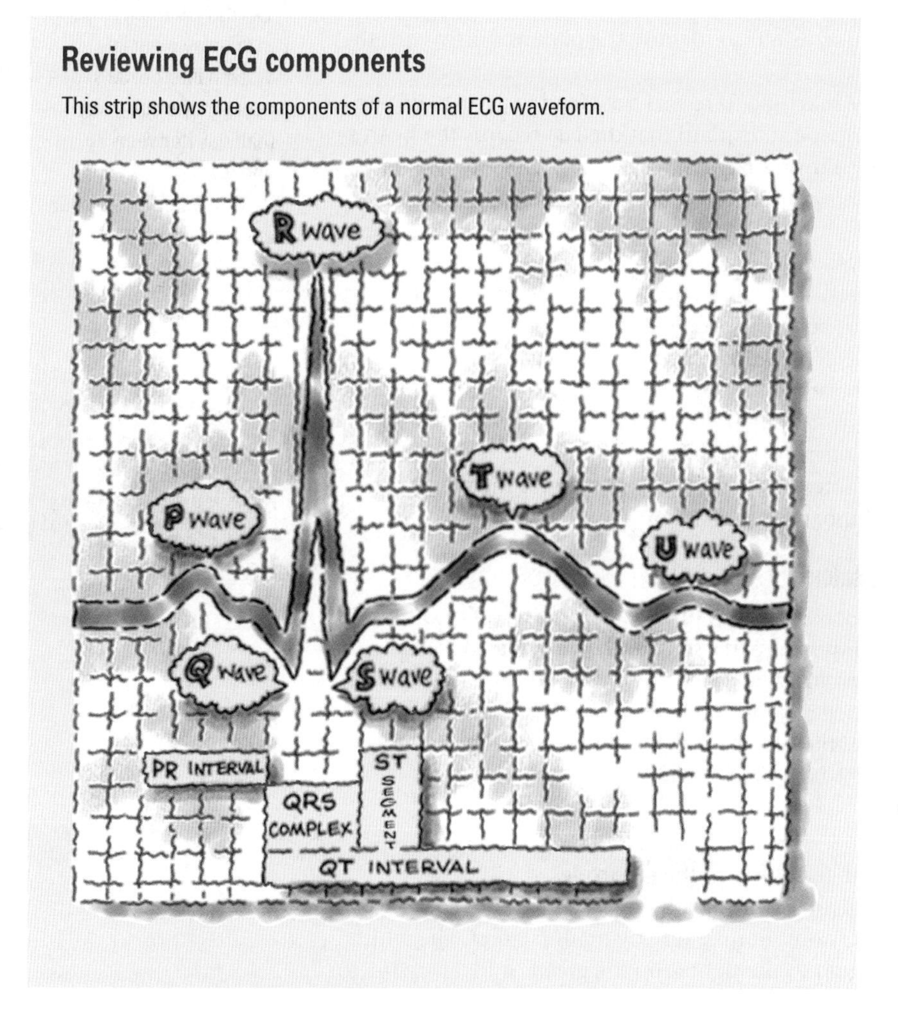

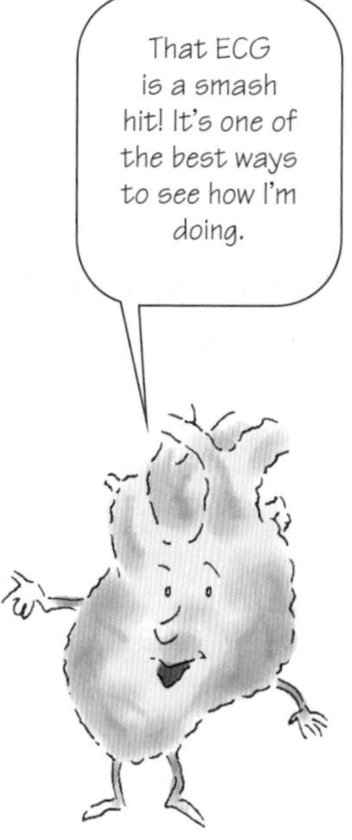
That ECG is a smash hit! It's one of the best ways to see how I'm doing.

What you need

ECG machine * recording paper * disposable pregelled electrodes (check expiration date) * 4″ × 4″ gauze pads * optional: clippers, alcohol swab or pad.

Getting ready

Place the ECG machine close to the patient's bed and plug the power cord into the wall outlet. Input the client information, referring to the medical record. Check that machine settings are standard.

How you do it

- Use two patient identifiers to identify the patient. Verify with the physician's order.
- As you set up the machine to record a 12-lead ECG, explain the procedure to the patient. Explain that the test records the heart's electrical activity. Emphasize that no electrical current will enter the body and it is painless. Tell the client the test typically takes about 5 minutes.
- Perform hand hygiene.
- Have the patient lie in a supine position in the center of the bed with his arms at his sides. You may raise the head of the bed *to promote comfort*. Expose his arms and legs and drape him appropriately. His arms and legs should be relaxed *to minimize muscle trembling, which can cause electrical interference*. Make sure the feet are not touching the bed board.
- Select flat, fleshy areas to place the electrodes. If the patient has an amputated limb, choose a site on the stump.

Need an appointment at the salon?

- If an area is excessively hairy, clip it. Clean excess oil or other substances from the skin with soap and water or alcohol *to enhance electrode contact. Apply the electrode to dry skin and ensure the pregelled electrodes are moist.*
- Apply the disposable pregelled electrodes to the patient's wrists and to the medial aspects of his ankles.

Colored for clarity

- Connect the limb leadwires to the electrodes.
- You'll see that the tip of each leadwire is lettered and color-coded for easy identification but may vary by manufacturer. The white or RA leadwire goes to the right arm; the green or RL leadwire, to

Positioning chest electrodes

To ensure accurate test results, position chest electrodes as follows:

V_1: Fourth intercostal space at right sternal border
V_2: Fourth intercostal space at left sternal border
V_3: Halfway between V_2 and V_4
V_4: Fifth intercostal space at midclavicular line
V_5: Fifth intercostal space at anterior axillary line (halfway between V_4 and V_6)
V_6: Fifth intercostal space at midaxillary line, level with V_4

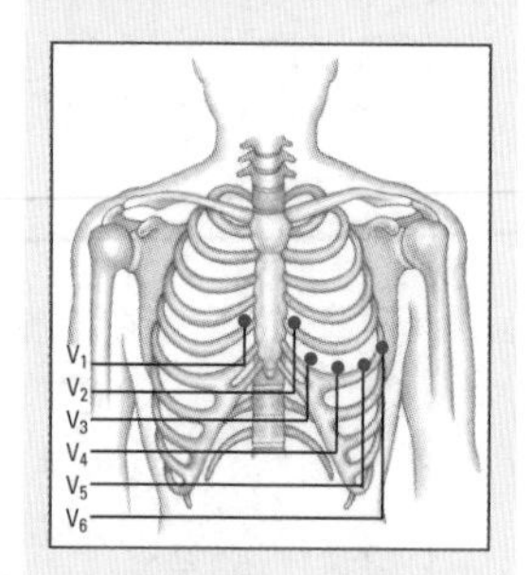

the right leg; the red or LL leadwire, to the left leg; the black or LA leadwire, to the left arm; and the brown or V_1 to V_6 leadwires, to the chest.

No time to be shy

- Now, expose the patient's chest. Place a disposable electrode at each electrode position. (See *Positioning chest electrodes*.)
- If your patient is a woman, be sure to place the chest electrodes below the breast tissue. In a large-breasted woman, you may need to displace the breast tissue laterally.
- Make sure that the paper speed selector is set to the standard 25 mm/second and the machine is set to full voltage. The machine will record a normal standardization mark—a square that's the height of two large squares or 10 small squares on the recording paper. If necessary, enter the appropriate patient identification data. Verify with the patient's chart.
- If any part of the waveform extends beyond the paper when you record the ECG, adjust the normal standardization to half-standardization. Note this adjustment on the ECG strip *because this will need to be considered in interpreting the results.*

Ready to roll

- Now you're ready to begin the recording. Ask the patient to relax and breathe normally. Tell him to lie still and not to talk. Then press the AUTO or RECORD button. Observe the tracing quality. The machine will record all 12 leads automatically, recording 3 consecutive leads simultaneously. Some machines have a display screen so you can preview waveforms before the machine records them.
- When the machine finishes recording the 12-lead ECG, remove the electrodes and clean the client's skin. Assist the client to a comfortable position. Ensure the bed is in a low position. Remove any remaining equipment.
- Perform hand hygiene.

Practice pointers

- If the patient's skin is exceptionally oily, scaly, or diaphoretic, rub the electrode site with a dry 4″ × 4″ gauze pad before applying the electrode *to help reduce interference in the tracing.*
- If the patient has a pacemaker, you can perform an ECG with or without a magnet, according to the physician's orders. Be sure to note the presence of a pacemaker and the use of the magnet (to turn off the pacemaker) on the strip. (See *Documenting ECG*.)

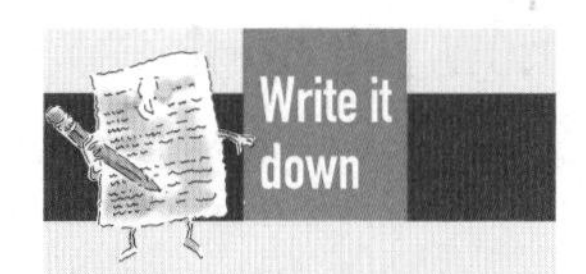

Documenting ECG

Label the ECG recording with the:

- patient's name
- medical record number
- date
- time.

Document in the chart:

- time and date the ECG was performed
- patient's tolerance to the procedure
- if copy was placed in the chart and/or sent for clinical interpretation.

- Note that the interpretation on the ECG printout is a machine interpretation. A physician must read and interpret the ECG and document the findings in the medical record.

Posterior chest lead ECG

Because of the location of the heart's posterior surface, myocardial damage to the side of the heart isn't apparent on a standard 12-lead ECG. To help identify posterior involvement, some practitioners recommend adding posterior leads to the 12-lead ECG.

Usually, the posterior lead ECG is performed with a standard ECG and involves recording only the additional posterior leads V_7, V_8, and V_9.

What you need

ECG machine with recording paper ✳ disposable pregelled electrodes (check the expiration date) ✳ 4″ × 4″ gauze pads ✳ marking pen ✳ optional: clippers, alcohol swab or pad.

How you do it

- Prepare the electrode sites according to the manufacturer's instructions. *To ensure good skin contact,* clip the site if the patient has considerable back hair. Make sure the skin is clean and dry (alcohol swab/pad as needed) and the electrode gel is moist.

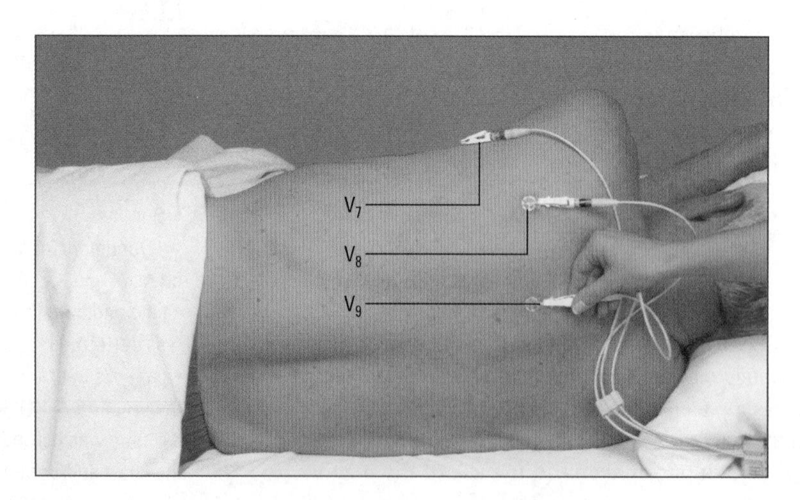

- Attach a disposable electrode to the V_7 position on the left posterior axillary line, fifth intercostal space. Then attach the V_4 leadwire to the V_7 electrode.
- Next, attach a disposable electrode to the patient's back at the V_8 position on the left midscapular line, fifth intercostal space, and attach the V_5 leadwire to this electrode.
- Finally, attach a disposable electrode to the patient's back at the V_9 position, just left of the spinal column at the fifth intercostal space (as shown in page 268). Then attach the V_6 leadwire to the V_9 electrode.

Recording time

Turn on the machine and make sure that the paper speed is set for 25 mm/second. If necessary, standardize the machine. Press AUTO or RECORD and the machine will record the waveforms.

Relabel . . .

All leads will print out as a straight line except those labeled V_4, V_5, and V_6. Relabel those leads V_7, V_8, and V_9, respectively.

. . . or reposition

When the ECG is complete, remove the electrodes and clean the patient's skin with a 4″ × 4″ gauze pad or a moist cloth. If you think you may need more than one posterior lead ECG, use a marking pen to mark the electrode sites on his skin *to permit accurate comparison for future tracings*.

Practice pointers

- The number of leads may vary according to the cardiologist's preference. (If right posterior leads are requested, position the patient on his left side. These leads, known as V_{7R}, V_{8R}, and V_{9R}, are located at the same landmarks on the right side of the patient's back.)
- Some ECG machines won't operate unless you connect all leadwires. In that case, you may need to connect the limb leadwires and the leadwires for V_1, V_2, and V_3.
- Note that the interpretation on the ECG printout is a machine interpretation. A physician must read and interpret the ECG and document the findings in the medical record. (See *Documenting posterior chest lead ECG*.)

Documenting posterior chest lead ECG

See "Relabel . . . " earlier.

Label the ECG recording with the:
- patient's name
- medical record number
- date
- time.

Document in the chart:
- time and date the ECG was performed
- patient's tolerance to the procedure
- if a copy was placed in the chart and/or sent for clinical interpretation.

Right chest lead ECG

Unlike a standard 12-lead ECG, used primarily to evaluate left ventricular function, a right chest lead ECG reflects right ventricular function and provides clues to damage or dysfunction in this chamber. You might need to perform a right chest lead ECG for a patient with an inferior wall myocardial infarction (MI) and suspected right ventricular involvement.

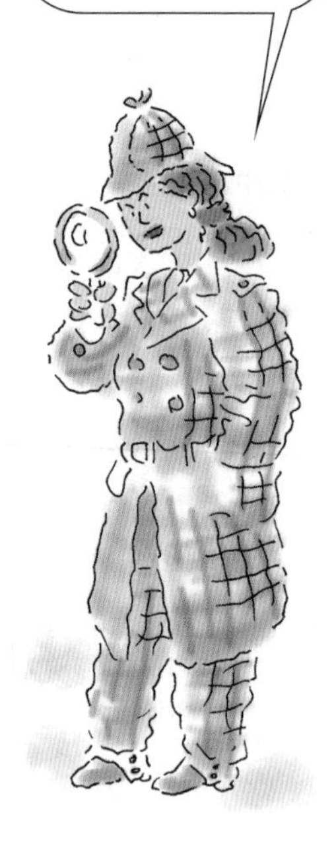
Suspect right ventricular MI? A right chest lead ECG can provide the clues you need to solve the case.

Because you need to know

Early identification of a right ventricular MI is essential because its treatment differs from that for other MIs. For instance, in left ventricular MI, treatment involves withholding intravenous (I.V.) fluids or administering them judiciously to prevent heart failure. Conversely, in right ventricular MI, treatment usually requires administration of I.V. fluids to maintain adequate filling pressures on the right side of the heart. This helps the right ventricle eject an adequate volume of blood at an adequate pressure.

What you need

Multichannel ECG machine ✻ paper ✻ pregelled disposable electrodes (check the expiration date) ✻ several 4″ × 4″ gauze pads.

How you do it

- Use two patient identifiers to identify the patient. Verify with the physician's order.
- Take the equipment to the patient's bedside.
- Set up the machine to record the ECG.
- Explain the procedure to the patient and/or patient representative. Explain the test records the heart's electrical activity. Emphasize that no electrical current will enter the body and it is painless. Tell the patient the test typically takes about 5 minutes. Ask if he has any allergies to adhesives.
- Perform hand hygiene.
- Make sure that the paper speed is set at 25 mm/second and the amplitude at 1 mV/10 mm.
- Place the patient in a supine position or, if he has difficulty lying flat, in semi-Fowler's position. Provide privacy and expose his arms, chest, and legs. (Cover a female patient's chest with her bed linens until you apply the chest leads.)

- Examine the patient's wrists and ankles for the best areas to place the electrodes. Choose flat, fleshy, hairless areas, such as the inner aspects of the wrists and medial aspects of the ankles. Clean the sites with the gauze pads *to promote good skin contact.* If the patient has an amputated limb, choose a site on the stump.
- Connect the leadwires to the electrodes. The leadwires are color-coded and lettered. Place the white or right arm (RA) wire on the right arm; the black or left arm (LA) wire on the left arm; the green or right leg (RL) wire on the right leg; and the red or left leg (LL) wire on the left leg.

Fingers and leads

Then examine the patient's chest *to locate the correct sites for chest lead placement* (as shown in the following figure). If the patient is a woman, place the electrodes under the breast tissue.

- Use your fingers to feel between the patient's ribs (the intercostal spaces). Start at the second intercostal space on the left (the notch felt at the top of the sternum, where the manubrium joins the body of the sternum). Count down two spaces to the fourth intercostal space. Then apply a disposable pregelled electrode to the site and attach leadwire V_{1R} to that electrode.
- Move your fingers across the sternum to the fourth intercostal space on the right side of the sternum. Apply a disposable electrode to that site and attach lead V_{2R}.
- Move your finger down to the fifth intercostal space and over to the midclavicular line. Place a disposable electrode here and attach lead V_{4R}.
- Visually draw a line between V_{2R} and V_{4R}. Apply a disposable electrode midway on this line and attach lead V_{3R}.

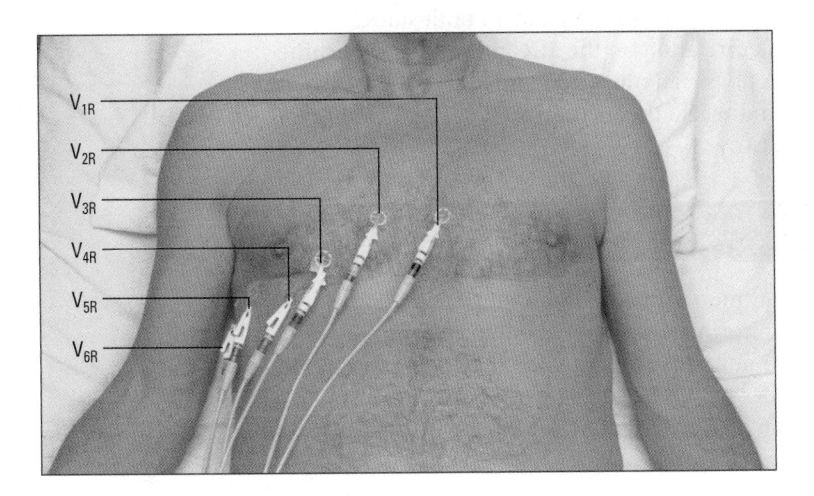

- Move your finger horizontally from V_{4R} to the right midaxillary line. Apply a disposable electrode to this site and attach lead V_{6R}.
- Move your fingers along the same horizontal line to the midpoint between V_{4R} and V_{6R}. This is the right anterior midaxillary line. Apply a disposable electrode to this site and attach lead V_{5R}.

Now we're ready

- Turn on the ECG machine. Ask the patient to breathe normally but to refrain from talking during the recording *so that muscle movement won't distort the tracing*. Enter any appropriate patient information required by the machine you're using. If necessary, standardize the machine. This will cause a square tracing of 10 mm (two large squares) to appear on the ECG paper when the machine is set for 1 mV (1 mV = 10 mm).
- Press the AUTO key or RECORD key. The ECG machine will record all 12 leads automatically.
- When you're finished recording the ECG, turn off the machine. Clearly label the ECG with the patient's name, medical record number, the date, and the time. Also, label the tracing "Right chest ECG" to distinguish it from a standard 12-lead ECG. Remove the electrodes and clean the client's skin. Assist the client to a comfortable position. Ensure the bed is in a low position. Remove any remaining equipment.
- Perform hand hygiene.

Documenting right chest lead ECG

Label the ECG recording with the:
- patient's name
- medical record number
- date
- time.

Document in the chart:
- time and date the ECG was performed
- patient's tolerance to the procedure
- if copy was placed in the chart and/or sent for clinical interpretation.

Practice pointers

For best results, place the electrodes symmetrically on the limbs. If the patient's wrist or ankle is covered by a dressing or if the patient is an amputee, choose an area that's available on both sides.

- Note that the interpretation on the ECG printout is a machine interpretation. A physician must read and interpret the ECG and document the findings in the medical record. (See *Documenting right chest lead ECG.*)

Cardiac monitoring

Because it allows continuous observation of the heart's electrical activity, cardiac monitoring is used in patients at risk for life-threatening dysrhythmias. Like other forms of ECG, cardiac monitoring uses electrodes placed on the patient's chest to transmit electrical signals that are converted into a cardiac rhythm tracing on an oscilloscope.

Hardwire vs. wireless

Continuous cardiac monitoring has two types of monitoring that may be performed: hardwire or telemetry. In *hardwire monitoring*, the patient is connected to a monitor at the bedside. The rhythm display appears at the bedside or it may be transmitted to a console at a remote location. *Telemetry* uses a small transmitter connected to the ambulatory patient to send electrical signals to another location, where they're displayed on a monitor screen.

Regardless of the type, cardiac monitors can display the patient's heart rate and rhythm, produce a printed record of cardiac rhythm, and sound an alarm if the heart rate exceeds or falls below specified limits. Monitors also recognize and count abnormal heartbeats as well as changes.

What you need

Cardiac monitor ✳ leadwires ✳ patient cable ✳ disposable pregelled electrodes (number of electrodes varies from three to five, depending on the patient's needs; check the expiration date) ✳ 4″ × 4″ gauze pads ✳ optional: clipper, washcloth.

For telemetry

Transmitter ✳ transmitter pouch ✳ telemetry battery pack, leads, and electrodes.

Getting ready

Turn on the cardiac monitor to warm up the unit while you prepare the equipment and the patient. Insert the cable into the appropriate monitor socket. Connect the leadwires to the cable. In some systems, the leadwires are permanently secured to the cable. Each leadwire should indicate the attachment location: right arm (RA), left arm (LA), right leg (RL), left leg (LL), and ground (C or V). This should appear on the leadwire—if it's permanently connected—or at the connection of the leadwires and cable to the patient. Then connect an electrode to each of the leadwires, carefully checking that each leadwire is in its correct outlet. Ensure all telemetry units and leadwires are cleaned according to hospital policy between patient use.

Keep on ticking

For telemetry monitoring, insert a new battery into the transmitter. Be sure to match the poles on the battery with the polar markings on the transmitter case. By pressing the button at the top of the unit, test the battery's charge and test the unit to ensure that the battery is operational. If the leadwires aren't permanently affixed to the telemetry unit, attach them securely.

How you do it

Explain the procedure to the patient and provide privacy. Perform hand hygiene.

For hardwire monitoring

- Expose the patient's chest and determine electrode placement, based on which system and lead you're using. (See *Positioning monitoring leads*.)
- If an area is excessively hairy, clip it and ensure skin is clean and dry.
- Remove the backing from the pregelled electrode. Check the gel for moistness. If the gel is dry, discard the electrode and replace it with a fresh one.

Press firmly

- Apply the electrode to the site and press firmly *to ensure a tight seal*. Repeat with the remaining electrodes.
- When all the electrodes are in place, check for a tracing on the cardiac monitor. Assess the quality of the ECG. (See *Identifying cardiac monitor problems*, page 276.)
- To verify that the monitor is detecting each beat, compare the digital heart rate display with your count of the patient's heart rate.
- If necessary, use the gain control to adjust the size of the rhythm tracing and use the position control to adjust the waveform position on the recording paper.
- Set the upper and lower limits of the heart rate alarm based on unit policy. Turn the alarm on.

For telemetry monitoring

- Perform hand hygiene. Explain the procedure to the patient and provide privacy.
- Expose the patient's chest and select the lead arrangement. Remove the backing from one of the pregelled electrodes. Check the gel for moistness. If it's dry, discard the electrode and obtain a new one.
- Apply the electrode to the appropriate site. Press your fingers in a circular motion around the electrode *to fix the gel and stabilize the electrode*. Repeat for each electrode.
- Attach an electrode to the end of each leadwire.

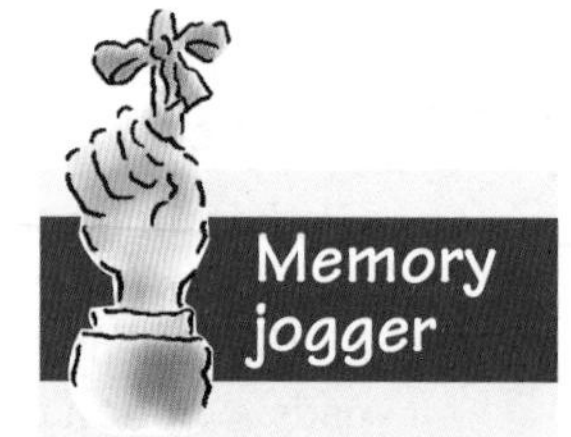

To help you remember where to place electrodes in a five-electrode configuration, think of the phrase "white to the upper right." Then think of snow over trees (white electrode over green electrode) and smoke over fire (black electrode above red electrode). And of course, chocolate (brown electrode) lies close to the heart.

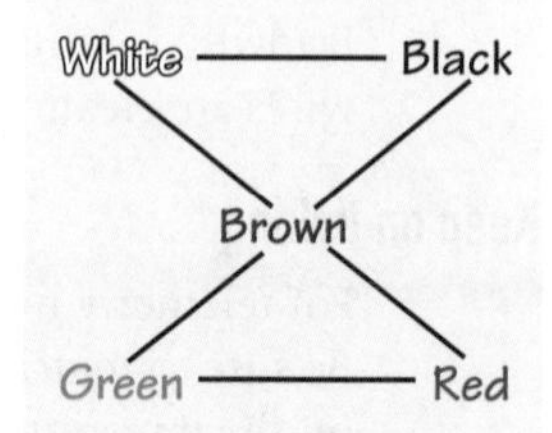

Positioning monitoring leads

These illustrations show correct electrode positions for some of the monitoring leads you'll use most often. For each lead, you'll see electrode placement for a five-leadwire system and a telemetry system.

In the hardwire system, the electrode position for one lead may be identical to the electrode position for another lead. In this case, simply change the lead selector switch to the setting that corresponds to the lead you want. In some cases, you'll need to reposition the electrodes.

In the telemetry system, you can create the same lead with two electrodes that you do with three simply by eliminating the ground electrode.

These illustrations use these abbreviations: RA, right arm; LA, left arm; RL, right leg; LL, left leg; C, chest; and G, ground.

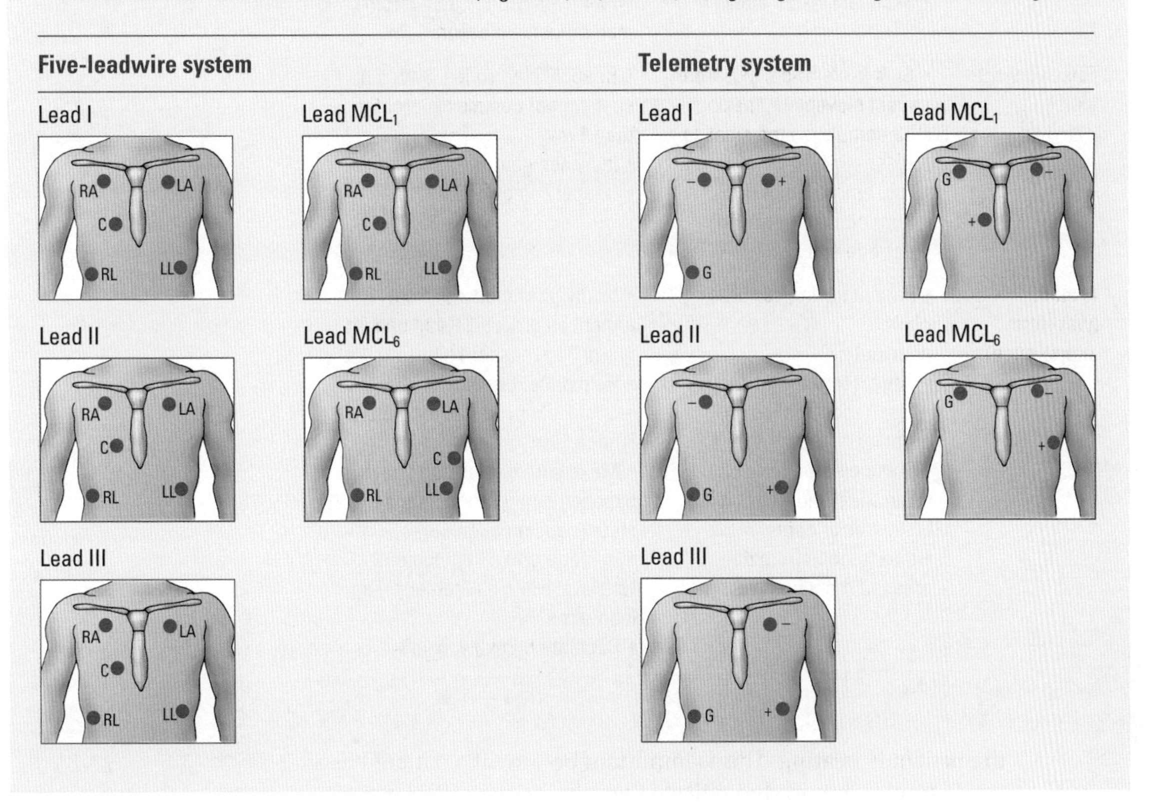

Walkie-talkie for the heart

- Place the transmitter in the pouch. Tie the pouch strings around the patient's neck and waist, making sure that the pouch fits snugly without causing him discomfort.
- Check the patient's waveform for clarity, position, and size. Adjust the gain and baseline as needed.
- At the central station, verify that the patient's name and room number is correct on the telemetry monitor and matches the unit

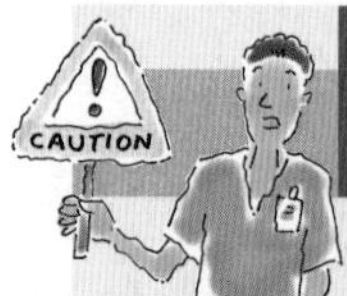

WARNING!

Identifying cardiac monitor problems

Problem	Possible causes	Solutions
False–high-rate alarm	• Monitor interpreting large T waves as QRS complexes, which doubles the rate • Skeletal muscle activity	• Reposition electrodes to lead where QRS complexes are taller than T waves. • Place electrodes away from major muscle masses.
False–low-rate alarm	• Shift in electrical axis from patient movement, making QRS complexes too small to register • Low amplitude of QRS • Poor contact between electrode and skin	• Reapply electrodes. Set gain so height of complex is greater than 1 mV. • Increase gain. • Reapply electrodes.
Artifact (waveform interference)	• Patient having seizures, chills, or anxiety • Patient movement • Electrodes applied improperly • Static electricity • Electrical short circuit in leadwires or cable • Interference from decreased room humidity	• Notify physician and treat patient as ordered. Keep patient warm and reassure him. • Help patient relax. • Check electrodes and reapply, if necessary. • Make sure cables don't have exposed connectors. Change static-causing bedclothes. • Replace broken equipment. Use stress loops when applying leadwires. • Regulate humidity to 40%.

the patient is wearing. This is important because if a patient has a dysrhythmia, you need to quickly identify and assess the patient.

- To obtain a rhythm strip, press the RECORD key at the central station. Label the strip with the patient's name and medical record number, date, and time. Also, identify the rhythm and place the rhythm strip in the patient's chart. (Practice rhythm interpretation at http://www.practicalclinicalskills.com/ekg.aspx.)

Practice pointers

- Make sure all electrical equipment and outlets are grounded *to avoid electric shock and interference (artifacts)*. Also ensure that the patient is clean and dry *to prevent electric shock.*
- If the patient's skin is very oily, scaly, or diaphoretic, rub the electrode site with a dry 4″ × 4″ gauze pad before applying the electrode *to help reduce interference in the tracing.*
- Assess skin integrity and reposition the electrodes every 24 hours or as necessary.

Important instructions

If the patient is being monitored by telemetry, tell him to remove the transmitter if he takes a shower or bath but stress that he should let you know before he removes the unit. However, some patients will need continual monitoring and will not be able to remove the monitor to bathe. (See *Documenting cardiac monitoring.*)

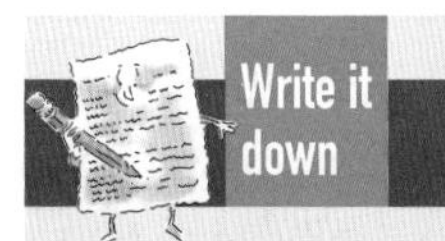

Documenting cardiac monitoring

In your notes, record the date and time monitoring began and the monitoring lead used. Note the patient's heart rate, rhythm, and any aberrancy. Document a rhythm strip at least every 8 hours and with changes in the patient's condition (or as specified by your facility's policy). Label the rhythm strip with the patient's name, medical record number, the monitored lead, date, and time.

Transducer system setup

There are several types of transducer systems, depending on the patient's needs and the physician's preference. Single-pressure transducers monitor only one type of pressure—for example, pulmonary artery pressure (PAP). Multiple-pressure transducers can monitor two or more types of pressure, such as PAP and central venous pressure (CVP).

What you need

Bag of flush solution (usually 500 mL normal saline solution, which may also contain 500 or 1,000 units heparin depending on facility policy) ✳ pressure infuser bag ✳ medication-added label ✳ preassembled disposable pressure tubing with flush device and disposable transducer ✳ monitor and monitor cable ✳ I.V. pole with transducer mount ✳ tubing label to identify the line type.

Getting ready

Turn the monitor on before gathering the equipment to give it sufficient time to warm up. Gather the equipment you'll need. Perform hand hygiene.

How you do it

To set up and zero a single-pressure transducer system, perform the following steps.

Setting up the system

Follow your facility's policy on whether to add heparin to the flush solution. If your patient has a history of bleeding or clotting problems, heparin most likely won't be added. In a circumstance where heparin is ordered, ensure a baseline platelet count is ordered. If appropriate, add the ordered amount of heparin to the solution—usually, 1 to 2 units of heparin per milliliter of solution—and then label the bag.

Connect and unwrap

- Put the pressure module into the monitor, if necessary, and connect the transducer cable to the monitor.
- Remove the preassembled pressure tubing from the package. If necessary, connect the pressure tubing to the transducer. Tighten all tubing connections.
- Position all stopcocks so the flush solution flows through the entire system. Then roll the tubing's flow regulator to the OFF position.

Spike and squeeze

- Spike the flush solution bag with the tubing, invert the bag, open the roller clamp, and squeeze all the air through the drip chamber. Then compress the tubing's drip chamber, filling it no more than halfway with the flush solution.
- Place the flush solution bag into the pressure infuser bag.
- Open the tubing's flow regulator, uncoil the tube if you haven't already done so and remove the protective cap at the end of the pressure tubing. Squeeze the continuous flush device slowly to prime the entire system, including the stopcock ports, with the flush solution.

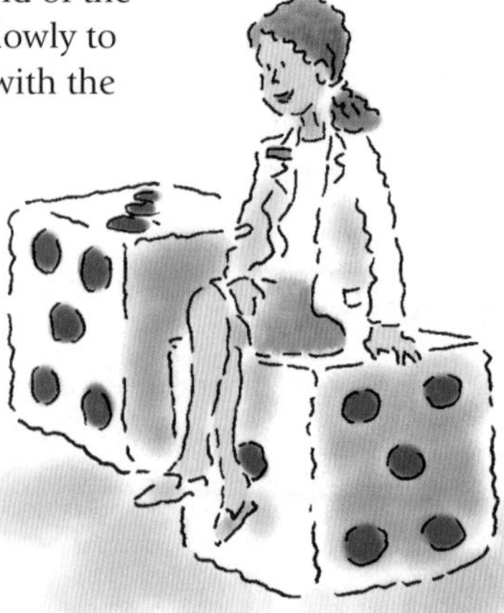
A dicey situation may arise if you fail to get all the air out of the system.

Angle and inflate

- As the solution nears the disposable transducer, hold the transducer at a 45-degree angle. *This forces the solution to flow upward to the transducer, pushing air out of the system.*
- When the solution nears a stopcock, open the stopcock to air, allowing the solution to flow into the stopcock. When the stopcock fills, close it to air and turn it open to the remainder of the tubing. Do this for each stopcock.

- After you've completely primed the system, replace the protective cap at the end of the tubing.
- Inflate the pressure infuser bag to 300 mm Hg. *This bag keeps the pressure in the arterial line higher than the patient's systolic pressure, preventing blood backflow into the tubing and ensuring a continuous flow rate.* Afterward, flush the system again *to remove all air bubbles.*
- Replace the vented caps on the stopcocks with sterile nonvented caps. If you're going to mount the transducer on an I.V. pole, insert the device into its holder.

Zeroing the system

- Now you're ready for a preliminary zeroing of the transducer. To ensure accuracy, position the patient flat in bed (if tolerated) and place the transducer on the same level each time you zero it or record a pressure.

A look at a transducer system setup

After you have set up the transducer system, it should look like the one shown below.

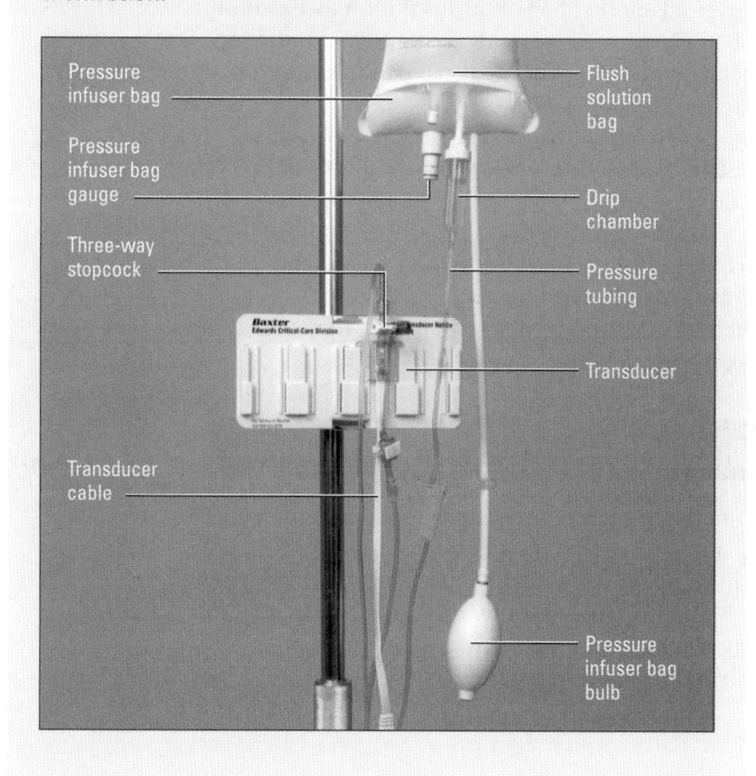

- Next, position the stopcock of the transducer level with the phlebostatic axis (midway between the posterior chest and the sternum at the fourth intercostal space, midaxillary line).
- After leveling the transducer, turn the stopcock next to the transducer off to the patient and open to air. Remove the cap to the stopcock port.
- Now zero the transducer. To do so, follow the manufacturer's directions. This will involve zeroing the waveform on the bedside monitor.
- When you've finished zeroing, turn the stopcock on the transducer so that it's open to the patient and closed to air. This is the monitoring position. Replace the cap on the stopcock. You're then ready to attach the single-pressure transducer to the patient's catheter. Now you've assembled a single-pressure transducer system. (See *A look at a transducer system setup*, page 279.)

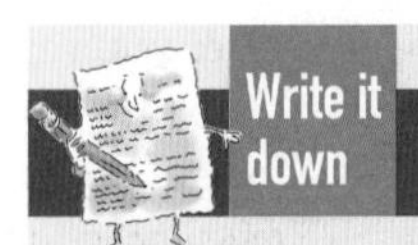

Documenting transducer system setup

Document the patient's position for zeroing so that other health care team members can replicate the placement.

Practice pointers

- You may use any of several methods to set up a multiple-pressure transducer system. The easiest way is to add to the single-pressure system. You'll also need another bag of flush solution in a second pressure infuser bag. Then you'll prime the tubing, mount the second transducer, and connect an additional cable to the monitor. Finally, you'll zero the second transducer.
- Alternatively, your facility may use a Y-type tubing setup with two attached pressure transducers. This method requires only one bag of heparin flush solution. To set up the system, proceed as you would for a single transducer, with this exception: First, prime one branch of the Y-type tubing and then the other. Next, attach two cables to the monitor in the modules for each pressure that you'll be measuring. Finally, zero each transducer. (See *Documenting transducer system setup*.)

Arterial pressure monitoring

Direct arterial pressure monitoring permits continuous measurement of systolic, diastolic, and mean pressures and allows arterial blood sampling. Because direct measurement reflects systemic vascular resistance as well as blood flow, it's generally more accurate than indirect methods (such as palpation and auscultation of audible pulse sounds), which are based on blood flow.

But what I really want to do is direct!

Direct monitoring is indicated when highly accurate or frequent blood pressure measurements are required—for example, in patients receiving titrated doses of vasoactive drugs.

What you need

Your equipment needs depend on which aspect of arterial pressure monitoring you'll be performing or assisting with: catheter insertion, blood sample collection, tubing changes, or catheter removal.

For catheter insertion

Gown ✳ mask ✳ protective eyewear ✳ sterile gloves ✳ 16G to 20G catheter (type and length depend on the insertion site, patient's size, and other anticipated uses of the line) ✳ preassembled preparation kit (if available) ✳ sterile drapes ✳ sheet protector ✳ prepared pressure transducer system ✳ ordered local anesthetic ✳ sutures ✳ syringe and needle (21G to 25G, 1″) ✳ I.V. pole ✳ tubing and medication labels ✳ site care kit (containing sterile dressing and hypoallergenic tape) ✳ arm board and soft wrist restraint (for a femoral site, an ankle restraint) ✳tubing label ✳ optional: clippers (for femoral artery insertion) ✳ bath towel for positioning, nonvented caps for stopcock.

For blood sample collection

If an *open system* is in place: nonsterile gloves ✳ gown ✳ mask ✳ protective eyewear ✳ sterile 4″ × 4″ gauze pads ✳ sheet protector ✳ 5- or 10-mL syringe for discard sample ✳ syringes of appropriate size and number for ordered laboratory tests ✳ laboratory requisition and labels ✳ Vacutainers ✳ sterile nonvented cap ✳ optional: bag of ice for blood specimen, blood gas sampling syringe

If a *closed system* is in place: nonsterile gloves ✳ gown ✳ mask ✳ protective eyewear ✳ syringes of appropriate size and number for ordered laboratory tests ✳ laboratory requisition and labels ✳ alcohol pad ✳ blood transfer unit ✳ Vacutainers ✳ sterile nonvented cap ✳ optional: bag of ice for blood specimen, blood gas sampling syringe.

For arterial line tubing changes

Gloves ✳ gown ✳ mask ✳ protective eyewear ✳ sheet protector ✳ preassembled arterial pressure tubing with flush device and disposable pressure transducer ✳ I.V. pole ✳ 500-mL bag of I.V. flush solution (such as normal saline solution) ✳ 500 or 1,000 units of heparin (if indicated, according to facility policy) ✳ alcohol pads ✳ medication label ✳ pressure bag ✳ site care kit ✳ tubing labels.

For arterial catheter removal

Gloves ✳ gown ✳ mask ✳ protective eyewear ✳ two sterile 4″ × 4″ gauze pads ✳ sheet protector ✳ sterile suture removal set ✳ dressing ✳ alcohol pads ✳ hypoallergenic tape.

For femoral line removal

Additional sterile 4″ × 4″ gauze pads ✳ small sandbag (which you may wrap in a towel or place in a pillowcase) ✳ adhesive bandage.

For a catheter-tip culture

Sterile scissors ✳ sterile container ✳ label.

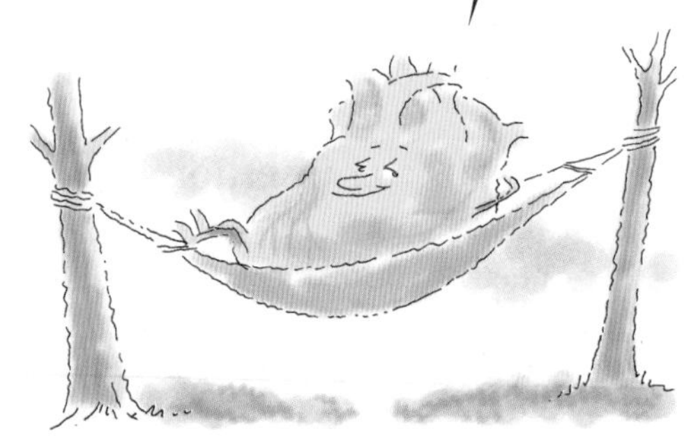
I'll just relax while you gather all that equipment.

Getting ready

Before setting up the transducer system, meticulously perform hand hygiene. Maintain asepsis and wear personal protective equipment (PPE) throughout preparation. (For instructions on setting up the system, see "Transducer system setup," page 277.)

When you have completed the equipment preparation, set the alarms on the bedside monitor according to your facility's policy.

How you do it

- The physician is responsible for obtaining consent from the patient or patient representative as determined by state law prior to the procedure. This includes explaining the procedure, risks, benefits, and alternatives to the procedure and answering their questions. The nurse should confirm with the patient/representative that the discussion has taken place and a consent form was signed. However, in emergency circumstances, time may not allow the form to be signed. Please refer to facility policy on informed consent.
- Explain the standard care including the insertion procedure, alarms, dressings, and length of time the catheter is expected to be in place and importance of keeping immobile. Instruct the patient to report any warmth, redness, pain, or wet feeling at the insertion site at any time, including after catheter removal.

- Check the patient's history for an allergy or a hypersensitivity to iodine or the ordered local anesthetic. If the patient is allergic to iodine, use an alternate skin prep to prevent line infection.
- Maintain asepsis and wear PPE throughout all procedures described in the following discussion.
- Position the patient for easy access to the catheter insertion site. Place a sheet protector under the site.
- If the catheter will be inserted into the radial artery, perform Allen's test *to assess collateral circulation in the hand.* (See chapter 2, Specimen collection.)

Inserting an arterial catheter

- Using a preassembled preparation kit, the physician prepares and anesthetizes the insertion site. He covers the surrounding area with sterile drapes. The catheter is then inserted into the artery and attached to the fluid-filled pressure tubing.
- While the physician holds the catheter in place, activate the fast-flush release *to flush blood from the catheter.* After each fast-flush operation, observe the drip chamber *to verify that the continuous flush rate is as desired.* A square waveform should appear on the bedside monitor.
- The physician may suture the catheter in place or you may secure it with hypoallergenic tape. Cover the insertion site with a transparent dressing, as specified by facility policy.

No movement allowed

- Immobilize the insertion site. With a radial or brachial site, use an arm board and soft wrist restraint (if the patient's condition requires it). With a femoral site, assess the need for an ankle restraint; maintain the patient on bed rest, with the head of the bed raised no more than 15 to 30 degrees, *to prevent the catheter from kinking.* Level the zeroing stopcock of the transducer with the phlebostatic axis. Then zero the system to atmospheric pressure.
- Refer to chapter 1, "Restraint application" section, to properly apply and monitor a patient with a restraint.
- Activate monitor alarms, as appropriate.
- Discard used supplies and perform hand hygiene.
- Run a waveform strip and record baseline pressures.
- Record the manual (noninvasive) blood pressure and compare with the arterial (invasive) blood pressure.

Obtaining a blood sample from an open system

- Assemble the equipment in the order of use in close proximity to the line. Turn off or temporarily silence the monitor alarms, depending on your facility's policy. (However, some facilities require that alarms be left on.)

- Identify the patient using two patient identifiers per facility policy.
- Perform hand hygiene.
- Don nonsterile gloves, mask, gown, and protective eyewear.
- Place the sheet protector under the affected extremity.
- Verify that you have the arterial line before proceeding.
- Locate the stopcock nearest the patient. Open a sterile 4″ × 4″ gauze pad. Remove the dead-end cap from the stopcock and place it on the gauze pad.

Just practicing

- Insert the syringe for the discard sample into the stopcock. (This sample is discarded because it's diluted with flush solution.) Follow your facility's policy on how much discarded blood to collect. In most cases, you'll withdraw 5 to 10 mL through a 5- or 10-mL syringe. If the patient's hemoglobin and hematocrit are low, check with the physician to determine if a smaller sample should be taken.
- Next, turn the stopcock off to the flush solution. Slowly retract the syringe to withdraw the discard sample. If you feel resistance, reposition the affected extremity and check the insertion site for obvious problems (such as catheter kinking). After correcting the problem, resume blood withdrawal. Then turn the stopcock halfway back to the open position to close the system in all directions.
- Remove the discard syringe and dispose of the blood in the syringe, observing standard precautions.

Now for real

- Place the syringe for the laboratory sample in the stopcock, turn the stopcock off to the flush solution, and slowly withdraw the required amount of blood. For each additional sample required, repeat this procedure. If drawing arterial blood gases (ABGs), use a blood gas sampling syringe and draw the sample slowly *to prevent contamination of the mixed venous sample with arterial blood from the pulmonary capillaries, which will falsely elevate the* SvO_2. Expel any air bubbles from the syringe and cap the syringe and place in ice. If the physician has ordered coagulation tests, obtain blood for this sample from the final syringe *to prevent dilution from the flush device.*
- After you've obtained blood for the final sample, turn the stopcock off to the syringe and remove the syringe. Activate the fast-flush release *to clear the tubing*. Then turn off the stopcock to the patient and repeat the fast flush *to clear the stopcock port.*
- Turn the stopcock off to the stopcock port and replace the dead-end cap. Reactivate the monitor alarms. Attach needleless devices to the filled syringes and transfer the blood samples to the appropriate specimen collection tubes or Vacutainer, labeling them

Understanding the arterial waveform

Normal arterial blood pressure produces a characteristic waveform, representing ventricular systole and diastole. The waveform has five distinct components: anacrotic limb, systolic peak, dicrotic limb, dicrotic notch, and end diastole.

Going up . . .

The *anacrotic limb* marks the waveform's initial upstroke, which results as blood is rapidly ejected from the ventricle through the open aortic valve into the aorta. Rapid ejection causes a sharp rise in arterial pressure, which appears as the waveform's highest point, called the *systolic peak*.

. . . and coming down

As blood continues into the peripheral vessels, arterial pressure falls and the waveform begins a downward trend, called the *dicrotic limb*. Arterial pressure usually continues to fall until pressure in the ventricle is less than pressure in the aortic root. When this occurs, the aortic valve closes. This event appears as a small notch (the *dicrotic notch*) on the waveform's downside. When the aortic valve closes, diastole begins, progressing until aortic root pressure gradually descends to its lowest point. On the waveform, this appears as *end diastole*.

Normal arterial waveform

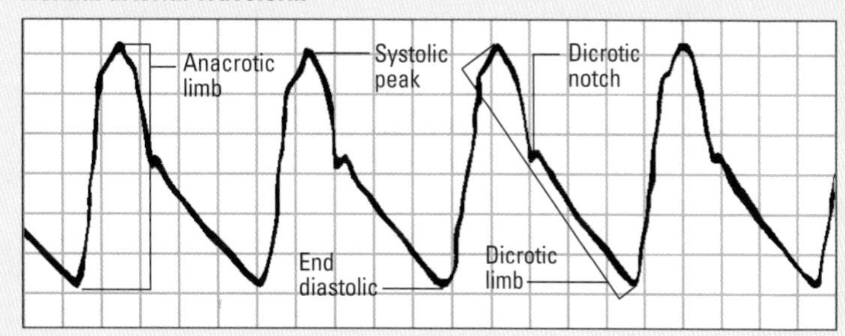

according to facility policy. **Verify that the information on the labels matches the requisition.** Send all samples to the laboratory with appropriate documentation.

- Remove PPE and discard according to facility policy.
- Perform hand hygiene.
- Check the monitor for return of the arterial waveform and pressure reading. (See *Understanding the arterial waveform*.)

Obtaining a blood sample from a closed system

- Identify the patient using two patient identifiers per facility policy.
- Perform hand hygiene.
- Don nonsterile gloves, mask, gown, and protective eyewear.
- Place the sheet protector under the affected extremity.
- Verify that you have the arterial line before proceeding.
- Assemble the equipment in the order of use in close proximity to the site, maintaining aseptic technique. Locate the closed-system reservoir and blood sampling site. Deactivate or temporarily silence monitor alarms. (However, some facilities require that alarms be left on.)
- Clean the sampling site with an alcohol pad.
- Holding the reservoir upright, grasp the flexures and slowly fill the reservoir with blood over 3 to 5 seconds. (*This blood serves*

as discard blood.) If you feel resistance, reposition the affected extremity and check the catheter for obvious problems (such as kinking). Then resume blood withdrawal.

- Turn the one-way valve off to the reservoir by turning the handle perpendicular to the tubing. Using a syringe with an attached cannula, insert the cannula into the sampling site. (Make sure the plunger is depressed to the bottom of the syringe barrel.) Slowly fill the syringe. Then grasp the cannula near the sampling site and remove the syringe and cannula as one unit. Repeat the procedure as needed to fill the required number of syringes. If drawing ABGs, use a blood gas sampling syringe and draw the sample slowly to prevent contamination of the mixed venous sample with arterial blood from the pulmonary capillaries, which will falsely elevate the SvO_2. Expel any air bubbles from the syringe and cap the syringe and place in ice. If the physician has ordered coagulation tests, obtain blood for those tests from the final syringe *to prevent dilution from the flush solution*.
- After filling the syringes, turn the one-way valve to its original position, parallel to the tubing. Now smoothly and evenly push down on the plunger until the flexures lock in place in the fully closed position and all fluid has been reinfused. The fluid should be reinfused over 3 to 5 seconds. Then activate the fast-flush release to clear blood from the tubing and reservoir.
- Clean the sampling site with an alcohol pad. Reactivate the monitor alarms. Using the blood transfer unit, transfer blood samples to the appropriate specimen collection tubes, labeling them according to facility policy. **Verify that the information on the labels matches the requisition.** Send all samples to the laboratory with appropriate documentation.
- Remove PPE and dispose per facility policy.
- Perform hand hygiene.

Changing arterial line tubing

- Wash your hands and follow standard precautions. Assemble the new pressure monitoring system.
- Consult your facility's policy and procedure manual to determine how much tubing length to change.
- Inflate the pressure bag to 300 mm Hg and check it for air leaks. Then release the pressure.
- Prepare the I.V. flush solution; ensure that accurate amount of heparin is in the flush solution, if ordered; and prime the pressure tubing and transducer system. At this time, add the medication label and tubing label, include the date and time the tubing was changed. Apply 300 mm Hg of pressure to the system. Then hang the I.V. bag on a pole.

Sound off

- Place the sheet protector under the affected extremity. Remove the dressing from the catheter insertion site, taking care not to dislodge the catheter or cause vessel trauma. Turn off or temporarily silence the monitor alarms. (However, some facilities require that alarms be left on.)
- Turn off the flow clamp of the tubing segment that you'll change. Disconnect the tubing from the catheter hub, taking care not to dislodge the catheter. Immediately insert new tubing into the catheter hub. Secure the tubing and then activate the fast-flush release to clear it.

Sound on

- Reactivate the monitor alarms. Clean the site using a site care kit (if available) or an alcohol pad. Apply an appropriate dressing.
- Level the zeroing stopcock of the transducer with the phlebostatic axis and zero the system to atmospheric pressure.

Removing an arterial line

- Consult facility policy to determine whether you're permitted to perform this procedure.
- Identify the patient using two patient identifiers and verify with the order.
- Assess the patient's coagulation profile (prothrombin time [PT], partial thromboplastin time [PTT], international normalized ratio [INR], platelets). *If abnormal, pressure will need to be applied for a longer period to achieve hemostasis.*
- Explain the procedure to the patient.
- Assemble all equipment.
- Observe standard precautions.
- Turn off the monitor alarms. Then turn off the flow clamp to the flush solution.
- Carefully remove the dressing over the insertion site. Remove any sutures using the suture removal kit and then carefully check that all sutures have been removed.

Steady withdrawal

- Attach a 3- to 5-mL syringe to the blood sampling port, turn the stopcock off to the flush solution, and draw blood back through the tubing.
- Apply pressure one to two fingerwidths above the insertion site.
- Withdraw the catheter using a sterile 4″ × 4″ gauze pad to cover the site as the catheter is being removed *to prevent splashing blood.* Use a gentle, steady motion. Continue to hold proximal pressure and immediately apply firm pressure over the insertion site as the catheter is removed.

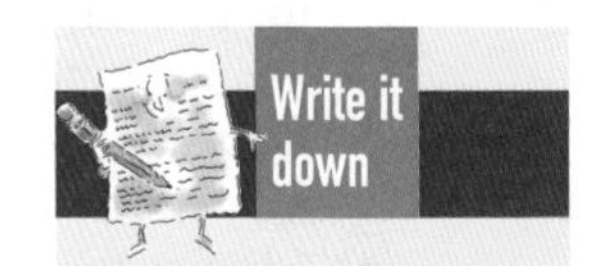

Documenting arterial pressure monitoring

In your notes, record:
- patient and family education
- peripheral vascular assessment before and after the procedure and catheter removal
- date and time of insertion with the size of catheter and site of placement
- assessment of insertion site
- patient response to insertion procedure
- status of the patient alarms and parameters
- type of flush solution used
- intake of flush solution on Intake and Output sheet and systolic and diastolic pressures
- time of arterial catheter removal
- unexpected outcomes
- additional nursing interventions.

- Maintain pressure for at least 10 minutes (longer if bleeding or oozing persists). Apply additional pressure to a femoral site or if the patient has coagulopathy or is receiving anticoagulants.
- Cover the site with an appropriate dressing and secure the dressing with tape. If stipulated by facility policy, make a pressure dressing for a femoral site by folding four sterile 4″ × 4″ gauze pads in half and apply the dressing. Cover the dressing with a tight adhesive bandage. Some hospital policies may include the use of a sandbag at the removal site to help control bleeding. Maintain the patient on bed rest for 6 hours with the sandbag in place and include frequent vascular assessments of the extremity where the sandbag is applied.
- Observe the site for bleeding. Assess circulation in the extremity distal to the site by evaluating color, pulses, and sensation. Repeat this assessment every 15 minutes for the first 4 hours, every 30 minutes for the next 2 hours, then hourly for the next 6 hours.
- Check the arterial flush line system every 4 hours to ensure the pressure bag is inflated to 300 mm Hg and fluid is present in the flush system.
- Monitor for overdamped or underdamped waveform.

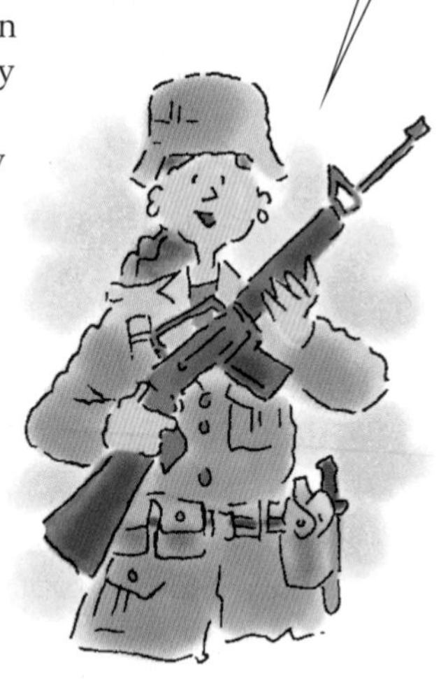
Attention! Immediately after withdrawing the catheter, apply pressure to the site for at least 10 minutes.

Collecting tips

If the physician has ordered a culture of the catheter tip (to diagnose a suspected infection), gently place the catheter tip on a 4″ × 4″ sterile gauze pad. When the bleeding is under control, hold the catheter over the sterile container. Using sterile scissors, cut the tip so it falls into the sterile container. Label the specimen, **verify that it matches the requisition**, and send it to the laboratory.

- Remove PPE and dispose per facility policy. Perform hand hygiene.

Practice pointers

- Observing the pressure waveform on the monitor can enhance arterial pressure assessment. An abnormal waveform may reflect an arrhythmia (such as atrial fibrillation) or other cardiovascular problems, such as aortic stenosis, aortic insufficiency, pulsus alternans, or pulsus paradoxus.
- Run an arterial pressure strip and obtain measurement of the arterial pressure during end-expiration. *This eliminates the effect of the respiratory cycle on the arterial pressure waveform.*
- Change the pressure tubing every 96 hours or according to hospital policy and immediately upon suspected contamination or when the integrity of the system has been compromised. Change the dressing at the catheter site according to facility

policy. Regularly assess the site for signs of infection, such as redness and swelling. Notify the physician immediately if you note such signs.
- Direct arterial pressure monitoring can cause such complications as arterial bleeding, infection, air embolism, arterial spasm, or thrombosis. (See *Documenting arterial pressure monitoring,* page 287.)

Temporary transcutaneous (external) pacing

A temporary pacemaker consists of an external, battery-powered pulse generator and a lead or electrode system. In a life-threatening situation, when time is critical, a transcutaneous pacemaker is the best choice. This device works by sending an electrical impulse from the pulse generator to the patient's heart by way of two electrodes, which are placed on the front and back of the patient's chest. Transcutaneous pacing is quick and effective. This is a short-term management of life-threatening dysrhythmias until the physician can institute transvenous pacing.

What you need

Transcutaneous pacing generator ✻ transcutaneous pacing electrodes (check expiration date) ✻ cardiac monitor ✻ optional: clippers, sedation or analgesia for conscious patients.

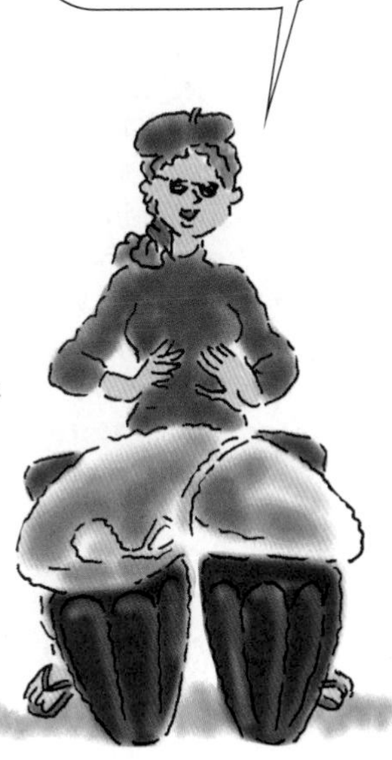
Need rhythm in a hurry? A transcutaneous pacemaker is the best choice.

How you do it

- Identify the patient using two patient identifiers per the facility policy.
- If applicable, explain the procedure to the patient or patient representative.
- Perform hand hygiene.
- Administer sedation or analgesia for the conscious patient to decrease discomfort with external cardiac pacing.
- If necessary, clip the hair over the areas of electrode placement. However, don't shave the area. *If you nick the skin, the current from the pulse generator could cause discomfort.*
- *Plug in the pulse generator and monitor to ensure the equipment is functional.*
- Attach monitoring electrodes to the patient in the lead I, II, or III position. Do this even if the patient is already on telemetry monitoring *because you'll need to connect the electrodes to the pacemaker.* If you select the lead II position, adjust

the LL electrode placement to accommodate the anterior pacing electrode and the patient's anatomy.

Get plugged in

- Plug the patient cable into the ECG input connection on the front of the pacing generator. Set the selector switch to the MONITOR ON position.
- You should see the ECG waveform on the monitor. Adjust the R-wave beeper volume to a suitable level and activate the alarm by pressing the ALARM ON button. Set the alarm for 10 to 20 beats lower and 20 to 30 beats higher than the intrinsic rate.
- Adjust the ECG size to the maximum R-wave size for proper demand pacing. Lead II usually provides the most prominent R wave.
- Press the START/STOP button for a printout of the waveform.
- Now you're ready to apply the two pacing electrodes. First, make sure the patient's skin is clean and dry *to ensure good skin contact.*

One for the back . . .

Pull off the protective strip from the posterior electrode (marked BACK) and apply the electrode on the left side of the back, just below the scapula and to the left of the spine. Avoid placement over bone because it increases the level of energy needed to pace, patient discomfort, and the possibility of noncapture.

. . . one for the front

- The anterior pacing electrode (marked FRONT) has two protective strips—one covering the gelled area and one covering the outer rim. Expose the gelled area and apply it to the skin in the anterior position—to the left side of the precordium in the usual V_2 to V_5 position. Move this electrode around to get the best waveform. Then expose the electrode's outer rim and firmly press it to the skin. (See *Proper electrode placement.*)
- Now you're ready to pace the heart. After making sure the energy output in milliamperes (mA) is on 0, connect the electrode cable to the monitor output cable.
- Check the waveform, looking for a tall QRS complex in lead II.
- Next, turn the selector switch to PACER ON. Tell the patient that he may feel a thumping or twitching sensation. Reassure him that you'll give him medication if he can't tolerate the discomfort. The pacemaker is set in either asynchronous or demand modes. Some devices permit demand pacing only. In the asynchronous mode, the pacemaker will generate a rhythm regardless of the patient's own rhythm. In demand mode, the pacemaker will fire only if the heart rate drops below a certain level.

Proper electrode placement

Place the two pacing electrodes for a noninvasive temporary pacemaker at heart level on the patient's chest and back (as shown). This placement ensures that the electrical stimulus must travel only a short distance to the heart.

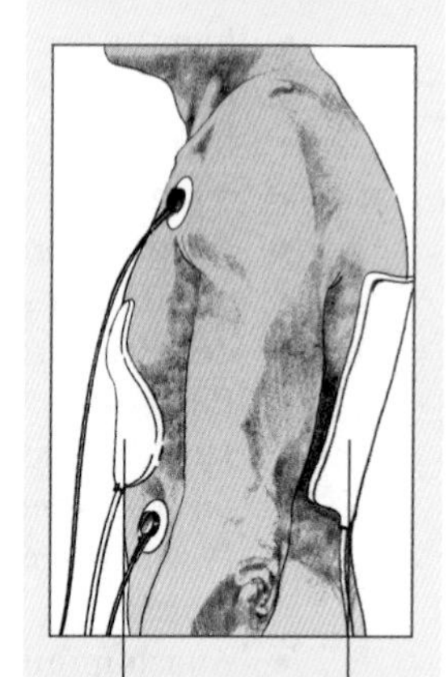

Feel the rhythm

- Now set the rate dial to 10 to 20 beats higher than the patient's intrinsic rhythm. Look for pacer artifact or spikes, which will appear as you increase the rate. If the patient doesn't have an intrinsic rhythm, set the rate at 60.
- Slowly increase the amount of energy delivered to the heart by adjusting the OUTPUT mA dial. Do this until capture is achieved—you'll see a pacer spike followed by a widened QRS complex that resembles a premature ventricular contraction. This is the pacing threshold. To ensure consistent capture, increase output by 10%. *Use the lowest amount of energy that consistently results in myocardial capture and contraction to minimize discomfort.*
- With full capture, the patient's heart rate should be approximately the same as the pacemaker rate set on the machine. The usual pacing threshold is between 40 and 80 mA.
- Discard used supplies and perform hand hygiene.

Monitoring the patient

- Assess the patient's vital signs, skin color, level of consciousness (LOC), and peripheral pulses hourly and as needed *to determine the effectiveness of the paced rhythm.*
- Perform a 12-lead ECG to serve as a baseline, and then perform additional ECGs daily or with clinical changes.
- Initially, obtain a rhythm strip before, during, and after pacemaker placement. Continue to monitor and record rhythm strips to document pacing function every 4 to 8 hours, any time pacemaker settings are changed, and whenever the patient receives treatment as a result of a pacemaker complication.

Practice pointers

- If the patient needs emergency defibrillation, make sure the pacemaker can withstand the procedure. If you're unsure, disconnect the pulse generator *to avoid damage.*
- With female patients, place the anterior electrode under the patient's breast but not over her diaphragm.
- Continuously monitor the ECG reading, noting capture, sensing, rate, intrinsic beats, and competition of paced and intrinsic rhythms. If the pacemaker is sensing correctly, the sense indicator on the pulse generator should flash with each beat.
- American Association of Critical-Care Nurses (AACN) recommends changing the electrodes at least every 24 hours.
- If the pacemaker is working as expected, the patient should have adequate tissue perfusion and cardiac output as evidenced by blood pressure greater than 90 systolic and alert and oriented

patient who has an absence of dizziness, shortness of breath, and chest pain.

The shocking truth

Take care to prevent microshock. All electrical equipment the patient is exposed to must be grounded, such as telephones, electric shavers, televisions, or lamps. (See *Documenting transcutaneous pacemaker use.*)

Documenting transcutaneous pacemaker use

In your notes, record:
- patient and family education
- reason for pacemaker use
- date and time cardiac pacing is initiated
- electrode locations
- medication administered
- pacemaker settings (rate, mode, milliampere)
- patient's response to the procedure and to temporary pacing
- complications and nursing actions taken.

Initially, obtain a rhythm strip before, during, and after pacemaker placement. Continue to monitor and record rhythm strips to document pacing function every 4 to 8 hours, any time pacemaker settings are changed, and whenever the patient receives treatment as a result of a pacemaker complication.

Temporary transvenous pacemaker

In addition to being more comfortable for the patient, a transvenous pacemaker is more reliable than a transcutaneous pacemaker. Transvenous pacing involves threading an electrode catheter percutaneously into the right ventricle where it contacts the endocardium near the ventricular septum. The electrode then attaches to an external pulse generator. As a result, the pulse generator can provide an electrical stimulus directly to the endocardium.

What you need

Temporary pacemaker gloves ✻ sterile dressings ✻ adhesive tape ✻ povidone-iodine solution or designated skin prep ✻ nonconducting tape or rubber surgical glove ✻ pouch for external pulse generator ✻ emergency cardiac drugs ✻ intubation equipment ✻ defibrillator ✻ cardiac monitor with strip-chart recorder ✻ equipment to start a peripheral I.V. line, if appropriate ✻ I.V. fluids ✻ sedative ✻ bridging cable ✻ percutaneous introducer tray or venous cutdown tray ✻ sterile gowns ✻ sterile gloves ✻ mask ✻ goggles or face shield ✻ surgical caps ✻ linen-saver pad ✻ antimicrobial soap ✻ alcohol pads ✻ vial of 1% lidocaine ✻ 5-mL syringe ✻ fluoroscopy equipment including lead apron, if necessary ✻ fenestrated drape ✻ prepackaged cutdown tray (for antecubital vein placement only) ✻ sutures ✻ receptacle for infectious wastes ✻ optional: elastic bandage or gauze strips, restraints, clippers.

How you do it

- Identify the patient using two patient identifiers per the facility policy.
- Explain the procedure to the patient and/or patient representative. Discuss the basic facts about the normal conduction system, temporary pacemaker insertion procedure, precautions and

restrictions while the temporary pacemaker is in place, and when to notify the nurse.

- Perform hand hygiene.
- Check the patient's history for hypersensitivity to local anesthetics and latex. Then attach the cardiac monitor to the patient and obtain a baseline assessment, including the patient's vital signs, skin color, LOC, heart rate and rhythm, and emotional state.
- Next, insert a peripheral I.V. line if the patient doesn't already have one. Begin an I.V. infusion of the specified I.V. fluid at a keep-vein-open rate.
- Insert a new battery into the external pacemaker generator and test it to make sure it has a strong charge. Connect the bridging cable to the generator and align the positive and negative poles. *This cable allows slack between the electrode catheter and the generator, reducing the risk of accidental catheter displacement.*

Clean entry

- Place the patient in the supine position. If necessary, clip the hair around the insertion site.
- All personnel performing and assisting with the procedure should don masks, caps, goggles or face shields, sterile gowns, and gloves.
- Next, open the supply tray while maintaining a sterile field. Using sterile technique, the physician will clean the insertion site with antimicrobial soap and then wipe the area with povidone-iodine solution. He'll cover the insertion site with a fenestrated drape. *Because fluoroscopy may be used during the placement of leadwires*, put on a protective apron.
- Provide the physician with the local anesthetic to numb the insertion site.
- After anesthetizing the insertion site, the physician will puncture the brachial, femoral, subclavian, or jugular vein. Then he'll insert a guide wire or an introducer and advance the electrode catheter.

Map to the heart

- As the catheter advances, watch the cardiac monitor. When the electrode catheter reaches the right atrium, you'll notice large P waves and small QRS complexes. Then, as the catheter reaches the right ventricle, the P waves become smaller while the QRS complexes enlarge. When the catheter touches the right ventricular endocardium, expect to see elevated ST segments, premature ventricular contractions, or both.

- When the electrode catheter is in the right ventricle, it will send an impulse to the myocardium, causing depolarization. If the patient needs atrial pacing, either alone or with ventricular pacing, the physician may place an electrode in the right atrium.

All fired up and ready to go

- Meanwhile, continuously monitor the patient's cardiac status and treat any dysrhythmias, as appropriate.
- When the electrode catheter is in place, attach the catheter leads to the bridging cable. Ensure that the positive and negative electrodes are connected to the respective positive and negative terminals.
- Check the battery's charge by pressing the BATTERY TEST button.
- Set the pacemaker as ordered. Pacing thresholds will be determined by each individual patient.
- The physician will then suture the catheter to the insertion site. Afterward, put on sterile gloves and apply a sterile occlusive dressing to the site. Label the dressing with the date and time of application.

Practice pointers

- Take care to prevent microshock. This includes warning the patient to only use grounded electrical equipment, such as telephones, electric shavers, televisions, or lamps. (See *Transvenous pacemaker complications.*)
- Other safety measures you'll want to take include placing a plastic cover supplied by the manufacturer over the pacemaker controls *to avoid an accidental setting change.* If the patient is disoriented or uncooperative, use restraints *to prevent accidental removal of pacemaker wires.* (See chapter 1, "Restraint application" section.) If the patient needs emergency defibrillation, make sure the pacemaker can withstand the procedure.
- If the physician inserts the electrode through the brachial or femoral vein, immobilize the patient's arm or leg *to avoid putting stress on the pacing wires.*

Check these . . .

After insertion, assess the patient's vital signs, skin color, LOC, and peripheral pulses *to determine the effectiveness of the paced rhythm.* Perform a 12-lead ECG to serve as a baseline and then perform additional ECGs daily or with clinical changes. Also, if possible,

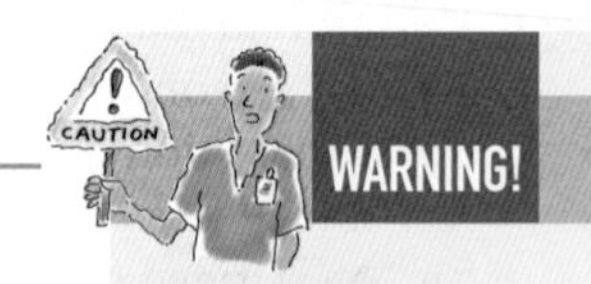

Transvenous pacemaker complications

Complications associated with transvenous pacemaker therapy include:

- cardiac perforation and tamponade
- competitive or fatal dysrhythmias
- diaphragmatic stimulation
- equipment failure
- infection
- microshock
- pneumothorax or hemothorax
- pulmonary embolism
- thrombophlebitis.

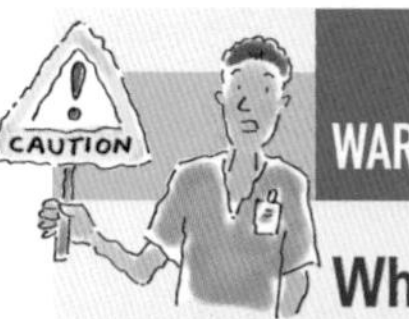
CAUTION

WARNING!

When a temporary pacemaker malfunctions

Occasionally, a temporary pacemaker may fail to function appropriately. When this occurs, you'll need to quickly identify the problem. The strips below illustrate problems that can occur with a temporary pacemaker.

Failure to pace

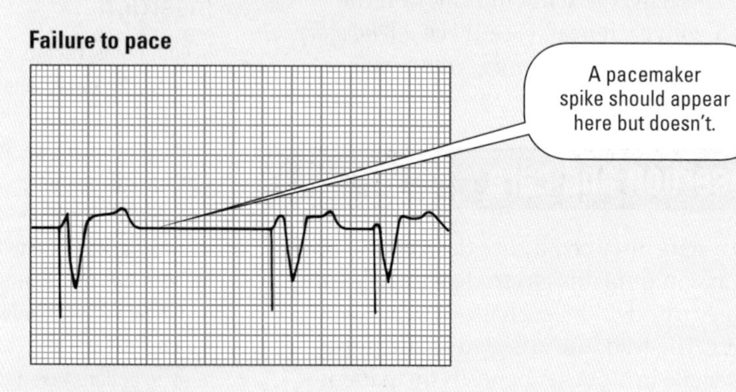
A pacemaker spike should appear here but doesn't.

Failure to capture

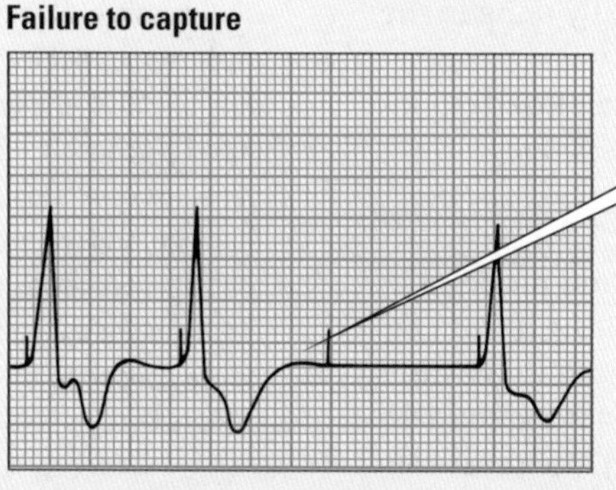
This strip shows a pacemaker spike but no response from the heart.

Failure to sense intrinsic beats

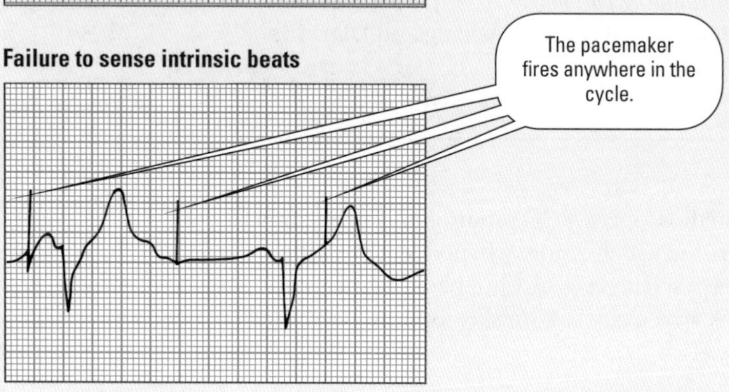
The pacemaker fires anywhere in the cycle.

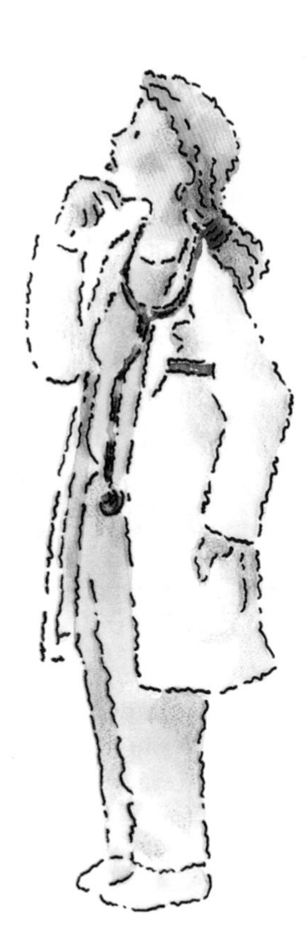

obtain a rhythm strip before, during, and after pacemaker placement; any time that pacemaker settings are changed; and whenever the patient receives treatment because of a complication caused by the pacemaker.

. . . and monitor these

Continuously monitor the ECG reading, noting capture, sensing, rate, intrinsic beats, and competition of paced and intrinsic rhythms. If the pacemaker is sensing correctly, the sense indicator on the pulse generator should flash with each beat. (See *When a temporary pacemaker malfunctions*, page 295, and *Documenting transvenous pacemaker insertion*.)

Documenting transvenous pacemaker insertion

In your notes, record:
- reason for pacemaker use
- time that pacing began
- electrode locations
- pacemaker settings
- patient's response to the insertion procedure and to temporary pacing
- complications and nursing actions taken.

If possible, obtain rhythm strips before, during, and after pacemaker placement; when pacemaker settings are changed; and when the patient receives treatment for a complication caused by the pacemaker.

Permanent pacemaker insertion and care

A permanent pacemaker is a self-contained device designed to operate for 3 to 20 years. The surgeon implants electrode wires that are typically placed transvenously through the cephalic or subclavian vein into the heart chambers. The leads are attached to the pulse generator and the pacemaker sits in a pocket beneath the patient's skin just below the patients left clavicle. This is usually done in the operating room or cardiac catheterization laboratory.

Nursing responsibilities for permanent pacemaker insertion involve monitoring the ECG and caring for the insertion site.

Only when needed

Today, permanent pacemakers function in the demand mode, allowing the patient's heart to beat on its own but preventing it from falling below a preset rate. Pacing electrodes can be placed in the atria, in the ventricles, or in both chambers (atrioventricular sequential, dual chamber). (See *Understanding pacemaker codes*.) The most common pacing codes are VVI for single-chamber pacing and DDD for dual-chamber pacing.

What you need

Sphygmomanometer ✳ stethoscope ✳ ECG monitor and strip-chart recorder ✳ clippers ✳ sterile gauze dressing ✳ hypoallergenic tape ✳ antibiotics ✳ analgesics ✳ sedatives ✳ alcohol pads ✳ emergency resuscitation equipment ✳ sterile gown ✳ mask ✳ optional: I.V. line for emergency medications.

Understanding pacemaker codes

A permanent pacemaker's three-letter (or sometimes five-letter) code indicates how it's programmed. The first letter represents the chamber being paced; the second letter, the chamber being sensed; and the third letter, how the pulse generator responds.

First letter	Second letter	Third letter
A = atrium	A = atrium	I = inhibited
V = ventricle	V = ventricle	T = triggered
D = dual (both chambers)	D = dual (both chambers)	D = dual (inhibited and triggered)
O = not applicablev	O = not applicable	O = not applicable

How you do it

- The physician is responsible for obtaining consent from the patient or patient representative as determined by state law prior to the procedure. This includes explaining the procedure, risks, benefits, and alternatives to the procedure and answering their questions. The nurse should confirm with the patient/representative that the discussion has taken place and a consent form was signed. However, in emergency circumstances, time may not allow the form to be signed. Please refer to facility policy on informed consent.
- Ask the patient if he's allergic to anesthetics or iodine.

Preoperative care

- For pacemaker insertion, clip the patient's chest hair from the axilla to the midline and from the clavicle to the nipple line on the side selected by the physician.
- Establish an I.V. line at a keep-vein-open rate *so that you can administer emergency drugs if the patient experiences ventricular arrhythmia.*
- Obtain baseline vital signs and a baseline ECG.
- Provide sedation as ordered.

In the operating room

- If you'll be present to monitor dysrhythmias during the procedure, put on a gown and mask.
- Connect the ECG monitor to the patient and run a baseline rhythm strip. Make sure that the machine has enough paper to run additional rhythm strips during the procedure.

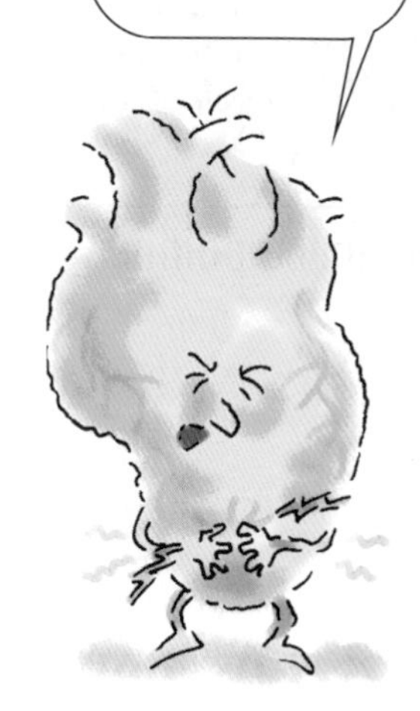
In case I go into ventricular arrhythmia, establish an I.V. line at a keep-vein-open rate.

- In *transvenous* placement, the physician, guided by a fluoroscope, passes the electrode catheter through the cephalic or external jugular vein and positions it in the right ventricle. He attaches the catheter to the pulse generator, inserts this into the chest wall, and sutures it closed, leaving a small outlet for a drainage tube. In some cases, he applies a sterile dressing over the incision.

Postoperative care

- Monitor the patient's ECG *to check for dysrhythmias and to ensure correct pacemaker functioning.*
- Make sure emergency resuscitation equipment is readily available in case a dysrhythmia develops or the pacemaker malfunctions.
- Monitor the I.V. flow rate; the I.V. line is usually kept in place for 24 hours postoperatively *to allow for possible emergency treatment of dysrhythmias.*
- Check the incision for signs of bleeding and infection (swelling, redness, or exudate).
- Administer antibiotics, if ordered.

I will follow you

- If a dressing was applied postoperatively, remove it after 24 hours.
- Check vital signs and LOC every 15 minutes for the first hour, every hour for the next 4 hours, every 4 hours for the next 24 hours, and then once every shift.
- Administer analgesics as needed.

Houston we have a problem

Watch for signs and symptoms of a perforated ventricle, with resultant cardiac tamponade: persistent hiccups, distant heart sounds, pulsus paradoxus, hypotension with narrow pulse pressure, increased venous pressure, cyanosis, distended neck veins, decreased urine output, restlessness, or complaints of fullness in the chest. If the patient develops any of these, **notify the physician immediately**.

Practice pointers

- If the patient wears a hearing aid, the pacemaker battery is placed on the opposite side accordingly.
- Provide the patient with an identification card that lists the pacemaker type and manufacturer, serial number, pacemaker rate setting, date implanted, and physician's name. (See *Teaching the patient who has a permanent pacemaker.*)
- Watch for signs of pacemaker malfunction. (See *Documenting permanent pacemaker insertion.*)

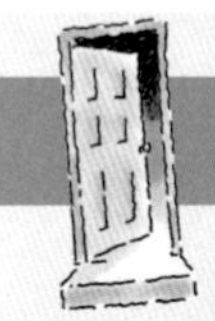

Home care connection

Teaching the patient who has a permanent pacemaker

If your patient is going home with a permanent pacemaker, be sure to cover these teaching points.

Daily care

- ☑ Clean the incision with soap and water.
- ☑ Notify the physician if swelling, redness, or drainage occurs.
- ☑ Perform a 1-minute pulse check and notify the physician of heart rate changes.

Safety and activity

- ☑ Carry your pacemaker identification card at all times.
- ☑ Avoid heavy lifting for at least 4 weeks.
- ☑ Check with the physician before strenuous activities.
- ☑ Avoid direct contact with large running motors, high-powered CB radios, and similar equipment.
- ☑ Avoid magnetic resonance imaging.

Special precautions

- ☑ Report a fast or slow heartbeat, dizziness, shortness of breath, or swollen ankles or feet to the physician.
- ☑ Keep regular physician appointments.

Write it down

Documenting permanent pacemaker insertion

In your notes, document:

- type of pacemaker used
- serial number
- manufacturer's name
- pacing rate
- implantation date
- physician's name
- whether the pacemaker successfully treated the patient's dysrhythmias
- condition of the incision.

Defibrillation

The standard treatment for ventricular fibrillation, defibrillation involves using electrode paddles to direct an electric current through the patient's heart. The current causes the myocardium to depolarize, which in turn encourages the sinoatrial node to resume control of the heart's electrical activity. The electrode paddles delivering the current may be placed on the patient's chest or, during cardiac surgery, directly on the myocardium.

Can't be soon enough

Because ventricular fibrillation leads to death if not corrected, the success of defibrillation depends on early recognition and quick treatment of this arrhythmia. In addition to treating ventricular fibrillation, defibrillation may also be used to treat ventricular tachycardia that doesn't produce a pulse.

Patients with a history of ventricular fibrillation may be candidates for an implantable cardioverter-defibrillator, a sophisticated device that automatically discharges an electric current when it senses a ventricular tachyarrhythmia. (See *Understanding the ICD*.)

What you need

Defibrillator ✳ external paddles ✳ conductive medium pads or gel ✳ ECG monitor with recorder ✳ oxygen therapy equipment ✳ handheld resuscitation bag ✳ endotracheal tube ✳ emergency pacing equipment ✳ emergency cardiac medications.

How you do it

Assess the patient *to determine if he lacks a pulse*. Call for help and perform cardiopulmonary resuscitation (CPR) until the defibrillator and other emergency equipment arrive.

Quick look if you can

- If the defibrillator has "quick-look" capability, place the paddles on the patient's chest *to quickly view his cardiac rhythm*. Otherwise, connect the monitoring leads of the defibrillator to the patient and assess his cardiac rhythm.

Understanding the ICD

The implantable cardioverter-defibrillator (ICD) has a programmable pulse generator and lead system that monitors the heart's activity, detects ventricular bradydysrhythmias and tachydysrhythmias, and responds with appropriate therapies. Its range of therapies includes antitachycardia and bradycardia pacing, cardioversion, and defibrillation. Some defibrillators also have the ability to pace the atrium and the ventricle.

Implantation of the ICD is similar to that of a permanent pacemaker. The cardiologist positions the lead (or leads) transvenously in the endocardium of the right ventricle (and the right atrium, if both chambers require pacing). The lead connects to a generator box, which is implanted in the right or left upper chest near the clavicle.

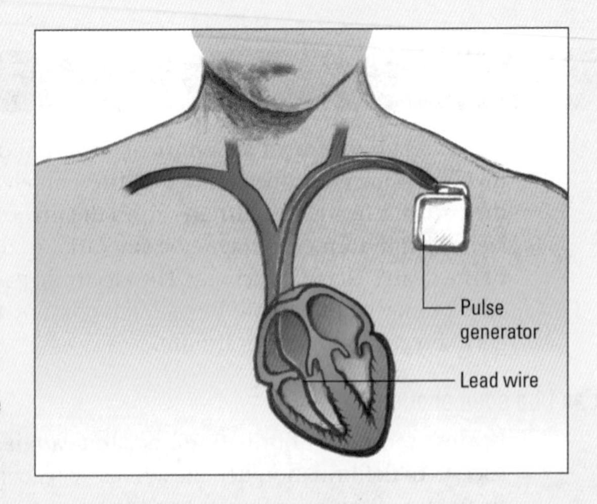

- Expose the patient's chest and apply conductive pads at the paddle placement positions or apply gel to the paddles.
  For anterolateral placement, place one paddle to the right of the upper sternum, just below the right clavicle, and the other over the fifth or sixth intercostal space at the left anterior axillary line.
  For anteroposterior placement, place the anterior paddle directly over the heart at the precordium, to the left of the lower sternal border. Place the flat posterior paddle under the patient's body beneath the heart and immediately below the scapulae (but not under the vertebral column).

Get ready for defibrillation

- Turn on the defibrillator and, if performing external defibrillation, set the energy level. The amount of energy delivered is referred to as joules. For monophasic defibrillation, 360 joules is used for all shocks. For biphasic defibrillation, refer to the manufacturer's instructions for the amount of joules to be delivered to the patient. If the recommended dose is unknown, use the maximum dose available.
- Charge the paddles by pressing the charge buttons, which are located either on the machine or on the paddles themselves.
- Place the paddles over the conductive pads (if used) and press firmly against the patient's chest, using 25 lb (11 kg) of pressure. Before delivering the shock, the person performing the defibrillation ensures that all personnel are standing clear of the bed and visually checks to see that no one is in contact with the patient or bed. The announcement "I'm clear, you're clear, oxygen clear" or "one, two, three, shocking" is announced as the shock is delivered.
- CPR is resumed immediately, beginning with chest compressions for five cycles or 2 minutes. Then the patient's rhythm and pulse are checked. Rhythm strips are recorded during the procedure to document response.

This is a shocking way to snap me out of a bad rhythm!

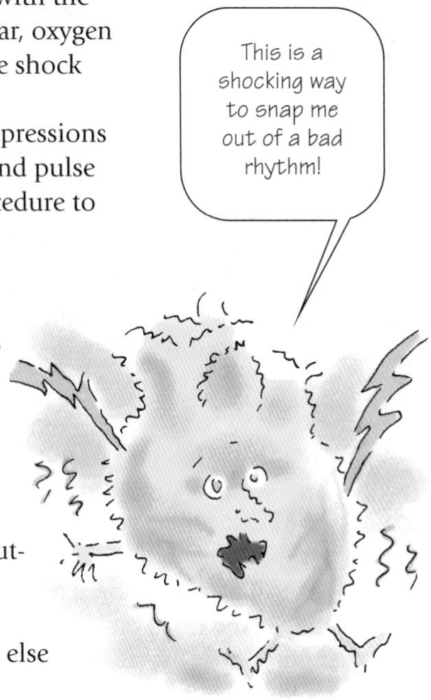

Everyone step back . . .

If the patient remains in ventricular fibrillation or pulseless ventricular tachycardia after five cycles or 2 minutes of CPR, another shock is indicated; instruct all personnel to stand clear of the patient and the bed.

. . . while I shock

- Discharge the current by pressing both paddle charge buttons simultaneously.
- Leaving the paddles in position on the patient's chest, reassess the patient's cardiac rhythm and have someone else assess the pulse.

Repeat if no change after five cycles of CPR

- If necessary, prepare to defibrillate a second time.
- Reassess the patient. If defibrillation is again necessary, instruct someone to reset the energy level to 360 joules. Then follow the same procedure as before.

If no success, reassess

- If the patient still has no pulse after three defibrillations followed by five rounds or 2 minutes of CPR, continue CPR and other advanced cardiac life support measures.
- If defibrillation restores a normal rhythm, assess the patient. Obtain baseline ABG levels and a 12-lead ECG. Provide supplemental oxygen, ventilation, and medications, as needed. (Endotracheal tube insertion may be necessary to ensure ventilation.) Check the patient's chest for electrical burns and treat them, as ordered. Also prepare the defibrillator for immediate reuse. A temporary pacemaker may be inserted.

Documenting defibrillation

In your notes, document:
- onset of arrest
- that the procedure was performed
- patient's ECG rhythms before and after defibrillation
- number of times defibrillation was performed
- voltage used during each attempt
- whether a pulse returned
- dosage, route, and time of drug administration
- whether CPR was used
- means of airway maintenance
- patient's outcome.

Practice pointers

- Defibrillators vary from one manufacturer to the next, so familiarize yourself with your facility's equipment. Defibrillator operation should be checked at least every 8 hours and after each use. (See *Documenting defibrillation*.)

Automated external defibrillation

Automated external defibrillators (AEDs) are commonly used today to meet the need for early defibrillation, which is currently considered the most effective treatment for ventricular fibrillation. Some facilities now require an AED in every noncritical care unit. Their use is also becoming common in such public places as shopping malls, sports stadiums, and airplanes. Instruction in using the AED is already required as part of basic life support (BLS) and advanced cardiac life support (ACLS) training.

All-in-one package

The AED is equipped with a microcomputer that senses and analyzes a patient's heart rhythm at the push of a button. Then it audibly or visually prompts you to deliver a shock. The AED eliminates the need for rhythm recognition because these devices analyze the ECG. The AED charges the device and instructs the operator through step-by-step instructions including when to defibrillate. The automated AED requires that the operator attach the pads and turn on the device, making them ideal for public settings.

All devices record your interactions with the patient during defibrillation, either on a cassette tape or in a solid-state memory module. Some AEDs have an integral printer for immediate event documentation.

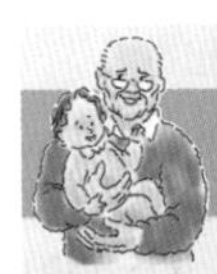

Ages and stages

For children younger than 8 years, AED pads designed for children should be used. If child pads are not available, use adult AED pads.

What you need

AED ✳ two prepackaged electrodes.

How you do it

- After discovering that your patient is unresponsive to your questions, pulseless, and apneic, activate the emergency response system in the facility and follow BLS and ACLS protocols. Then ask a colleague to bring the AED into the patient's room and set it up before the code team arrives.
- Open the foil packets containing the two electrode pads. Attach the white electrode cable connector to one pad and the red electrode cable connector to the other.
- Expose the patient's chest. Remove the plastic backing film from the electrode pads and place the electrode pad attached to the white cable connector on the right upper portion of the patient's chest, just beneath his clavicle.

White to the right, red to the ribs

Place the pad attached to the red cable connector to the left of the heart's apex. To help remember where to place the pads, think "white—right, red—ribs." (Placement for both electrode pads is the same as for manual defibrillation or cardioversion.)

The machine talks

- Firmly press the device's ON button and wait while the machine performs a brief self-test. Most AEDs signal their readiness by a computerized voice stating "Stand clear" or by emitting a series of loud beeps. (If the AED isn't functioning properly, it will convey the message "Don't use the AED. Remove and continue CPR.") Report AED malfunctions in accordance with facility procedure.
- The machine is ready to analyze the patient's heart rhythm. Have everyone stand clear and press the ANALYZE button when the machine prompts you to. Don't touch or move the patient while the AED is in analysis mode. (If the message "Check electrodes" appears, verify correct electrode placement and a secure patient cable attachment; then press the ANALYZE button again.)
- In 15 to 30 seconds, the AED will analyze the patient's rhythm. When the patient needs a shock, the AED displays a "Stand clear" message and emits a beep that changes to a steady tone as it charges.

Safety alert

Do not attach pads to a wet surface, over a medication patch, or over a pacemaker or implanted defibrillator because they reduce the effectiveness of the defibrillation attempt and result in complications.

Just press the button

- When fully charged and ready to deliver a shock, the AED will prompt you to press the SHOCK button. (Some fully automatic AED models automatically deliver a shock within 15 seconds after analyzing the patient's rhythm. If a shock isn't needed, the AED displays "No shock indicated" and prompts you to "Check patient.")
- Make sure that no one is touching the patient or his bed and call out "Stand clear." Then press the SHOCK button on the AED. Most AEDs are ready to deliver a shock within 15 seconds.
- After the first shock, the AED automatically instructs the user to resume CPR. After 2 minutes, the AED will prompt you to check the patient. If the patient is still in ventricular fibrillation, the AED will automatically begin recharging to prepare for a second shock. Repeat the steps you performed before shocking the patient. According to the AED algorithm, the patient can be shocked up to three times with each shock followed by 2 minutes or five rounds of CPR.

Shock three, then start over

- If ventricular fibrillation persists, resume and continue BLS and ACLS and continue the algorithm sequence until the code team leader arrives.
- After the code, remove and transcribe the AED's computer memory module or tape or prompt the AED to print a rhythm strip with code data. Follow your facility's policy for analyzing and storing code data.

Documenting AED use

After using an AED, give a synopsis to the code team leader. Remember to report:

- patient's name, age, medical history, and reason for seeking care
- when you found the patient in cardiac arrest
- when you started CPR
- when you applied the AED
- how many shocks the patient received
- when the patient regained a pulse at any point
- what postarrest care was given, if any
- physical assessment findings.

Later, be sure to document the code on the appropriate form.

Practice pointers

- Defibrillators vary from one manufacturer to the next, so be sure to familiarize yourself with your facility's equipment. Defibrillator operation should be checked at least every 8 hours and after each use. (See *Documenting AED use*.)

Synchronized cardioversion

Synchronized cardioversion is the treatment of choice for dysrhythmias that don't respond to vagal maneuvers or drug therapy, such as atrial tachycardia, atrial flutter, atrial fibrillation, and symptomatic ventricular tachycardia.

Cardioversion works by delivering an electric charge to the myocardium at the peak of the R wave. This causes immediate depolarization, interrupting reentry circuits and allowing the sinoatrial node to resume control. Synchronizing the electric charge with the R wave ensures the current won't be delivered on the vulnerable T wave and thus disrupt repolarization.

What you need

Cardioverter-defibrillator ✻ conductive medium pads or gel ✻ anterior, posterior, or transverse paddles ✻ ECG monitor with recorder ✻ sedative ✻ oxygen therapy equipment ✻ airway ✻ handheld resuscitation bag ✻ emergency pacing equipment ✻ emergency cardiac medications ✻ automatic blood pressure cuff (if available) ✻ pulse oximeter (if available).

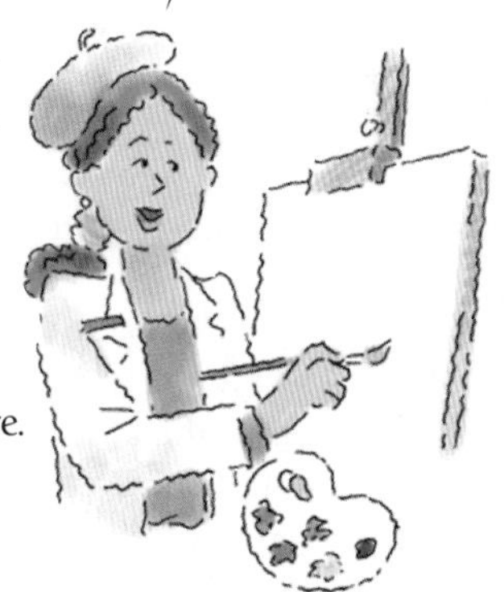
Here's the picture. Use cardioversion to treat certain dysrhythmias that don't respond to drugs or vagal massage.

How you do it

- Explain the procedure to the patient and make sure he has signed a consent form.
- Check the patient's recent serum potassium and magnesium levels and ABG results. Also check recent digoxin levels if indicated. Although patients taking digoxin may undergo cardioversion, they tend to require lower energy levels to convert. If the patient takes digoxin, withhold the dose on the day of the procedure.

Close the kitchen

- Withhold all food and fluids for 6 to 12 hours before the procedure. If the cardioversion is urgent, withhold the previous meal.
- Obtain a 12-lead ECG to serve as a baseline.
- Check to see if the physician has ordered administration of cardiac drugs before the procedure. Also verify that the patient has a patent I.V. site in case drug administration becomes necessary.

Attend to oxygen

- Connect the patient to a pulse oximeter and automatic blood pressure cuff, if available.
- Consider administering oxygen for 5 to 10 minutes before the cardioversion *to promote myocardial oxygenation.* If the patient wears dentures, remove them.
- Place the patient in the supine position. Assess vital signs, LOC, cardiac rhythm, and peripheral pulses.
- Remove an oxygen delivery device just before cardioversion *to avoid possible combustion.*

Bring your backup

- Have a handheld resuscitation bag, an airway, epinephrine, lidocaine, and atropine at the patient's bedside.
- Administer sedation medications, as ordered. The patient should be sedated but still able to breathe adequately.
- Press the POWER button to turn on the defibrillator. Next, push the SYNC button *to synchronize the machine with the patient's QRS*

complexes. Make sure the SYNC button flashes with each of the patient's QRS complexes. You should also see a bright green flag flash on the monitor.

Turn the dial

- Turn the ENERGY SELECT dial to the ordered amount of energy. The purpose of cardioversion is to disrupt the rhythm opposed to defibrillation, which is used to completely depolarize the heart. Because of this, cardioversion requires less energy. The provider can use energy levels as low as 50 joules that is gradually increased until the rhythm is converted.
- Remove the paddles from the machine and prepare them as you would for defibrillation. Place the conductive gel pads or paddles in the same positions as for defibrillation.

Now do it

- Make sure everyone stands away from the bed; then push the discharge buttons. Hold the paddles in place and wait for the energy to be discharged—the machine has to synchronize the discharge with the QRS complex.
- Check the monitor's waveform. If the dysrhythmia persists, repeat the procedure two or three more times at 3-minute intervals, gradually increasing the energy level with each countershock.
- After cardioversion, frequently assess the patient's vital signs, LOC, and respiratory status, including airway patency, respiratory rate and depth, and the need for supplemental oxygen. *The patient will be heavily sedated and may require airway support.*
- Record a postcardioversion 12-lead ECG and monitor the patient's ECG for 2 hours. Check his chest for electrical burns.

Practice pointers

- If the patient is attached to a bedside or telemetry monitor, disconnect the unit before cardioversion. *The electric current it generates could damage the equipment.*
- Although the electric shock of cardioversion won't usually damage an implanted pacemaker, avoid placing the paddles directly over the pacemaker.
- Common complications following cardioversion include transient, harmless dysrhythmias such as atrial, ventricular, and junctional premature beats. Serious ventricular dysrhythmias, such as ventricular fibrillation, may also occur. However, this type of arrhythmia is more likely to result from high amounts of electrical energy, digoxin toxicity, severe heart disease, electrolyte imbalance, or improper synchronization with the R wave. (See *Documenting synchronized cardioversion*.)

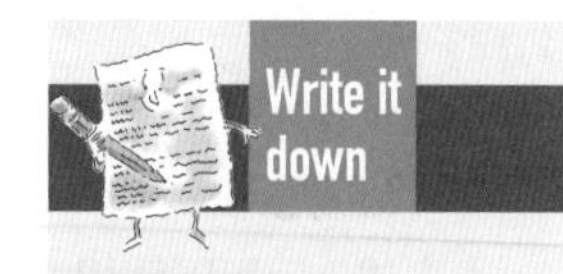

Documenting synchronized cardioversion

In your notes, record:

- that the procedure was performed
- voltage delivered with each attempt
- patient's tolerance of the procedure.

In the patient's chart, place rhythm strips recorded before and after the procedure.

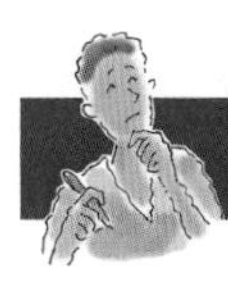

Quick quiz

1. Which information should the nurse include when teaching a patient who is scheduled to have a permanent pacemaker inserted for symptomatic bradycardia?
   - A. The pacemaker will pace the atria up to 400 impulses per minute to keep up with ventricular contractions.
   - B. The pacemaker automatically discharges if ventricular fibrillation and cardiac arrest occur.
   - C. The pacemaker stimulates the heart to contract if the patient's heart rate drops too low.
   - D. The pacemaker battery must be replaced every 2 years to make certain it is functioning.

Answer: C. A permanent pacemaker will discharge when the ventricular rate drops below the preset rate. The pacemaker does not discharge if the patient develops ventricular fibrillation and does not prevent ventricular irritability.

2. The nurse is caring for a patient who has had an arterial line placed. To reduce the risk of complications, what is the priority nursing intervention?
   - A. Restrain the limb affected for the duration of the line placement.
   - B. Ensure all tubing and connections are tightened.
   - C. Apply a pressure dressing at the insertion site.
   - D. Clean insertion site twice a day.

Answer: B. You should ensure all tubing is tightly connected to ensure no complications of bleeding, infection, or thrombosis. Applying a pressure dressing at the site will be done after the line is removed, not during line placement; there is also no clinical need to restrain the affected limb unless the patient's condition warrants.

3. The nurse caring for a patient with a pulmonary artery catheter notices the pulmonary artery occlusion pressure (PAOP) is significantly higher than previous values. The nurse assesses the patient and finds respirations are 14 and unlabored with oxygen saturation of 99% on 2 L nasal cannula, lungs are clear, and the patient appears hemodynamically stable. What is the priority nursing action?
   - A. Increase the supplemental oxygen by 2 L of oxygen.
   - B. Obtain a stat chest X-ray to verify catheter placement.
   - C. Zero reference and level the catheter at the phlebostatic axis.
   - D. Position the patient in high Fowler's and reassess the PAOP.

Answer: C. With any reading that does not match the clinical condition of the patient, level and zero at the phlebostatic axis and reevaluate your readings.

4. When does the dicrotic notch appear on a normal arterial waveform?

A. Blood is ejected from the ventricle.
B. The aortic valve closes.
C. Arterial pressure rises sharply.
D. Opening of the mitral valve

Answer: B. The dicrotic notch appears on the arterial waveform's downside when the aortic valve closes.

Scoring

☆☆☆ If you answered all four items correctly, splendid! You have certainly learned the procedure for acing a quick quiz.

☆☆ If you answered three items correctly, fabulous! You're making solid contact with cardiovascular procedures.

☆ If you answered fewer than three items correctly, don't miss a beat. Just review the chapter and try again.

Selected References

Bickley, L. S., & Hoekelman, R. A. (1999). *Bates' guide to physical examination and history taking* (7th ed.). Philadelphia, PA: Lippincott Williams & Wilkins.

Centers for Disease Control and Prevention. (2011). Vital signs: Central line-associated bloodstream infections—United States, 2001, 2008, and 2009. *Annals of Emergency Medicine, 58*(5), 450.

Elkin, M. K., Perry, A. G., & Potter, P. A. (2000). *Nursing interventions and clinical skills* (2nd ed.). St. Louis, MO: Mosby.

Ellis, J. R., & Hartley, C. L. (2000). *Managing and coordinating nursing care* (3rd ed.). Philadelphia, PA: Lippincott Williams & Wilkins.

Fortunato, N. H. (2000). *Berry & Kohn's operating room technique* (9th ed.). St. Louis, MO: Mosby.

Goldman, L., & Bennett, J. C. (2000). *Cecil textbook of medicine* (21st ed.). Philadelphia, PA: W.B. Saunders.

Hadaway, L. C. (1999). I.V. infiltration. Not just a peripheral problem. *Nursing Management, 29*(9), 41–47.

Herrmann, C. (2014). Cardiac advanced life support-surgical guideline: Overview and implementation. *AACN Advanced Critical Care, 25*(2), 123–129.

Hess, C. T. (2002). *Clinical guide to wound care* (4th ed.). Spring House, PA: Springhouse.

Horne, C., & Derrico, D. (1999). Mastering ABGs. The art of arterial blood gas measurement. *The American Journal of Nursing, 99*(8), 26–32.

Ignatavicius, D. D., & Workman, M. L. (2001). *Medical-surgical nursing: Critical thinking for collaborative care* (4th ed.). Philadelphia, PA: W.B. Saunders.

Jagger, J., & Perry, J. (1999). Power in numbers: Reducing your risk of bloodborne exposures. *Nursing, 29*(1), 51–52.

Joint Commission on Accreditation of Healthcare Organizations. (2001). *Comprehensive accreditation manual for hospitals*. Oakbrook Terrace, IL: Author.

Lanken, P. N., Hanson, C. W., & Manaker, S. (2001). *The intensive care unit manual.* Philadelphia, PA: W.B. Saunders.

Maklebust, J., & Sieggreen, M. (2001). *Pressure ulcers: Guidelines for prevention and management* (3rd ed.). Spring House, PA: Springhouse.

Nicol, M., Bavin, C., Bedford-Turner, S., et al. (2000). *Essential nursing skills.* St. Louis, MO: Mosby.

Phillips, L. D. (2001). *Manual of I.V. therapeutics* (3rd ed.). Philadelphia, PA: F.A. Davis.

Phippen, M. L., & Wells, M .P. (2000). *Patient care during operative and invasive procedures.* Philadelphia, PA: W.B. Saunders.

Pierson, F. M. (1999). *Principles and techniques of patient care* (2nd ed.). Philadelphia, PA: W.B. Saunders.

Shoemaker, W. C., Ayres, S. M., Grenvik, A., et al. (2000). *Textbook of critical care* (4th ed.). Philadelphia, PA: W.B. Saunders.

Smeltzer, S. C., & Bare, B. G. (2000). *Brunner and Suddarth's textbook of medical-surgical nursing* (9th ed.). Philadelphia, PA: Lippincott Williams & Wilkins.

Sole, M. L., Klein, D. G., & Mosely, M. J. (2013). *Introduction to critical care nursing* (6th ed.). St. Louis, MO: Elsevier.

Springhouse. (2001). *Diagnostics: An A-to-Z guide to laboratory tests & diagnostic procedures.* Spring House, PA: Author.

Springhouse. (2008). *Lippincott's nursing procedures* (5th ed.). Philadelphia, PA: Lippincott Williams & Wilkins.

Wiegand, D. J. (Ed.). (2010). *AACN procedure manual for critical care* (6th ed.). Philadelphia, PA: W.B. Saunders.

Wright, R. S., Anderson, J. L., Adams, C. D., et al. (2011). ACCF/AHA focused update of the guidelines for the management of patients with unstable angina/non-ST-elevation myocardial infarction: A report of the American College of Cardiology Foundation/American Heart Association Task Force on Practice Guidelines. *Journal of the American College of Cardiology, 57*(19), 215–367.

Chapter 6

Respiratory care

Just the facts

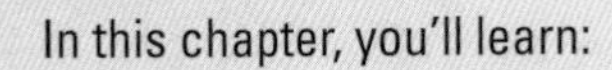

In this chapter, you'll learn:

- about respiratory monitoring and treatment procedures
- what patient care and patient teaching are associated with each procedure
- how to manage complications associated with each procedure
- about essential documentation for each procedure.

Pulse oximetry

Pulse oximetry is a relatively simple, noninvasive procedure used to monitor arterial oxygen saturation. It can be performed continuously or intermittently.

Light reading

In this procedure, two diodes send red and infrared light through a pulsating arterial vascular bed such as the one in the fingertip. A photodetector slipped over the finger measures the transmitted light as it passes through the vascular bed, detects the relative amount of color absorbed by arterial blood, and calculates the exact mixed venous oxygen saturation without interference from surrounding venous blood, skin, connective tissue, or bone.

Another method, ear oximetry, works by monitoring the transmission of light waves through the vascular bed of a patient's earlobe. Results will be inaccurate if the patient's earlobe is poorly perfused, as from a low cardiac output.

Symbolically speaking

Pulse oximeters usually denote arterial oxygen saturation values with the symbol Spo_2. Invasively measured arterial oxygen saturation values, on the other hand, are denoted by the symbol Sao_2.

What you need

Oximeter ✳ finger or ear probe ✳ alcohol pads ✳ nail polish remover, if necessary.

Getting ready

Review the manufacturer's instructions for assembling the oximeter.

How you do it

Explain the procedure to the patient.

For pulse oximetry

- Select a finger for the test. Although the index finger is commonly used, a smaller finger may be selected if the patient's fingers are too large for the equipment. Make sure the patient isn't wearing false fingernails and remove any nail polish from the test finger. Place the transducer (photodetector) probe over the patient's finger so that light beams and sensors oppose each other. If the patient has long fingernails, position the probe perpendicular to the finger, if possible, or clip the fingernail. Always position the patient's hand at heart level *to eliminate venous pulsations and to promote accurate readings.* (See *Pediatric pulse oximetry.*)
- Turn on the power switch. If the device is working properly, a beep will sound, a display will light momentarily, and the pulse searchlight will flash. The SpO_2 and pulse rate displays will show stationary zeros. After four to six heartbeats, the SpO_2 and pulse rate displays will supply information with each beat and the pulse amplitude indicator will begin tracking the pulse.

For ear oximetry

- Using an alcohol pad, massage the patient's earlobe for 10 to 20 seconds. Mild erythema indicates adequate vascularization. Following the manufacturer's instructions, attach the ear probe to the patient's earlobe or pinna. Use the ear probe stabilizer for prolonged or exercise testing. Be sure to establish good contact on the ear; *an unstable probe may set off the low-perfusion alarm.* After the probe has been attached for a few seconds, a saturation reading and pulse waveform will appear on the oximeter's screen.
- Leave the ear probe in place for 3 or more minutes until readings stabilize at the highest point or take three separate readings and average them. Make sure you revascularize the patient's earlobe each time.

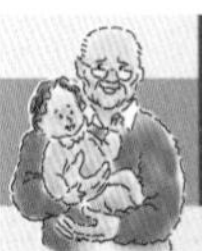

Ages and stages

Pediatric pulse oximetry

If you need to monitor arterial oxygen saturation in a neonate or a small infant, wrap the oximeter's probe around the infant's foot so that light beams and detectors oppose each other. For a large infant, use a probe that fits on the great toe and secure it to the foot.

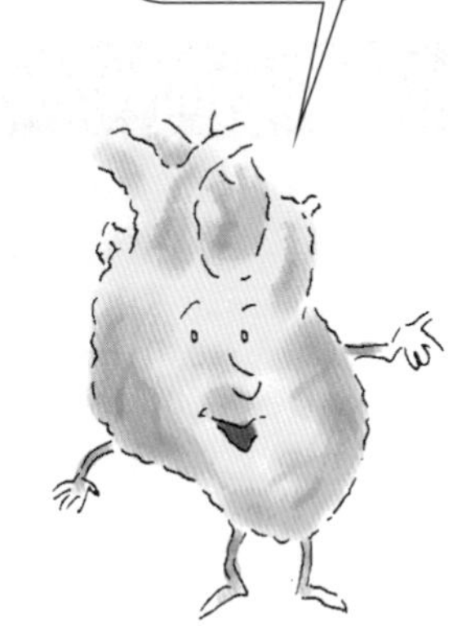
For best pulse oximetry results, keep the patient's hand at my level.

- Remove the probe, turn off and unplug the unit, and clean the probe by gently rubbing it with an alcohol sponge.

Documenting pulse oximetry

In your notes, document the procedure, including the date, time, procedure type, oximetric measurement, and actions taken. Record the readings on appropriate flowcharts, if indicated.

Practice pointers

If oximetry has been performed properly, readings are typically accurate. However, certain factors (such as hypothermia or hypotension) may interfere with accuracy.

Detour over the bridge

- If the patient has compromised circulation in his extremities, you can place a photodetector across the bridge of his nose.
- If SpO_2 is used to guide weaning the patient from mechanical ventilation, obtain arterial blood gas (ABG) analysis occasionally to correlate SpO_2 readings with SaO_2 levels.
- If an automatic blood pressure cuff is used on the same extremity that's used for measuring SpO_2, the cuff will interfere with SpO_2 readings during inflation. The SpO_2 measurements can be lower than the actual SaO_2 if there is reduced perfusion to the site where the sensor is placed. For example, this can occur with limb ischemia or an inflated blood pressure cuff.

Problem solving

Normal SpO_2 levels for ear and pulse oximetry are 95% to 100% for adults and 93.8% to 100% by 1 hour after birth for healthy, full-term neonates. Lower levels may indicate hypoxemia, which warrants intervention. For such patients, follow your facility's policy, notify the doctor, or resuscitate the patient immediately, if necessary. (See *Documenting pulse oximetry*.)

Oropharyngeal airway use

The tongue is the most common cause of airway obstruction in an unconscious person. Keeping the tongue from blocking the airway passage (pharynx) is a high priority. It can be accomplished by using an oropharyngeal airway or a nasopharyngeal airway.

An oropharyngeal airway (OPA), a curved rubber or plastic device, is inserted into the mouth to the posterior pharynx to establish or maintain a patent airway. It also facilitates oropharyngeal suctioning. The OPA is intended for short-term use, as in the postanesthesia or postictal stage. It may be left in place longer as an airway adjunct to prevent the orally intubated patient from biting the endotracheal tube.

The OPA should not be used in patients with loose or avulsed teeth or recent oral surgery. Inserting an OPA in a conscious or semiconscious patient may stimulate vomiting and laryngospasm; therefore, **only insert the airway in unconscious, unresponsive patients with NO gag reflex.**

What you need

For inserting

Oral airway of appropriate size ✱ tongue blade ✱ padded tongue blade ✱ gloves ✱ mask ✱ goggles or face shield ✱ optional: suction equipment, handheld resuscitation bag or oxygen-powered breathing device.

For cleaning

Hydrogen peroxide ✱ water ✱ basin ✱ optional: pipe cleaner.

For reflex testing

Cotton-tipped applicator.

Getting ready

Select an airway of appropriate size for your patient; *an oversized airway can obstruct breathing by depressing the epiglottis into the laryngeal opening.* To determine the appropriate size, measure the OPA from the patient's earlobe to the corner of the mouth. Usually, you'll select a small size (size 1 or 2) for an infant or child, a medium size (size 4 or 5) for an average adult, and a large size (size 6) for a large adult.

How you do it

- Identify the patient using two patient identifiers.
- Explain the procedure to the patient even though he may not appear to be alert. Provide privacy and follow standard precautions. If the patient is wearing dentures, remove them *so they don't cause further airway obstruction.*
- Suction the patient if necessary.
- Place the patient in the supine position.

Best techniques

For an adult

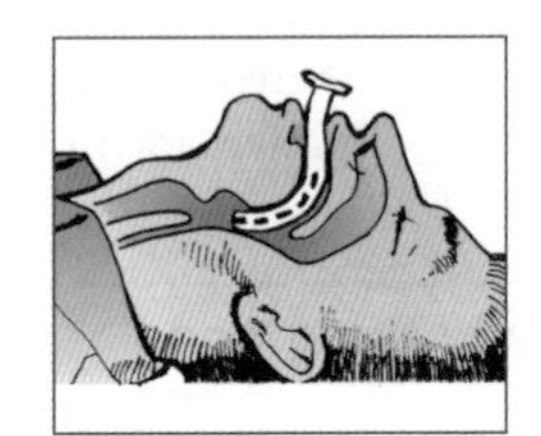

- *Use the cross-finger technique to open the patient's mouth by* placing your thumb on the patient's lower teeth and your index finger on his upper teeth and open his mouth.
- Grasp the patient's lower jaw and tongue and lift upward or use a head-tilt/chin-lift or a modified jaw thrust.
- Insert the OPA into the patient's mouth with the curved end along the roof of the mouth. As the airway is inserted, it is rotated 1/2 turn (180 degrees) with the curvature of the tongue until the flange comes to rest on the patient lips and or teeth.
- The OPA can also be inserted with the pharyngeal curve if a tongue blade is used to depress the tongue.

For child or infant

- Use a tongue blade or a tongue depressor and insert with the tip of the device pointing toward the back of the tongue and throat in the position it will rest in after insertion.

OR

- Insert the OPA sideways and then rotate it 90 degrees.
- The flange should rest on the patient's lips.

For all patients . . .

- If the patient begins to gag or vomit, remove the OPA and suction the airway, ensuring all debris are removed from the airway. Thoroughly clean the device and reinsert the OPA only if the patient is still unconscious and does not have a gag reflex.
- Auscultate the lungs to ensure adequate ventilation.
- After the airway is inserted, position the patient on his side *to decrease the risk of aspiration of vomitus.*
- Perform mouth care every 2 to 4 hours as needed. Begin by holding the patient's jaws open with a padded tongue blade and gently removing the airway. Place the airway in a basin and rinse it with hydrogen peroxide and then water. If secretions remain, use a pipe cleaner to remove them. Complete standard mouth care and reinsert the airway.
- While the airway is removed for mouth care, observe the mouth's mucous membranes *because tissue irritation or ulceration can result from prolonged airway use.*
- Frequently check airway position *to ensure correct placement.* (See "Oropharyngeal airway insertion" at http://www.youtube.com/watch?v=vgqOrmBskaw.)

Awakenings

- When the patient regains consciousness and can swallow, remove the airway by pulling it outward and downward, following the mouth's natural curvature. After the airway is removed, test the patient's cough and gag reflexes *to ensure that removal of the airway wasn't premature and that the patient can maintain his own airway.*

Documenting oral airway use

In your notes, record:
- date and time of airway insertion
- airway size
- airway removal and cleaning
- mucous membrane condition
- suctioning
- adverse reactions and nursing actions taken
- patient's tolerance of the procedure.

Practice pointers

- Avoid taping the airway in place *because untaping it could delay airway removal, thus increasing the risk of aspiration.*

Next stop, the dentist

- Tooth damage or loss, tissue damage, and bleeding may result from insertion.
- If the airway is too long, it may press the epiglottis against the entrance of the larynx, producing complete airway obstruction.
- To prevent traumatic injury, make sure that the patient's lips and tongue aren't between his teeth and the airway.
- If placed improperly, it can depress the tongue into the back of the throat, further blocking the airway.
- Immediately after inserting the airway, check for respirations. If respirations are absent or inadequate, initiate artificial positive pressure ventilation by using a mouth-to-mask technique, a hand-held resuscitation bag, or an oxygen-powered breathing device. (See "Manual ventilation," page 342, and *Documenting oral airway use.*)

Nasopharyngeal airway use

Insertion of a nasopharyngeal airway (NPA)—a soft rubber or latex uncuffed catheter—establishes or maintains a patent airway. This airway is the typical choice for patients who have had recent oral surgery or facial trauma and for patients with loose, cracked, or avulsed teeth. It's also used to protect the nasal mucosa from injury when the patient needs frequent nasotracheal suctioning. NPAs are better tolerated in a conscious patient but come with a higher risk for infection.

Bypassing the mouth

The airway follows the curvature of the nasopharynx, passing through the nose and extending from the nostril to the posterior pharynx. The bevel-shaped pharyngeal end of the airway facilitates insertion and its funnel-shaped nasal end helps prevent slippage.

An NPA is contraindicated if the patient is receiving anticoagulant therapy or has a hemorrhagic disorder, head trauma, skull fracture, sepsis, or a pathologic nasopharyngeal deformity.

What you need

For insertion

NPA of proper size ✳ water-soluble lubricant ✳ gloves ✳ mask ✳ goggles or face shield ✳ handheld resuscitation bag ✳ optional: suction equipment.

For cleaning

Hydrogen peroxide ✳ water ✳ basin ✳ optional: pipe cleaner.

Getting ready

Measure the diameter of the patient's nostril and the distance from the tip of his nose to his earlobe. Select an airway of slightly smaller diameter than the nostril and of slightly longer length (1″ [2.5 cm] more) than measured. The sizes for this type of airway are labeled according to their internal diameter.

The recommended size for a large adult is 8 to 9 mm; for a medium adult, 7 to 8 mm; and for a small adult, 6 to 7 mm. Lubricate the distal half of the airway's surface with a water-soluble lubricant *to prevent traumatic injury during insertion.*

How you do it

- Follow standard precautions.
- In nonemergency situations, explain the procedure to the patient.
  - Measure the NPA from the patient's earlobe to the tip of the nostril. The diameter should be slightly smaller than the diameter of the nostril. (See *Inserting a nasopharyngeal airway.*)
  - Use a water-soluble lubricant prior to insertion.
  - When you insert the airway, remember to use a chin-lift or jaw-thrust technique to anteriorly displace the patient's mandible. With the bevel toward the septum (center of the nose), advance the NPA gently, straight in, following the floor of the nose.(See *Keeping a clear airway.*)

Inserting a nasopharyngeal airway

Hold the airway beside the patient's face to make sure it's the proper size. It should be slightly smaller than the nostril diameter and slightly longer than the distance from the tip of the nose to the earlobe.

To insert the airway, hyperextend the patient's neck (unless contraindicated). Push up the tip of his nose and pass the airway into his nostril (as shown below).

To check for correct airway placement, first close the patient's mouth. Then place your finger over the tube's opening to detect air exchange. Also, depress the patient's tongue with a tongue blade and look for the airway tip behind the uvula.

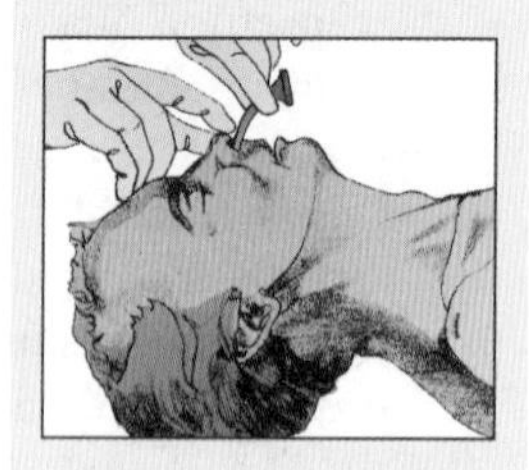

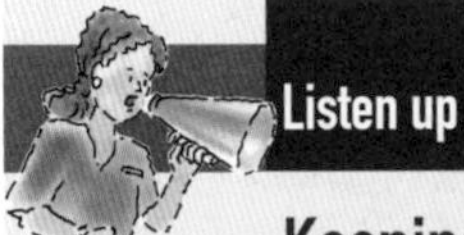

Listen up

Keeping a clear airway

Deep breathing and coughing are vital for removing lung secretions. Other methods to help clear the airway include diaphragmatic breathing and forced expiration. Here's how to teach these methods to your patients.

Diaphragmatic breathing

First, tell the patient to lie supine, with his head elevated 15 to 20 degrees on a pillow. Tell him to place one hand on his abdomen and then inhale so that he can feel his abdomen rise. Explain that this is known as "breathing with the diaphragm."

Next, instruct the patient to exhale slowly through his nose—or, better yet, through pursed lips—while letting his abdomen collapse. Explain that this action decreases his respiratory rate and increases his tidal volume.

Suggest that the patient perform this exercise for 30 minutes several times per day. After he becomes accustomed to the position and has learned to breathe using his diaphragm, he may apply abdominal weights of 8.8 to 11 lb (4 to 5 kg). The weights enhance the movement of the diaphragm toward the head during expiration.

To enhance the effectiveness of exercise, the patient also may manually compress the lower costal margins, perform straight-leg lifts, and coordinate the breathing technique with a physical activity such as walking.

Forced expiration

Tell the patient that forced expiration helps clear secretions while causing less traumatic injury than does a cough. To perform the technique, tell the patient to forcefully expire without closing his glottis, starting with a mid to low lung volume. Tell him to follow this expiration with a period of diaphragmatic breathing and relaxation.

Inform the patient that if his secretions are in the central airways, he may have to use a more forceful expiration or a cough to clear them.

- If resistance is felt, do not force it. Remove and try the other nostril.
- The flange should be at the patient's nostril. (See the following text.)

To check for correct airway placement, first, close the patient's mouth. Then place your finger over the tube's opening to detect air exchange. Also depress the patient's tongue with a tongue blade and look for the airway tip behind the uvula.

- After the airway is inserted, check it regularly *to detect dislodgment or obstruction.*
- When the patient's natural airway is patent, remove the airway in one smooth motion.

Practice pointers

- Immediately after insertion, assess the patient's respirations. If absent or inadequate, initiate artificial ventilation using a mouth-to-mask technique or a handheld resuscitation bag.
- If the patient coughs or gags, the tube may be too long. If so, remove the airway and insert a shorter one. If the tube is too long, it may enter the esophagus and cause gastric distention and hypoventilation during artificial ventilation.
- At least once every 8 hours, remove the airway *to check nasal mucous membranes for irritation or ulceration.*
- Sinus infection may result from obstruction of sinus drainage. Insertion of the airway may injure the nasal mucosa and cause bleeding and possibly aspiration of blood into the trachea. Suction as necessary to remove secretions or blood.
- Although semiconscious patients usually tolerate NPAs better than conscious patients, they may still experience laryngospasm and vomiting. (See *Documenting nasopharyngeal airway use.*)

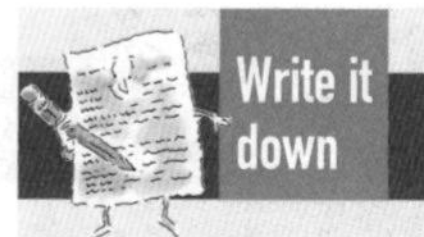

Documenting nasopharyngeal airway use

In your notes, record:
- date and time of airway insertion
- airway size
- airway removal and cleaning
- shifts from one nostril to the other
- mucous membrane condition
- suctioning
- complications and nursing actions taken
- patient's tolerance of the procedure.

Suctioning—nasopharyngeal, nasotracheal, and artificial airway

Oropharyngeal suctioning removes secretions from the back of the throat. Tracheal suctioning goes down further to the lower airway to remove secretions and maintain optimum ventilation and oxygenation in patients who are not able to remove the secretions independently. Some patients require suctioning as often as every 1 to 2 hours, whereas others only once or twice a day. One indicator of the need for suctioning is when the oxygen saturation falls below 90%.

What you need

- Appropriate size suction catheter (smallest diameter to remove secretions effectively) ✳ nasal or oral airway as needed ✳ two sterile or one sterile and one clean glove ✳ clean towel or drape ✳ suction machine ✳ mask ✳ goggles or face shield ✳ connecting tubing (6 ft) ✳ small Y-adapter (if catheter does not have a suction port) ✳ water-soluble lubricant ✳ sterile basin ✳ sterile normal saline or water, about 100 mL ✳ pulse oximeter and stethoscope.

Getting ready

Assess the patient for signs and symptoms of upper and lower airway obstruction requiring suctioning (wheezes, crackles, gurgling on inspiration or expiration, restlessness, decreased breath sounds, cyanosis, tachypnea, hypertension, or hypotension) before and after suctioning. Determine the presence of anxiety, apprehension, change in level of consciousness, behavioral changes, dyspnea, or use of accessory muscles.

Assess factors that affect volume and consistency of secretions—fluid balance, lack of humidity, infection, and allergies/sinus drainage.

To do or not to do

Weigh the patient's need for suctioning along with contraindications for nasotracheal suctioning including facial or neck trauma/surgery, bleeding disorders, nasal bleeding, epiglottis or croup, laryngospasm, irritable airway, gastric surgery, and acute head injuries.

How you do it

Nasopharyngeal and nasotracheal suctioning

- Identify patient with two identifiers.
- Place pulse oximeter on patient's finger. Take reading and leave oximeter in place.
- Perform hand hygiene and apply mask, goggles, or face shield.
- Attach one end of connecting tubing to suction machine and other in a location near the patient. Turn suction device on and set suction pressure to the lowest level while still effectively clearing secretions: less than 150 mm Hg in adults. Check the pressure by putting your thumb over the tubing.
- Using aseptic technique, open the catheter or suction kit. Place on a sterile drape if it is available. Do not let the catheter touch any nonsterile surfaces.
- Unwrap or open the sterile bowl and pour 100 mL of sterile normal saline in bowl, being careful not to touch the inside.
- Open lubricant and squeeze onto the open sterile catheter package.
- Don sterile gloves to both hands or clean glove to nondominant hand and sterile glove to dominant hand.

Getting connected . . .

- Pick up the catheter with the dominant hand and the connector tubing with the nondominant hand. Secure catheter to tubing.

- Suction a small amount of the normal saline to confirm the equipment is functioning properly.
- Suction airway. Hyperoxygenate for 30 to 60 seconds prior to suctioning by increasing oxygen to face mask. Have the patient breathe slowly and deeply if able.
- Lightly coat distal catheter with water-soluble lubricant.
- Remove the oxygen delivery device, then quickly insert catheter into the nares. Instruct the patient to deep breathe. Slightly slant the catheter downward or through the mouth. Do *not* force through nares. If you feel resistance after insertion of the catheter, use caution; it has probably hit the carina. Pull the catheter back 1 to 2 cm before applying suction.

Come on baby, let's do the twist

- Apply intermittent suction for no more than 15 seconds by putting finger over the catheter vent. Carefully rotate or twirl the catheter as you are withdrawing it from the airway.
- Rinse catheter and connecting tubing with normal saline until clear. Assess for need to repeat suctioning.
- Allow 1 minute to pass between suction passes to allow for oxygenation.

Artificial airway suctioning (endotracheal tube or tracheostomy tube)

- Hyperoxygenate patient with 100% oxygen for 30 to 60 seconds prior to suctioning. Either adjust the FIO_2 on the ventilator or use an oxygen-enrichment program on microprocessor ventilators. Manual ventilation is not recommended because it cannot deliver an FIO_2 of 1.0.
- If on mechanical ventilation, open the swivel adapter.
- Without applying suction, insert catheter quickly into the artificial airway using your dominant thumb and forefinger until you meet resistance. (Try to time the catheter insertion with inspiration.) Pull back 1 cm and apply suction by placing nondominant thumb over the vent; withdraw catheter while rotating it back and forth to *avoid trauma to the tracheal tissue.*
- Encourage patient to cough. Watch for respiratory distress.
- If patient is on mechanical ventilation, close the swivel adapter.
- Encourage patient to deep breathe and hyperoxygenate for at least 1 minute.
- Rinse catheter and connect tubing with normal saline until clear.
- Assess patient's vital signs, cardiopulmonary status, and ventilator measurements to determine if secretions are clear. Repeat steps once or twice as necessary to remove secretions. Suction oropharynx as needed.
- Readjust oxygen to original level as indicated.

Suctioning—closed (in-line)

Some facilities use an in-line or closed-system suction catheter device to minimize infections for patients with an ETT or tracheostomy tube. It allows for quicker lower airway suctioning without donning sterile gloves or a mask and does not interrupt oxygenation. Another advantage of a closed-system is the patient's artificial airway remains connected to the ventilator.

What you need

Closed-system or in-line suction catheter ✳ suction machine ✳ connecting tubing ✳ mask, goggles, or face shield ✳ pulse oximeter ✳ stethoscope ✳ optional: two clean gloves.

How you do it

- Identify the patient using two identifiers.
- Assess breath sounds, SpO_2, and vital signs.
- Explain the procedure to the patient.
- Place the patient in semi- or high-Fowler's position.
- Perform hand hygiene and follow standard precautions.
- The respiratory therapist often attaches the catheter to the mechanical ventilator. If catheter is not attached, open the suction catheter package using aseptic technique and attach to the ventilator circuit by removing swivel adapter and placing closed-system suction catheter apparatus on ETT or tracheostomy tube. Connect Y on mechanical ventilator circuit to closed-system suction catheter with flex tubing.
- Connect the end of the tubing to the suction machine; connect the other end to the closed-system or in-line suction catheter. Turn suction on, set vacuum regulator to appropriate negative pressure, and check pressure. It may require a slightly higher pressure (check manufacturer's guidelines).
- Hyperoxygenate with 100% oxygen by changing the FIO_2 to 1.0. Manual ventilation is not recommended.
- Pick up suction catheter in plastic sleeve with dominant hand.

Smooth move

- Wait until the patient inhales and insert the catheter. Use a repeating maneuver of pushing the catheter and sliding the plastic sheath back with the thumb and forefinger until resistance is met or the patient coughs. Pull back 1 cm before applying continuous suction for no more than 10 seconds. Be sure to withdraw the catheter completely into sheath. Reassess the patient and repeat steps as needed. Lock suction mechanism and turn off suction.

- Hyperoxygenate the patient and return the FIO_2 to previous setting.
- Perform oral suctioning as needed.
- Reposition patient. Remove personal protective equipment (PPE) and discard in appropriate receptacle.
- Compare patient's respiratory assessment pre- and postprocedure.

Practice pointers

- Have the patient turn his head to the side to help you suction more effectively. Turning to the right helps to suction the left mainstem bronchus and to the left the right mainstem bronchus.
- Preoxygenation converts large proportions of resident lung gas to 100% oxygen to supplement the volume lost during the interruption of ventilation.

An "aah" moment

- When there is difficulty passing the catheter, ask the patient to take a deep breath, cough, or say "aah" and try to advance the catheter. These measures help to open the glottis to permit the passage of the suction catheter into the trachea. (See *All about tracheal suctioning.*)

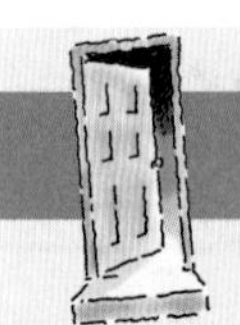

Home care connection

All about tracheal suctioning

If a patient can't mobilize secretions effectively by coughing, he may have to perform tracheal suctioning at home using either clean or aseptic technique. Most patients use clean technique, which consists of thorough hand washing and possibly wearing a clean glove.

Because the cost of disposable catheters can be prohibitive, many patients reuse disposable catheters. Consult your facility's policy regarding the care and cleaning of nondisposable suction catheters in the home setting.

Making the grade

Before discharge, the patient and his family should demonstrate the suctioning procedure. They also need to recognize the indications for suctioning; the signs and symptoms of infection; the importance of adequate hydration; and when to use adjunct therapy, such as aerosol therapy, chest physiotherapy, oxygen therapy, or a handheld resuscitation bag. At discharge, arrange for a home health care provider and a durable medical equipment vendor to follow up with the patient.

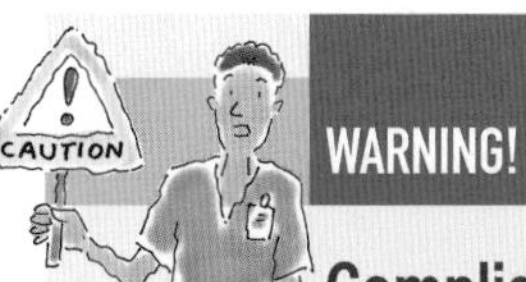

WARNING!

Complications of tracheal suctioning

Common complications of tracheal suctioning include:

- hypoxemia and dyspnea, from removal of oxygen along with secretions
- altered respiratory patterns, from anxiety
- cardiac arrhythmias, from hypoxia and vagus nerve stimulation
- tracheal or bronchial trauma, from traumatic or prolonged suctioning
- hypoxemia, arrhythmias, hypertension, and hypotension, in patients with compromised cardiovascular or pulmonary status
- bleeding, in patients with a history of nasopharyngeal bleeding, those receiving anticoagulants, those who have undergone a recent tracheostomy, and those with blood dyscrasias
- further rise in intracranial pressure (ICP), in patients with increased ICP.

Rare complications

Rare complications of suctioning include laryngospasm and bronchospasm. If either occurs, disconnect the suction catheter from the connecting tubing and let the catheter act as an airway. Discuss with the doctor whether the patient should receive bronchodilators or lidocaine to reduce the risk of the complication.

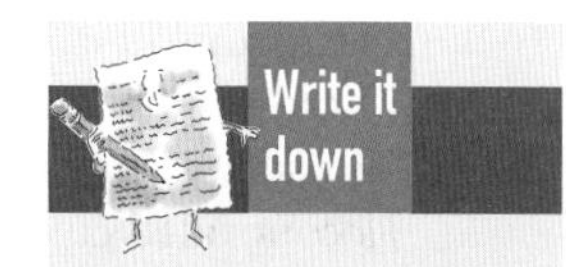

Write it down

Documenting tracheal suctioning

In your notes, document:

- date and time of the procedure
- suctioning technique used
- reason for suctioning
- amount, color, consistency, and odor of secretions
- complications and nursing actions taken
- patient's tolerance of the procedure.

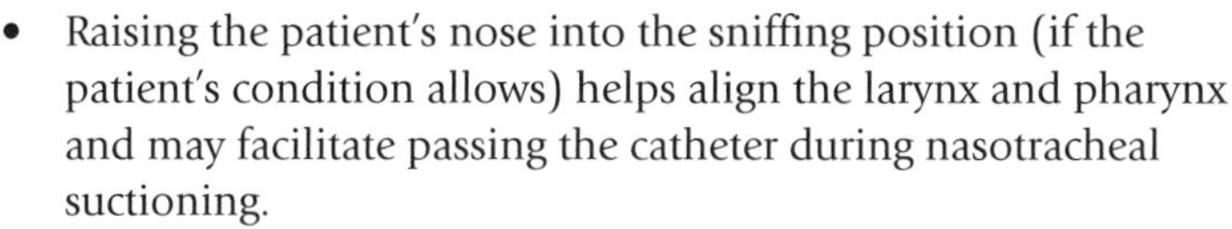

- Raising the patient's nose into the sniffing position (if the patient's condition allows) helps align the larynx and pharynx and may facilitate passing the catheter during nasotracheal suctioning.
- Don't allow the collection container on the suction machine to become more than three-quarters full *to keep from damaging the machine.*
- Assess the patient for complications of tracheal suctioning. See *Complications of tracheal suctioning* for details. (Also see *Documenting tracheal suctioning.*)
- Upper airway is considered "clean" and lower airway is considered "sterile." You can use the same catheter to suction from sterile to clean (e.g., tracheal suctioning to oropharyngeal suctioning) but not from clean to sterile areas.

Assisting with endotracheal tube intubation

An endotracheal tube (ETT) is an artificial airway inserted to relieve airway obstruction, provide a route for mechanical ventilation, protect the airway from aspiration, and allow for easy removal of secretions. It is inserted through the mouth or nares past the epiglottis and vocal cords and down into the trachea. This procedure is usually done in an emergency situation but can also be done in a controlled environment such as the operating room for general anesthesia.

It is indicated when there is an inability to oxygenate the patient (Spo_2 <95% or Pao_2 <55 mm Hg), inability to ventilate the patient (respiratory acidosis, mental status change, or other symptoms), or the patient is unable to protect the airway (loss of gag reflex or impaired cough).

A physician or respiratory therapist in most instances will perform this procedure; however, nurses with advanced cardiac life support certification are able to insert an ETT. Refer to the facility policies and procedures to determine who can perform ETT intubation in your facility.

What you need

PPE, including eye protection ✱ ETT with intact cuff and 15-mm connector (general sizes are a 7- to 8-mm tube for women and 8- to 9-mm tube for men) ✱ laryngoscope handle with fresh batteries ✱ laryngoscope blades (straight and curved) ✱ spare bulb for laryngoscope blades (check to see if it is working prior to procedure) ✱ flexible stylet ✱ self-inflating resuscitation bag with mask connected to supplemental oxygen (greater than or equal to 15 L/minute) ✱ oxygen source and connecting tubes ✱ swivel adapter (to attach to resuscitation bag or ventilator) ✱ suction apparatus (wall or portable) ✱ suction catheters ✱ rigid suction tip catheter (Yankauer) ✱ suction tubing ✱ bite block or OPA ✱ ETT securing apparatus (commercially available ETT holders and tube securement, adhesive tape, and twill tape cut into 30″ lengths) ✱ stethoscope ✱ monitoring equipment (continuous oxygen saturation and cardiac rhythm) ✱ secondary confirmation device: disposable end-tidal detector, continuous end-tidal CO_2 monitoring device or esophageal detection device ✱ drugs for intubation, as indicated ✱ additional equipment includes the following: anesthetic spray, local anesthetic jelly, Magill forceps (foreign body removal if obstructing airway), ventilator.

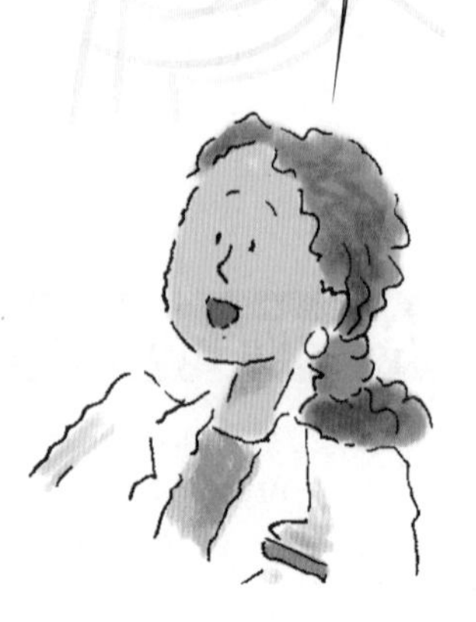
Even on a sunny day, the laryngoscope needs a working light bulb.

Getting ready

- Identify the patient with two identifiers.
- Explain the procedure to the patient and family. Explain that the patient will be unable to talk with the ETT in place but that other means of communication will be provided. Explain that the patient's hands may be restrained to prevent dislodgement of the ETT.

- Have crash cart available.
- Assess the patient's respiratory status, vital signs, oxygenation (Spo_2), mental status, and level of consciousness.
- Check the laryngoscope blade to ensure the light is working.
- Perform hand hygiene and don PPE.
- Insert oropharyngeal in the unconscious patient. (See "Oropharyngeal airway insertion.")
- Place the patient on cardiac monitor and pulse oximetry.
- Set up the suction apparatus and attach rigid suction tip catheter to tubing—test to ensure it is working appropriately.
- Assist in positioning the patient's head by flexing the neck forward and extending the head (sniffing position). *It allows for visualization of the vocal cords.*
- Check the mouth for dentures and remove if present (put in labeled container); suction the mouth as needed. *Dentures can remain in for nasal intubation.*

How you do it

- Insert OPA in the unconscious patient only.
- Premedicate the patient per physician order. Do not give medications until the physician is at the bedside and is ready to intubate the patient.
- Hyperoxygenate and ventilate the patient with 100% oxygen prior to intubation and between attempts. *Attempts should not take longer than 30 seconds.*

Sherlock Holmes at your service

- When the ETT has been placed, assist to confirm tube placement while bagging with 100% oxygen. Use a *disposable CO_2 detector or esophageal detector device to confirm proper tube placement.*
- Auscultate over epigastrium *to identify esophageal intubation.*
- Auscultate lung bases and apices for bilateral breath sounds and observe for symmetric chest wall movement. *Assists in verification of correct tube placement.*
- Evaluate the oxygen saturation by pulse oximetry. *It will decrease with esophageal intubation; it may or may not change with right mainstem bronchus intubation.*
- If the physician determines the tube is not placed correctly, assist with reintubation. Hyperoxygenate with 100% oxygen for 3 to 5 minutes and reattempt intubation.
- If breath sounds are absent on the left, the cuff will be deflated and the tube pulled back. Reevaluate for correct tube placement as above.
- Connect ETT to oxygen source or mechanical ventilator using swivel adapter.

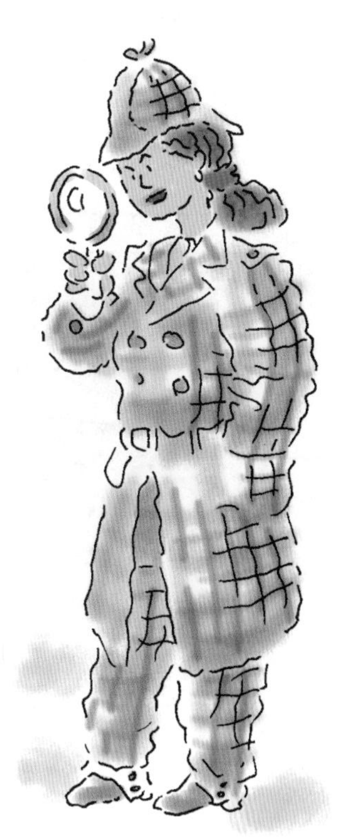

Securing an ETT

Before taping an ETT in place, make sure the patient's face is clean, dry, and free from beard stubble. If possible, suction his mouth and dry the tube just before taping. Also check the reference mark on the tube to ensure correct placement. After taping, always check for bilateral breath sounds to ensure that the tube hasn't been displaced by manipulation.

Method 1

Cut one piece of 1″ cloth adhesive tape long enough to wrap around the patient's head and overlap in front. Then cut an 8″ (20.3 cm) piece of tape and center it on the longer piece, sticky sides together. Next, cut a 5″ (12.7 cm) slit in each end of the longer tape (as shown below).

Apply benzoin tincture to the patient's cheeks, under his nose, and under his lower lip. (Don't spray benzoin directly on his face because the vapors can be irritating if inhaled and can also harm the eyes.)

Place the top half of one end of the tape under the patient's nose and wrap the lower half around the ETT. Place the lower half of the other end of the tape along his lower lip and wrap the top half around the tube (as shown below).

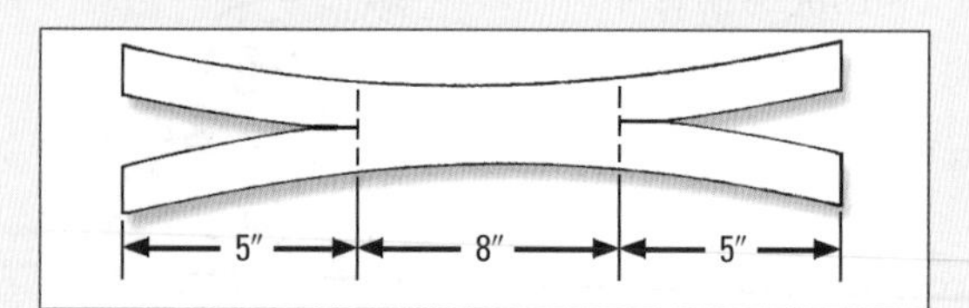

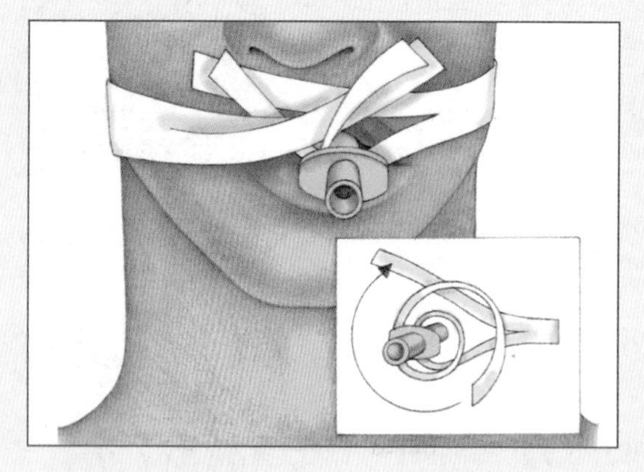

Method 2

Cut a tracheostomy lie in two pieces, one a few inches longer than the other, and cut two 6″ (15.2 cm) pieces of 1″ cloth adhesive tape. Then cut a 2″ (5 cm) slit in one end of both pieces of tape. Fold back the other end of the tape ½″ (1.3 cm) so that the sticky sides are together and cut a small hole in it (as shown below).

Apply benzoin tincture to the part of the ETT that will be taped. Wrap the split ends of each piece of tape around the tube, one piece on each side. Overlap the tape to secure it.

Apply the free ends of the tape to both sides of the patient's face. Then insert tracheostomy ties through the holes in the tape and knot the ties (as shown below).

Bring the longer tie behind the patient's neck. Knotting the ties on the side prevents the patient from lying on the knot and developing a pressure ulcer.

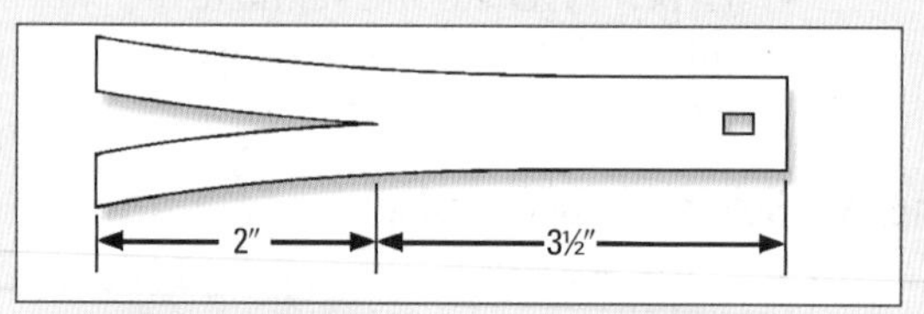

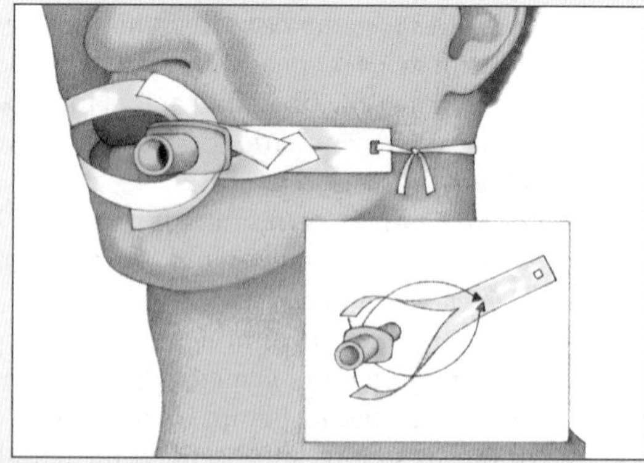

- Insert a bite block or OPA as indicated to prevent dislodgement of the tube.
- Secure the ETT in place according to facility standard. (See *Securing an ETT.*)

Monitoring

- Auscultate breath sounds every 2 to 4 hours.
- Monitor tube stability.
- Monitor and record the tube position at teeth or nose to *identify if tube is migrating.*
- Maximum tube cuff pressure should be 20 to 25 mm Hg. *This decreases the risk of aspiration and prevents overinflation of cuff to avoid tracheal damage.*
- Hyperoxygenate and suction as needed.

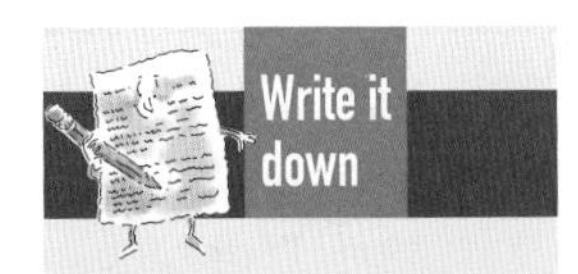

Documentation of ETT intubation

In your notes, document:

- patient and family education
- vital signs; SpO_2 before, during, and after procedure
- type of intubation (oral or nasal)
- use of any medications
- size of ETT
- depth of ETT insertion (centimeters at teeth or nose)
- measurement of cuff pressure
- assessment of breath sounds
- confirmation of tube placement and how confirmed including imaging
- secretions
- any unexpected outcomes
- patient response to the procedure
- any nursing interventions.

Practice pointers

- Always ensure the oxygen and suction equipment is fully functioning prior to the procedure. This should be part of your routine as you assess your patients at the beginning of the shift. Always be prepared. (See *Documentation of ETT intubation.*)

Should I stay or should I go

- The length of time the ETT stays in place is controversial; commonly, the ETT tube is replaced with a tracheostomy in 2 to 4 weeks if the artificial airway is still needed. It is more comfortable for the patient and allows the patient to talk.

ETT and oral care

ETT and oral care is performed to prevent buccal, oropharyngeal, and tracheal trauma from the tube; to provide oral hygiene; to promote ventilation; and to decrease the risk of associated ventilator pneumonia.

What you need

Gloves ✳ goggles ✳ mask ✳ bite block or oral airway if needed ✳ adhesive, twill tape, or commercial ETT tube holder ✳ normal saline solution ✳ soft adult/pediatric toothbrush or suction toothbrush ✳ toothettes/oral swab/suction swab ✳ oral cleansing solution or toothpaste ✳ stethoscope ✳ optional: closed-suction setup with a catheter, Yankauer, two sources of suction.

How you do it

- Identify the patient with two identifiers.
- Perform hand hygiene and don PPE.
- Ensure the ETT is connected to the ventilator using a swivel adapter.
- Suction the patient if clinically indicated; hyperoxygenate prior to suctioning.
- Loosen and remove old tape and ties.
- If patient is nasally intubated, clean around the ETT with saline-soaked gauze or swabs.
- If patient is orally intubated, remove bite block or oral airway.
- Suction oral cavity to remove secretions frequently.

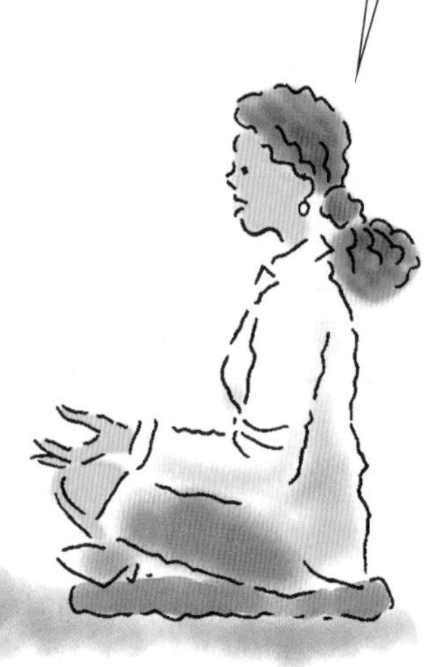
Periodic position changes for the ETT promote comfort and prevent pressure ulcers.

Move it, move it, move it

- Move oral tube to the other side of the mouth. Replace bite block or oral airway along the ETT if necessary to prevent biting. *It prevents or minimizes pressure areas on lips, tongue, and oral cavity.*
- Ensure proper cuff inflation using minimum leak volume or minimum occlusion volume.
- Reconfirm tube placement and note position of tube on teeth or nares.
- Secure the tube according to facility policy. (See *Documenting ETT care.*)

Practice pointers

- Suctioning of airways should be performed only for a clinical indication and not on a routine schedule.
- Report an inability to pass the suction catheter; changes in quantity or character of secretions; purulent drainage; mouth sores; and any breakdown of lip, tongue, or oral cavity.
- Only leave suction catheter in ETT for 10 seconds.

Tracheal cuff pressure measurement

An endotracheal (ET) or tracheostomy cuff provides a closed system for mechanical ventilation, allowing a desired tidal volume to be delivered to the patient's lungs. To function properly, the cuff must exert enough pressure on the tracheal wall to seal the airway without compromising the blood supply to the tracheal mucosa.

A nurse or a respiratory therapist can measure cuff pressure. The ideal pressure (known as minimal occlusive volume) is the lowest amount needed to seal the airway. Many authorities recommend maintaining a cuff pressure lower than venous perfusion pressure—usually 16 to 24 cm H_2O. Actual cuff pressure will vary with each patient, however. To keep pressure within safe limits, measure minimal occlusive volume at least once each shift or as directed by facility policy.

Documenting ETT care

In your notes, document:
- patient response to suctioning
- aspirate type, amount, and color
- presence of nasal drainage
- repositioning and re-taping of ETT
- oral care, moisturization, and oral suctioning
- condition of lips, tongue and mouth
- presence of cuff leak
- amount of air used to inflate cuff
- centimeter mark on ETT
- which nares tube is in.

What you need

10-mL syringe ✳ three-way stopcock ✳ cuff pressure manometer ✳ stethoscope ✳ suction equipment ✳ gloves.

Getting ready

Assemble all equipment at the patient's bedside. If measuring with a blood pressure manometer, attach the syringe to one stopcock port; then attach the tubing from the manometer to another port of the stopcock. Turn off the stopcock port where you'll be connecting the pilot balloon cuff *so that air can't escape from the cuff*. Use the syringe to instill air into the manometer tubing until the pressure reaches 10 mm Hg. *This will prevent sudden cuff deflation when you open the stopcock to the cuff and the manometer.*

How you do it

Explain the procedure to the patient. Put on gloves and suction the ET or tracheostomy tube and the patient's oropharynx *to remove accumulated secretions above the cuff*. Then attach the cuff pressure manometer to the pilot balloon port.

Smooth + hollow = sealed

- Place the diaphragm of the stethoscope over the trachea and listen for an air leak.
- If you don't hear an air leak, press the red button under the dial of the cuff pressure manometer to slowly release air from the balloon on the tracheal tube (as shown in the following figure). Auscultate for an air leak.
- As soon as you hear an air leak, release the red button and gently squeeze the handle of the cuff pressure manometer to inflate the cuff. Continue to add air to the cuff until you no longer hear an air leak.
- When the air leak ceases, read the dial on the cuff pressure manometer. This is the minimal pressure required to effectively occlude the trachea around the tracheal tube. In many cases, this

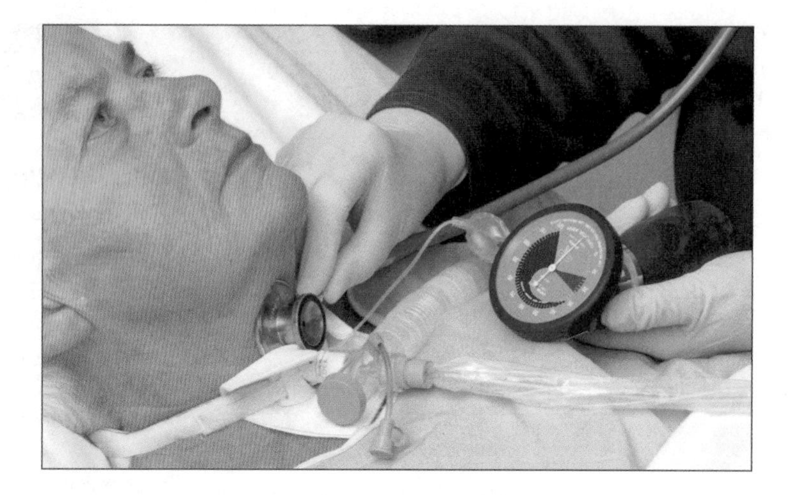

pressure will fall within the green area (16 to 24 cm H_2O) on the manometer dial.

- Disconnect the cuff pressure manometer from the pilot balloon port.

Ideally, cuff pressure should be kept at the lowest amount needed to seal the patient's airway.

Practice pointers

- Measure cuff pressure at least every 8 hours *to avoid overinflation.*
- When measuring cuff pressure, note the volume of air needed to inflate the cuff. A gradual increase in this volume indicates tracheal dilation or erosion. A sudden increase in volume indicates cuff rupture and requires immediate reintubation if the patient is being ventilated. (See *Documenting tracheal cuff pressure measurement.*)

Tracheostomy care

Whether a tracheotomy is performed in an emergency situation or after careful preparation, as a permanent measure or as temporary therapy, tracheostomy care has identical goals: to ensure airway patency by keeping the tube free from mucus buildup, to maintain mucous membrane and skin integrity, to prevent infection, and to provide psychological support.

Simple, medium, and complex

The patient may have one of three types of tracheostomy tube:

1. An uncuffed tube, which may be plastic or metal, allows air to flow freely around the tracheostomy tube and

through the larynx, reducing the risk of tracheal damage. Used primarily for long-term airway management.

2. A cuffed tube, made of plastic, is disposable. The cuff and the tube won't separate accidentally inside the trachea because the cuff is bonded to the tube. Also, it doesn't require periodic deflating to lower pressure because cuff pressure is low and evenly distributed against the tracheal wall. Although cuffed tubes may cost more than other tubes, they reduce the risk of tracheal damage. The cuffed tube is frequently used in critically ill patients who need mechanical ventilation and to prevent aspiration.
3. A plastic fenestrated tube permits speech through the upper airway when the external opening is capped and the cuff is deflated. It also allows easy removal of the inner cannula for cleaning. However, a fenestrated tube may become occluded.

Whichever tube is used, tracheostomy care should be performed using aseptic technique until the stoma has healed to prevent infection. For recently performed tracheotomies, use sterile gloves for all manipulations at the tracheostomy site. When the stoma has healed, clean gloves may be substituted for sterile ones.

Documenting tracheal cuff pressure measurement

After cuff pressure measurement, record:
- date and time of the procedure
- cuff pressure
- total volume of air in the cuff after the procedure
- complications and nursing actions taken
- patient's tolerance of the procedure.

What you need

For aseptic stoma and outer cannula care

Waterproof trash bag * two sterile solution containers * normal saline solution * hydrogen peroxide * sterile cotton-tipped applicators * sterile 4″ × 4″ gauze pads * sterile gloves * prepackaged sterile tracheostomy dressing (or 4″ × 4″ gauze pad) * equipment and supplies for suctioning and mouth care * materials as needed for cuff procedures and for changing tracheostomy ties (see the following text) * mask, goggles, or face shield.

For aseptic inner cannula care

All of the preceding equipment plus a prepackaged commercial tracheostomy care set or sterile forceps * sterile nylon brush * sterile 6″ (15.2 cm) pipe cleaners * clean gloves * a third sterile solution container * disposable temporary inner cannula (for a patient on a ventilator) * mask, goggles, or face shield.

For changing tracheostomy ties

30″ (76.2 cm) length of tracheostomy twill tape * bandage scissors * sterile gloves * hemostat * mask, goggles, or face shield.

For emergency tracheostomy tube replacement

Sterile tracheal dilator or sterile hemostat ✳ sterile obturator that fits the tracheostomy tube in use ✳ extra sterile tracheostomy tube and obturator in appropriate size ✳ suction equipment and supplies ✳ mask, goggles, or face shield.

Keep these supplies in full view in the patient's room at all times for easy access in case of an emergency. Consider taping an emergency sterile tracheostomy tube in a sterile wrapper to the head of the bed for easy access.

For cuff procedures

5- or 10-mL syringe ✳ padded hemostat ✳ stethoscope.

Getting ready

Perform hand hygiene, and assemble all equipment and supplies in the patient's room. Open the waterproof trash bag and place it next to you *so that you can avoid reaching across the sterile field or the patient's stoma when discarding soiled items.*

Establish a sterile field near the patient's bed (usually on the overbed table) and place equipment and supplies on it. Pour normal saline solution, hydrogen peroxide, or a mixture of equal parts of both solutions into one of the sterile solution containers; then pour normal saline solution into the second sterile container for rinsing. For inner-cannula care, you may use a third sterile solution container to hold the gauze pads and cotton-tipped applicators saturated with cleaning solution. If you'll be replacing the disposable inner cannula, open the package containing the new inner cannula while maintaining sterile technique. Obtain or prepare new tracheostomy if indicated.

Unless you create a sterile field for supplies, I'll invade your patient's space.

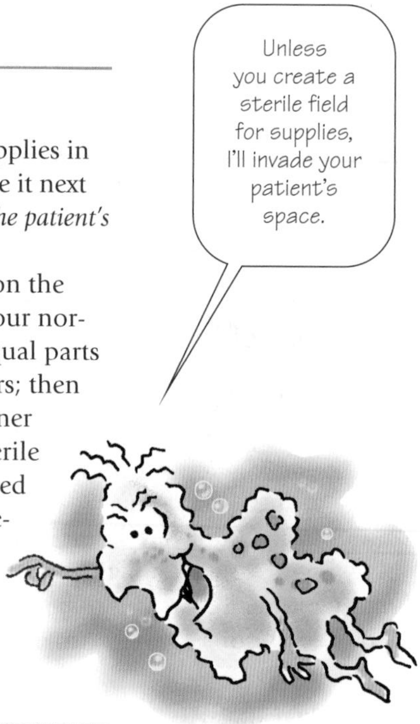

How you do it

- Identify the patient using two patient identifiers.
- Assess the patient's condition *to determine his need for care.*
- Explain the procedure to the patient even if he's unresponsive. Provide privacy.
- Place the patient in semi-Fowler's position (unless it's contraindicated) *to decrease abdominal pressure on the diaphragm and promote lung expansion.*
- Remove humidification or ventilation devices.
- Don PPE and sterile gloves.

- Using sterile technique, suction the entire length of the tracheostomy tube *to clear the airway of any secretions that may hinder oxygenation.*
- Reconnect the patient to the humidifier or ventilator, if necessary.

Cleaning a stoma and outer cannula

- With your dominant hand, saturate a cotton-tipped applicator or sterile gauze pad with the cleaning solution. Squeeze out the excess liquid *to prevent accidental aspiration.* Then wipe the patient's neck under the tracheostomy tube flanges and twill tapes.
- Use more pads or cotton-tipped applicators to clean the stoma site and the tube's flanges. Wipe only once with each pad or applicator and then discard it *to prevent contamination of a clean area with a soiled pad.*
- Rinse debris and peroxide (if used) with one or more sterile 4″ × 4″ gauze pads dampened in normal saline solution. Dry the area thoroughly with additional sterile gauze pads, then apply a new sterile tracheostomy dressing.
- Remove and discard your gloves.

Cleaning a nondisposable inner cannula

- Put on sterile gloves and follow standard precautions.
- Using your nondominant hand, remove and discard the patient's tracheostomy dressing. Then, with the same hand, disconnect the ventilator or humidification device and unlock the tracheostomy tube's inner cannula by rotating it counterclockwise. Place the inner cannula in the container of hydrogen peroxide.
- Working quickly, use your dominant hand to scrub the cannula with the sterile nylon brush. If the brush doesn't slide easily into the cannula, use a sterile pipe cleaner.
- Immerse the cannula in the container of normal saline solution and agitate it for about 10 seconds *to rinse it thoroughly.*
- Inspect the cannula for cleanliness. Repeat the cleaning process if necessary. If it's clean, tap it gently against the inside edge of the sterile container *to remove excess liquid and prevent aspiration.* Don't dry the outer surface *because a thin film of moisture acts as a lubricant during insertion.*
- Reinsert the inner cannula into the patient's tracheostomy tube. Lock it in place and then gently pull on it *to make sure it's positioned securely.* Reconnect the mechanical ventilator. Apply a new sterile tracheostomy dressing.
- If the patient can't tolerate being disconnected from the ventilator for the time it takes to clean the inner cannula, replace the existing inner cannula with a clean one and reattach the

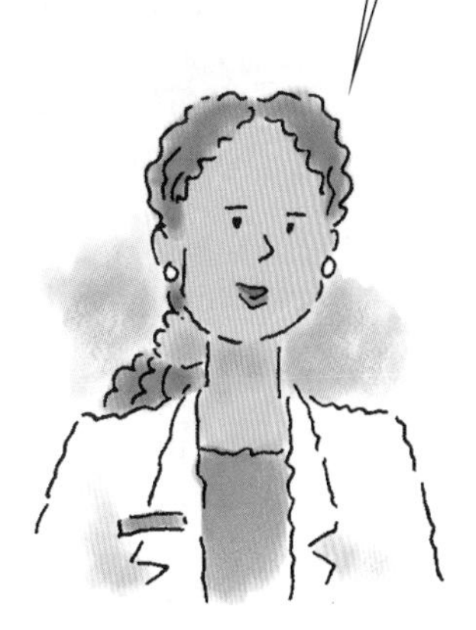
If the patient can't breathe while you clean the cannula, change it for a new one and then clean it.

mechanical ventilator. Then clean the cannula just removed from the patient and store it in a sterile container for the next time.

Caring for a disposable inner cannula

- Put on clean gloves and follow standard precautions.
- Using your dominant hand, remove the patient's inner cannula. After evaluating the secretions in the cannula, discard it properly.
- Pick up the new inner cannula, touching only the outer locking portion. Insert the cannula into the tracheostomy and, following the manufacturer's instructions, lock it securely.

Changing tracheostomy ties

- Obtain assistance from another nurse or a respiratory therapist *because of the risk of accidental tube expulsion during this procedure.* Patient movement or coughing can dislodge the tube.
- Wash your hands thoroughly and put on sterile gloves if you aren't already wearing them.
- If you aren't using commercially packaged tracheostomy ties, prepare new ties from a 30" (76.2 cm) length of twill tape by folding one end back 1" (2.5 cm) on itself. Then, with the bandage scissors, cut a ½" (1.3 cm) slit down the center of the tape from the folded edge.
- Prepare the other end of the tape the same way.

Cut to order

- Hold both ends together and using scissors, cut the resulting circle of tape so that one piece is approximately 10" (25 cm) long and the other is about 20" (50 cm) long.
- Help the patient into semi-Fowler's position if possible.
- After your assistant puts on gloves, instruct her to hold the tracheostomy tube in place *to prevent its expulsion during replacement of the ties.* If you must perform the procedure without assistance, fasten the clean ties in place before removing the old ties *to prevent tube expulsion.*
- With the assistant's gloved fingers holding the tracheostomy tube in place, cut the soiled tracheostomy ties with the bandage scissors or untie them and discard the ties. Be careful not to cut the tube of the pilot balloon.
- Thread the slit end of one new tie a short distance through the eye of one tracheostomy tube flange from the underside; use the hemostat, if needed, to pull the tie through. Then thread the other end of the tie completely through the slit end and pull it taut so it loops firmly through the flange. *This avoids knots that can cause throat discomfort, tissue irritation, pressure, and necrosis at the patient's throat.*
- Fasten the second tie to the opposite flange in the same manner.

Just like the boy (or girl) scouts

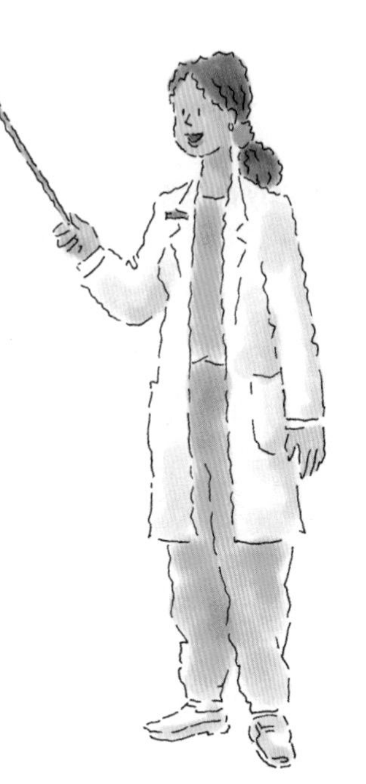

- Instruct the patient to flex his neck while you bring the ties around to the side and tie them together with a square knot. *Flexion produces the same neck circumference as coughing and helps prevent an overly tight tie.* Instruct your assistant to place one finger under the tapes as you tie them *to ensure that they're tight enough to avoid slippage but loose enough to prevent choking or jugular vein constriction.*
- After securing the ties, cut off the excess tape with the scissors and instruct your assistant to release the tracheostomy tube.
- Make sure the patient is comfortable and can reach the call button easily.
- Check tracheostomy-tie tension often on patients with traumatic injury, radical neck dissection, or cardiac failure *because neck diameter can increase from swelling and cause constriction;* also, check neonatal or restless patients frequently *because ties can loosen and cause tube dislodgement.*

Nearing the finishing line

- Replace the humidification device.
- Provide oral care as needed *because the oral cavity can become dry and malodorous or develop sores from encrusted secretions.*
- Observe soiled dressings and suctioned secretions for amount, color, consistency, and odor.
- Properly clean or dispose of all equipment, supplies, solutions, and trash according to policy.
- Take off and discard your gloves.
- Make sure that the patient is comfortable.
- Make sure all necessary supplies are readily available at the bedside.
- Repeat the procedure at least once every 8 hours or as needed. Change the dressing as often as necessary regardless of whether you also perform the entire cleaning procedure *because a wet dressing with exudate or secretions predisposes the patient to skin excoriation, breakdown, and infection.*

Deflating and inflating a tracheostomy cuff

- Read the cuff manufacturer's instructions *because cuff types and procedures vary widely.*
- Assess the patient's condition, explain the procedure to him, and reassure him. Wash your hands thoroughly.

Sit up . . .

Help the patient into semi-Fowler's position, if possible, or place him in a supine position so secretions above the cuff site will be pushed up into his mouth if he's receiving positive-pressure ventilation.

. . . and suction

- Suction the oropharyngeal cavity *to prevent pooled secretions from descending into the trachea after cuff deflation.*
- Release the padded hemostat, clamping the cuff inflation tubing if a hemostat is present.

Slowly deflate . . .

- Insert a 5- or 10-mL syringe into the cuff pilot balloon and very slowly withdraw all air from the cuff. Leave the syringe attached to the tubing for later reinflation of the cuff. *Slow deflation allows positive lung pressure to push secretions upward from the bronchi. Cuff deflation may also stimulate the patient's cough reflex, producing additional secretions.*
- Remove any ventilation device. Suction the lower airway through any existing tube *to remove all secretions*. Then reconnect the patient to the ventilation device.
- Maintain cuff deflation for the prescribed time. Observe the patient for adequate ventilation and suction as necessary. If the patient has difficulty breathing, reinflate the cuff immediately by depressing the syringe plunger very slowly. Inject the least amount of air necessary to achieve an adequate tracheal seal.

. . . then pump back up

- When inflating the cuff, you may use the minimal-leak technique or the minimal occlusive volume technique *to help gauge the proper inflation point.* (For more information, see "Assisting with endotracheal tube intubation," page 323, and "ETT and oral care," page 327.)
- If you're inflating the cuff using cuff pressure measurement, be careful not to exceed 25 mm Hg. Note the exact amount of air needed to inflate the cuff. If pressure exceeds 25 mm Hg, notify the doctor *because you may need to change to a larger size tube, use higher inflation pressures, or permit a larger air leak.* Recommended cuff pressure is about 18 mm Hg.
- After you have inflated the cuff, if the tubing doesn't have a one-way valve at the end, clamp the inflation line with a padded hemostat (to protect the tubing) and remove the syringe.

Did you hear that?

- Check for a minimal-leak cuff seal. You shouldn't feel air coming from the patient's mouth, nose, or tracheostomy site, and a conscious patient shouldn't be able to speak.
- Be alert for air leaks from the cuff itself. Suspect a leak if injection of air fails to inflate the cuff or increase cuff pressure,

if you're unable to inject the amount of air you withdrew, if the patient can speak, if ventilation fails to maintain adequate respiratory movement with pressures or volumes previously considered adequate, or if air escapes during the ventilator's inspiratory cycle.
- Make sure the patient is comfortable.
- Properly clean or dispose of all equipment, supplies, and trash according to facility policy.
- Replenish any used supplies and make sure all necessary emergency supplies are at the bedside.

Practice pointers

- Make sure the patient can easily reach the call button and communication aids.
- Keep appropriate equipment at the patient's bedside for immediate use in an emergency.
- Follow facility policy regarding procedure if a tracheostomy tube is expelled or if the outer cannula becomes blocked. Use extreme caution when attempting to reinsert an expelled tracheostomy tube *because of the risk of tracheal trauma, perforation, compression, and asphyxiation.*

What not to do

Refrain from changing tracheostomy ties unnecessarily during the immediate postoperative period before the stoma track is well formed (usually 4 days) *to avoid accidental dislodgment and expulsion of the tube.* Unless secretions or drainage is a problem, ties can be changed once per day.

Class time

- If the patient is being discharged with a tracheostomy, start self-care teaching as soon as he's receptive. Teach the patient and family how to change and clean the tube using simulation. Include a return demonstration to check for understanding.
- Assess for the following complications, which can occur within the first 48 hours after tracheostomy tube insertion: hemorrhage at the operative site, causing drowning; bleeding or edema in tracheal tissue, causing airway obstruction; aspiration of secretions; introduction of air into the pleural cavity, causing pneumothorax; hypoxia or acidosis, triggering cardiac arrest; and introduction of air into surrounding tissues, causing subcutaneous emphysema. (See *Documenting tracheostomy care.*)

Documenting tracheostomy care

In your notes, record:
- date and time of the procedure
- type of procedure
- amount, consistency, color, and odor of secretions
- stoma and skin condition
- patient's respiratory status
- tracheostomy tube changes made by the doctor
- duration of cuff deflation
- amount of cuff inflation
- cuff pressure readings, with patient's body position during reading
- complications and nursing actions taken
- patient's tolerance of the procedure
- patient or family teaching and their comprehension and progress.

Oxygen administration

A patient needs oxygen therapy when hypoxemia (lack of oxygen) results from a respiratory or cardiac emergency or an increase in metabolic function.

ABG analysis (for pediatric patients, capillary blood gases), oximetry monitoring, and clinical examinations are used to determine if the patient is receiving enough oxygen.

There are several ways to administer oxygen. The patient's disease, physical condition, and age will help determine the most appropriate method.

What you need

The equipment needed depends on the type of delivery system ordered. (See *Oxygen delivery systems*.) Equipment includes selections from the following list: oxygen source (wall unit, cylinder, liquid tank, or concentrator) ✳ flowmeter ✳ adapter, if using a wall unit, or a pressure-reduction gauge, if using a cylinder ✳ sterile humidity bottle and adapters ✳ sterile distilled water ✳ OXYGEN PRECAUTION sign ✳ appropriate oxygen delivery system (a nasal cannula, simple mask, partial rebreather mask, or nonrebreather mask for low-flow and variable oxygen concentrations; a Venturi mask, aerosol mask, T tube, tracheostomy collar, tent, or oxygen hood for high-flow and specific oxygen concentrations) ✳ small-diameter and large-diameter connection tubing ✳ flashlight (for nasal cannula) ✳ water-soluble lubricant ✳ gauze pads and tape (for oxygen masks) ✳ jet adapter for Venturi mask (if adding humidity) ✳ optional: oxygen analyzer.

Getting ready

Although a respiratory therapist typically is responsible for setting up, maintaining, and managing the equipment, you'll need a working knowledge of the oxygen system being used.

Check the oxygen outlet port *to verify flow*. Pinch the tubing near the prongs *to ensure that an audible alarm will sound if the oxygen flow stops*.

How you do it

- Assess the patient's condition. In an emergency situation, verify that he has an open airway before administering oxygen.
- Explain the procedure to the patient and let him know why he needs oxygen *to ensure his cooperation*.

Oxygen delivery systems

Patients may receive oxygen through one of several administration systems.

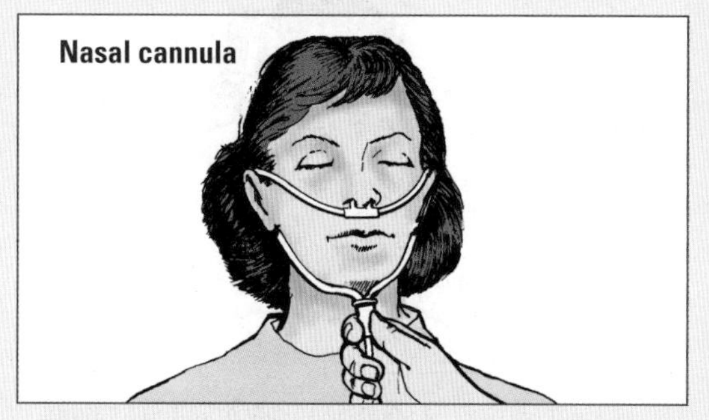

Oxygen is delivered in concentrations of less than 40% through a plastic cannula in the patient's nostrils.

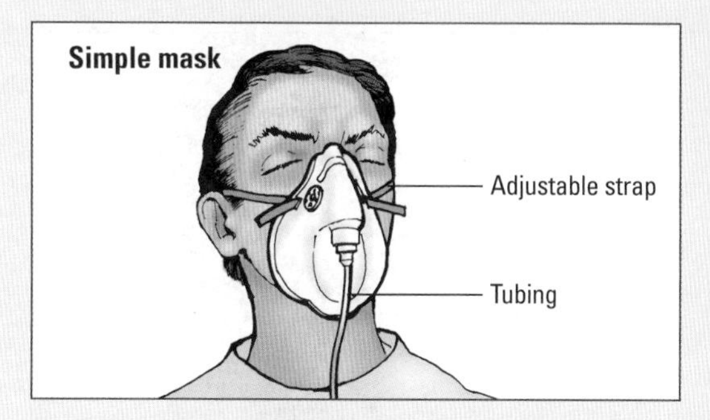

Oxygen flows through an entry port at the bottom of the mask and exits through large holes on the sides of the mask. It delivers oxygen in concentrations of 40% to 60%.

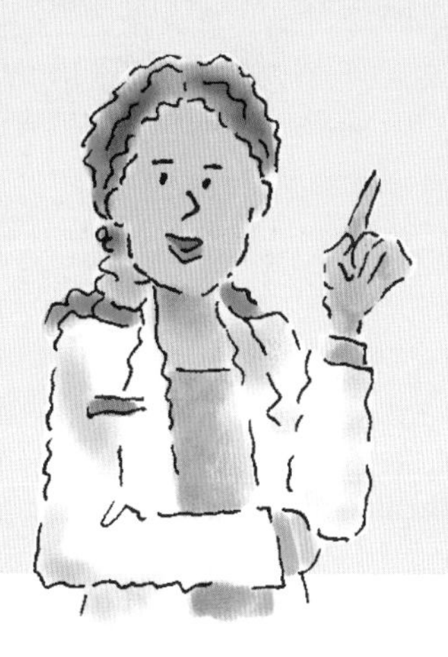

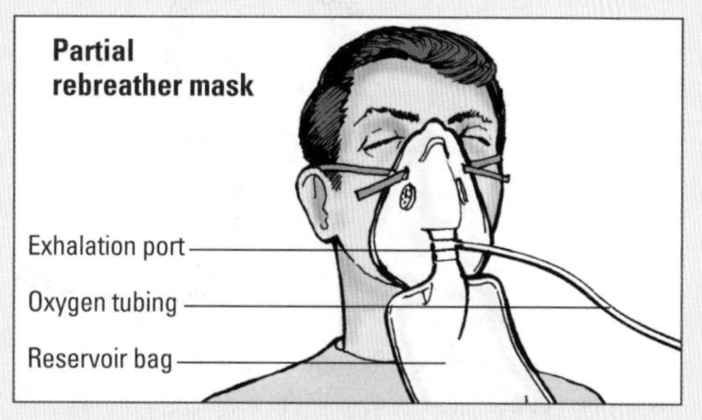

The patient inspires oxygen from a reservoir bag along with atmospheric air and oxygen from the mask. The first third of exhaled tidal volume enters the bag; the rest exits the mask. Because air entering the reservoir bag comes from the trachea and bronchi, where no gas exchange occurs, the patient rebreathes the oxygenated air he just exhaled. Oxygen can be administered in concentrations of 40% to 60%.

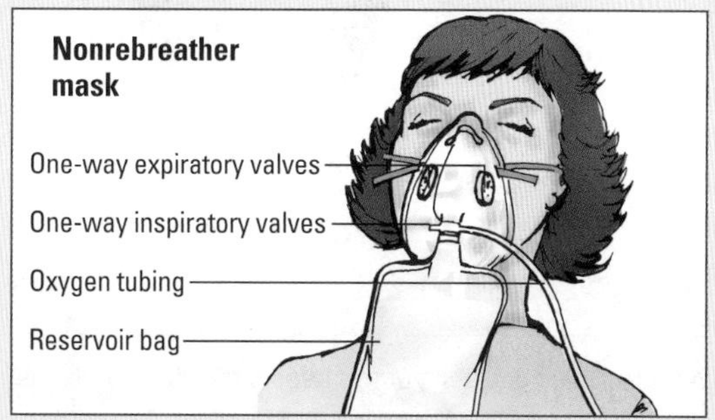

On inhalation, the one-way inspiratory valve opens, directing oxygen from a reservoir bag into the mask. On exhalation, gas exits the mask through the one-way expiratory valves and enters the atmosphere. The patient breathes air only from the bag. It delivers the highest possible oxygen concentration (60% to 90%) short of intubation and mechanical ventilation.

Oxygen delivery systems *(continued)*

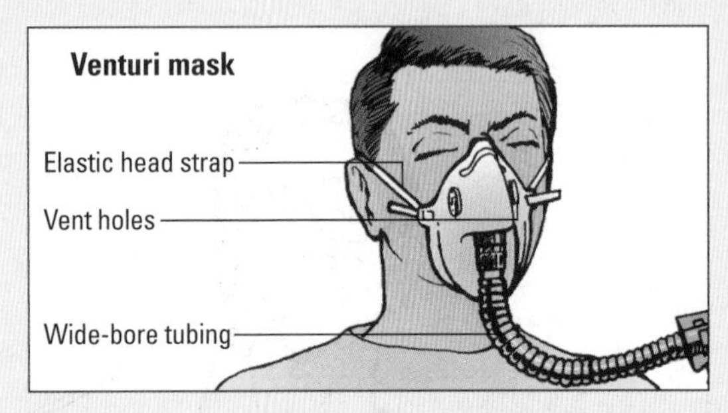

The mask is connected to a Venturi device, which mixes a specific volume of air and oxygen. It delivers highly accurate oxygen concentration despite the patient's respiratory pattern. This is commonly used in hypoxic chronic obstructive pulmonary disease (COPD) patients where excessive oxygen can decrease the respiratory drive of the patient.

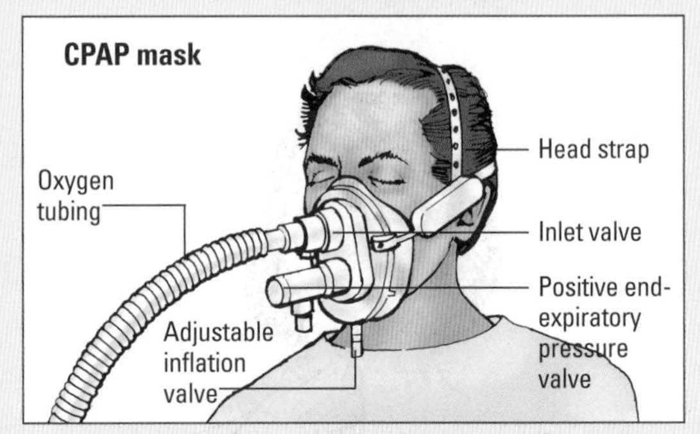

This system allows the spontaneously breathing patient to receive continuous positive airway pressure (CPAP) with or without an artificial airway.

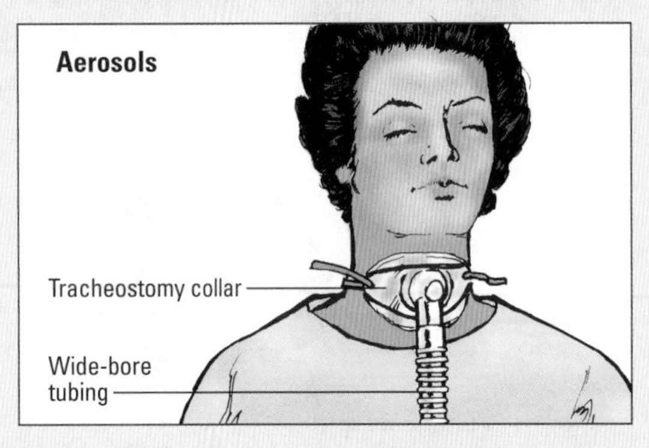

A face mask, hood, tent, or tracheostomy tube or collar is connected to wide-bore tubing that receives aerosolized oxygen from a jet nebulizer. It delivers high-humidity oxygen.

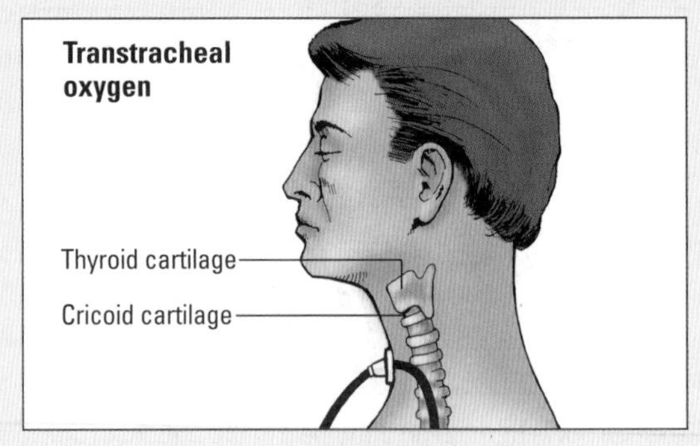

The patient receives oxygen through a catheter inserted into the base of his neck in a simple outpatient procedure.

Safety first

- Check the patient's room *to make sure it's safe for oxygen administration*. Whenever possible, replace electrical devices with nonelectric ones and post a NO SMOKING sign in the patient's room. (See *Caution: Oxygen in use.*)

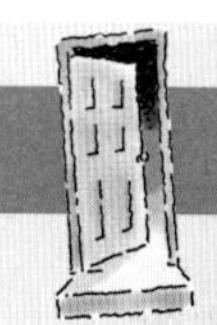

Home care connection

Home oxygen therapy

If your patient will receive oxygen therapy after discharge, make sure he's familiar with the types of oxygen therapy, the services available, and the service schedules offered by local home suppliers. Together with the doctor and patient, help choose the device that's best suited to the patient.

If the patient will be receiving transtracheal oxygen therapy, teach him how to clean and care for the catheter. Advise him to keep the skin around the insertion site clean and dry to prevent infection.

Safety and supplies

No matter which device the patient uses, you'll need to evaluate his and his caregivers' ability and motivation to administer oxygen therapy at home. Make sure they understand the reason the patient is receiving oxygen and the safety issues involved. Teach them how to properly use and clean the equipment and supplies.

Paperwork points

If the patient will be discharged with oxygen for the first time, make sure his health insurance covers home oxygen. If it doesn't, find out what criteria he must meet to obtain coverage. Without a third-party payer, he may not be able to afford home oxygen therapy.

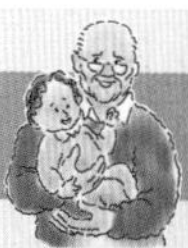

Ages and stages

Caution: Oxygen in use

If a child is receiving oxygen through an oxygen mist tent, remove all toys that may produce a spark, including those that are battery-powered. Oxygen supports combustion, and the smallest spark can cause a fire.

- Place an OXYGEN PRECAUTION sign over the patient's bed and on the door to his room.
- Help place the oxygen delivery device on the patient. Make sure it fits properly and is stable.

Measure your success

- Monitor the patient's response to oxygen therapy. Check his ABG values during initial adjustments of oxygen flow. When the patient is stabilized, you may use pulse oximetry instead. Check the patient frequently for signs of hypoxia, such as a decreased level of consciousness; increased heart rate; arrhythmias; restlessness; perspiration; dyspnea; use of accessory muscles; yawning or flared nostril; cyanosis; and cool, clammy skin.
- Observe the patient's skin integrity *to prevent skin breakdown on pressure points from the oxygen delivery device.* Wipe moisture or perspiration from the patient's face and from the mask as needed.
- If the patient will be receiving oxygen at a concentration above 60% for more than 24 hours, watch carefully for signs of oxygen toxicity.

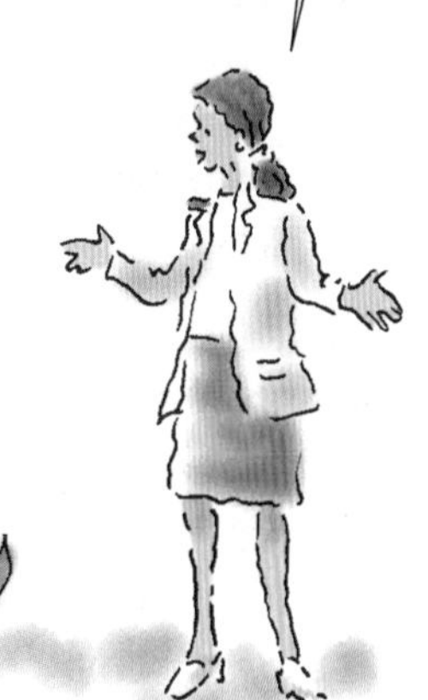
Hey! Oxygen is highly flammable. Use nonelectric devices and make sure no one smokes.

Practice pointers

- Use caution when administering oxygen by nasal cannula at more than 2 L/minute to a patient with chronic lung disease. *Some patients with chronic lung disease become dependent on a state of hypercapnia and hypoxia to stimulate their respirations and supplemental oxygen could cause them to stop breathing.*
- When monitoring a patient's response to a change in oxygen flow, check the pulse oximetry monitor or measure ABG values 20 to 30 minutes after adjusting the flow. In the interim, monitor the patient closely for an adverse response to the change in oxygen flow.
- Teaching and planning for home oxygen therapy should begin as soon as possible. (See *Home oxygen therapy*, page 341, and *Documenting oxygen administration*.)

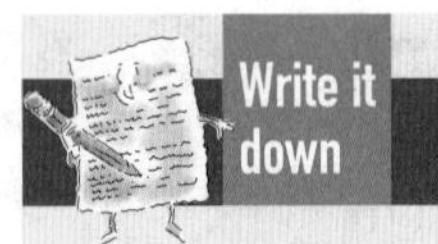

Documenting oxygen administration

In your notes, record:
- date and time of oxygen administration
- type of delivery device used
- oxygen flow rate
- patient's vital signs, skin color, respiratory effort, and breath sounds
- patient's response to oxygen therapy
- patient or family teaching provided.

Manual ventilation

A handheld resuscitation bag is an inflatable device that can be attached to a face mask or directly to an ETT or tracheostomy tube. It allows manual delivery of oxygen or room air to the lungs of a patient who can't breathe by himself.

Hey! We've been disconnected

Usually used in an emergency, manual ventilation can also be performed while the patient is disconnected temporarily from a mechanical ventilator, such as during a tubing change, during transport, or before suctioning. In such instances, use of the handheld resuscitation bag maintains ventilation. Oxygen administration with a resuscitation bag can help improve a compromised cardiorespiratory system.

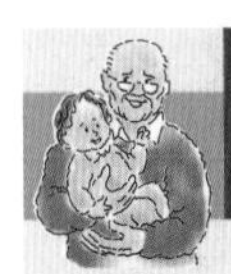

Pediatric manual ventilation

Make sure you have the proper bag and mask size. For a child, deliver 15 breaths/minute or one compression of the bag every 4 seconds; for an infant, 20 breaths/minute or one compression every 3 seconds. Infants and children should receive 250 to 500 cc of air with each bag compression.

What you need

Handheld resuscitation bag * mask * oxygen source (wall unit or tank) * oxygen tubing * nipple adapter attached to oxygen flowmeter * suction equipment * optional: oxygen accumulator, positive end-expiratory pressure (PEEP) valve.

Getting ready

Unless the patient is intubated or has a tracheostomy, select a mask that fits snugly over the mouth and nose. (See *Pediatric manual ventilation*.) Attach the mask to the resuscitation bag.

If oxygen is readily available, connect the handheld resuscitation bag to the oxygen. Attach one end of the tubing to the bottom of the bag and the other end to the nipple adapter on the flowmeter of the oxygen source.

Turn on the oxygen and adjust the flow rate according to the patient's condition. If time allows, set up suction equipment.

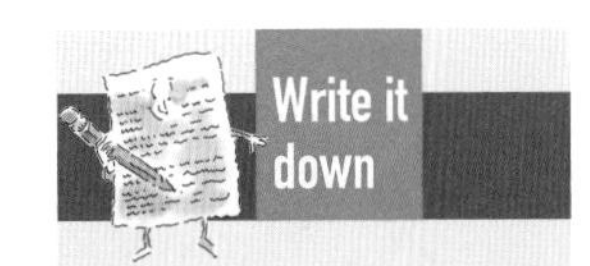

Documenting manual ventilation

In your notes, record:

- date and time of manual ventilation efforts
- reason for the procedure
- length of time the patient received manual ventilation
- patient's response
- complications and nursing actions taken.

How you do it

- Before using the handheld resuscitation bag, check the patient's upper airway for foreign objects. If present, remove them. Suction the patient *to remove any secretions that may obstruct the airway.* If necessary, insert an oropharyngeal or nasopharyngeal airway *to maintain airway patency.* If the patient has a tracheostomy or ETT in place, suction the tube.
- If appropriate, remove the bed's headboard and stand at the head of the bed *to help keep the patient's neck extended and to free space at the side of the bed for other activities such as cardiopulmonary resuscitation.*

Head back, jaw forward

- Tilt the patient's head backward, if not contraindicated, and pull his jaw forward *to move the tongue away from the base of the pharynx and prevent airway obstruction.* (See *How to apply a handheld resuscitation bag and mask.*)

How to apply a handheld resuscitation bag and mask

Place the mask over the patient's face so that the apex of the triangle covers the bridge of his nose and the base lies between his lower lip and chin (as shown below left). Hold the mask on, taking care to avoid soft tissue by keeping your fingers on the bony part of the jaw.

Make sure the patient's mouth remains open beneath the mask. Attach the bag to the mask and to the tubing leading to the oxygen source.

Alternatively, if the patient has a tracheostomy tube or an ETT in place, remove the mask from the bag and attach the handheld resuscitation bag directly to the tube (as shown below right).

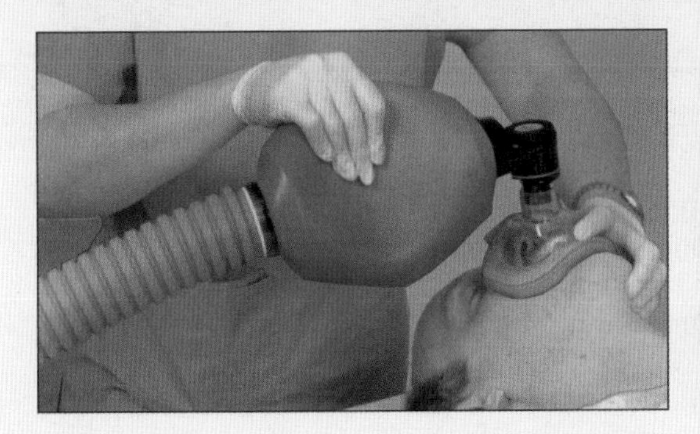

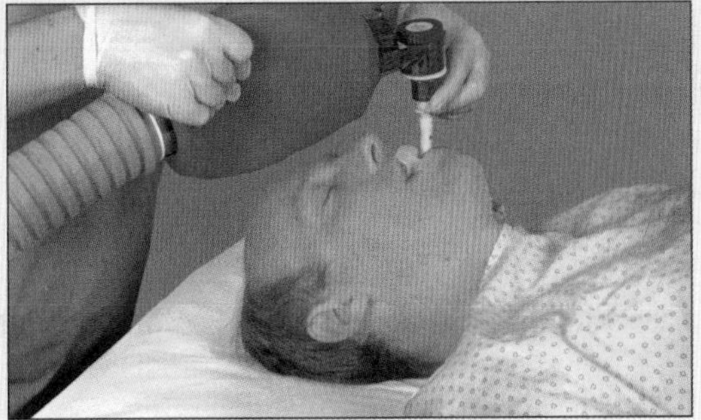

- Keeping your nondominant hand on the patient's mask, exert downward pressure *to seal the mask against his face*. For an adult patient, use your dominant hand to compress the bag every 5 seconds to deliver approximately 1,000 cc of air.
- Deliver breaths with the patient's own inspiratory effort, if present. Don't attempt to deliver a breath as the patient exhales.

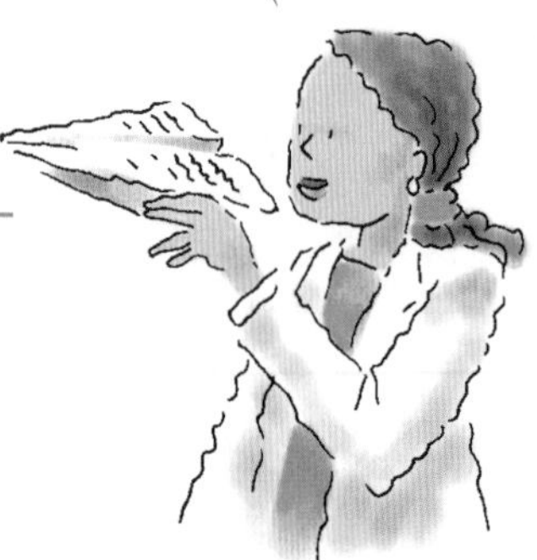
Read this note. It says to squeeze the ventilation bag every 5 seconds.

Rise and fall

Observe the patient's chest *to ensure that it rises and falls with each compression*. If ventilation fails to occur, check the fit of the mask and the patency of the patient's airway; if necessary, reposition his head and ensure patency with an oral airway.

Practice pointers

- Avoid neck hyperextension if the patient has a possible cervical injury; instead, use the jaw-thrust technique to open the airway. If you need both hands to keep the patient's mask in place and maintain hyperextension, use the lower part of your arm to compress the bag against your side.
- Observe for vomiting through the clear part of the mask. If vomiting occurs, stop the procedure immediately, lift the mask, wipe and suction the vomitus, and resume resuscitation. Aspiration of vomitus can result in pneumonia. (See *Documenting manual ventilation*, page 343.)

Mechanical ventilation

A mechanical ventilator moves air in and out of a patient's lungs. Although the equipment serves to ventilate a patient, it doesn't ensure adequate gas exchange. Mechanical ventilators may use either positive or negative pressure to ventilate patients.

What you need

Oxygen source ✳ air source that can supply 50 psi ✳ mechanical ventilator ✳ humidifier ✳ ventilator circuit tubing, connectors, and adapters ✳ condensation collection trap ✳ spirometer, respirometer, or electronic device to measure flow and volume ✳ in-line thermometer ✳ probe for gas sampling and measuring airway pressure ✳ gloves ✳ handheld resuscitation bag with reservoir ✳ suction equipment ✳ sterile distilled water ✳ equipment for ABG analysis ✳ soft restraints, if indicated ✳ optional: oximeter, ordered sedative, ordered neuromuscular blocking agent.

Getting ready

In most facilities, respiratory therapists assume responsibility for setting up the ventilator. If necessary, check the manufacturer's instructions for setting it up.

How you do it

- Verify the doctor's order for ventilator support. If the patient isn't already intubated, prepare him for intubation. (See "Assisting with endotracheal tube intubation," page 323.)
- Identify the patient using two patient identifiers.
- When possible, explain the procedure to the patient and his family *to help reduce anxiety and fear.*
- Perform a complete physical assessment and draw blood for ABG analysis *to establish a baseline.*

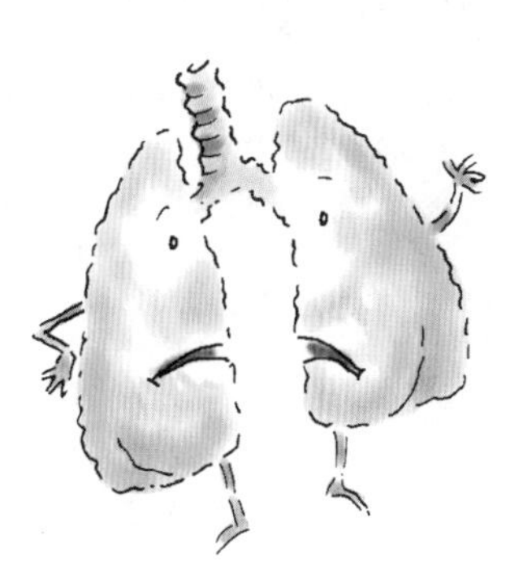

Adjust as necessary

- Plug the ventilator into the electrical outlet and turn it on. Adjust the settings on the ventilator as ordered.
- Make sure that the ventilator's alarms are set as ordered and that the humidifier is filled with sterile distilled water.
- Ensure that suction equipment is readily available and functioning properly.

Is it working?

- Put on gloves if you haven't already. Connect the ETT to the ventilator. Observe for chest expansion and auscultate for bilateral breath sounds *to verify that the patient is being ventilated.*
- Monitor the patient's ABG values after the initial ventilator setup (usually 20 to 30 minutes), after changes in ventilator settings, and as the patient's clinical condition indicates *to determine whether the patient is being adequately ventilated and to avoid oxygen toxicity.* Be prepared to adjust ventilator settings based on ABG analysis.
- Monitor pulse oximetry values.

Water, temperature, breathing

- Check the ventilator tubing frequently for condensation, *which can cause resistance to airflow and may also be aspirated by the patient.* As needed, drain the condensate into a collection trap or briefly disconnect the patient from the ventilator (ventilating him with a handheld resuscitation bag if necessary) and empty the water into a receptacle. Don't drain the condensate into the humidifier *because the condensate may be contaminated with the patient's secretions.*

- Check the in-line thermometer to make sure that the temperature of the air delivered to the patient is close to body temperature.
- When monitoring the patient's vital signs, count spontaneous breaths as well as ventilator-delivered breaths.

Time for a change

- Change, clean, or dispose of the ventilator tubing and equipment according to your facility's policy *to reduce the risk of bacterial contamination*. Typically, ventilator tubing should be changed every 48 to 72 hours and sometimes more often.
- When ordered, begin to wean the patient from the ventilator. (See *Weaning a patient from the ventilator*.)

Practice pointers

- Provide emotional support to the patient during all phases of mechanical ventilation *to reduce his anxiety and promote successful treatment*. Even if the patient is unresponsive, continue to explain all procedures and treatments to him.
- Be aware that some patients may require soft restraints *to prevent extubation*.
- Make sure that the ventilator alarms are on at all times. *These alarms alert the nursing staff to potentially hazardous conditions and changes in patient status.* If an alarm sounds and the problem can't be identified easily, disconnect the patient from the ventilator and use a handheld resuscitation bag to ventilate him. (See *Responding to ventilator alarms*.)

Get a move on

- If the patient's condition permits, position him upright at regular intervals *to increase lung expansion*. When moving the patient or the ventilator tubing, be careful to prevent condensation

Weaning a patient from the ventilator

A patient is ready to be weaned if he has a spontaneous respiratory effort that can keep him ventilated, a stable cardiovascular system, and sufficient respiratory muscle strength and level of consciousness to sustain spontaneous breathing.

Support for each breath

Weaning usually is accomplished by switching the ventilator to pressure support ventilation (PSV) with or without intermittent mandatory ventilation (IMV). That way, the ventilator augments each spontaneous breath. As the patient's own respirations improve, IMV and PSV can be decreased. Eventually, the patient will be able to breathe on his own all day.

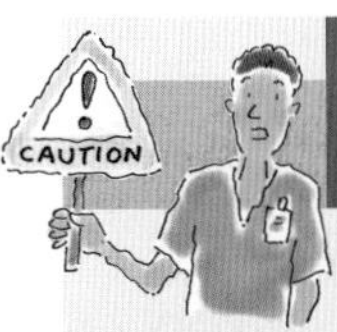

WARNING!

Responding to ventilator alarms

Signal	Possible cause	Interventions
Low-pressure alarm	• Tube disconnected from ventilator	• Reconnect the tube to the ventilator.
	• ETT tube displaced above vocal cords or tracheostomy tube extubated	• Check tube placement and reposition if needed. If extubation or displacement has occurred, ventilate the patient manually and call the doctor immediately.
	• Leaking tidal volume from low cuff pressure (from an underinflated or ruptured cuff or a leak in the cuff or one-way valve)	• Listen for a whooshing sound around the tube, indicating an air leak. If you hear one, check cuff pressure. If you can't maintain pressure, call the doctor; he may need to insert a new tube.
	• Ventilator malfunction	• Disconnect the patient from the ventilator and ventilate him manually if necessary. Obtain another ventilator.
	• Leak in ventilator circuitry (from loose connection or hole in tubing, loss of temperature-sensitive device, or cracked humidification jar)	• Make sure all connections are intact. Check for holes or leaks in the tubing and replace if necessary. Check the humidification jar and replace it if it's cracked.
High-pressure alarm	• Increased airway pressure or decreased lung compliance caused by worsening disease	• Auscultate the lungs for evidence of increasing lung consolidation, barotrauma, or wheezing. Call the doctor if indicated.
	• Patient biting on oral ETT	• Insert a bite block if needed.
	• Secretions in airway	• Look for secretions in the airway. To remove them, suction the patient or have him cough.
	• Condensate in large-bore tubing	• Check tubing for condensate and remove fluid.
	• Intubation of right mainstem bronchus	• Check tube position. If it has slipped, call the doctor; he may need to reposition it.
	• Patient coughing, gagging, or attempting to talk	• If the patient fights the ventilator, the doctor may order a sedative or neuromuscular blocker.
	• Chest wall resistance	• Reposition the patient to see if doing so improves chest expansion. If repositioning doesn't help, administer the prescribed analgesic.
	• Failure of high-pressure relief valve	• Have the faulty equipment replaced.
	• Bronchospasm	• Assess the patient for the cause. Report to the doctor and intervene as ordered.

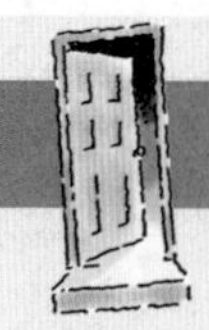

Home care connection

Using a mechanical ventilator at home

If the patient will be discharged on a ventilator, evaluate the family's or caregiver's ability and motivation to provide care. Involve case management or social services to identify additional resources to assist the patient at home including home health care.

Step 1: Teach
Well before discharge, develop a teaching plan that will address the patient's needs. For example, teaching should include information about ventilator care and settings, artificial airway care, suctioning, respiratory therapy, communication, nutrition, therapeutic exercise, signs and symptoms of infection, and ways to troubleshoot minor equipment malfunctions.

Step 2: Evaluate
Evaluate the patient's need for adaptive equipment, such as a hospital bed, wheelchair or walker with a ventilator tray, patient lift, and bedside commode. Determine whether the patient needs to travel; if so, select appropriate portable and backup equipment.

Step 3: Demonstrate
Before discharge, have the patient's caregiver demonstrates his ability to use the equipment. At discharge, contact a durable medical equipment vendor and a home health nurse to follow up with the patient. Plan for backup equipment in case of a power failure or equipment failure. Also, refer the patient to community resources, if available.

in the tubing from flowing into the lungs *because aspiration of this contaminated moisture can cause infection.*

- Place the call light within the patient's reach, and establish a method of communication, such as a communication board, *because intubation and mechanical ventilation impair the patient's ability to speak.*

This will help you relax

- Administer a sedative or neuromuscular blocking agent as ordered *to relax the patient or eliminate spontaneous breathing efforts that can interfere with the ventilator's action.* Remember that the patient receiving a neuromuscular blocking drug requires close observation *because of his inability to breathe or communicate.*
- If the patient is receiving a neuromuscular blocking agent, make sure that he also receives a sedative. *Neuromuscular blocking agents cause paralysis without altering the patient's level of consciousness.* Reassure the patient and his family that the paralysis is temporary.

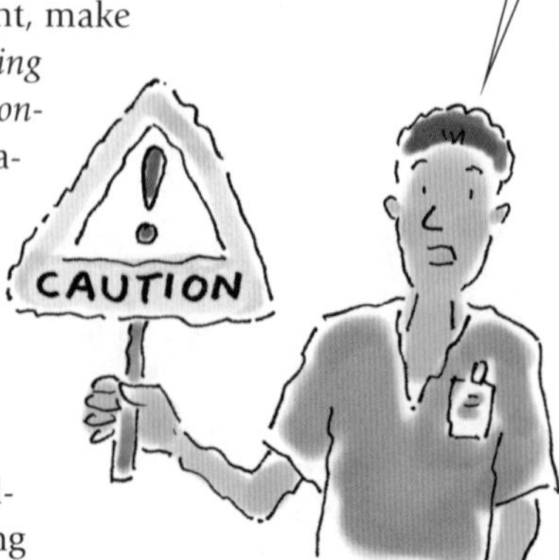
Be careful! If the patient is receiving a neuromuscular blocker, make sure he also receives a sedative and observe him closely because he'll be unable to breathe or communicate.
CAUTION

Shhh! Someone's sleeping

- Ensure that the patient gets adequate rest and sleep *because fatigue can delay weaning from the ventilator.*
- When weaning the patient, continue to observe for signs of hypoxia. Schedule weaning to fit comfortably and realistically with the patient's daily regimen. Avoid scheduling

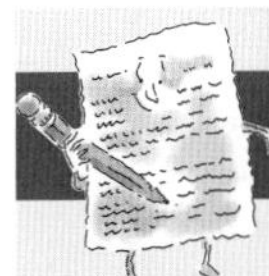

Write it down

Documenting mechanical ventilation

In your notes, document:
- date and time that mechanical ventilation was initiated
- type of ventilator used
- ventilator settings
- patient's subjective and objective response to ventilation, including vital signs, breath sounds, and accessory muscle use
- fluid intake and output
- body weight
- complications and nursing actions taken
- pertinent laboratory data, including ABG analysis results and oxygen saturation levels.

During weaning from the ventilator, record:
- date and time of each weaning session
- weaning method used
- baseline and subsequent vital signs, oxygen saturation levels, and ABG values
- patient's subjective and objective responses, including level of consciousness, respiratory effort, arrhythmias, skin color, and need for suctioning
- complications and nursing actions taken.

What else?

If the patient has been receiving PSV or using a T piece or tracheostomy collar, note the duration of spontaneous breathing and the patient's ability to maintain the weaning schedule. If he has been using intermittent mandatory ventilation (with or without PSV), record the control breath rate, the time of each breath reduction, and the rate of spontaneous respirations.

sessions after meals, baths, or lengthy therapeutic or diagnostic procedures. Have the patient help you set up the schedule *to give him some sense of control over a frightening procedure*. As the patient's tolerance for weaning increases, help him sit up out of bed *to improve his breathing and sense of well-being*. Suggest diversionary activities *to take his mind off breathing*.

- If the patient will be discharged on a ventilator, start teaching early in his hospital stay. (See *Using a mechanical ventilator at home*.)
- Assess the patient for complications of mechanical ventilation, such as tension pneumothorax, decreased cardiac output, oxygen toxicity, fluid volume excess caused by humidification, infection, and such gastrointestinal (GI) complications as distention or bleeding from stress ulcers. (See *Documenting mechanical ventilation*.)

Incentive spirometry

Incentive spirometry involves using a breathing device to help promote lung expansion after prolonged bedrest or surgery. The device requires that the patient take a deep breath and hold it for several seconds.

Performing incentive spirometry increases lung volume, boosts alveolar inflation, and promotes venous return, which helps prevent atelectasis and pneumonia.

What you need

Flow or volume incentive spirometer, as indicated, with sterile disposable tube and mouthpiece (the tube and mouthpiece are sterile on first use and clean on subsequent uses) ✳ stethoscope ✳ watch.

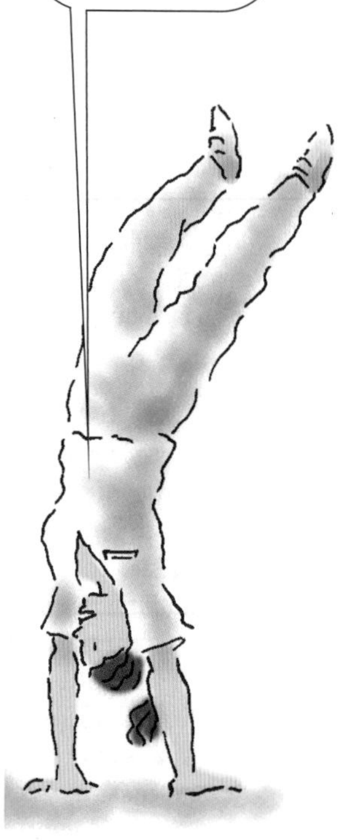

The patient can perform incentive spirometry from any position . . . but remember to keep the device perfectly upright.

Getting ready

Assemble the ordered equipment at the patient's bedside. Read the manufacturer's instructions for spirometer setup and operation.

Remove the sterile flow tube and mouthpiece from the package and attach them to the device. Set the flow rate or volume goal as determined by the doctor or respiratory therapist and based on the patient's preoperative performance.

How you do it

- Assess the patient's condition.
- Identify the patient using two patient identifiers.
- Perform hand hygiene.
- Explain the procedure to the patient, making sure that he understands the importance of performing incentive spirometry regularly *to maintain alveolar inflation*. Wash your hands.
- Help the patient into a comfortable sitting or semi-Fowler's position *to promote optimal lung expansion*. If you're using a flow incentive spirometer and the patient can't assume or maintain this position, he can perform the procedure in any position as long as the device remains upright. *Tilting a flow incentive spirometer decreases the required patient effort and reduces the exercise's effectiveness.*

First, listen

- Auscultate the patient's lungs *to provide a baseline for comparison with posttreatment auscultation.*
- Instruct the patient to insert the mouthpiece and close his lips tightly around it *because a weak seal may alter flow or volume readings.*

Here's where it happens

- Instruct the patient to exhale normally and then inhale as slowly and as deeply as possible. If he has difficulty with this step, tell him to suck as he would through a straw but more slowly. Ask the patient to retain the entire volume of air he inhaled for 3 seconds.

Only nine more to go

- Tell the patient to remove the mouthpiece and exhale normally. Allow him to relax and take several normal breaths before attempting another breath with the spirometer. Repeat this sequence 5 to 10 times during every waking hour. Note tidal volumes.

- Evaluate the patient's ability to cough effectively and encourage him to cough after each effort *because deep lung inflation may loosen secretions and facilitate their removal.* Observe expectorated secretions.
- Auscultate the patient's lungs and compare findings with the first auscultation.

Now you're done

- Instruct the patient to remove the mouthpiece. Wash the device in warm water and shake it dry. Avoid immersing the spirometer itself *because this enhances bacterial growth and impairs the internal filter's effectiveness in preventing inhalation of extraneous material.*
- Place the mouthpiece in a plastic storage bag between exercises and label it and the spirometer, if applicable, with the patient's name *to avoid inadvertent use by another patient.*

Practice pointers

- If the patient is scheduled for surgery, make a preoperative assessment of his respiratory pattern and capability *to ensure the development of appropriate postoperative goals.* Teach the patient how to use the spirometer before surgery *so that he can concentrate on your instructions and practice the exercise.* A preoperative evaluation will also help in establishing a postoperative therapeutic goal.
- Immediately after surgery, monitor the exercise frequently *to ensure compliance and assess achievement.* (See *Documenting incentive spirometry.*)

Write it down

Documenting incentive spirometry

In your notes, record:

- preoperative flow or volume levels
- preoperative teaching provided
- date and time of the procedure
- type of spirometer used
- flow or volume levels achieved
- number of breaths taken
- patient's condition before and after the procedure
- patient's tolerance of the procedure
- results of both auscultations.

Chest physiotherapy

Chest physiotherapy (PT) includes postural drainage, chest percussion and vibration, and coughing and deep-breathing exercises. Together, these techniques mobilize and eliminate secretions, reexpand lung tissue, and promote efficient use of respiratory muscles. The goal is to improve the patient's respiratory status and speed recovery by improving airway clearance and reducing the work of breathing. Patients may find this therapy uncomfortable and undesirable.

Chest PT is critical to the bedridden patient because it helps prevent or treat atelectasis and may also help prevent pneumonia, two respiratory complications that can seriously impede recovery. It is often used in combination with other treatments such as bronchodilators, hydration, mucolytic agents, and antibiotics.

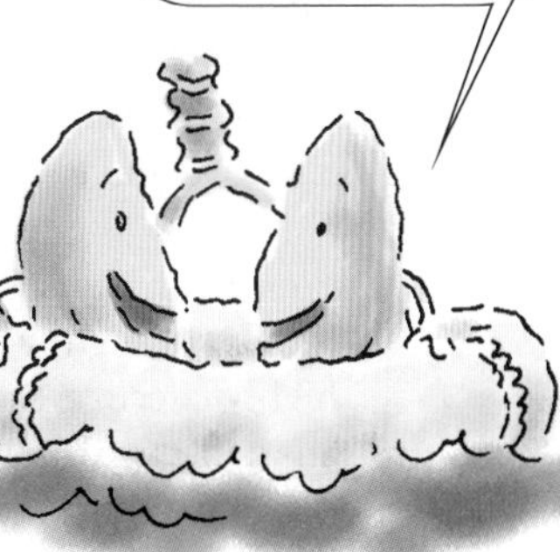
Chest PT can prevent pneumonia. Thanks for the help!

What you need

Stethoscope * pillows * tilt or postural drainage table (if available) or adjustable hospital bed * emesis basin * facial tissues * suction equipment as needed * equipment for oral care * towel * trash bag * optional: sterile specimen container, supplemental oxygen.

Getting ready

Gather the equipment at the patient's bedside. Set up suction equipment, if needed, and test its function.

How you do it

- Identify the patient using two patient identifiers.
- Determine the patient's understanding and explain to the patient and family: patient positioning, sensations, how procedure is performed, how long it takes, or side effects that may occur. Explain the frequency will depend on the patient's need and tolerance. Explain the best time to perform the procedure is in the morning before breakfast and bedtime.
- Perform hand hygiene and don gloves.
- Auscultate the patient's lungs to determine baseline respiratory status. Assess the patient's breathing pattern, including chest wall movement, use of accessory muscles, rate and depth of respirations.
- Position the patient as ordered. The lung's lower lobes commonly require drainage because the upper lobes drain during normal activity. (See *Positioning the patient for postural drainage*.)

Wanted: Drum players

Instruct the patient to remain in each position for 10 to 15 minutes. During this time, perform percussion and vibration as ordered. (See *Performing percussion and vibration*, page 354.)

Coughs—I'll take three

- After percussion or vibration, instruct the patient to cough *to remove loosened secretions.* Give him an emesis basin and facial tissues to dispose of secretions; if a sputum specimen is necessary, also give him a sterile specimen container. To begin the procedure, tell him to inhale deeply through his nose and then exhale in three short huffs. Then have him inhale deeply again and cough through a slightly open mouth. Three consecutive coughs are highly effective. An effective cough sounds deep, low, and hollow; an ineffective one, high-pitched. Have the patient perform exercises for about 1 minute and then rest for 2 minutes. Gradually progress to a 10-minute exercise period four times daily.

Positioning the patient for postural drainage

Postural drainage most commonly is required for the lower lobes of the lung. These illustrations show various postural drainage positions and the lung areas affected by each position.

Lower lobes: Posterior basal segments
Elevate the foot of the bed 30 degrees. Have the patient lie prone with his head lowered. Position pillows under his chest and abdomen. Percuss his lower ribs on both sides of his spine.

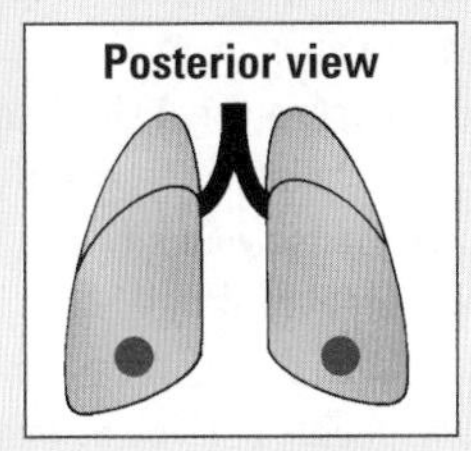

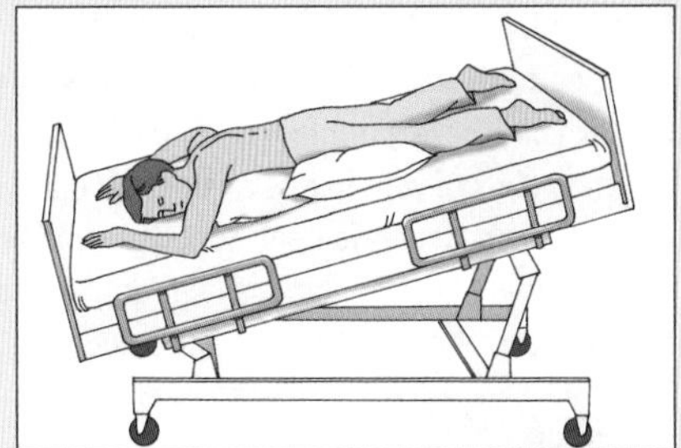

Lower lobes: Lateral basal segments
Elevate the foot of the bed 30 degrees. Instruct the patient to lie on his abdomen with his head lowered and his upper leg flexed over a pillow for support. Then have him rotate a quarter turn upward. Percuss his lower ribs on the uppermost portion of his lateral chest wall.

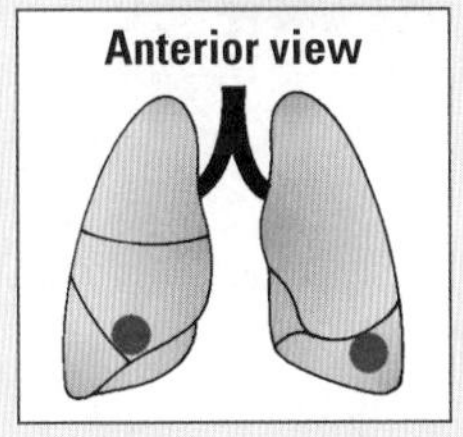

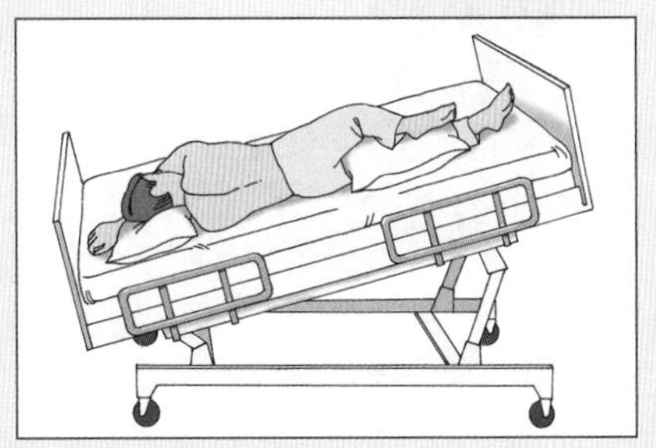

Lower lobes: Anterior basal segments
Elevate the foot of the bed 30 degrees. Instruct the patient to lie on his side with his head lowered. Then place pillows as shown. Percuss with a slightly cupped hand over his lower ribs just beneath the axilla. If an acutely ill patient has trouble breathing in this position, adjust the bed to an angle he can tolerate. Then begin percussion.

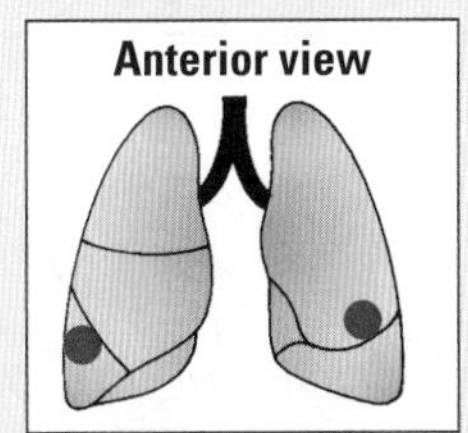

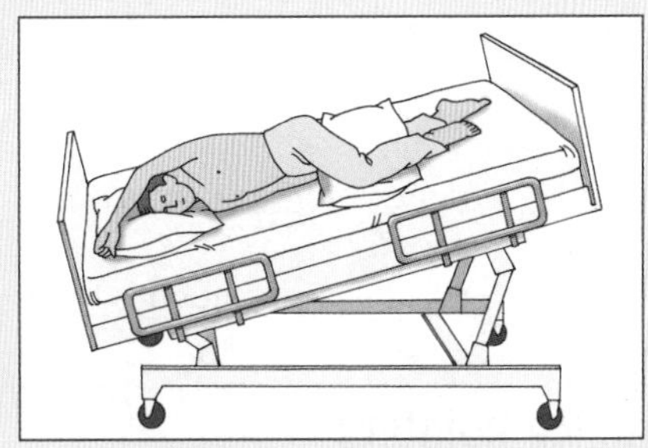

Lower lobes: Superior segments
With the bed flat, have the patient lie on his abdomen. Place two pillows under his hips. Percuss on both sides of his spine at the lower tip of his scapulae.

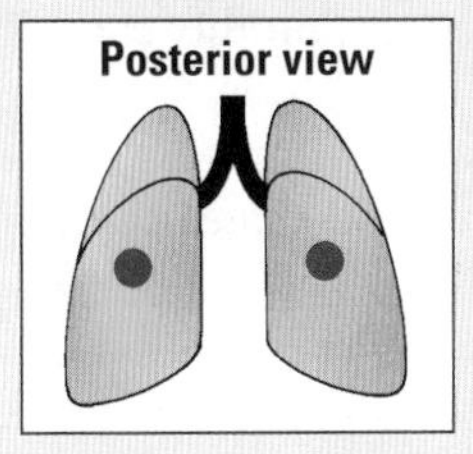

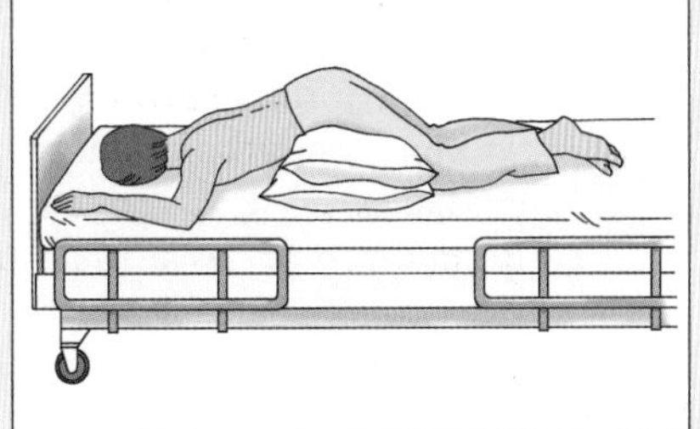

Performing percussion and vibration

To perform *percussion*, hold your hands in a cupped shape, with fingers flexed and thumbs pressed tightly against your index fingers. Percuss each segment for 1 to 2 minutes by alternating your hands against the patient in a rhythmic manner. Listen for a hollow sound on percussion to verify correct technique.

To perform *vibration*, ask the patient to inhale deeply and hold for 2 seconds before exhaling slowly through pursed lips. During exhalation, firmly press your fingers and the palms of your hands against his chest wall. Tense your arm and shoulder muscles in an isometric contraction to send fine vibrations through the chest wall. Vibrate during five exhalations over each chest segment. Perform a total of three or four sets of three vibrations and coughing in each patient position as tolerated.

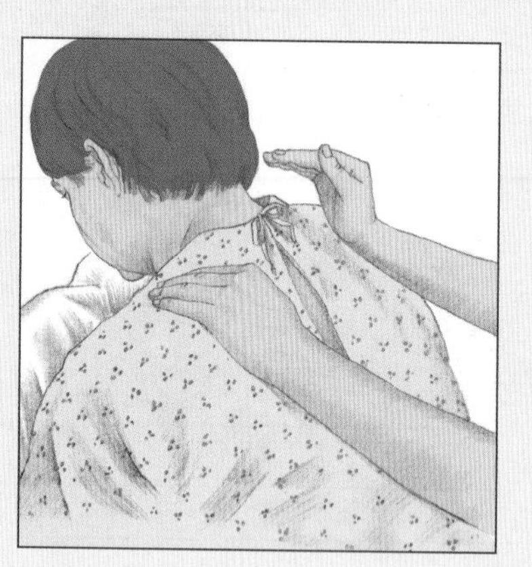

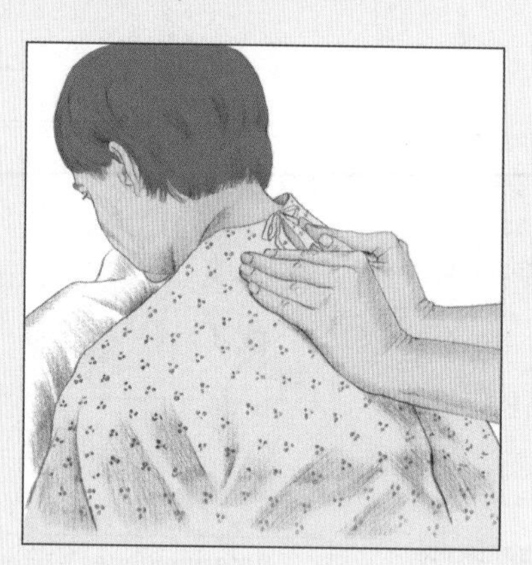

- Provide oral hygiene *because secretions may have a foul taste or a stale odor.*
- Auscultate the patient's lungs *to evaluate the effectiveness of therapy.*

Documenting chest PT

In your notes, record:
- patient and family education
- respiratory assessment before and after procedure
- date and time of chest PT
- positions used for secretion drainage and the duration each position is maintained
- chest segments percussed or vibrated
- color, amount, odor, and viscosity of secretions produced
- presence of blood
- complications and nursing actions taken
- patient's tolerance of the procedure.

Practice pointers

- For optimal effectiveness and safety, modify chest PT according to the patient's condition.
- Avoid performing postural drainage immediately before or within 1½ hours after meals *to avoid nausea and aspiration of food or vomitus.*
- *Because chest percussion can induce bronchospasm,* adjunct treatment (for example, aerosol or nebulizer therapy) should precede chest PT.

Hey! That hurts!

- Refrain from percussing over the spine, liver, kidneys, or spleen *to avoid injury to the spine or internal organs.* Also, avoid performing percussion on bare skin or the female patient's breasts. Percuss

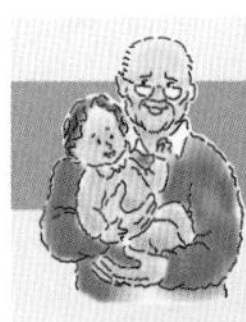

Ages and stages

Pediatric

- Handheld percussors may be used when a child is in an oxygen-rich environment.
- Chest PT should be used cautiously in infants because it may cause distress.
- Airway clearance techniques are recommended for all children with cystic fibrosis to clear airway secretions.
- To prevent vomiting and aspiration, chest PT should not be performed for at least 1 hour after feedings or meals, and continuous drip feeds should be turned off at least 30 minutes before therapy.

Geriatric

- Percussion, vibration, and shaking should be performed more gently in the elderly.
- In frail older adults, a mechanical percussor should be used instead of manual chest PT.

over soft clothing (but not over buttons, snaps, or zippers) or place a thin towel over the chest wall. Remember to remove jewelry that might scratch or bruise the patient.

- Be aware that chest PT is contraindicated in patients with active pulmonary bleeding, rib fracture, lung contusion, pulmonary tuberculosis, untreated pneumothorax, acute asthma, or bronchospasm.
- Explain coughing and deep-breathing exercises preoperatively *so that the patient can practice them when he's pain-free and better able to concentrate*. Postoperatively, splint the patient's incision using your hands or, if possible, teach the patient to splint it himself *to minimize pain during coughing*. (See *Documenting chest PT*.)
  - If long-term therapy is needed, the family should be instructed on performing chest PT.
  - If the family is unable to do chest PT, refer to outpatient therapy or home health care.

Think of a chest tube as a life preserver for the lungs.

Assisting with chest tube insertion

Chest tube insertion allows drainage of air or fluid from the pleural space. The pleural space normally contains a thin layer of lubricating fluid that allows the lungs to move without friction during respiration. Excess fluid (hemothorax or pleural effusion), air (pneumothorax), or both in this space alters intrapleural pressure and causes partial or complete lung collapse. If this occurs, chest tube insertion is necessary to help reinflate the lungs.

Selecting a site

Usually performed by a doctor with a nurse assisting, this procedure requires sterile technique. The insertion site varies depending on the patient's condition and the doctor's judgment.

After insertion, one or more chest tubes are connected to a thoracic drainage system that removes air, fluid, or both from the pleural space and prevents backflow into that space, thus promoting lung reexpansion. (See "Thoracic drainage," page 359.)

What you need

Two pairs of sterile gloves ✳ mask and goggles or face shield ✳ gowns ✳ sterile drape ✳ linen saver pad ✳ sterile towels ✳ safety pin ✳ vial of 1% lidocaine ✳ povidone-iodine solution ✳ 0-mL syringe ✳ alcohol pad ✳ 22G 1" needle ✳ 25G ⅜" needle ✳ sterile scalpel (usually with #11 blade) ✳ sterile forceps ✳ two rubber-tipped clamps for each chest tube inserted ✳ sterile 4" × 4" gauze pads ✳ two sterile 4" × 4" drain dressings (gauze pads with slit) ✳ 3" or 4" sturdy, elastic tape ✳ 1" adhesive tape for connections ✳ chest tube of appropriate size (#16 to #20 French catheter for air or serous fluid; #28 to #40 French catheter for blood, pus, or thick fluid), with or without a trocar ✳ two sterile Kelly clamp ✳ curved clamps ✳ suture material (usually 2-0 silk with cutting needle) ✳ thoracic drainage system ✳ suction source ✳ sterile drainage tubing, 6" (15.2 cm) long, and connector ✳ sterile Y connector (for two chest tubes on the same side) ✳ optional: petroleum gauze.

Getting ready

Check the expiration date on the sterile packages and inspect for tears. In a nonemergency situation, make sure that the patient has signed the appropriate consent form. Then assemble all equipment in the patient's room and set up the thoracic drainage system. Place it next to the patient's bed below the chest level *to facilitate drainage.*

How you do it

- Identify the patient using two patient identifiers.
- Explain the procedure to the patient.
- Perform hand hygiene and don PPE.
- Record baseline vital signs and respiratory assessment.
- Position the patient to allow for adequate breathing. If he has a *pneumothorax,* place him in high Fowler's, semi-Fowler's, or the supine position. The doctor will insert the tube in the anterior chest at the

midclavicular line in the second to third intercostal space. If the patient has a *hemothorax*, have him lean over the overbed table or straddle a chair with his arms dangling over the back. The doctor will insert the tube in the fourth to sixth intercostal space at the midaxillary line. For either pneumothorax or hemothorax, the patient may lie on his unaffected side with arms extended over his head.

- When you've positioned the patient properly, place the chest tube tray on the overbed table. Open it using sterile technique. Provide supplemental oxygen if needed.
- The doctor dons sterile gloves and prepares the insertion site by cleaning the area with povidone-iodine solution.
- Wipe the rubber stopper of the lidocaine vial with an alcohol pad. Then invert the bottle and hold it for the doctor to withdraw the anesthetic.

We're going in

- After the doctor anesthetizes the site, he makes a small incision and inserts the chest tube.
- Connect the chest tube to the closed chest drainage system and check for respiratory variation of the H_2O column. Apply ordered amount of suction.
- Assist with suturing of the tube to the chest wall.
- Apply an occlusive dressing to the site. *This provides an airtight seal around the chest tube.*
  - Petrolatum gauze is used around the chest tube or follow institutional standard.
  - Split drain sponges are placed around the chest tube, one from top, one underneath.
  - Cover with 4″ × 4″ gauze.
  - Tape dressing completely.

Stick around

- Tape the chest tube to the patient's chest distal to the insertion site *to help prevent accidental tube dislodgment.*
- Tape the junction of the chest tube and the drainage tube *to prevent their separation and prevent air leaks into the pleural space.*
- Coil the drainage tubing and secure it to the bed linen with tape and a safety pin, leaving enough slack for the patient to move and turn. *These measures prevent the tubing from getting kinked or dropping to the floor and they help prevent accidental chest tube dislodgement.*

Everyone has a job

- Immediately after the drainage system is connected, instruct the patient to take a deep breath, hold it momentarily, and slowly exhale *to assist drainage of the pleural space and lung reexpansion.*

- A portable chest X-ray is then done *to check tube position.*
- Take the patient's vital signs every 15 minutes for 1 hour, then as his condition indicates. Auscultate his lungs at least every 4 hours following the procedure *to assess air exchange in the affected lung.* Diminished or absent breath sounds indicate that the lung hasn't reexpanded.

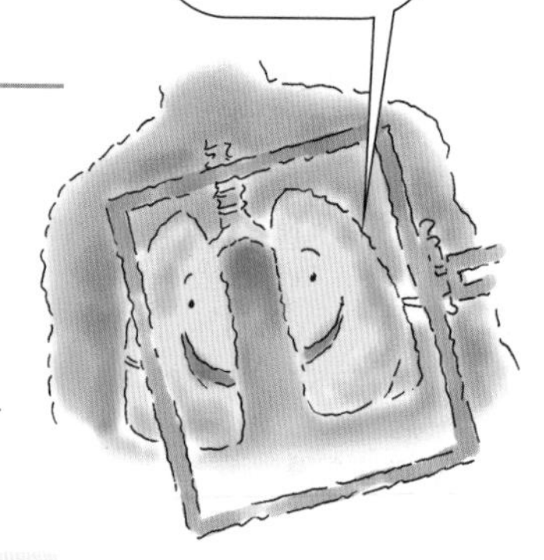

An X-ray tells you whether the chest tube is in the right place.

Practice pointers

- If the chest tube comes out, cover the site immediately with 4″ × 4″ gauze pads and tape them in place. Stay with the patient and monitor his vital signs every 10 minutes. Observe him for signs of tension pneumothorax (hypotension, distended neck veins, absent breath sounds, tracheal shift, hypoxemia, weak and rapid pulse, dyspnea, tachypnea, diaphoresis,

Removing a chest tube

After the patient's lung has reexpanded, you may assist the doctor in removing the chest tube. To do so, first obtain the patient's vital signs and perform a respiratory assessment. After explaining the procedure to the patient, administer an analgesic, as ordered. Then follow the steps below:

- Place the patient in semi-Fowler's position or on his unaffected side.
- Place a linen-saver pad under the affected side to protect the linen from drainage.
- Put on clean gloves and remove the chest tube dressings, being careful not to dislodge the chest tube. Discard soiled dressings.

The value of Valsalva

- The doctor dons sterile gloves, holds the chest tube in place with sterile forceps, and cuts the suture anchoring the tube.
- Make sure the chest tube is securely clamped, and then instruct the patient to perform Valsalva's maneuver by exhaling fully and bearing down. Valsalva's maneuver effectively increases intrathoracic pressure.
- The doctor holds an airtight dressing, usually petroleum gauze, so that he can cover the insertion site with it immediately after removing the tube. After he removes the tube and covers the insertion site, secure the dressing with tape. Be sure to cover the dressing completely with tape to make it as airtight as possible.
- Dispose of the chest tube, soiled gloves, and equipment according to your facility's policy.
- Take vital signs as ordered and assess the depth and quality of the patient's respirations. Assess the patient carefully for signs and symptoms of pneumothorax, subcutaneous emphysema, or infection.

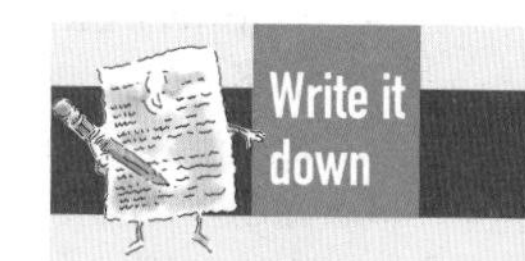

Documenting chest tube insertion

In your notes, document:

- patient and family education
- date and time of chest tube insertion
- insertion site
- drainage system used
- presence of drainage and bubbling
- amount and type of drainage if present
- amount of suction
- patient's vital signs and auscultation findings before and after procedure
- complications and nursing actions taken.

and chest pain). Have another staff member notify the doctor and gather the equipment needed to reinsert the tube.

- Place the rubber-tipped clamps at the bedside. If a drainage system cracks or if a tube disconnects, clamp the chest tube momentarily as close to the insertion site as possible. *Because no air or liquid can escape from the pleural space while the tube is clamped,* observe the patient closely for signs of tension pneumothorax while the clamp is in place.
- Petroleum gauze may be wrapped around the tube at the insertion site *to make an airtight seal.*
- A chest tube is usually removed within 7 days of insertion *to prevent infection along the tube tract.* (See *Removing a chest tube* and *Documenting chest tube insertion.*)

Thoracic drainage

Thoracic drainage uses gravity (and occasionally suction) to restore negative pressure, remove material that collects in the pleural cavity, or to reexpand a partially or totally collapsed lung. An underwater seal in the drainage system allows air and fluid to escape from the pleural cavity but doesn't allow air to reenter.

Rare sighting

The system is a self-contained, disposable system that collects drainage, creates a water seal, and controls suction. (See *Disposable drainage systems,* page 360.)

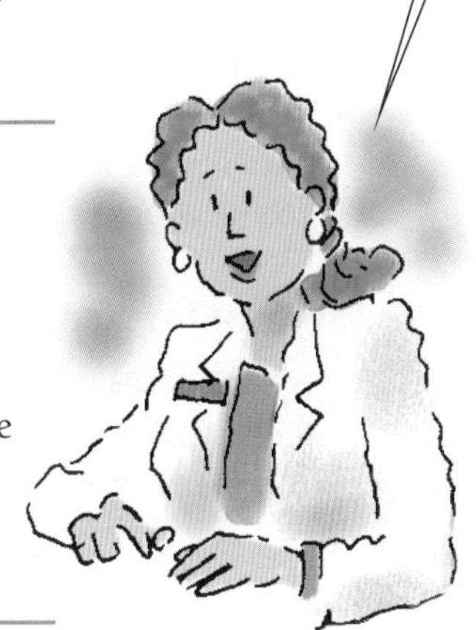
Thoracic drainage systems have an underwater seal that allows air and fluid to leave the pleural cavity—but doesn't let them back in.

What you need

Thoracic drainage system (Pleur-evac, Argyle, Ohio, or Thora-Klex system, which can function as gravity drainage systems or be connected to suction to enhance chest drainage) ✻ sterile distilled water (usually 1 L) ✻ adhesive tape ✻ sterile clear plastic tubing ✻ bottle or system rack ✻ two rubber-tipped Kelly clamps ✻ sterile 50-mL catheter-tip syringe ✻ suction source, if ordered ✻ pain medication, if ordered.

Getting ready

Check the doctor's order to determine the type of drainage system to be used and specific procedural details. If appropriate, request the drainage system and suction system from the central supply department. Collect the appropriate equipment and take it to the patient's bedside.

Disposable drainage systems

Commercially prepared disposable drainage systems combine drainage collection, water seal, and suction control in one unit (as shown here). These systems, which have a prominent air leak indicator, ensure patient safety with positive and negative pressure relief valves. Some systems produce no bubbling sound.

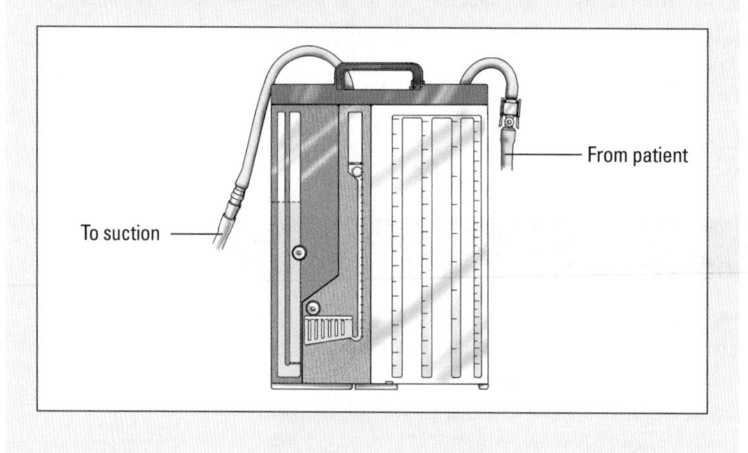

How you do it

- Identify the patient with two patient identifiers.
- Explain the procedure to the patient and perform hand hygiene.
- Maintain sterile technique throughout the entire procedure and whenever you make changes in the system or alter any of the connections *to avoid introducing pathogens into the pleural space.*

Setting up a commercially prepared disposable system

Open the packaged system and place it on the floor in the rack supplied by the manufacturer *to avoid accidentally knocking it over or dislodging the components.* After the system is prepared, it may be hung from the side of the patient's bed.

Just add water

- Remove the plastic connector from the short tube attached to the water-seal chamber. Using a 50-mL catheter-tip syringe, instill sterile distilled water into the water-seal chamber until it reaches the 2-cm mark or the mark specified by the manufacturer. The Ohio and Thora-Klex systems are ready to use, but with the Thora-Klex system, 15 mL of sterile water may be added to help detect air leaks. Replace the plastic connector.

- If suction is ordered, remove the cap (also called the muffler or atmosphere vent cover) on the suction control chamber *to open the vent*. Next, instill sterile distilled water until it reaches the 20-cm mark or the ordered level, and recap the suction control chamber.
- Using the long tube, connect the patient's chest tube to the closed drainage collection chamber. Secure the connection with tape.
- Connect the short tube on the drainage system to the suction source and turn on the suction. Gentle bubbling should begin in the suction chamber, *indicating that the correct suction level has been reached*.

CAUTION

WARNING!

Clamping alert

Never leave a chest tube clamped for more than 1 minute. Keeping it clamped too long can cause a tension pneumothorax, which may occur when clamping stops air and fluid from escaping.

Managing closed-chest underwater seal drainage

- Repeatedly note the character, consistency, and amount of drainage in the drainage collection chamber.
- Mark the drainage level in the drainage collection chamber by noting the time and date at the drainage level on the chamber every 8 hours (or more often if there's a large amount of drainage).

Look for the level

- Check the water level in the water-seal chamber every 8 hours. If necessary, carefully add sterile distilled water until the level reaches the 2-cm mark indicated on the water-seal chamber of the commercial system.
- Check for fluctuation in the water-seal chamber as the patient breathes. Normal fluctuations of 2″ to 4″ (5 to 10 cm) reflect pressure changes in the pleural space during respiration.
  To check for fluctuation when a suction system is being used, momentarily disconnect the suction system so the air vent is opened and observe for fluctuation.
- Check for intermittent bubbling in the water-seal chamber. This occurs normally when the system is removing air from the pleural cavity. If bubbling isn't readily apparent during quiet breathing, have the patient take a deep breath or cough. Absence of bubbling indicates that the pleural space has sealed.
- Check the water level in the suction control chamber. Detach the chamber from the suction source; when bubbling ceases, observe the water level. If necessary, add sterile distilled water to bring the level to the −20-cm line or as ordered.
- Check for gentle bubbling in the suction control chamber *because it indicates that the proper suction level has been reached*. Vigorous bubbling in this chamber increases the rate of water evaporation.

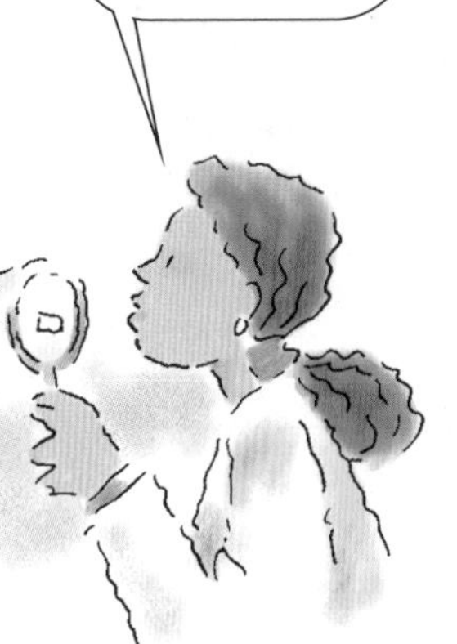
What can I say? One of your jobs with thoracic drainage is to check for bubbling.

- Periodically check that the air vent in the system is working properly. Occlusion of the air vent results in a buildup of pressure in the system that could cause the patient to develop a tension pneumothorax.

Always ready to clamp down

- Be sure to keep two rubber-tipped clamps at the bedside *to clamp the chest tube if the system cracks or to locate an air leak in the system.* (See *Clamping alert,* page 361.)
- Encourage the patient to cough frequently and breathe deeply *to help drain the pleural space and expand the lungs.*
- Tell him to sit upright *for optimal lung expansion* and to splint the insertion site while coughing *to minimize pain.*
- Check the rate and quality of the patient's respirations and auscultate his lungs periodically *to assess air exchange in the affected lung.* Diminished or absent breath sounds may indicate that the lung hasn't reexpanded.

Cause for alarm

- Tell the patient to report breathing difficulty immediately. **Notify the doctor immediately** if the patient develops cyanosis, rapid or shallow breathing, subcutaneous emphysema, chest pain, or excessive bleeding.
- Check the chest tube dressing at least every 8 hours. Palpate the area surrounding the dressing for crepitus or subcutaneous emphysema, which indicates that air is leaking into the subcutaneous tissue surrounding the insertion site. Change the dressing if necessary or according to policy. (See *To strip or not to strip.*)
- Give ordered pain medication as needed *for comfort and to help with deep breathing and coughing.*

Practice pointers

- Avoid lifting the drainage system above the patient's chest *because fluid may flow back into the pleural space.*
- If excessive continuous bubbling is present in the water-seal chamber, especially if suction is being used, rule out a leak in the drainage system. Try to locate the leak by clamping the tube momentarily at various points along its length. Begin clamping at the tube's proximal end and work down toward the drainage system, paying special attention to the seal around the connections. If a connection is loose, push it back together and tape it securely. *The bubbling will stop when a clamp is placed between the air leak and the water seal.* If you clamp along the tube's entire length and the bubbling doesn't stop, the drainage unit may be cracked and needs replacement.

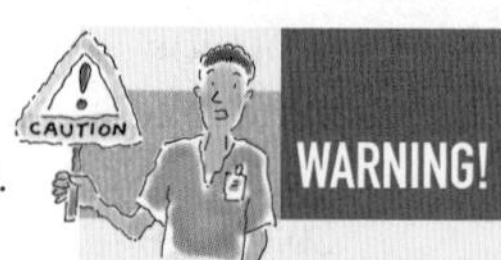

To strip or not to strip

When clots are visible, you may be able to strip (or milk) the tubing, depending on your facility's policy. This procedure is controversial because it creates high negative pressure that could suck viable lung tissue into the tube's drainage ports, with subsequent ruptured alveoli and pleural air leak.

If you're ready for the challenge . . .
Strip the tubing only when clots are visible. Use an alcohol pad or lotion as a lubricant on the tube and pinch it between your thumb and index finger about 2" (5 cm) from the insertion site. Using the other thumb and index finger, compress the tubing as you slide your fingers down the tube or use a mechanical stripper. After stripping, release the thumb and index finger pinching the tube near the insertion site.

- If the drainage collection chamber fills, replace it. To do this, double-clamp the tube close to the insertion site (use two clamps facing in opposite directions), exchange the system, remove the clamps, and retape the bottle connection.

If there's a crack

- If the commercially prepared system cracks, clamp the chest tube momentarily with the two rubber-tipped clamps at the bedside (placed there at the time of tube insertion). Place the clamps close to each other near the insertion site; they should face in opposite directions *to provide a more complete seal.* Observe the patient for altered respirations while the tube is clamped. Then replace the damaged equipment. (Prepare the new unit before clamping the tube.)
- Tension pneumothorax may result from excessive accumulation of air, drainage, or both and eventually may exert pressure on the heart and aorta, causing a precipitous fall in cardiac output. (See *Documenting thoracic drainage.*)

Documenting thoracic drainage

In your notes, record:
- date and time thoracic drainage began
- type of system used
- amount of suction applied to the pleural cavity
- presence or absence of bubbling or fluctuation in the water-seal chamber
- initial amount and type of drainage
- patient's respiratory status.

At the end of each shift, record:
- frequency of system inspection
- amount, color, and consistency of drainage
- presence or absence of bubbling or fluctuation in the water-seal chamber
- patient's respiratory status
- condition of chest dressings
- administration of pain medication
- complications and nursing actions taken.

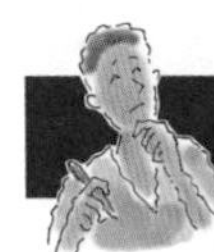

Quick quiz

1. The nurse is caring for a patient with respiratory failure who is hypoxemic even though he is on mechanical ventilation. Despite sedation and analgesia, the patient remains restless and appears to be in discomfort. The nurse informs the physician of this assessment and anticipates which order for this patient?

A. Prone positioning
B. Neuromuscular blockade
C. Guided imagery
D. Muscle relaxants

Answer: B. The patient will need a neuromuscular blockade to decrease restlessness and overall oxygen demand and requirements.

2. PEEP is a mode of ventilator assistance that produces which situation?

A. The patient must have a respiratory drive for PEEP to be effective and support ventilation.
B. For each spontaneous breath taken, the tidal volume is determined by the patient's ability to generate negative pressure.
C. There is pressure remaining in the lungs at the end of expiration that is measured in centimeters of water.
D. The lung pressure is completely diminishes to establish a new baseline for the lung pressure.

Answer: C. PEEP is effective by keeping the alveoli open at the end of expiration to promote gas exchange.

3. The nurse is caring for a patient who is mechanically ventilated. What must the nurse understand in providing care to this patient?

A. Communication with intubated patients is often difficult.
B. Controlled ventilation is the preferred mode for most patients.
C. Wrist restraints are applied to all patients to avoid self-extubation.
D. The patient's nutritional needs are decreased while being ventilated.

Answer: A. Communication with intubated patients can be challenging, and the nurse needs to ensure to explain procedures to the patient to decrease anxiety.

4. After ETT placement, the nurse should measure cuff pressure every 8 hours to avoid overinflation, which can cause tracheal erosion and necrosis. What is normal cuff pressure?

A. 10 mm Hg
B. 18 mm Hg
C. 20 mm Hg
D. 25 mm Hg

Answer: B. Normal cuff pressure is 18 mm Hg.

5. Which type of tracheostomy tube permits speech through the upper airway?

A. Uncuffed tube
B. Cuffed tube
C. Fenestrated tube
D. No tracheostomy tube allows for speech.

Answer: C. The fenestrated tube permits speech through the upper airway when the external opening is capped and the cuff is deflated.

6. The nurse is caring for a mechanically ventilated patient and notes the high pressure alarm sounding. The nurse cannot identify the cause of the alarm and the patient's oxygen saturation is decreasing and heart rate and respiratory rate are increasing. What is the priority action by the nurse?

A. Ask the respiratory therapist to switch out the ventilator.
B. Manually ventilate the patient while calling for a respiratory therapist.
C. Call a code blue so the nurse will have help in resuscitating the patient.
D. With assistance, move the patient to a room closer to the nurses' station.

Answer: B. The priority is ensuring the patient is getting oxygenated so the nurse will need to manually ventilate the patient until respiratory therapy can get there and assess if a new ventilator is needed.

Scoring

☆☆☆ If you answered all six questions correctly, feel pumped! You're terrific with tubes and cuffs.

☆☆ If you answered four or five questions correctly, great! You're A-OK with airways and oxygen.

☆ If you answered three or fewer questions correctly, no need to hyperventilate. Just take a deep breath and give this chapter another try.

Selected References

American Red Cross. (2011). *Administering emergency oxygen*. Retrieved from http://www.redcross.org/images/MEDIA_CustomProductCatalog/m3240082_AdministeringEmergencyOxygenFactandSkill.pdf

Happ, M. B., Tuite, P., Dobbin, K., et al. (2004). Communication ability, method, and content among nonspeaking nonsurviving patients treated with mechanical ventilation in the intensive care unit. *American Journal of Critical Care, 13*(3), 210–218.

Kacmarek, R. M., Dimas, S., & Mack, C. W. (2005). *The essentials of respiratory care*. St. Louis, MO: Mosby.

Perry, A., & Potter, P. (2015). *Mosby's pocket guide to nursing skills and procedures* (8th ed.). St. Louis, MO: Mosby.

Shilling, A., & Durbin, C. G. (2010). Airway management devices. In J. Cairo (Ed.), *Mosby's respiratory care equipment* (8th ed., pp. 168–212). St. Louis, MO: Mosby.

Simmons, K. F., & Scanlan, C. L. (2009). Airway management. In R. L. Wilkins, J. K. Stoller, C. L. Scanlan, et al. (Eds.), *Egan's fundamentals of respiratory care* (9th ed., pp. 694–765). St. Louis, MO: Mosby.

Skillings, K., & Curtis, B. (2010). Tracheal tube cuff care. In D. J. Wiegand (Ed.), *AACN procedure manual for critical care* (6th ed., pp. 88–95). Philadelphia, PA: Saunders.

Sole, M. L., Klein, D. G., & Mosely, M. J. (2013). *Introduction to critical care nursing* (6th ed.). St. Louis, MO: Elsevier.

St. John, R. E., & Seckel, M. A. (2007). Airway management. In S. M. Burns (Ed.), *AACN protocols for practice: Care of the mechanically ventilated patient* (2nd ed., pp. 1–58). Boston, MA: Jones & Bartlett.

Wiegand, D. J. (Ed.). (2010). *AACN procedure manual for critical care* (6th ed.). Philadelphia, PA: W.B. Saunders.

Chapter 7

Neurologic care

Just the facts

In this chapter, you'll learn:

- about neurologic monitoring and treatment procedures
- what patient care and patient teaching are associated with each procedure
- how to manage complications associated with each procedure
- about essential documentation for each procedure.

Halo-vest traction

Halo-vest traction immobilizes and stabilizes the cervical spine. It can be used alone or in conjunction with spine surgery for patients with an unstable cervical spine as a result of a spinal fracture of dislocation, traumatic cervical spine injury, inflammatory disease, degenerative disease, or an infection. This procedure is performed by an orthopedic surgeon, with nursing assistance, in the emergency department, a specially equipped room, or in the operating room after surgical reduction of vertebral injuries. (See *A look at the halo-vest traction device.*)

A halo ring device is attached using four to six stabilizing pins that are screwed into the skull. A vest is applied once the cervical spine is aligned. The advantage to this method versus cervical tongs is the patient can sit up, get up to a chair, and ambulate if able. It also carries less risk of infection because it doesn't require skin incisions and drill holes to position skull pins.

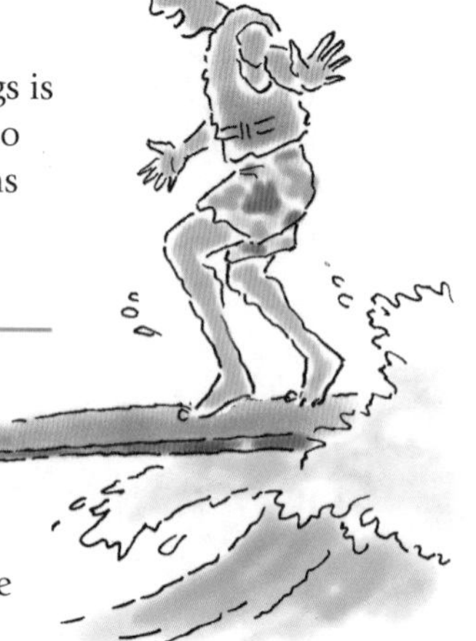
Halo-vest traction allows greater mobility than skull tongs—but surfing is still out.

What you need

Halo-vest traction unit * halo ring * cervical collar or sandbags (if needed) * plastic vest * board or padded headrest * tape measure * halo ring conversion chart * scissors * 4″ × 4″ gauze pads * povidone-iodine solution * sterile gloves ✱ Allen wrench ✱ four positioning pins ✱ multiple-dose vial of 1% lidocaine (with or without epinephrine) ✱ alcohol pads ✱ 3-mL syringe ✱ 25G needles ✱ five sterile skull pins (one more than needed) ✱ torque screwdriver ✱ sheepskin liners ✱ cotton-tipped applicators ✱ ordered cleaning solution ✱ medicated powder or cornstarch ✱ sterile water or normal saline solution ✱ optional: hair dryer, pain medication (such as an analgesic).

Full package

Most facilities supply packaged halo-vest traction units that include software (jacket and sheepskin liners), hardware (halo, head pins, upright bars, and screws), and tools (torque screwdriver, two conventional wrenches, Allen wrench, and screws and bolts). These units don't include sterile gloves, povidone-iodine solution, sterile drapes, cervical collars, or equipment for local anesthetic injection.

A look at the halo-vest traction device

The halo-vest traction device consists of a metal ring that fits over the patient's head and metal bars that connect the ring to a plastic vest that distributes the weight of the entire apparatus around the chest.

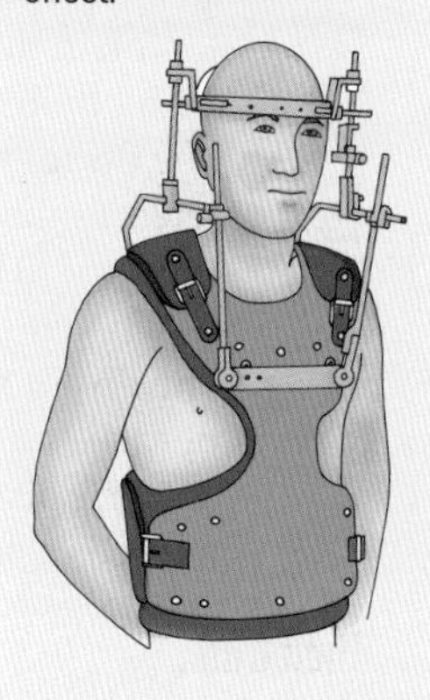

Getting ready

Obtain a halo-vest traction unit with halo rings and plastic vests in several sizes. Check the expiration date of the prepackaged tray and check the outside covering for damage *to ensure the sterility of the contents*. Then assemble the equipment at the patient's bedside. Check to see that a consent form was signed and in the chart.

How you do it

Check the order and verify the correct patient using two patient identifiers. Check the support that was applied to the patient's neck on the way to the hospital. If necessary, apply the cervical collar immediately or immobilize the head and neck with sandbags. Keep the cervical collar or sandbags in place until the halo is applied. This support will then be carefully removed *to facilitate application of the vest. Because the patient is likely to be frightened,* try to reassure him.

Time to redecorate

- Remove the headboard and any furniture at the head of the bed *to provide ample working space*. Then carefully place the patient's head on a board or on a padded headrest that extends beyond the edge of the bed.
- Never put the patient's head on a pillow before applying the halo *to avoid further injury to the spinal cord*.
- Elevate the bed to a working level that gives the doctor easy access to the front and back of the halo unit.

All ducks in a row

Stand at the head of the bed and see if the patient's chin lines up with his midsternum, indicating proper alignment. If ordered, support the patient's head in your hands and gently rotate the neck into alignment without flexing or extending it.

Assisting with halo application

- Ask another nurse to help you with the procedure.
- Explain the procedure to the patient and family, perform hand hygiene, and provide privacy.

Start with support . . .

- Have the assisting nurse hold the patient's head and neck stable while the doctor removes the cervical collar or sandbags. Maintain this support until the halo is secure while you assist with pin insertion.
- The doctor measures the patient's head with a tape measure and refers to the halo ring conversion chart to determine the correct ring size. (The ring should clear the head by ⅔″ [1.5 cm] and fit ½″ [1.3 cm] above the bridge of the nose.)
- The doctor selects four pin sites: ½″ above the lateral one-third of each eyebrow and ½″ above the top of each ear in the occipital area. He also takes into account the degree and type of correction needed to provide proper cervical alignment.

. . . Then trim . . .

- Trim the hair at the pin sites with scissors *to facilitate subsequent care and help prevent infection*. Then use 4″ × 4″ gauze pads soaked in povidone-iodine solution to clean the sites.
- Open the halo-vest unit using sterile technique *to avoid contamination*. The doctor puts on the sterile gloves and removes the halo and the Allen wrench. He then places the halo over the patient's head and inserts the four positioning pins *to hold the halo in place temporarily*.

. . . And prepare for pain relief

- Help the doctor prepare the anesthetic. First, clean the injection port of the multiple-dose vial of lidocaine with the alcohol pad. Then, invert the vial so the doctor can insert a 25G needle attached to the 3-mL syringe and withdraw the anesthetic.
- The doctor injects the anesthetic at the four pin sites. He may change needles on the syringe after each injection.
- The doctor removes four of the five skull pins from the sterile setup and firmly screws in each pin at a 90-degree angle to the skull. When the pins are in place, he removes the positioning pins. He then tightens the skull pins with the torque screwdriver.

Applying the vest

After the doctor measures the patient's chest and abdomen, he selects a vest of appropriate size.

Sounds stylish

- Place the sheepskin liners inside the front and back of the vest *to make it more comfortable to wear and to help prevent pressure ulcers.*
- Help the doctor carefully raise the patient while the other nurse supports the head and neck. Slide the back of the vest under the patient and gently lay him down. The doctor then fastens the front of the vest on the patient's chest using Velcro straps.
- The doctor attaches the metal bars to the halo and vest and tightens each bolt in turn *to avoid tightening any single bolt completely, causing maladjusted tension.* When halo-vest traction is in place, X-rays should be taken immediately *to check the depth of the skull pins and verify proper alignment.* (See *Complications of halo-vest traction,* page 370.)

Caring for the patient

- Take routine and neurologic vital signs at least every 2 hours for 24 hours (preferably every hour for 48 hours) and then every 4 hours until stable.
- Notify the doctor immediately if you observe loss of motor function or decreased sensation; *these findings could indicate spinal cord trauma.*

Infection protection

- Check the order. Perform hand hygiene and don gloves. Verify the patient with two patient identifiers.
- Gently clean the pin sites every 4 hours with cotton-tipped applicators dipped in cleaning solution. Rinse the sites with sterile water or normal saline solution *to remove excess cleaning solution.* Then clean the pin sites with povidone-iodine solution or another ordered solution. *Meticulous pin site care prevents infection and removes debris that might block drainage and lead to abscess formation.* Watch for signs of infection—a loose pin, swelling or redness, purulent drainage, pain at the site—and notify the doctor if these signs develop. (See *Homeward bound with halo-vest traction,* page 370.)
- The doctor retightens the skull pins with the torque screwdriver 24 and 48 hours after the halo is applied. If the patient complains of a headache after the pins are tightened, obtain an order for an analgesic. If pain occurs with jaw movement, notify the doctor *because this may indicate that pins have slipped onto the thin temporal plate.*

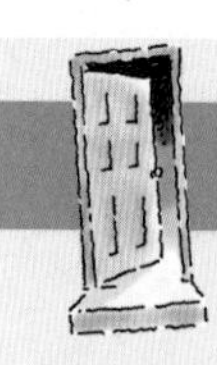

Home care connection

Homeward bound with halo-vest traction

Before the patient goes home in his halo-vest traction, teach him to turn slowly—in small increments—to avoid losing his balance. Remind him to avoid bending forward because the extra weight of the halo apparatus could cause him to fall. Teach him to bend at the knees rather than the waist.

One size up
Have a physical therapist teach the patient how to use assistive devices to extend his reach and to help him put on socks and shoes. Suggest that he wear shirts that button in front and that are larger than usual to accommodate the halo vest.

Rinse, lather, repeat
Most important, teach the patient about pin site care and about shampooing and hair care.

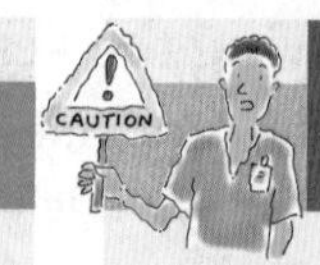

WARNING!

Complications of halo-vest traction

Manipulating the patient's neck during application of halo-vest traction may cause subluxation of the spinal cord. Or it could push a bone fragment into the spinal cord, possibly compressing the cord and causing paralysis below the break.

And that's not all
Inaccurate positioning of the skull pins can lead to a puncture of the dura mater, causing loss of cerebrospinal fluid and a serious central nervous system infection. Nonsterile technique during halo-vest application or inadequate pin site care can lead to infection at the pin sites. Pressure ulcers can develop if the vest fits poorly or chafes the skin.

Two-finger test

Examine the halo-vest unit every shift *to make sure that everything is secure and that the patient's head is centered within the halo*. If the vest fits correctly, you should be able to insert one or two fingers under the jacket at the shoulder and chest when the patient is lying supine.

Wash and wear

- Wash the patient's chest and back daily.
- Perform hand hygiene and don gloves. Verify the correct patient using two patient identifiers.
- Place the patient on his back or side.
- Unbuckle one side of the vest while maintaining cervical spine alignment if permitted per facility policy.
- Assess the patient's skin and ensure the sheepskin lining is not wrinkled or wet *because it can cause skin breakdown*. As you press the liner down on the vest, use a flashlight to assess the skin. *Patients with decreased sensation are at greater risk skin breakdown.*
- Bathe the skin with soap and water. If you are not permitted to unbuckle the vest, slide a damp towel between the liner and the skin to wash all skin surfaces. Dry the skin thoroughly. *Avoid lotion or powder because it can cause matting of the sheepskin.* However, if the patient is itching, a light dusting or cornstarch can be used.
- Rebuckle the vest then turn the patient on the other side and repeat the bathing procedure.

- Discard supplies, remove gloves, and perform hand hygiene. (See *Documenting halo-vest traction.*)
- If your facility's policy allows, change the vest lining as necessary.
- Be careful not to put any stress on the apparatus, *which could knock it out of alignment and lead to subluxation of the cervical spine.*

Practice pointers

Never lift the patient up by the vertical bars. This could strain or tear the skin at the pin sites or misalign the traction.

Mr. (or Ms.) Goodwrench

- Keep two conventional wrenches available at all times. In case of cardiac arrest, use them to remove the distal anterior bolts. Pull the two upright bars outward. Unfasten the Velcro straps and remove the front of the vest. Use the sturdy back of the vest as a board for cardiopulmonary resuscitation (CPR). *To prevent subluxating the cervical injury,* start CPR with the jaw-thrust maneuver, which avoids hyperextension of the neck. Pull the patient's mandible forward while maintaining proper head and neck alignment. *This pulls the tongue forward to open the airway.*
- *To prevent falls,* walk with the ambulatory patient. Remember, he'll have trouble seeing objects at or near his feet and the weight of the halo-vest unit (about 10 lb [4.5 kg]) may throw him off balance. If the patient is in a wheelchair, lower the leg rests *to prevent the chair from tipping backward.*

Breath check

Because the vest limits chest expansion, routinely assess pulmonary function, especially in a patient with pulmonary disease. (See *Documenting halo-vest traction.*)

Patient and family education

- Educate the patient and family that pins transmit vibration and can cause a cold sensation to the head.
- Teach the family how to do pin care and have them perform a return demonstration.
- Instruct the patient/family to notify the physician immediately if the halo vest or pins become loose and *not* to try and fix it themselves.
- Instruct the family to notify the physician immediately if there is a change in neurologic function, difficulty swallowing, or an increase in pain.

Documenting halo-vest traction

In your notes, document:
- date and time of halo-vest traction application and physician who performed the procedure
- type, model, and size of halo vest
- length of the procedure
- patient's response to the procedure
- patient education
- X-ray obtained.

Post procedure—monitoring and care
- routine and neurologic vital signs
- neurologic and spinal cord assessment per facility policy
- pin site care
- bathing and skin care
- skin assessment
- signs and symptoms of infection
- integrity of the halo vest and ring
- liner changes
- pain assessment and medications
- complications and nursing actions
- patient teaching provided for home care.

Pain management

Several interventions can be used to manage pain. These include analgesic administration, emotional support, comfort measures, and cognitive techniques to distract the patient. Severe pain usually requires a narcotic analgesic. Invasive measures, such as epidural analgesia or patient-controlled analgesia (PCA), may also be required.

What you need

Pain assessment tool or scale ✳ oral hygiene supplies ✳ water ✳ nonnarcotic analgesic (such as acetaminophen or aspirin) ✳ optional: PCA device, mild narcotic (such as oxycodone or codeine), strong narcotic (such as methadone, levorphanol, morphine, or hydromorphone), muscle relaxants, antidepressants.

How to assess pain

To assess pain properly, you must consider both the patient's description and your observations of his physical and behavioral responses. Start by asking him to rank his pain on a scale of 0 to 10, with 0 denoting lack of pain and 10 denoting the worst pain imaginable. Besides establishing a baseline, this will help him evaluate pain therapies verbally. In children, use a FACES pain scale to rate their pain. The child can point to the face, with a frown a 10 and a large smile a 0. For children who aren't able to select a face, the nurse should rate them based on their facial expressions and body language using the FACES scale.

Key questions

Next, ask the patient the following questions:

- Where is the pain located?
- How long does the pain last?
- How often does it occur?
- Can you describe the pain?
- What relieves the pain?
- What makes the pain worse?

Bear in mind that his experiences, self-image, and beliefs about his condition will influence his answers to these questions.

Other clues

Observe the patient's behavioral responses to pain. Also note physiologic responses, which may be sympathetic or parasympathetic.

Behavioral responses include altered body position, moaning, sighing, grimacing, withdrawal, crying, restlessness, muscle twitching, and immobility.

Sympathetic responses—commonly associated with mild to moderate pain—include pallor, elevated blood pressure, dilated pupils, skeletal muscle tension, dyspnea, tachycardia, and diaphoresis.

Parasympathetic responses—commonly associated with severe, deep pain—include pallor, decreased blood pressure, bradycardia, nausea and vomiting, weakness, dizziness, and loss of consciousness.

How you do it

- Verify the correct patient with two patient identifiers.
- Explain to the patient how pain medications work together with other pain management therapies to provide relief. Also explain that management aims to keep pain at a low level to permit optimal bodily function.
- Assess the patient's pain by asking to rate his pain on a scale of 1 to 10, in which 10 is the worst pain imaginable. Note his response to the pain and ask him to describe its duration, severity, and source. Look for physiologic or behavioral clues to the pain's severity. (See *How to assess pain.*)

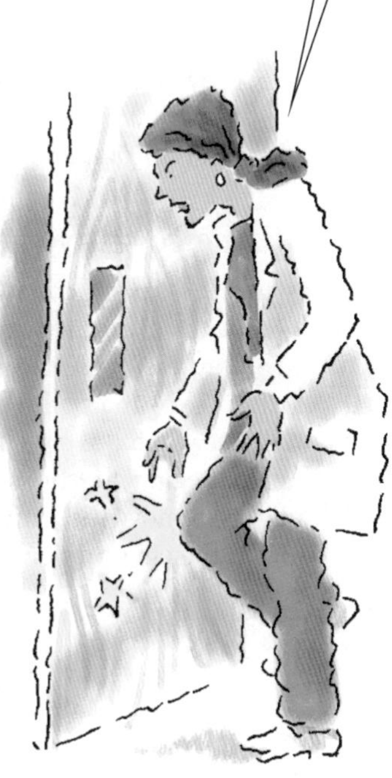
On a scale of 0 to 10, I'd give it an OUCH!

Partners in pain management

- Work with the patient to develop a plan of care that uses interventions that fit the patient's lifestyle. These may include prescribed medications, emotional support, comfort measures, cognitive techniques, and education about pain and its management. Emphasize the importance of maintaining good bowel habits, respiratory function, and mobility *because pain increases problems in these areas.*
- Implement your plan of care. Because individuals respond to pain differently, you'll find that what works for one person may not work for another.

Giving medications

- Check the patient's orders.
- If the patient is allowed oral intake, begin with a nonnarcotic analgesic, such as acetaminophen or aspirin, every 4 to 6 hours as ordered.
- If the patient needs more relief than a nonnarcotic analgesic provides, you may give a mild narcotic (such as oxycodone or codeine) as ordered.
- If the patient needs still more pain relief, you may administer a strong narcotic (such as morphine) as prescribed. Administer oral medications if possible. Check the appropriate drug information for each medication given.
- If ordered, teach the patient how to use a PCA device. *Such a device can help the patient manage his pain and decrease his anxiety.*
- If ordered, use antidepressants as adjuvants for pain control and muscle relaxants for muscle spasms.

Providing emotional support

Show your concern by spending time talking with the patient. Because of his pain and his inability to manage it, the patient may be anxious and frustrated. Such feelings can worsen his pain.

Performing comfort measures

- Periodically reposition the patient *to reduce muscle spasms and tension and to relieve pressure on bony prominences*. Increasing the angle of the bed can reduce pull on an abdominal incision, diminishing pain. If appropriate, elevate a limb *to reduce swelling, inflammation, and pain*.
- Give the patient a back massage *to help relax tense muscles*.
- Perform passive range-of-motion exercises *to prevent stiffness and further loss of mobility, relax tense muscles, and provide comfort*.
- Provide oral hygiene. Keep a fresh water glass or cup at the bedside *because many pain medications tend to dry the mouth*.
- Wash the patient's face and hands.

Using cognitive therapy

Help the patient enhance the effect of analgesics by using such techniques as distraction, guided imagery, deep breathing, and relaxation. You can easily use these "mind-over-pain" techniques at the bedside. Choose the method the patient prefers. If possible, start these techniques when the patient feels little or no pain. If he feels persistent pain, begin with short, simple exercises. Before beginning, dim the lights, remove the patient's restrictive clothing, and eliminate noise from the environment.

A brief get-away

For *distraction*, have the patient recall a pleasant experience or focus his attention on an enjoyable activity. For instance, he can use music as a distraction by turning on the radio when the pain begins. Have him close his eyes and concentrate on listening, raising or lowering the volume as his pain increases or subsides. Note, however, that distraction is usually effective only against brief pain episodes lasting less than 5 minutes.

Hey! This guided imagery is really powerful!

Without ever leaving the house

- For *guided imagery*, help the patient concentrate on a peaceful, pleasant image such as a walk on the beach. Encourage him to concentrate on the details of the image he has selected by asking about its sight, sound, smell, taste, and touch. If available, use audiotapes of sounds to help with guided imagery. The positive emotions evoked by this exercise minimize pain.
- For *deep breathing*, have the patient stare at an object and then slowly inhale and exhale as he counts aloud to maintain a comfortable rate and rhythm. Have him concentrate on the rise and fall of his abdomen. Encourage him to feel more and more weightless with

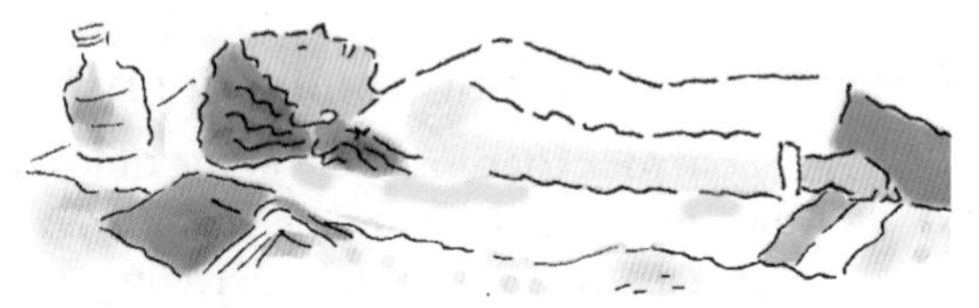

each breath while he concentrates on the rhythm of his breathing or on any restful image.

Focus, tense, relax

For *muscle relaxation*, have the patient focus on a particular muscle group. Then ask him to tense the muscles and note the sensation. After 5 to 7 seconds, tell him to relax the muscles and concentrate on the relaxed state. Have him note the difference between the tense and relaxed states. After he tenses and relaxes one muscle group, have him proceed to another and another until he has covered his entire body.

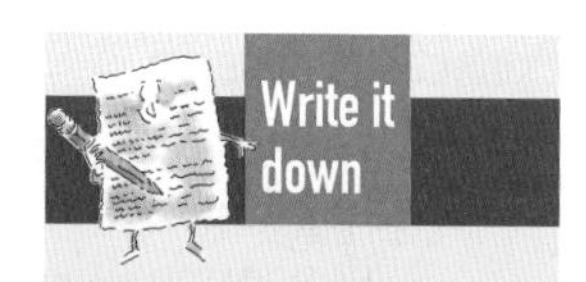

Documenting pain management

Document pain as a fifth vital sign, recording it as frequently as other vital signs. In your notes, record:

- each step of the nursing process
- subjective information elicited from the patient, using his own words
- location, quality, and duration of pain
- precipitating factors
- pain relief method used
- nursing interventions and patient's responses
- alternative treatments to consider the next time pain occurs (if pain wasn't relieved)
- complications of drug therapy.

Practice pointers

- Evaluate your patient's response to pain management. If he's still in pain, reassess him and alter your plan of care as appropriate.
- Remember that patients receiving narcotic analgesics could develop tolerance, dependence, or addiction. Patients with acute pain may have a smaller risk of dependence or addiction than patients with chronic pain.

Danger signs

- If a patient receiving a narcotic analgesic experiences abstinence syndrome when the drug is withdrawn abruptly, suspect physical dependence. The signs and symptoms include anxiety, irritability, chills and hot flashes, excessive salivation and tearing, rhinorrhea, sweating, nausea, vomiting, and seizures. These signs and symptoms are likely to begin in 6 to 12 hours and to peak in 24 to 72 hours. *To reduce the risk of dependence*, discontinue a narcotic analgesic by decreasing the dose gradually each day. Also, you may switch to an oral narcotic and decrease its dose gradually.
- The most common adverse effects of analgesics include respiratory depression (the most serious), sedation, constipation, nausea, and vomiting. (See *Documenting pain management*.)

Seizure management

Seizures are paroxysmal events associated with abnormal electrical discharges of neurons in the brain in response to a stimulus. Partial seizures are usually unilateral, involving a localized or focal area of the brain. Generalized seizures involve the entire brain.

Symptoms can vary widely based on the area of the brain that is affected. Seizures can result in an alteration in sensation, behavior, movement, perception, or consciousness lasting from a few seconds to several minutes.

Protect and observe

When a patient has a generalized seizure, nursing care aims to protect him from injury and prevent serious complications such as aspiration. Appropriate care also includes observation of seizure characteristics to help determine the area of the brain involved.

One step ahead

Certain conditions predispose patients to seizures. These conditions include metabolic abnormalities, such as hypocalcemia, hypoglycemia, and pyridoxine deficiency; brain tumors or other space-occupying lesions; infections, such as meningitis, encephalitis, and brain abscess; traumatic injury, especially if the dura mater was penetrated; ingestion of toxins, such as mercury, lead, or carbon monoxide; genetic abnormalities, such as tuberous sclerosis and phenylketonuria; perinatal injuries; and cerebrovascular accident.

If your patient has a history of seizures or has a condition that increases his risk, take precautionary measures (such as padding

Seizure precautions

By taking appropriate precautions, you can help protect the patient from injury, aspiration, and airway obstruction in the event of a seizure. Plan your precautions using information obtained from his history. For instance, what types of seizures has he previously had? Can he identify exacerbating factors? (Sleep deprivation, missed anticonvulsant doses, and even upper respiratory infections can increase seizure frequency in some seizure-prone patients.)

Gathering equipment

- Based on the patient's history, tailor your precautions to his needs. Start by gathering the appropriate equipment, including a hospital bed with full-length side rails, commercial side rail pads, or six bath blankets (four for a crib). Also gather adhesive tape, an oral airway, and oral or nasal suction equipment.

Preparing the bedside

- Carry out the precautions the patient requires. Keep in mind that a seizure-prone patient admitted for a medication change, infection treatment, or detoxification may be at increased risk for seizures.
- Explain to the patient why the precautions are necessary.
- To protect the patient's arms, legs, head, and feet from injury caused by a seizure while he's in bed, cover the side rails, headboard, and footboard with side rail pads or bath blankets. If you use blankets, secure them with adhesive tape. To prevent falls, always keep the side rails raised while the patient is in bed. Keep the bed in a low position to minimize injuries that may occur if he climbs over the rails.
- Place an airway at the bedside or tape it to the wall above the bed according to your facility's protocol. Keep suction equipment nearby in case you need to establish a patent airway. Explain to the patient how the airway will be used.
- If the patient has a history of frequent or prolonged seizures, prepare an intravenous (I.V.) saline lock to promote emergency medication administration.
- After a seizure, place the patient in a side-lying position to prevent aspiration of oral secretions resulting from a diminished level of consciousness.

the side rails) to help prevent injury if a seizure occurs. (See *Seizure precautions.*)

What you need

Oral airway ✳ suction equipment ✳ side rail pads ✳ optional: normal saline solution, I.V. insertion equipment, oxygen, endotracheal intubation equipment.

How you do it

If you're with a patient when he experiences an aura (a subjunctive sensation preceding a seizure), help him into bed, raise the side rails, and adjust the bed flat. If he's away from his room, lower him to the floor and place a pillow, blanket, or other soft material under his head *to keep it from hitting the floor.*

Keep company

- Stay with the patient during the seizure and be ready to intervene if complications such as airway obstruction develop. A soft plastic airway can be inserted if it's possible to do so without forcing the teeth apart. If necessary, have another staff member obtain the appropriate equipment and notify the doctor of the obstruction.
- Provide privacy, if possible.

No holding back

- Don't forcibly restrain the patient or restrict his movements during the seizure *because the force of the patient's movements against restraints could cause muscle strain or even joint dislocation.*
- Move hard or sharp objects out of the patient's way and loosen his clothing.

Tell the story

- Continually assess the patient during the seizure. Observe the earliest symptom, such as head or eye deviation, as well as how the seizure progresses, what form it takes, and how long it lasts. *Your description may help determine the seizure's type and cause.*
- Following the seizure, the patient may require suctioning *to maintain a patent airway.* Traditionally, nurses have inserted an airway during the seizure; however, it is no longer recommended to force an airway into the patient's mouth. Insert an airway only when there is clear access. If the patient's teeth are clenched, do not attempt to open his mouth *because you can damage teeth or lacerate the mucous membranes.* Never put your fingers in the patient's mouth and do not use a tongue depressor.

First time?

If this is the patient's first seizure, notify the doctor immediately. If the patient has had seizures before, notify the doctor only if the seizure activity is prolonged or if the patient fails to regain consciousness. (See *Understanding status epilepticus*.)

When it's done

- If ordered, establish an I.V. line and infuse normal saline solution at a keep-vein-open rate.
- If the seizure is prolonged and the patient becomes hypoxemic, administer oxygen as ordered. Some patients may require endotracheal intubation.
- For a patient known to be diabetic, administer 50 mL of dextrose 50% in water by I.V. push as ordered.
- For the first few minutes following the seizure (postictal phase), the person may be limp and unresponsive. The pupils will begin to react to light and return to their normal size. After about 5 minutes, the patient will be sleepy, confused, and have difficulty speaking clearly.
- After the seizure, turn the patient on his side and apply suction if necessary *to facilitate drainage of secretions and maintain a patent airway*. Insert an oral airway if needed. Check for injuries and reorient and reassure the patient as necessary.
- After the seizure, monitor vital signs and mental status every 15 to 20 minutes for 2 hours.

Understanding status epilepticus

A state of continuous seizure without intervening periods of consciousness, status epilepticus can occur in any seizure type. The most life-threatening form of status epilepticus is generalized tonic-clonic status epilepticus.

Let's name the causes

Always an emergency, status epilepticus is accompanied by respiratory distress. It can result from abrupt withdrawal of anticonvulsant medications, hypoxic or metabolic encephalopathy, acute head trauma, or septicemia secondary to encephalitis or meningitis. Brain injury can occur in 20 to 30 minutes and irreversible damage can occur in 60 minutes. Death may follow.

Stop the seizure

Emergency treatment usually consists of diazepam, phenytoin, and dextrose 50% I.V. (when seizures result from hypoglycemia).

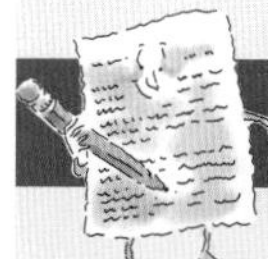

Write it down

Documenting seizure management

In your notes, record:

- patient's need for seizure precautions
- seizure precautions taken
- date and time the seizure began
- seizure duration
- precipitating factors
- sensations the patient reported or experienced before the seizure (possibly part of an aura)
- involuntary behavior at seizure onset, such as lip smacking, chewing movements, or hand and eye movements
- where body movements began and body parts involved
- progression or pattern to body movements
- deviation of the eyes to one side
- change in pupil size, shape, equality, or reaction to light
- whether the patient's teeth were clenched or open
- incontinence, vomiting, or salivation during the seizure
- patient's response to the seizure (for instance, whether he was aware of what happened, fell into a deep sleep afterward, or was upset or ashamed)
- medications given
- complications during the seizure and nursing actions
- patient's postseizure mental status.

- Ask the patient about his aura and activities preceding the seizure. The type of aura (auditory, visual, olfactory, gustatory, or somatic) helps pinpoint the site in the brain where the seizure originated.

Ask the patient what he experienced just before the seizure. That information can provide clues to the seizure's cause.

Practice pointers

- Because a seizure commonly indicates an underlying disorder, such as meningitis or a metabolic or electrolyte imbalance, a complete diagnostic workup will be ordered if the cause of the seizure isn't evident.
- Changes in respiratory function may include aspiration, airway obstruction, and hypoxemia. After the seizure, complete a respiratory assessment and notify the doctor if you suspect a problem. Expect most patients to experience a postictal period of decreased mental status lasting 30 minutes to 24 hours. Reassure the patient that this doesn't indicate incipient brain damage. (See *Documenting seizure management.*)

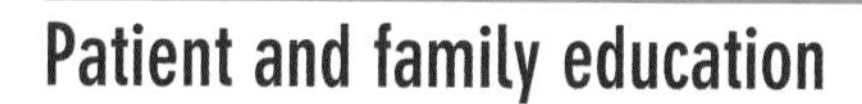

Patient and family education

- Instruct the patient to avoid triggers.
- Explain that stress, fatigue, and illness can potentiate seizures.
- Instruct the patient to stay on his antiepileptic drugs (AEDs).

- Explain that certain medications including herbals and some foods such as grapefruit juice can interact with the medication.
- Tell the family not to force anything into the mouth during a seizure.
- Advise the patient to wear a medical alert bracelet identifying the seizure disorder.
- Advise the patient to contact the state department of motor vehicles to determine driving limitations.
- Teach the patient to avoid caffeine and alcohol and overhydration, which can precipitate a seizure.

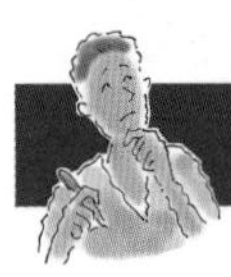

Quick quiz

1. Which intracranial pressure (ICP) waveform is an ominous sign of intracranial decompensation and poor compliance?
   A. A waves
   B. B waves
   C. C waves
   D. D waves

Answer: A. A waves, the most clinically significant ICP waveforms, are an ominous sign of intracranial decompensation and poor compliance.

2. Which is true about caring for a patient with skull tongs?
   A. You can add or subtract weight to enhance patient comfort, and likewise this will increase the patient's recovery time.
   B. If a pin becomes dislodged, immobilize the patient, apply manual traction, and have someone call the doctor immediately.
   C. You may remove the patient from traction for transport to another department, although continuous monitoring is required.
   D. The patient should not be turned or mobilized in order to keep the tongs intact and undisturbed.

Answer: B. If a pin becomes dislodged, this interrupts traction and the patient must receive immediate attention to prevent further injury.

3. When performing CPR on a patient in halo traction, the nurse knows which action should be performed?
   A. Begin CPR using the jaw-thrust maneuver.
   B. Avoid removing the halo vest.
   C. Keep all upright bars intact.
   D. Stabilize patient with the free hand.

Answer: A. For a patient in halo traction, you should begin CPR using the jaw-thrust maneuver to avoid hyperextending the patient's neck, which can cause further injury.

Scoring

☆☆☆ If you answered all three items correctly, super! You're seeing the aura of success.

☆☆ If you answered two items correctly, great! Even a halo vest couldn't slow you down.

☆ If you answered just one item correctly, don't get upset—it only increases ICP. Give the quiz another shot, and all readings are likely to improve.

Selected References

American Association of Neuroscience Nurses. (2011). *Care of the patient undergoing intracranial pressure monitoring/external ventricular drainage of lumbar drainage.* AANN Clinical Practice Guideline Series. Retrieved from http://www.aann.org/pubs/content/guidelines.html

Bickley, L. S. (2012). *Bates' guide to physical examination and history taking* (11th ed.). Philadelphia, PA: Lippincott Williams & Wilkins.

Centers for Disease Control and Prevention. (2010). *Central line insertion practices (CLIP) adherence monitoring.* Retrieved from http://www.cdc.gov/nhsn/PDFs/pscManual/5psc_CLIPcurrent.pdf

Cheever, K. H., & Hinkle, J. L. (2013). *Brunner and Suddarth's textbook of medical-surgical nursing* (13th ed.). Philadelphia, PA: Lippincott Williams & Wilkins.

Ellis, J. R., & Hartley, C. L. (2008). *Managing and coordinating nursing care* (5th ed.). Philadelphia, PA: Lippincott Williams & Wilkins.

Fairchild, S. L. (2013). *Principles and techniques of patient care* (5th ed.). Philadelphia, PA: Elsevier.

Goldman, L., & Schafer, A. I. (2012). *Goldman's Cecil medicine* (24th ed.). Philadelphia, PA: Elsevier.

Gozal, Y., Farley, C., Hanseman, D., et al. (2014). Ventriculostomy-associated infection: A new, standardized reporting definition and institutional experience. *Neurocritical Care, 21*(1), 147–151. doi:10.1007/s12028-013-9936-9

Hadaway, L .C. (1999). I.V. infiltration: Not just a peripheral problem. *Nursing, 29*(9), 41–47.

Hess, C. T. (2007). *Clinical guide to wound care* (6th ed.). Philadelphia, PA: Lippincott Williams & Wilkins.

Hill, M., Baker, G., Carter, D., et al. (2012). A multidisciplinary approach to end external ventricular drain infections in the neurocritical care unit. *Journal of Neuroscience Nursing, 44*(4), 188–193.

Horne, C., & Derrico, D. (1999). Mastering ABGs. The art of arterial blood gas measurement. *American Journal of Nursing, 99*(8), 26–32.

Ignatavicius, D. D., & Workman, M. L. (2012). *Medical-surgical nursing: Patient-centered collaborative care* (7th ed.). St. Louis, MO: Elsevier.

Jagger, J., & Perry, J. (1999). Power in numbers: Reducing your risk of bloodborne exposures. *Nursing, 29*(1), 51–52.

Joint Commission on Accreditation of Healthcare Organizations. (2014). 2015 *Comprehensive accreditation manuals.* Oakbrook Terrace, IL: Author.

Lanken, P. N., Manaker, S., Kohl, B. A., et al. (2013). *The intensive care unit manual.* Philadelphia, PA: Elsevier.

Lippincott. (2012). *Lippincott's nursing procedures* (6th ed.). Philadelphia, PA: Author.

Nicol, M., Bavin, C., Cronin, P., et al. (2012). *Essential nursing skills* (4th ed.). St. Louis, MO: Elsevier.

Perry, A. G., Potter, P. A., & Elkin, M. K. (2011). *Nursing interventions and clinical skills* (5th ed.). St. Louis, MO: Elsevier.

Phillips, L. D., & Gorski, L. (2014). *Manual of I.V. therapeutics* (6th ed.). Philadelphia, PA: F.A. Davis.

Phillips, N. (2013). *Berry & Kohn's operating room technique* (12th ed.). St. Louis, MO: Mosby.

Phippen, M. L., & Wells, M. P. (2000). *Patient care during operative and invasive procedures.* Philadelphia, PA: W.B. Saunders.

Springhouse. (2001). *Diagnostics: An A-to-Z guide to laboratory tests & diagnostic procedures.* Spring House, PA: Author.

Vincent, J., Abraham, E., Kochanek, P., et al. (2011). *Textbook of critical care.* Philadelphia, PA: W.B. Saunders.

Wiegand, D. J. (Ed.). (2010). *AACN procedure manual for critical care* (6th ed.). Philadelphia, PA: Elsevier.

Wound, Ostomy, and Continence Nurses Society. (2010). *Guideline for prevention and management of pressure ulcers.* Mount Laurel, NJ: Author.

Chapter 8

Gastrointestinal care

Just the facts

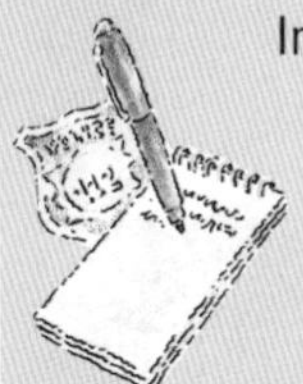

In this chapter, you'll learn:

- about GI procedures and how to perform them
- what patient care is associated with each procedure
- how to manage complications associated with each procedure
- about essential documentation for each procedure.

NG tube insertion and removal

A nasogastric (NG) tube is usually inserted to decompress the stomach and to prevent vomiting after major surgery. It also allows bile and saliva to be removed from the stomach in the event of a bowel obstruction or gastric outlet obstruction. This can occur from adhesions or "scar tissue" from a prior operation, a healed peptic ulcer, or a mass. An NG tube typically is in place for 48 to 72 hours after surgery, by which time peristalsis usually resumes.

And that isn't all

The NG tube can also be used to assess and treat upper gastrointestinal (GI) bleeding, collect gastric contents for analysis, perform gastric lavage, aspirate gastric secretions, and administer medications and nutrients.

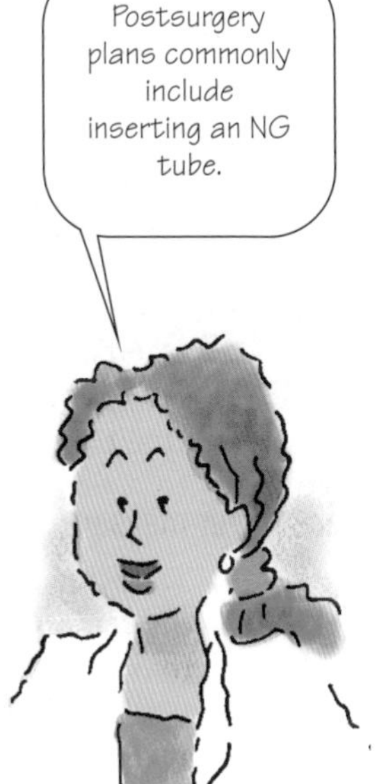
Postsurgery plans commonly include inserting an NG tube.

What you need

For NG tube insertion

Tube (usually #12, #14, #16, or #18 French for a normal adult) ✳ towel or linen-saver pad ✳ penlight ✳ 1″ or 2″ hypoallergenic tape or Opsite ✳ liquid skin barrier ✳ gloves ✳ water-soluble lubricant ✳ cup or glass of water with straw (if appropriate) ✳ stethoscope ✳ tongue blade ✳ catheter-tip or bulb syringe or irrigation set ✳

safety pin ✻ ordered suction equipment ✻ lidocaine hydrochloride topical solution USP 4% (prescribed by a health care provider) ✻ pH strip ✻ optional: metal clamp, ice, alcohol pad, warm water, large basin or plastic container, rubber band.

For NG tube removal

Stethoscope ✻ gloves ✻ catheter-tip syringe ✻ normal saline solution ✻ towel or linen-saver pad ✻ adhesive remover ✻ optional: clamp.

Getting ready

To ease insertion, increase a stiff tube's flexibility by coiling it around your gloved fingers for a few seconds or by dipping it into warm water. Stiffen a limp rubber tube by briefly chilling it in ice or the refrigerator.

How you do it

- **First check the patient's chart for any notation regarding esophageal stricture or varices. Varices are not considered a contraindication, but a stricture usually is.**
- Verify the order in the patient's chart.
- Identify the patient with two patient identifiers per facility policy.
- Provide privacy, perform hand hygiene, and don gloves.

Inserting an NG tube

- Explain the procedure to the patient. Tell him that he may experience some discomfort and swallowing will ease the tube's advancement. Be sure to tell him you will numb the inside (mucosa) of his nostril to eliminate some of the discomfort. Check for any allergies or sensitivity to lidocaine.
- Help the patient into high Fowler's position unless contraindicated.
- Stand at the patient's right side if you're right-handed or at his left side if you're left-handed *to ease insertion*.
- Drape the towel or linen-saver pad over the patient's chest.

Measure for measure

- *To determine how long the NG tube must be to reach the stomach,* hold the end of the tube at the tip of the patient's nose. Extend the tube to the patient's earlobe and then down to the xiphoid process.
- Mark this distance on the tubing with the tape.
- *To determine which nostril will allow easier access,* use a penlight and inspect for a deviated septum or other abnormalities. Generally, it

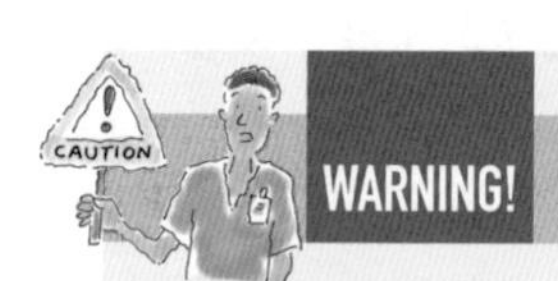

Lidocaine hydrochloride topical solution 4%

Excessive dosage, or short intervals between doses, can result in high plasma levels and severe adverse reactions. Excessive blood levels may cause changes in cardiac output, total peripheral resistance, and mean arterial pressure. The manifestations are hypotension, bradycardia, and cardiovascular collapse and lead to cardiac arrest.

The central nervous system can also be affected and can result in convulsions, confusion, light-headedness, drowsiness, vomiting, tinnitus, blurred or double vision, and respiratory depression and arrest.

is best to use the wider nostril or one that is free from any lesions or mucosal interruptions.

- Apply 1 to 5 mL (40 to 200 mg) of the lidocaine hydrochloride topical solution 4% to a sterile cotton-tipped applicator. The maximum dose should be less than 300 mg or 0.6 to 3.0 mg/kg *to prevent toxicity*. (See *Lidocaine hydrochloride topical solution 4%*.) The lowest dosage to produce the desired anesthesia should be used to prevent high plasma levels and adverse effects. Throw the cotton-tipped applicator out and do *not* use it again. Wait for 5 minutes before inserting the NG tube. Note that the numbness can last from 15 to 60 minutes following application.

- Lubricate the first 3" (7.6 cm) of the tube with a water-soluble gel.
- Instruct the patient to hold his head straight and upright.

Down the hatch

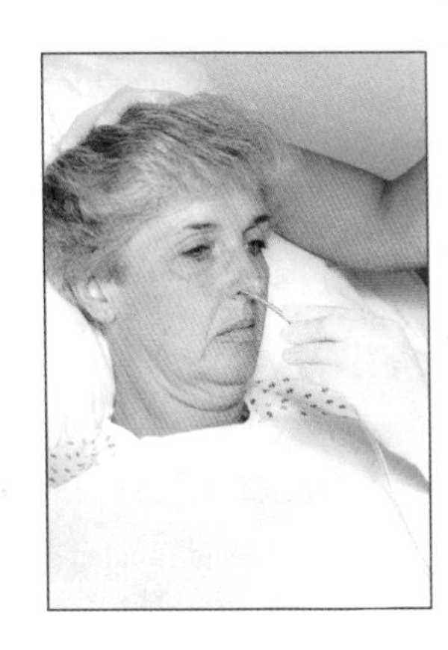

- Grasp the tube with the end pointing downward, curve it if necessary, and carefully insert it into the more patent nostril (as shown at right).
- Aim the tube downward and toward the ear closest to the chosen nostril. Advance it slowly *to avoid pressure on the turbinates and resultant pain and bleeding*.
- When the tube reaches the nasopharynx, you'll feel resistance. Instruct the patient to lower his head slightly *to close the trachea and open the esophagus*. Then rotate the tube 180 degrees toward the opposite nostril *to redirect it so that the tube won't enter the patient's mouth*.

Take a sip

- Unless contraindicated, offer the patient a cup of water with a straw. Direct him to sip and swallow as you slowly advance the tube. *This helps the tube pass to the esophagus.* (If you aren't using water, ask the patient to swallow.)

Ensuring proper tube placement

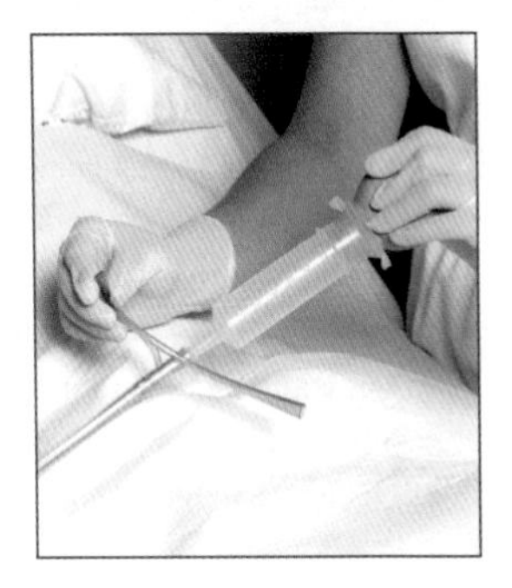

- As you carefully advance the tube and the patient swallows, watch for respiratory distress signs, *which may mean the tube is in the bronchus and must be removed immediately*.
- Stop advancing the tube when the tape mark reaches the patient's nostril.
- Attach a catheter-tip or bulb syringe to the tube and try to aspirate stomach contents (as shown at right). If you don't obtain stomach contents, position the patient on his left side *to move the contents into the stomach's greater curvature* and aspirate again. (See *Confirming NG tube placement*, page 386.)

- If you still can't aspirate stomach contents, advance the tube 1" to 2" (2.5 to 5 cm). Then inject 10 cc of air into the tube. At the same time, auscultate for air sounds with your stethoscope placed over the epigastric region. You should hear a whooshing sound if the tube is patent and properly positioned in the stomach.

  There has been much debate about whether the "auscultatory method" or listening for the whoosh of injected air with your stethoscope is a reliable method. The "whooshing sound" can still be heard if the NG tube is in the distal esophagus, small bowel, or lungs. Upward displacement into the esophagus increases the risk for aspiration and downward displacement increases the risk for feeding intolerance.

  There are many studies that advocate the use of pH paper to confirm the NG tube's placement. A drop of aspirate, after NG tube placement, is placed on an approximate 3" pH strip. A visual reading is made after immediately the aspirate comes in contact with the pH paper. The pH should be documented. The color the aspirate turns the pH paper is compared to a color-coded chart (similar to urinalysis "dip stick"). pH readings using color-coded pH paper were often effective in differentiating between gastric and intestinal placement. A fasting pH of 5 or less means that it is in the stomach,

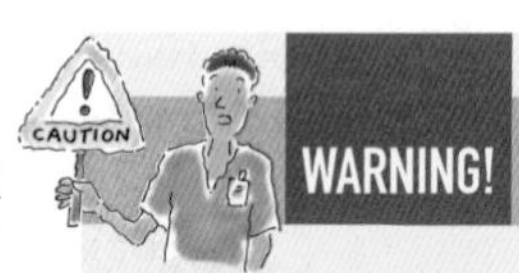

Confirming NG tube placement

When confirming NG tube placement, never place the tube's end in a container of water. If the tube is malpositioned in the trachea, the patient may aspirate water. Besides, water without bubbles doesn't confirm proper placement. Instead, the tube may be coiled in the trachea or the esophagus.

American Association of Critical Care Nurses Practice Alert

Verification of Feeding Tube Placement

- Use a variety of bedside methods to predict tube location ***during*** the insertion procedure:
  - Observe for signs of respiratory distress.
  - Use capnography if available.
  - Measure pH of aspirate from tube if pH-strips are available.
  - Observe visual characteristics of aspirate from the tube.
  - Recognize that auscultatory (air bolus) and water bubbling methods are unreliable. [Level B]
- Obtain radiographic confirmation of correct placement of any blindly inserted tube prior to its initial use for feedings or medication administration.
  - The radiograph should visualize the entire course of the feeding tube in the gastrointestinal tract and should be read by a radiologist to avoid errors in interpretation. Mark and document the tube's exit site from the nose or mouth immediately after radiographic confirmation of correct tube placement. [Level A]
- Check tube location at 4-hour intervals after feedings are started:
  - Observe for a change in length of the external portion of the feeding tube (as determined by movement of the marked portion of the tube).
  - Review routine chest and abdominal x-ray reports to look for notations about tube location.
  - Observe changes in volume of aspirate from feeding tube.
  - If pH strips are available, measure pH of feeding tube aspirates if feedings are interrupted for more than a few hours.
  - Observe the appearance of feeding tube aspirates if feedings are interrupted for more than a few hours.
  - Obtain an x-ray to confirm tube position if there is doubt about the tube's location. [Level B]

Revised 12/2009

and a pH of 6 and above indicates a small bowel placement. Please keep in mind that if a patient is on a proton pump inhibitor, antacid, or a H2 receptor antagonist, the patient's pH may be altered, but studies suggest that it still tests at 5 or below on pH paper. Respiratory secretions have a pH of 6 that is why X-ray confirmation of placement is recommended. pH testing is not a reliable method for eliminating esophageal placement either but is urged to be used to eliminate repeat X-rays to see if the tube is advancing from the stomach to small bowel before a final confirmatory X-ray is ordered. An example of the brand of pH paper used is pHydrion but varies with institution. It is important to check your nursing unit's guidelines for the collection procedure for fluid to be tested.

- If these tests don't confirm proper tube placement, you'll need X-ray verification. X-ray verification is best in patients who are confused, comatose, intubated, in the intensive care unit (ICU), or who have swallowing problems. (See *American Association of Critical Care Nurses Practice Alert.*)

Nobody move

- Secure the NG tube to the patient's nose with hypoallergenic tape (or other designated tube holder). If the patient's skin is oily, wipe the bridge of his nose with an alcohol pad and allow to dry. Apply liquid skin barrier, or benzoin, *to make the tape more adherent to the skin*. You'll need about 4" (10 cm) of 1" tape. Split one end of the tape up the center about 1½" (3.8 cm). Make tabs on the split ends (by folding sticky sides together). Stick the uncut tape end on the patient's nose so that the split in the tape starts about ½" (1.3 cm) to 1½" from the tip of his nose. Crisscross the tabbed ends around the tube. Then apply another piece of tape over the bridge of the nose to secure the tube.
- Alternatively, stabilize the tube with Opsite or a prepackaged product that secures and cushions it at the nose.
- *To reduce discomfort from the weight of the tube*, tie a slipknot around the tube with a rubber band and then secure the rubber band to the patient's gown with a safety pin or wrap another piece of tape around the end of the tube and leave a tab. Then fasten the tape tab to the patient's gown.
- Attach the tube to suction equipment, if ordered, and set the designated suction pressure.

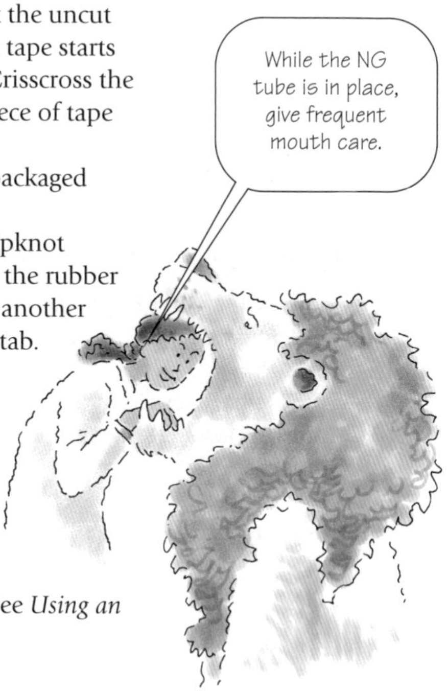

While the NG tube is in place, give frequent mouth care.

I'll be back

- Provide frequent nose and mouth care while the tube is in place.
- An NG tube may be inserted or removed at home. (See *Using an NG tube at home*, page 388.)

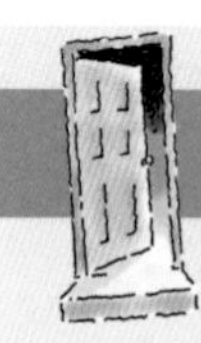

Home care connection

Using an NG tube at home

If your patient will have an NG tube in place at home, find out who will insert the tube. If he will have a home care nurse, tell him when to expect her.

Make a list; check it twice

If the patient or a family member will perform the procedure, you'll need to provide additional instruction and supervision. Use this checklist to prepare teaching topics:

- ☑ how and where to obtain equipment needed for home intubation
- ☑ how to insert the tube
- ☑ how to verify tube placement by aspirating stomach contents
- ☑ how to correct tube misplacement
- ☑ how to prepare formula for tube feeding
- ☑ how to store formula, if appropriate
- ☑ how to administer formula through the tube
- ☑ how to remove and dispose of an NG tube
- ☑ how to clean and store a reusable NG tube
- ☑ how to use the NG tube for gastric decompression, if appropriate
- ☑ how to set up and operate suctioning equipment
- ☑ how to troubleshoot suctioning equipment
- ☑ how to perform mouth care and other hygienic procedures.

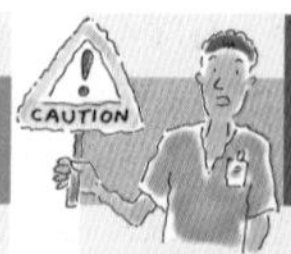

WARNING!

Complications of NG intubation

Although NG intubation is a common procedure, it does carry risks.

Long-term concerns

Potential complications of prolonged intubation include the following:

- esophagitis
- esophagotracheal fistula
- gastric ulceration
- gastritis
- vocal cord paralysis
- pulmonary and oral infection
- sinusitis
- epistaxis
- skin erosion at the nostril.

Suction reactions

Additional complications of suction include electrolyte imbalances and dehydration. Vigorous suction may damage the gastric mucosa and cause significant bleeding, possibly interfering with endoscopic assessment and diagnosis.

- Correct intragastric positioning should be confirmed, in addition to initial placement, before each feed, if there is suggestion of tube misplacement (loose tape or portion of visible tube appears longer), following vomiting/coughing, observing decreased oxygen saturation, and if the patient complains of discomfort or dislodgment.

Removing an NG tube

- Verify the order in the patient's medical record.
- Identify the patient using two patient identifiers per the facility policy.
- Explain the procedure to the patient and that it may cause some discomfort.
- Assess bowel function by auscultating for peristalsis or flatus.
- Help the patient into semi-Fowler's position. Then drape a towel or linen-saver pad across her chest *to protect her from spills.*
- *Get a few pieces of dry gauze to wipe the patient's nose after tube removal.*
- Don gloves. Using a catheter-tip syringe, flush the tube with 10 mL of normal saline solution *to ensure that the tube doesn't contain stomach contents that could irritate tissues during tube removal.*

- Untape the tube from the patient's nose and then unpin it from her gown.
- Clamp the tube by folding it in your hand.

Pull slowly, then quickly

- Ask the patient to hold her breath *to close the epiglottis*. Then withdraw the tube gently and steadily. (When the distal end of the tube reaches the nasopharynx, you can pull it quickly.)
- Assist the patient with thorough mouth care and clean the tape residue from her nose with adhesive remover.
- Monitor the patient for signs of GI dysfunction.

Documenting NG tube insertion and removal

In your notes, record:

- patient education
- type and size of the NG tube
- anesthetic medication and amount—also needs documented on the medication administration record (MAR)
- insertion date and time
- type and amount of suction, if used
- drainage characteristics, including amount, color, character, consistency, and odor
- pH of the aspirate
- patient's tolerance of the procedure.

Do it again

When you remove the tube, record:

- removal date and time
- color, consistency, and amount of gastric drainage
- patient's tolerance of the procedure.

Practice pointers

- If the patient has a nasal condition that prevents nasal insertion, pass the tube orally after removing any dentures, if necessary. First, coil the end of the tube around your hand. *This helps curve and direct the tube downward at the pharynx.*

Down the wrong pipe

- While advancing the tube, observe for signs that it has entered the trachea, such as choking or breathing difficulties in a conscious patient and cyanosis in an unconscious patient or a patient without a cough reflex. If these signs occur, remove the tube immediately. Allow the patient time to rest; then try to reinsert the tube. If you use the opposite nostril and want to numb the area, you need to determine what dosage was already given and subtract from the maximum dosage for the amount you can give the patient. The total dosage cannot exceed the maximum dose. If you gave 5 mL (200 mg) the first time, you can only give up to 100 mg in the second nostril.
- After tube placement, vomiting suggests tubal obstruction or incorrect position. Assess immediately to determine the cause. (See *Complications of NG intubation* and *Documenting NG tube insertion and removal*.)

Nasogastric tube care

Providing effective NG tube care requires meticulous monitoring of both the patient and the equipment.

Monitoring the patient involves checking drainage from the NG tube and assessing GI function. Monitoring the equipment involves verifying correct tube placement and irrigating the tube to ensure patency and to prevent mucosal damage.

What you need

Irrigant (usually normal saline solution) ✳ irrigant container ✳ 60-mL catheter-tip syringe or bulb syringe ✳ suction equipment ✳ toothbrush and toothpaste ✳ petroleum jelly ✳ ½″ or 1″ hypoallergenic tape ✳ water-soluble lubricant ✳ gloves ✳ stethoscope ✳ linen-saver pad ✳ pH paper ✳ optional: emesis basin.

Getting ready

Make sure the suction equipment works properly. When using a Salem sump tube with suction, connect the larger, primary lumen (for drainage and suction) to the suction equipment and select the appropriate setting, as ordered (usually low constant suction). If the physician doesn't specify the setting, follow the manufacturer's directions. A Levin tube usually calls for intermittent low suction.

How you do it

- Identify the patient using two patient identifiers per facility policy.
- Explain the procedure to the patient and provide privacy.
- Perform hand hygiene and don gloves.

Irrigating an NG tube

- Inject 10 cc of air and auscultate the epigastric area with a stethoscope and aspirate stomach contents *to check correct positioning.*
- Measure the amount of irrigant in the syringe (usually 10 to 20 mL) *to maintain an accurate intake and output record.*
- When using suction with a Salem sump tube or a Levin tube, unclamp and disconnect the tube from the suction equipment.
- Slowly instill the irrigant into the NG tube.
- Gently aspirate the solution with the syringe or connect the tube to the suction equipment, as ordered. Report any bleeding.
- Reconnect the tube to suction after completing irrigation.

Instilling a solution through an NG tube

- If the physician orders *instillation,* inject the solution—don't aspirate it—and record the amount as "intake" on the intake and output record. Ensure the solution is at room temperature *to avoid abdominal cramping.*
- Reattach the tube to suction as ordered.

Documenting NG tube care

- Regularly record NG tube placement confirmation (usually every 4 to 8 hours).
- Keep a precise record of fluid intake and output, including the instilled irrigant in fluid input.
- Track the irrigation schedule and note the actual time of each irrigation.
- Describe drainage color, consistency, odor, and amount.
- Note tape change times and the condition of the nares.

- After attaching the Salem sump tube's primary lumen to suction, instill 10 to 20 cc of air into the vent lumen *to verify patency*. Listen for a soft hiss in the vent. If you don't hear this sound, suspect a clogged tube; recheck patency by instilling 10 mL of normal saline solution and 10 to 20 cc of air in the vent.

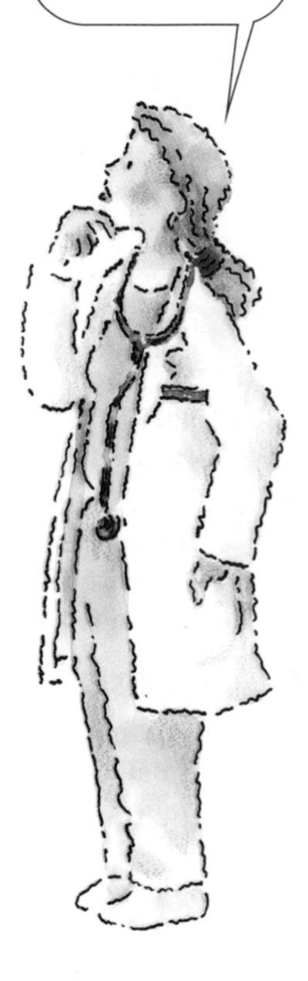
Do you hear
a hiss? If not,
the tube may be
clogged.

Monitoring patient comfort and condition

- Provide mouth care once per shift or as needed.
- Change the tape securing the tube daily or as needed. Clean the skin, apply fresh tape, and dab water-soluble lubricant on the nostrils as needed.
- Assess bowel sounds regularly (every 4 to 8 hours) *to verify GI function*.
- Measure the drainage amount and update the intake and output record every 8 hours. Be alert for electrolyte imbalances with excessive gastric output.
- Inspect gastric drainage and note its color, consistency, odor, and amount. Normal gastric secretions have no color or appear yellow-green from bile and have a mucoid consistency. Immediately report any drainage with a coffee-bean color; *this may indicate bleeding*. If you suspect that the drainage contains blood, use a screening test (such as Hematest) for occult blood according to your facility's policy.

Practice pointers

- Irrigate the NG tube with 30 mL of irrigant before and after instilling medication. Ensure the irrigant is at room temperature. Wait about 30 minutes, or as ordered, after instillation before reconnecting the suction equipment *to allow sufficient time for the medication to be absorbed*. (See chapter 4, "Nasogastric tubes.")

Suction function

- If no drainage appears, check the suction equipment for proper function. Then, holding the NG tube over a linen-saver pad or an emesis basin, separate the tube and the suction source. Check the suction equipment by placing the suction tubing in an irrigant container. If the apparatus draws the water, check the NG tube for proper function. Be sure to note the amount of water drawn into the suction container on the intake and output record.
- If the patient ambulates, disconnect the NG tube from the suction equipment. Clamp the tube *to prevent stomach contents from draining out of the tube*. (See *Documenting NG tube care*.)

Feeding tube insertion and removal

Inserting a feeding tube into the stomach or duodenum allows a patient who can't or won't eat to receive nourishment. The feeding tube also permits administration of supplemental feedings to a patient who has high nutritional requirements, such as an unconscious patient or one with extensive burns. The preferred feeding tube route is nasal, but the oral route may be used for patients with such conditions as deviated septum or a head or nose injury. Research has shown that if a patient needs tube feeds longer than 30 days, a percutaneous endoscopic gastrostomy (PEG) tube is preferred, but this needs to be placed by an endoscopist under conscious sedation. (See "PEG-ing the patient," page 400.)

Feeding tubes can help patients with high nutritional requirements. Waitress!

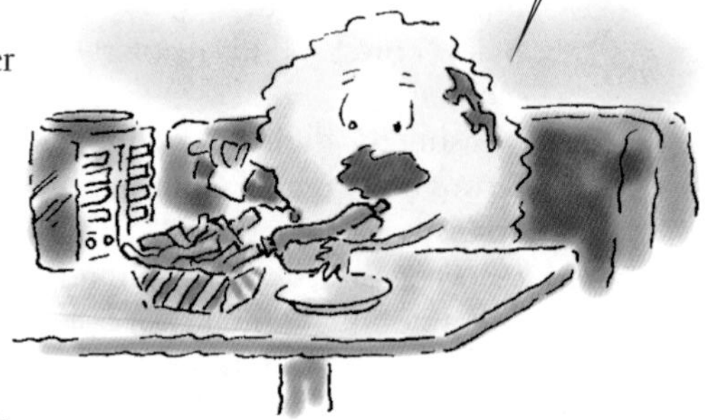

Can't stomach this

The physician may order duodenal feeding when the patient can't tolerate gastric feeding or when he expects gastric feeding to produce aspiration. Absence of bowel sounds or possible intestinal obstruction contraindicates using a feeding tube.

Flexibility rules!

Feeding tubes are made of silicone, rubber, or polyurethane and have small diameters and great flexibility. To ease passage, some feeding tubes are weighted with tungsten, and some need a guide wire to keep them from curling in the back of the throat. These small-bore tubes usually have radiopaque markings and a water-activated coating, which provides a lubricated surface. NG tubes for feeding have a smaller bore than NG tubes used for drainage.

What you need

For insertion

Feeding tube (#6 to #8 French, with or without guide) ✱ linen-saver pad ✱ gloves ✱ hypoallergenic tape ✱ water-soluble lubricant ✱ cotton-tipped applicators ✱ skin preparation (such as tincture of benzoin) ✱ facial tissues ✱ penlight ✱ small cup of water with straw or ice chips ✱ emesis basin ✱ 60-mL syringe ✱ stethoscope ✱ order for lidocaine hydrochloride aqueous solution from the health care provider to enhance patient comfort.

During use

Mouthwash or saltwater solution ✱ toothbrush.

For removal

Gloves ✳ linen-saver pad ✳ tube clamp ✳ bulb syringe.

Getting ready

Have the proper size tube available. Usually, the physician orders the smallest bore tube that will allow free passage of the liquid feeding formula. Read the instructions on the tubing package carefully *because tube characteristics vary according to the manufacturer.*

Check for cracks

Examine the tube to make sure it's free from defects, such as cracks or rough or sharp edges. Next, run water through the tube. This checks for patency, activates the coating, and facilitates guide removal.

How you do it

- Explain the procedure to the patient and show him the tube *so that he knows what to expect and can cooperate more fully.*
- Provide privacy. Perform hand hygiene and put on gloves.
- Assist the patient into semi-Fowler's or high Fowler's position *to prevent aspiration.*
- Place a linen-saver pad across the patient's chest *to protect him from spills.*

When I say so, tuck your chin to your chest. That will close your trachea—and help the tube go into the esophagus.

Inner tube

- *To determine the tube length needed to reach the stomach,* first extend the distal end of the tube from the tip of the patient's nose to his earlobe. Coil this portion of the tube around your fingers *so the end will remain curved until you insert it.* Then extend the uncoiled portion from the earlobe to the xiphoid process. Use a small piece of hypoallergenic tape to mark the total length of the two portions.

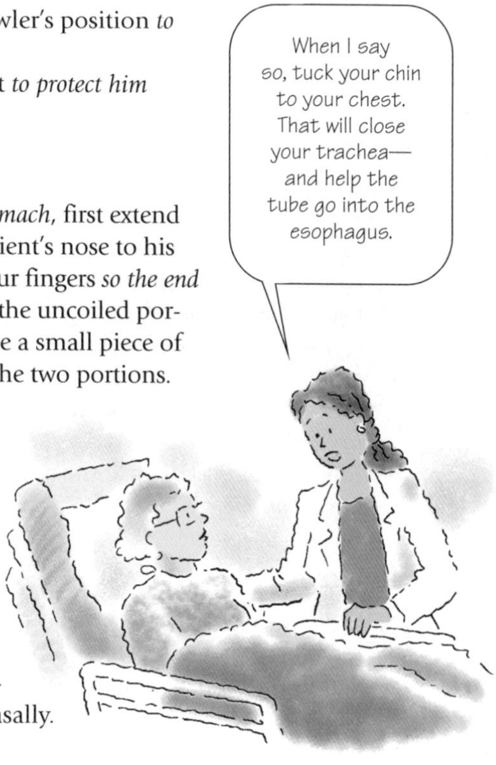

Inserting the tube nasally

- See "Inserting an NG tube," page 384.

Inserting the tube orally

- Have the patient lower his chin *to close his trachea* and ask him to open his mouth.
- Place the tip of the tube at the back of the patient's tongue, give water, and instruct the patient to swallow, as described when inserting nasally. Advance the tube as he swallows.

Positioning the tube

- Keep passing the tube until the tape marking the appropriate length reaches the patient's nostril or lips.

Listen for the whoosh

- *To check tube placement,* attach the syringe filled with 10 cc of air to the end of the tube. Gently inject the air into the tube as you auscultate the patient's abdomen with the stethoscope about 3″ (7.6 cm) below the sternum. Listen for a whooshing sound, *which signals that the tube has reached its target in the stomach.* If the tube remains coiled in the esophagus, you'll feel resistance when you inject the air or the patient may belch.
- If you hear the whooshing sound, gently try to aspirate gastric secretions. Successful aspiration confirms correct tube placement. You can also place a small drop of the gastric aspirate on a 3″ strip of pH paper to check the pH. Any number less than 5.5 means that the contents are acidic and therefore in the stomach. If no gastric secretions return, the tube may be in the esophagus. You'll need to advance the tube or reinsert it before proceeding.

Tale of the tape

- After confirming proper tube placement, remove the tape marking the tube length.
- Tape the tube to the patient's nose and remove the guide wire. *Note:* X-rays should always be ordered to verify tube placement.

Gravity is your friend

- *To advance the tube to the duodenum,* position the patient on his right side. *This lets gravity assist tube passage through the pylorus.* Move the tube forward 2″ to 3″ (5 to 7.6 cm) hourly until X-rays confirm duodenal placement. (An X-ray must confirm placement before feeding begins *because duodenal feeding can cause nausea and vomiting if accidentally delivered to the stomach.*)
- Apply a skin preparation to the patient's cheek before securing the tube with tape. *This helps the tube adhere to the skin and also prevents irritation.*
- Tape the tube securely to the patient's cheek *to avoid excessive pressure on his nostrils.*

Removing the tube

- Verify the order in the patient's medical record.
- Identify the patient using two patient identifiers per facility policy.
- Perform hand hygiene, provide privacy, and don gloves.
- Explain the procedure to the patient.
- Protect the patient's chest with a linen-saver pad.

- Flush the tube with air, clamp or pinch it *to prevent fluid aspiration during withdrawal,* and withdraw it gently but quickly.
- Promptly cover and discard the used tube in the appropriate container per facility policy.
- Wipe the patient's nose with gauze to adsorb any fluid that might come out during withdrawal.

Documenting feeding tube insertion and removal

For tube insertion, record:

- insertion date and time
- patient education
- tube type and size
- insertion site
- placement area
- confirmation of proper placement by indicating two forms of verification; auscultatory (whooshing sound) and pH of aspirate
- name of the person who performed the procedure.

For tube removal, record:

- removal date and time
- patient education
- patient's tolerance of the procedure.

Practice pointers

- Flush the feeding tube every 8 hours with up to 60 mL of normal saline solution or water *to maintain patency*. Retape the tube daily and as needed. Alternate taping the tube toward the inner and outer side of the nose. Inspect the skin for redness and breakdown.
- Provide nasal hygiene daily using the cotton-tipped applicators and water-soluble lubricant *to remove crusted secretions*. Also help the patient brush his teeth, gums, and tongue with mouthwash or a mild saltwater solution at least twice daily.
- When aspirating gastric contents to check tube placement, pull gently on the syringe plunger *to prevent trauma to the stomach lining or bowel*. (See *Documenting feeding tube insertion and removal.*)

Tube feedings

This procedure involves delivery of a liquid feeding formula directly to the stomach (known as gastric gavage), duodenum, or jejunum. Gastric gavage typically is indicated for a patient who can't eat normally because of dysphagia or oral or esophageal obstruction or injury. Gastric feedings also may be given to an unconscious or intubated patient or to a patient recovering from GI tract surgery or patients who have severe GI disease such as inflammatory bowel disease (Crohn's and ulcerative colitis) who can't ingest food orally. It is very important to use the GI tract for feeds in patients who will need them long term to maintain the bowel's integrity, as opposed to total parenteral nutrition (TPN).

Warning: Don't (tube) feed these patients

Tube feeding is contraindicated in patients who have no bowel sounds or suspected intestinal obstructions.

What you need

For gastric feedings

Feeding formula ✳ graduated container ✳ 120 mL of water ✳ gavage bag with tubing and flow regulator clamp ✳ towel or linen-saver pad ✳

60-mL syringe ✱ stethoscope ✱ optional: infusion controller and tubing set (for continuous administration), adapter to connect gavage tubing to feeding tube.

For duodenal or jejunal feedings

Feeding formula ✱ enteral administration set containing a gavage container, drip chamber, roller clamp or flow regulator, and tube connector ✱ intravenous (I.V.) pole ✱ 60-mL syringe with adapter tip ✱ water ✱ optional: pump administration set (for an enteral infusion pump). In general, jejunal feeds will require a pump and may be continuous, whereas NG tube or PEGs usually use gravity and are intermittent, Y-connector.

For nasal and oral care

Cotton-tipped applicators ✱ water-soluble lubricant ✱ petroleum jelly ✱ sponge-tipped applicators.

Getting ready

Be sure to refrigerate formulas prepared in the dietary department or pharmacy. Refrigerate commercial formulas only after opening them. Check the date on all formula containers. Discard expired commercial formula. Use powdered formula within 24 hours of mixing. Always shake the container well to mix the solution thoroughly.

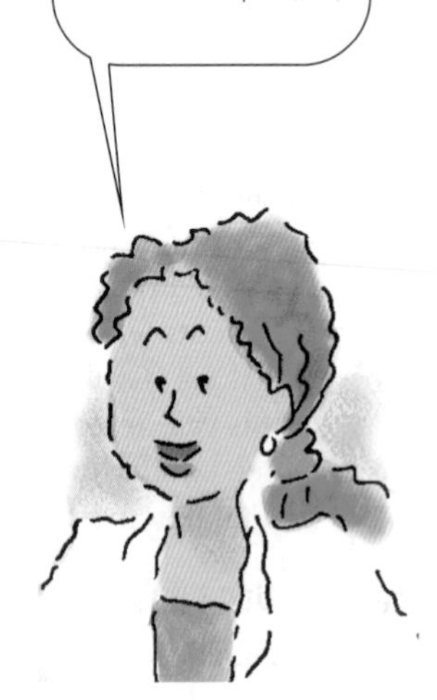
Always serve your powdered formula shaken, not stirred. Shake it up well!

Warm, not hot . . .

Let the formula warm to room temperature before administration. *Cold formula can increase the chance of diarrhea and abdominal cramping.*

Pour 60 mL of water into the graduated container. After closing the flow clamp on the administration set, pour the appropriate amount of formula into the gavage bag. Hang no more than a 4- to 6-hour supply at one time *to prevent bacterial growth.*

Letting the air out

Open the flow clamp on the administration set to remove air from the lines. *This keeps air from entering the patient's stomach and causing distention and discomfort.*

How you do it

- Verify the order in the patient's medical record.
- Identify the patient using two patient identifiers per facility policy.
- Provide privacy and perform hand hygiene.

- Explain the procedure to the patient.
- Cover his chest with a towel or linen-saver pad *to protect him and the bed linens from spills.*
- Assess the patient's abdomen for bowel sounds and distention.

Delivering a gastric feeding

- Elevate the bed to semi-Fowler's or high Fowler's position *to prevent aspiration by gastroesophageal reflux and to promote digestion.*

Tube check

- Check placement of the feeding tube *to be sure it hasn't slipped out since the last feeding.* (See *Before you give that tube feeding.*)
- *To check tube patency and position,* remove the cap or plug from the feeding tube and use the syringe to inject 5 to 10 cc of air through the tube. At the same time, auscultate the patient's stomach with the stethoscope. Listen for a whooshing sound to confirm tube positioning in the stomach. Also aspirate stomach contents and check pH to confirm tube patency and placement.
- *To assess gastric emptying,* aspirate and measure residual gastric contents. Withhold feedings if residual volume is greater than the predetermined amount specified in the physician's order (usually 50 to 100 mL). Reinstill any aspirate obtained.
- Connect the gavage bag tubing to the feeding tube. Depending on the type of tube used, you may need to use an adapter to connect the two.

Something blue

- If you're using a bulb or catheter-tip syringe, remove the bulb or plunger and attach the syringe to the pinched-off feeding tube *to prevent excess air from entering the patient's stomach, causing distention.* If you're using an infusion controller, thread the tube from the formula container through the controller according to the manufacturer's directions. Blue food dye can be added to the feeding *to quickly identify aspiration.* Purge the tubing of air and attach it to the feeding tube.
- Open the regulator clamp on the gavage bag tubing and adjust the flow rate appropriately. When using a bulb syringe, fill the syringe with formula and release the feeding tube *to allow formula to flow through it.* The height at which you hold the syringe will determine the flow rate. When the syringe is three-quarters empty, pour more formula into it. Remember, the syringe height should be *above* the level of the stomach.

No air allowed

- *To prevent air from entering the tube and the patient's stomach,* never allow the syringe to empty completely. Always administer

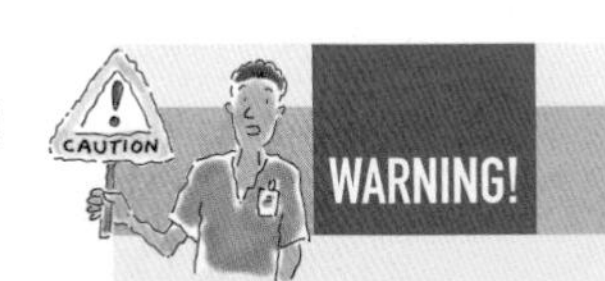

Before you give that tube feeding

Never give a tube feeding until you're sure the tube is properly positioned in the patient's stomach. Administering a feeding through a misplaced tube can cause formula to enter the patient's lungs.

a tube feeding slowly—typically 200 to 350 mL over 15 to 30 minutes, depending on the patient's tolerance and the physician's order—*to prevent sudden stomach distention, which can cause nausea, vomiting, cramps, or diarrhea*. If you're using an infusion controller, set the flow rate according to the manufacturer's directions. (See *Managing tube feeding problems*.)
- After administering the appropriate amount of formula, flush the tubing by adding about 60 mL of water to the gavage bag or bulb syringe or manually flush it using a barrel syringe. *This maintains the tube's patency by removing excess formula, which could occlude the tube.*
- If you're administering a continuous feeding, flush the feeding tube every 4 hours *to help prevent tube occlusion*. Monitor gastric emptying every 4 hours.

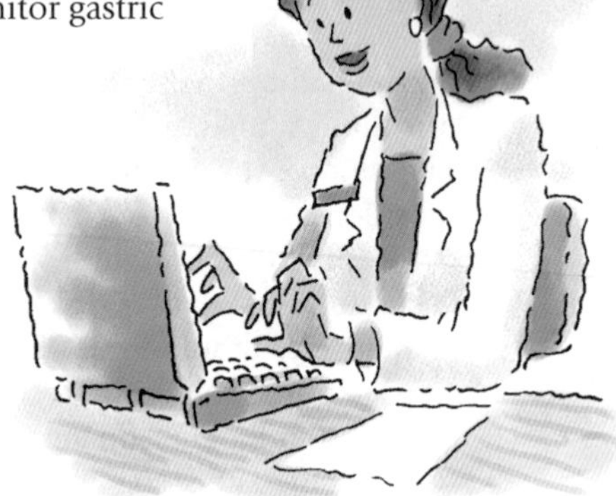
I may type fast, but I always administer tube feedings slowly.

When dinner is done

- To discontinue gastric feeding, close the regulator clamp on the gavage bag tubing, disconnect the syringe from the feeding tube, or turn off the infusion controller.
- Cover the end of the feeding tube with its plug or cap *to prevent leakage and contamination of the tube*.
- Leave the patient in semi-Fowler's or high Fowler's position for at least 30 minutes.
- Rinse all reusable equipment. Dry it and store it in a convenient place. Change equipment every 24 hours or according to your facility's policy.

Delivering a duodenal or jejunal feeding

- Elevate the head of the bed and place the patient in low Fowler's position.
- Open the enteral administration set and hang the gavage container on the I.V. pole.
- If you're using a nasoduodenal tube, measure its length *to check tube placement*. Remember that you may not get any residual when you aspirate the tube.
- Open the flow clamp and regulate the flow to the desired rate. To regulate the rate using a volumetric infusion pump, follow the manufacturer's directions for setting up the equipment. Most patients receive small amounts initially, with volumes increasing gradually once tolerance is established.
- Flush the tube every 4 hours with water *to maintain patency and provide hydration*.

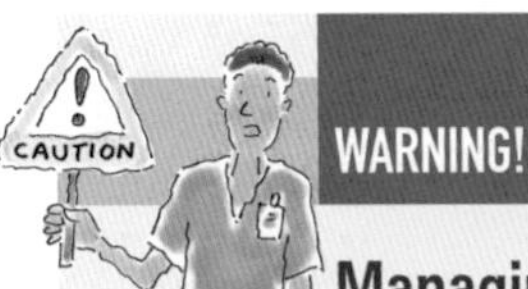

WARNING!

Managing tube feeding problems

Administering a tube feeding isn't always problem-free. If your patient develops complications, you'll need to intervene quickly to avoid serious problems.

Complication	Interventions
Aspiration of gastric secretions	• Discontinue feeding immediately. • Perform tracheal suction of aspirated contents, if possible. • Notify the physician. Prophylactic antibiotics and chest physiotherapy may be ordered. • Check tube placement before feeding to prevent complications.
Tube obstruction	• Flush the tube with warm water. If necessary, replace the tube. • Flush the tube with 50 mL of water after each feeding to remove excess sticky formula, which could occlude the tube. • Use Clog Zapper (it is commercially available and stocked by many pharmacies), which is a syringe with papain and digestive enzymes that requires reconstituting. Then it is instilled into the tube and allowed to "sit" for 30 to 60 minutes per package instructions. Then it is flushed with water to check for patency.
Oral, nasal, or pharyngeal irritation or necrosis	• Provide frequent oral hygiene using mouthwash or moist sponge-tipped swabs. Use petroleum jelly on cracked lips. • Change the tube's position. If necessary, replace the tube.

Practice pointers

- If the patient becomes nauseated or vomits, stop the feeding immediately.
- *To reduce oropharyngeal discomfort from the tube,* provide mouth care.

Something extra

- Drugs can be administered through the feeding tube. (See chapter 4, "Nasogastric tubes.") Keep in mind that some drugs may change the osmolarity of the feeding formula and cause diarrhea.
- For duodenal or jejunal feeding, most patients tolerate a continuous drip better than bolus feedings. *Bolus feedings can cause complications such as hyperglycemia, glucosuria, and diarrhea, which may result in dehydration.* (See *Documenting tube feedings,* page 400.)
- Glucose and electrolytes should be monitored for patients receiving tube feedings. The formulas are usually isotonic (or mimicking the body's natural fluid), but high calorie feeds, which may be

necessary in severe malnutrition or patients with high metabolic demands, are usually hypertonic and "pull water" into the intestine. These patients are typically receiving I.V. normal saline. If they are, while simultaneously getting high calorie, *hypertonic*, tube feeds, they can be at risk for *hypernatremia*. In addition, patients who are receiving I.V. fluids with a lot of *free water* (tube flushes) may be at risk for *hyponatremia*.

Transabdominal tube feedings

To access the stomach, duodenum, or jejunum, the physician may place a tube through the patient's abdominal wall. This procedure may be done surgically or percutaneously. The tube may be used for feeding during the immediate postoperative period or it may provide long-term enteral access. Typically, the physician will suture the tube in place to prevent gastric contents from leaking.

PEG-ing the patient

In contrast, a PEG or percutaneous endoscopic jejunostomy (PEJ) tube can be inserted endoscopically without the need for laparotomy or general anesthesia. A PEG or PEJ tube may be used for nutrition, drainage, and decompression. A PEG is sometimes referred to as a "stomach plug" or "buttons" by laypersons.

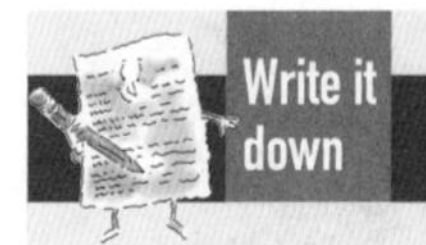

Documenting tube feedings

In your notes, document:

- amount, type, and time of feeding
- abdominal assessment findings (including tube exit site, if appropriate)
- amount of residual gastric contents
- tube placement verification
- tube patency
- patient's tolerance of the feeding, recording such problems as nausea, vomiting, cramping, diarrhea, and distention
- patient's hydration status
- drugs given through the tube
- date and time of administration set changes
- oral and nasal hygiene performed
- results of specimen collections
- blood and urine test results.

On the patient's intake and output sheet, record the date, volume of formula administered, and volume of water administered.

What you need

For feeding

Feeding formula ✳ large-bulb or catheter-tip syringe ✳ 120 mL of water ✳ 4″ × 4″ gauze pads ✳ soap ✳ skin protectant ✳ hypoallergenic tape ✳ gravity drip administration bags ✳ mouthwash, toothpaste, or mild salt solution ✳ gloves ✳ optional: enteral infusion pump.

For decompression

Suction apparatus with tubing and straight drainage collection set.

Getting ready

Always check the expiration date on commercially prepared feeding formulas. If the formula has been prepared by the dietitian or pharmacist, check the preparation time and date. Discard any opened formula that's more than 1 day old.

A winning formula

Commercially prepared administration sets and enteral pumps allow continuous formula administration. Place the desired amount of formula into the gavage container and purge air from the tubing. *To avoid contamination,* hang only a 4- to 6-hour supply of formula at a time.

How you do it

- Verify the order in the patient's medical record.
- Identify the patient with two patient identifiers.
- Provide privacy and perform hand hygiene.
- Explain the procedure to the patient. After he tolerates continuous feedings, he may progress to intermittent feedings, as ordered.
- Assess for bowel sounds before feeding and monitor for abdominal distention.

A sit-down dinner

- Ask the patient to sit, or assist him into semi-Fowler's position, for the entire feeding. *This helps to prevent esophageal reflux and pulmonary aspiration of the formula.* For an intermittent feeding, have him maintain this position throughout the feeding and for 30 minutes to 1 hour afterward.
- Don gloves. Before starting the feeding, measure residual gastric contents. Attach the syringe to the feeding tube and aspirate. If the contents measure more than twice the amount infused, hold the feeding and recheck in 1 hour. If residual contents still remain too high, notify the physician. Chances are the formula isn't being absorbed properly. Keep in mind that residual contents will be minimal with PEJ tube feedings.
- Allow 30 mL of water to flow into the feeding tube *to establish patency.*
- Be sure to administer formula at room temperature. *Cold formula may cause abdominal cramping.*

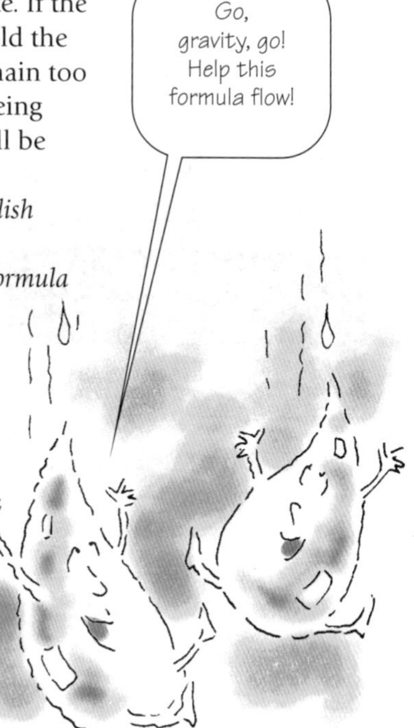
Go, gravity, go! Help this formula flow!

Intermittent feedings

- Allow gravity to help the formula flow over 30 to 45 minutes. *Faster infusions may cause bloating, cramps, or diarrhea.*
- Begin intermittent feeding with a low volume (200 mL) daily. According to the patient's tolerance, increase the volume per feeding as needed *to reach the desired calorie intake.*
- When the feeding finishes, flush the feeding tube with 30 to 60 mL of water. *This maintains patency and provides hydration.*

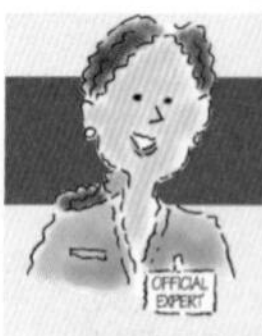

Advice from the experts

Caring for a PEG or PEJ site

The exit site of a PEG or PEJ tube requires routine observation and care. Follow these guidelines:

- Change the dressing daily while the tube is in place.
- After removing the dressing, carefully slide the tube's outer bumper away from the skin about ½″ (1.5 cm), as shown below left.
- Examine the skin around the tube. Look for redness and other signs of infection or erosion.
- Gently depress the skin around the tube and inspect for drainage, as shown below right. Expect minimal wound drainage initially after implantation. This should subside in about 1 week.
- Inspect the tube for wear and tear. A tube that wears out will need replacement.
- Clean the site with the prescribed cleaning solution. Then apply povidone-iodine ointment over the exit site according to your facility's guidelines.
- Rotate the outer bumper 90 degrees (to avoid repeating the same tension on the same skin area) and slide the outer bumper back over the exit site.
- If leakage appears at the PEG site or if the patient risks dislodging the tube, apply a sterile gauze dressing over the site. Don't put sterile gauze underneath the outer bumper. Loosening the anchor this way gives the feeding tube free play, which could lead to wound abscess.
- Record the date and time of the dressing change on the tape.

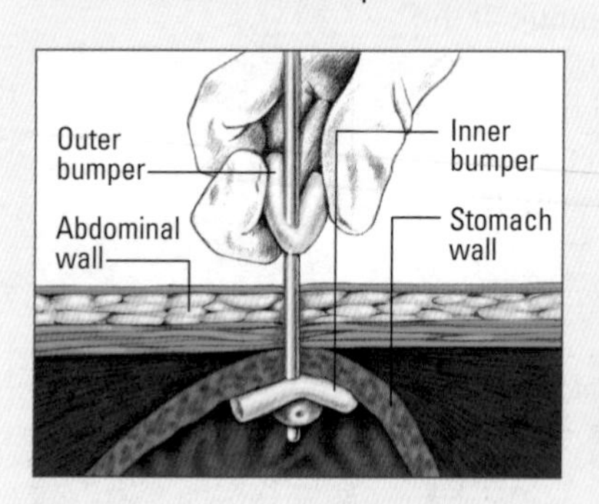

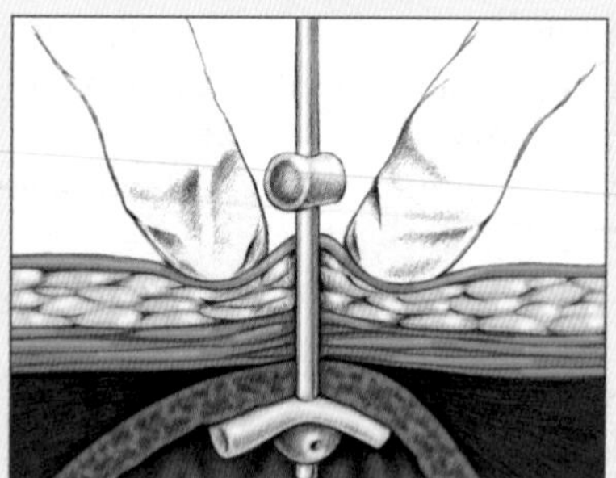

- Rinse the feeding administration set thoroughly with hot water *to avoid contaminating subsequent feedings*. Allow it to dry between feedings.

Continuous feedings

- Measure residual gastric contents every 4 hours.
- To administer the feeding with a pump, set up the equipment according to the manufacturer's guidelines and fill the feeding bag.

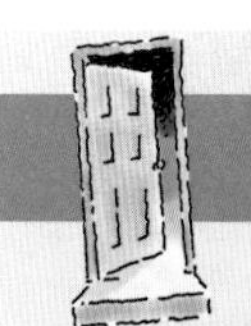

Home care connection

Teaching about syringe feedings

If the patient will feed himself by syringe when he returns home, you'll need to provide instructions about this procedure before discharge. Be sure to teach him how to:

- clamp the feeding tube
- place the syringe tip into the feeding tube
- flush the tube with water to verify patency
- pour the feeding solution into the syringe to begin the feeding
- tilt the syringe to let air bubbles escape
- flush the tube when feeding is completed
- clamp the tube
- care for the equipment.

Have the patient or family do a return demonstration to verify understanding. Give the patient a DVD if available that demonstrates the procedure so he can refer to it at home. If the patient and family are unable to do the procedure, consult case management for other options such as home health care.

To administer the feeding by gravity, fill the container with formula and purge air from the tubing.

- Monitor the gravity drip rate or pump infusion rate frequently *to ensure accurate delivery of formula.*
- Flush the feeding tube with 30 to 60 mL of water every 4 hours *to maintain patency and to provide hydration.*
- Monitor intake and output *to anticipate and detect fluid or electrolyte imbalances.*

Decompression

- To decompress the stomach, connect the PEG port to the suction device with tubing or straight gravity drainage tubing. Jejunostomy feeding may be given simultaneously through the PEJ port of the dual-lumen tube.

Tube exit site care

- Provide daily skin care.
- Gently remove the dressing.
- At least daily and as needed, clean the skin around the tube's exit site using a 4″ × 4″ gauze pad soaked in the prescribed cleaning solution. When healed, wash the skin around the exit site daily with soap. Rinse the area with water and pat dry. Apply skin protectant, if necessary, at the exit site *to prevent or treat skin maceration.*

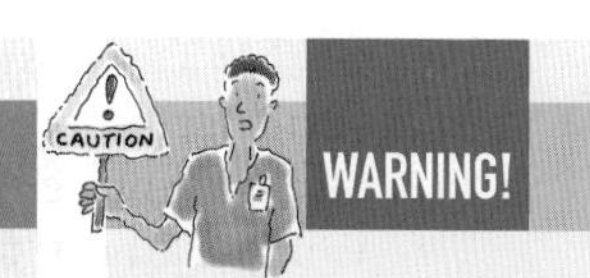

WARNING!

Danger signs during transabdominal feeding

If a patient who is receiving a transabdominal feeding vomits, regurgitates, or complains of nausea or feeling too full, stop the feeding immediately and assess his condition. Then flush the feeding tube. After 1 hour, try to restart the feeding (after measuring residual gastric contents). You may have to decrease the volume or rate of feedings.

Deter dumping

If the patient develops dumping syndrome, the feedings may have been given too quickly. This syndrome causes nausea, vomiting, cramps, flushing, dizziness, increased heart rate, sweating, and diarrhea.

- Anchor a gastrostomy or jejunostomy tube to the skin with hypoallergenic tape *to prevent peristaltic migration of the tube*. This also prevents tension on the suture anchoring the tube in place.
- Coil the tube, if necessary, and tape it to the abdomen *to prevent pulling and contamination of the tube*. PEG and PEJ tubes have toggle bolt–like internal and external bumpers that make tape anchors unnecessary. (See *Caring for a PEG or PEJ site*, page 402.)

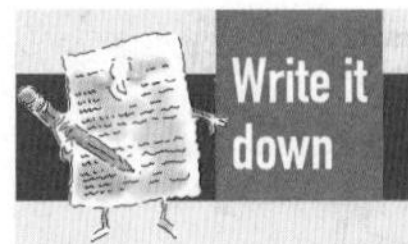

Documenting transabdominal tube feedings

On the patient's intake and output record, note the date, time, and amount of each feeding and the water volume instilled. Keep total volumes for nutrients and water separate to allow the calculation of nutrient intake.

In your notes, document:

- type of formula given
- infusion method
- infusion rate
- patient's tolerance of the procedure and formula
- amount of residual gastric contents
- abdominal assessment findings
- complications
- patient-teaching topics covered
- patient's self-care progress.

Practice pointers

- Assess for abdominal complications. (See *Danger signs during transabdominal feeding*, page 403.)
- Provide oral hygiene frequently.

To crush or not to crush?

- You can administer most tablets and pills through the tube by crushing them and diluting as necessary. (However, don't crush enteric-coated or sustained-release drugs, *which lose their effectiveness when crushed*.) Medications should be in liquid form for administration.

Take-out order

- If the patient is going home with tube feedings, instruct the patient and family members or other caregivers in all aspects of enteral feedings. If appropriate, teach him how to feed himself by the syringe method. (See *Teaching about syringe feedings*, page 403 and *Documenting transabdominal tube feedings*.)

Enema administration

Enema administration involves instilling a solution into the rectum and colon. In a retention enema, the patient holds the solution within the rectum or colon for 30 minutes to 1 hour. In an irrigating enema, the patient expels the solution almost completely within 15 minutes. Both types of enema stimulate peristalsis by mechanically distending the colon and stimulating rectal wall nerves.

Oil retention enemas act by lubricating the rectum and colon, so feces become softer from absorbing the oil. Medicated enemas can be prescribed to reduce high potassium levels (e.g., Kayexalate enema) or to reduce bacteria in the colon (e.g., neomycin enema) prior to bowel surgery.

Enem-ies

Enemas are contraindicated, however, after recent colon or rectal surgery or myocardial infarction and in a patient with an acute abdominal condition of unknown origin (such as suspected appendicitis). They should be administered cautiously to a patient with an arrhythmia.

What you need

Correct volume of warmed (tepid) solution ✳ bath (utility) thermometer ✳ enema administration bag with attached rectal tube and clamp ✳ I.V. pole ✳ gloves ✳ linen-saver pads ✳ bath blanket ✳ two bedpans with covers or bedside commode ✳ water-soluble lubricant ✳ toilet tissue ✳ bulb syringe or funnel ✳ plastic bag for equipment ✳ water ✳ gown ✳ washcloth ✳ soap and water ✳ if observing enteric precautions: plastic trash bags, labels ✳ optional (for patients who can't retain the solution): plastic rectal tube guard, indwelling urinary catheter or Verden rectal catheter with 30-mL balloon and syringe.

Prepackaged disposable enema sets are available, as are small-volume enema solutions in both irrigating and retention types and in pediatric sizes.

Getting ready

Prepare the prescribed type and amount of solution, as indicated. The standard volume of an irrigating enema for an adult is 750 to 1,000 mL. For an adult, warm the solution to 100° to 105° F (37.8° to 40.6° C) *to reduce patient discomfort.*

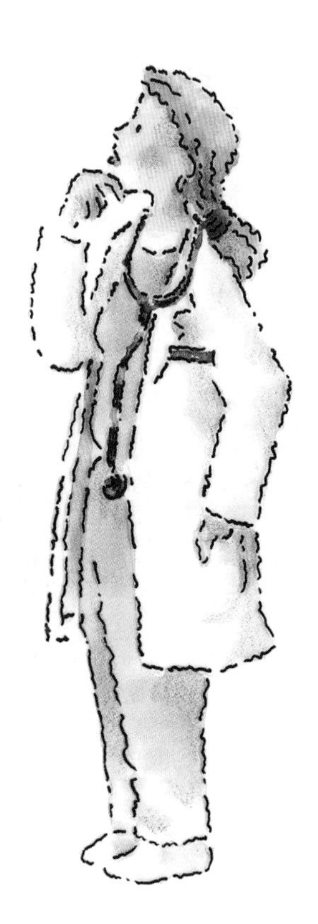

Working toward the right solution

Clamp the tubing and fill the solution bag with the prescribed solution. Unclamp the tubing, flush the solution through the tubing, and then reclamp it. *Flushing detects leaks and removes air that could cause discomfort if introduced into the colon.*

Hang the solution container on the I.V. pole and take all supplies to the patient's room. If you're using an indwelling urinary catheter or Verden catheter, fill the syringe with 30 mL of water.

Note: "Enemas until clear" order means that you repeat the enemas until the patient passes fluid that is clear of fecal material. Usually, you should not give more than three consecutive enemas *because it can cause an electrolyte imbalance.* It is essential to observe the results of the enema. Go slowly in elderly patients who may not tolerate the procedure and notify the physician if unable to proceed until clear.

How you do it

- Check the physician's order and assess the patient's condition.
- Identify the patient using two patient identifiers per facility policy.

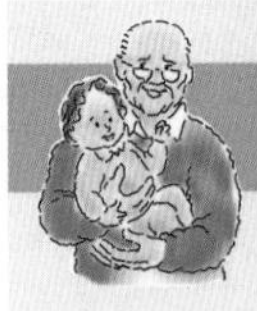

Ages and stages

Giving an enema to a child

Unless contraindicated, help the child into a dorsal recumbent position. After lubricating the end of the tube, separate the child's buttocks and push the tube gently into the anus, aiming it toward the umbilicus. Insert the tube 3″ to 4″ (7.5 to 10 cm) in an adolescent; for a child, 2″ to 3″ (5 to 7.5 cm); for an infant, insert it 1″ to 1½″ (2.5 to 4 cm).

Try this solution

Avoid forcing the tube to prevent rectal wall trauma. If it doesn't advance easily, let a little solution flow in to relax the inner sphincter enough to allow passage.

Standard irrigating enema volumes for pediatric patients are adolescent: 500 to 700 mL; school-age child: 300 to 500 mL; toddler: 250 to 300 mL; infant: 150 to 250 mL.

A matter of degree (and inches)

To avoid burning rectal tissues, don't administer an enema solution that's warmer than 100° F (37.8° C). Be sure not to raise the solution container higher than 12″ (30.5 cm) above bed level for a child or 6″ to 8″ (15 to 20.5 cm) for an infant. Excessive pressure can force colonic bacteria into the small intestine or cause the colon to rupture.

- Provide privacy and explain the procedure to the patient. If you're administering an enema to a child, familiarize him with the equipment and allow a parent or another relative to remain with him during the procedure *to provide reassurance.* (See *Giving an enema to a child.*)
- Instruct the patient to breathe through his mouth *to relax the anal sphincter, which will ease catheter insertion.*
- Perform hand hygiene and put on gloves. If there's a chance you could become soiled, put on a gown.
- Assist the patient into left-lateral Sims' position. *This will facilitate the solution's flow by gravity into the descending colon.* If contraindicated or if the patient reports discomfort, reposition him on his back or right side. If the patient has poor sphincter control, place them on a bedpan during the procedure.

Prep procedures

- Place linen-saver pads under the patient's buttocks *to prevent soiling the linens.* Cover the patient with a bath blanket only exposing the rectal area.
- Have a bedpan or commode nearby for the patient to use. If the patient can use the bathroom, make sure that it will be

available when the patient needs it. Have toilet tissue within the patient's reach.

- Lubricate the distal tip of the rectal catheter with water-soluble lubricant *to facilitate rectal insertion and reduce irritation.*

Contraction reaction

- Separate the patient's buttocks and observe for any abnormalities such as hemorrhoids, anal fissure, and rectal prolapse. *This will influence the approach for inserting the enema tip. An enema is contraindicated if there is a rectal prolapse.*
- Touch the anal sphincter with the rectal tube *to stimulate contraction.* Then, as the sphincter relaxes, tell the patient to breathe deeply through his mouth as you gently advance the tube.
- If the patient feels pain or the tube meets continued resistance, notify the physician. *This may signal an unknown stricture or abscess.*
- You can also use an indwelling urinary or Verden catheter as a rectal tube if your facility's policy permits. This is especially helpful in patients that have anal sphincter dysfunction or incontinence. Insert the lubricated catheter as you would a rectal tube. Then gently inflate the catheter's balloon with 20 to 30 mL of water. Gently pull the catheter back against the patient's internal anal sphincter *to seal off the rectum.* If leakage still occurs with the balloon in place, add more water to the balloon in small amounts. When using either catheter, avoid inflating the balloon above 45 mL *because overinflation can compromise blood flow to the rectal tissues and may cause necrosis from pressure on the rectal mucosa.*
- If you're using a rectal tube, hold it in place throughout the procedure *because bowel contractions and the pressure of the tube against the anal sphincter can promote tube displacement.*

Administer a retention enema at the slowest possible rate.

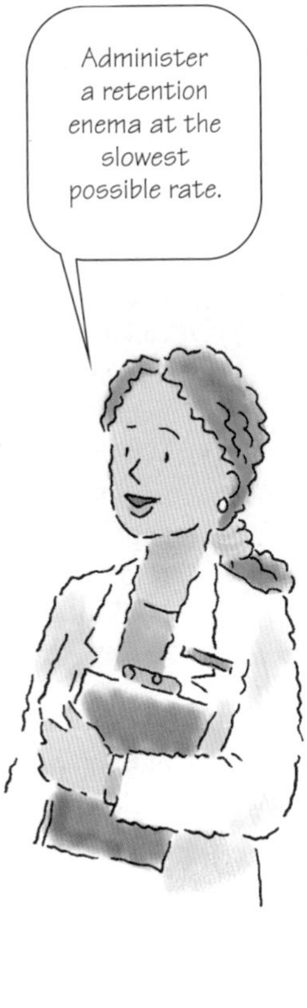

Go with the flow

- Hold the solution container slightly above bed level and release the tubing clamp. Then raise the container gradually to start the flow—usually at a rate of 75 to 100 mL/minute for an irrigating enema, but at the slowest possible rate for a retention enema *to avoid stimulating peristalsis and to promote retention.* Adjust the flow rate of an irrigating enema by raising or lowering the solution container according to the patient's retention ability and comfort. However, be sure not to raise it higher than 18" (46 cm) above bed level for an adult.
- Assess the patient's tolerance frequently during instillation. If he complains of discomfort, cramps, or the need to defecate, stop the flow by pinching or clamping the tubing. Instruct him to breathe slowly and deeply through their mouth *to help relax his abdominal muscles and promote retention.* Resume administration at a slower flow rate after a few minutes when discomfort passes but interrupt the flow any time the patient complains of discomfort.

Sudden slowdown

- If the flow slows or stops, the catheter tip may be clogged with feces or pressed against the rectal wall. Gently turn the catheter slightly *to free it without stimulating defecation*. If the catheter tip remains clogged, withdraw the catheter, flush it with solution, and reinsert it.
- After administering most of the prescribed amount of solution, clamp the tubing. Stop the flow before the container empties completely *to avoid introducing air into the bowel*.
- To administer a commercially prepared, small-volume enema, first remove the cap from the rectal tube. Insert the rectal tube into the rectum and squeeze the bottle *to deposit the contents in the rectum*. Remove the rectal tube, replace the used enema unit in its original container, and discard.
- For a flush enema, stop the flow by lowering the solution container below bed level and allowing gravity to siphon the enema from the colon. Continue to raise and lower the container until gas bubbles cease or the patient feels more comfortable and abdominal distention subsides. Don't allow the solution container to empty completely before lowering it *because this may introduce air into the bowel*.

Time frame

- For an irrigating enema, instruct the patient to retain the solution for 15 minutes, if possible.
- For a retention enema, instruct the patient to avoid defecation for the prescribed time or as follows: 30 minutes or longer for oil retention and 15 to 30 minutes for anthelmintic and emollient enemas. If you're using an indwelling catheter, leave the catheter in place *to promote retention*.
- Position the patient on the bedpan. Place the call signal within his reach. If he'll be using the bathroom or the commode, instruct him to call for help before attempting to get out of bed *because the procedure may make the patient—particularly an elderly patient—feel weak or faint*. Also instruct him to call you if he feels weak at any time.
- When the solution has remained in the colon for the recommended time or for as long as the patient can tolerate it, assist the patient onto a bedpan or to the commode or bathroom, as required.
- If an indwelling catheter is in place, deflate the balloon and remove the catheter, if applicable.

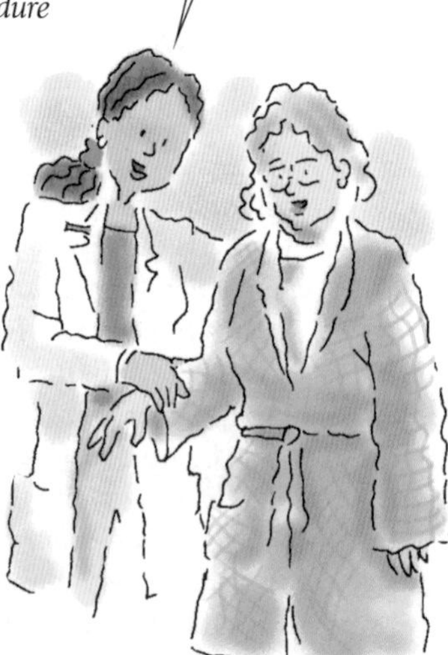
Your patient will need help getting out of bed because the procedure is tiring.

Wrapping it up

- Provide privacy. Instruct the patient not to flush the toilet.
- Assist the patient with cleaning, if necessary, and help him to bed. Place a clean linen-saver pad under him *to absorb rectal drainage, especially if a patient had a mineral oil enema; he may leak oil rectally*.

- Observe the contents of the toilet or bedpan. Carefully note fecal color, consistency, amount, and foreign matter, such as blood, rectal tissue, worms, pus, mucus, or other unusual matter.
- Send specimens to the laboratory, if ordered.
- Rinse and wash the bedpan or commode.
- Properly dispose of the enema equipment. Store clean, reusable equipment. Discard your gloves and gown and perform hand hygiene.

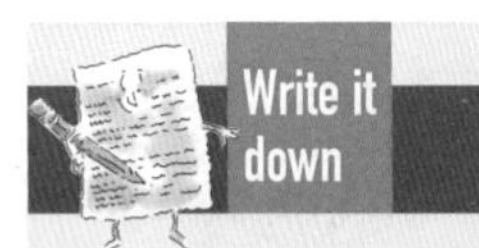

Documenting enema administration

If you have administered an enema, be sure to record:

- date and time of administration
- patient education
- type and amount of solution administered
- special equipment used
- retention time
- approximate amount returned
- color, consistency, and amount of the return
- abnormalities within the return
- complications.

Practice pointers

- Schedule a retention enema before meals *because a full stomach may stimulate peristalsis and make retention difficult*. Follow an oil-retention enema with a soap and water enema 1 hour later *to help expel the softened feces completely*.
- If the patient has hemorrhoids, instruct him to bear down gently during tube insertion. *This causes the anus to open and facilitates insertion*.

A failed solution

- If the patient fails to expel the solution within 1 hour, you may need to remove the enema solution. First, review your facility's policy *because you may need a physician's order*. Then inform the physician. To siphon the enema solution from the patient's rectum, assist him to a side-lying position on the bed. Place a bedpan on a bedside chair so that it rests below mattress level. Disconnect the tubing from the solution container, place the distal end in the bedpan, and reinsert the rectal end into the patient's anus. If gravity fails to drain the solution into the bedpan, instill 30 to 50 mL of warm water (105° F [40.6° C]) for an adult. Then quickly direct the distal end of the tube into the bedpan. In both cases, measure the return *to make sure all of the solution has drained*. (See *Documenting enema administration*.)

Disimpacting a patient

If an enema fails to yield stool or a bowel movement, it is usually necessary to disimpact a patient. This is the manual removal of hard stool from the rectum. Patients usually present with abdominal distention, nausea, vomiting, and constipation, *but* some patients, especially those with dementia, may present with watery stool after being constipated (liquid passes around the hard stool). A stool impaction is more common in the elderly, those on regular narcotics and other medications, such as anticholinergics, and patients who are immobile.

What you need

For stool disimpaction

Towel or linen-saver pad ✱ gown ✱ gloves ✱ water-soluble lubricant ✱ a basin to place the stool that is removed ✱ a stethoscope to listen for bowel sounds ✱ toilet tissue ✱ optional: mask ✱ hair net (surgical scrub caps) ✱ glycerine suppository to aid with the disimpaction prescribed by the health care provider.

How you do it

- Identify the patient using two patient identifiers per facility policy.
- Provide privacy, perform hand hygiene, and put on your gloves and gown.
- Explain the procedure to the patient. Tell him that he may experience some discomfort and that taking deep breaths and relaxing the abdominal musculature will help.
- Help the patient into a Sims' position and place a pillow under the right knee for comfort.
- Place the towel and linen saver under the patient's hips/buttocks.
- Place the basin next to the patient on the bed/exam table.

Going in

- Put water-soluble lubricant on the index finger of your dominant hand.
- Tell the patient that you are going to touch him before you do so and place your nondominant hand on his buttock to gently lift while you gently insert the lubricated index finger into his rectum.
- Ease your finger gently in, until you feel the hard stool. (If you don't, try to go a little farther, but if still nothing, the impaction may be farther up in the distal sigmoid colon and the physician may need to do the procedure with an anal retractor, or more diagnostic studies, such as an abdominal X-ray or computed tomography (CT) scan of the abdomen, may need to be done.)

Pulling it out

Assuming you feel the hard stool, you will need to "break it up" with your finger and remove fragments. First, curve your index finger, and with a "scooping" motion, start pulling stool out and placing it in the basin. Keep the scooping motion going, until all the hardened stool is removed.

Watch your patient

- Keep an eye on more than the rectum. Monitor your patient for sweating, flushing, nausea, or dizziness.

- When you are done, wipe the patient's rectum with toilet tissue and remove the towel and linen saver. As long as no stool cultures are ordered, dispose of the stool in the toilet bowl and wash the basin. (See *Document disimpaction of a patient.*)

Document disimpaction of a patient

In your notes, record:
- client's tolerance of procedure
- color, odor, and consistency of stool expelled or obtained.

Report immediately if patient is unable to expel impacted feces.

Colostomy and ileostomy care

A patient with a colostomy or an ileostomy must wear an external pouch to collect emerging fecal matter. Besides collecting waste matter, the pouch helps to control odor and protect the stoma and peristomal skin. Most disposable pouching systems can be used for 2 to 7 days; some models last even longer. Your responsibilities include caring for the colostomy or ileostomy and teaching the patient self-care.

What you need

Pouching system ✳ stoma measuring guide ✳ stoma paste (if drainage is watery to pasty or stoma secretes excess mucus) ✳ plastic bag ✳ water ✳ washcloth and towel ✳ closure clamp ✳ toilet or bedpan ✳ water or pouch cleaning solution ✳ gloves ✳ facial tissues ✳ optional: ostomy belt, paper tape, mild nonmoisturizing soap, skin shaving equipment, liquid skin sealant, pouch deodorant.

Catalog of choices

Pouching systems may be drainable or closed-bottomed, disposable or reusable, adhesive-backed, and one-piece or two-piece. (See *Comparing ostomy pouching systems*, page 412.)

How you do it

- Identify the patient using two patient identifiers per facility policy.
- Provide privacy and emotional support.
- Explain the procedure to the patient.

Fitting the pouch and skin barrier

- For a pouch with an attached skin barrier, measure the stoma with the stoma measuring guide. Select the opening size that matches the stoma.
- For an adhesive-backed pouch with a separate skin barrier, measure the stoma with the measuring guide and select the opening that matches the stoma. Trace the selected size opening onto the paper back of the skin barrier's adhesive side. Cut out the opening. (If the pouch has precut openings, which can be handy for

Comparing ostomy pouching systems

Available in many shapes and sizes, ostomy pouches are fashioned for comfort, safety, and easy application. A disposable closed-end pouch may meet the needs of a patient who irrigates, wants added security, or wants to discard the pouch after each bowel movement. Another patient may prefer a reusable, drainable pouch. Some commonly available pouches are described here.

One-piece disposable pouch

The patient who must empty his pouch often (because of diarrhea or a new colostomy or ileostomy) may prefer a one-piece, drainable, disposable pouch with a closure clamp attached to a skin barrier (below left).

This odor-proof, plastic pouch comes with an attached adhesive or Karaya seal. The bottom opening allows for easy draining. This pouch may be used permanently or temporarily, until stoma size stabilizes.

Also disposable and made of odor-proof plastic, a one-piece disposable closed-end pouch (below right) may come in a kit with adhesive seal, belt tabs, skin barrier, or carbon filter for gas release. A patient with a regular bowel elimination pattern may choose this style.

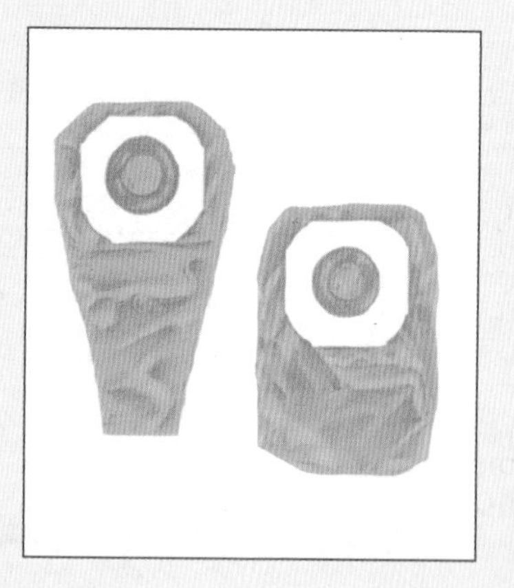

Two-piece disposable pouch

A two-piece disposable drainable pouch with separate skin barrier (below) permits frequent changes and minimizes skin breakdown. Also made of odor-proof plastic, this style comes with belt tabs and usually snaps to the skin barrier with a flange mechanism.

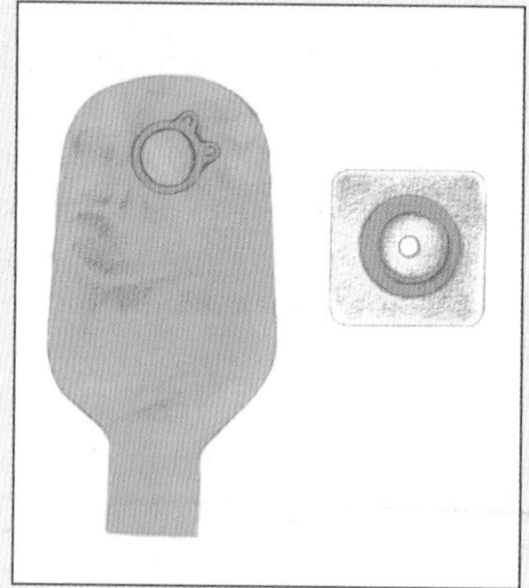

Reusable pouch

Typically made of sturdy, hypoallergenic plastic, the reusable pouch (below) comes with a separate custom-made faceplate and O-ring. Some reusable pouches have pressure valves for releasing gas. The device has a 1- to 2-month life span, depending on how frequently the patient empties the pouch.

Reusable equipment may benefit a patient who needs a firm faceplate or who wishes to minimize cost. However, many reusable ostomy pouches aren't odor-proof.

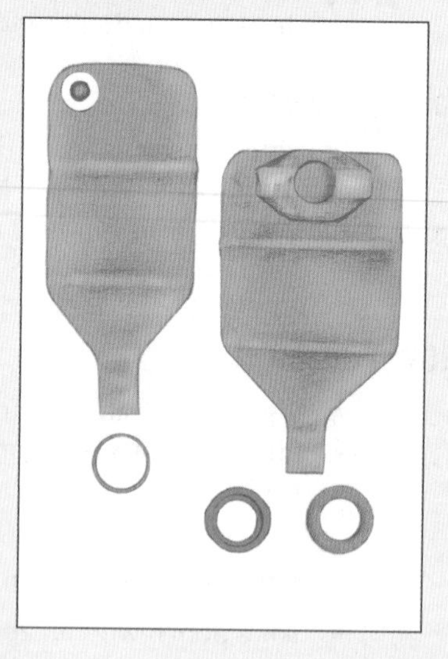

a round stoma, select an opening that's 1/8" [0.3 cm] larger than the stoma. If the pouch comes without an opening, cut the hole 1/8" wider than the measured tracing.) The cut-to-fit system works best for an irregularly shaped stoma.

- For a two-piece pouching system with flanges. (See *Applying a skin barrier and pouch*.)

Can't feel a thing

- Avoid fitting the pouch too tightly *because the stoma has no pain receptors. A constrictive opening could injure the stoma or skin tissue without the patient feeling warning discomfort.* Also avoid cutting the opening too big *because this may expose the skin to fecal matter and moisture. A normal stoma should be red and moist.*
- If the patient has a descending or sigmoid colostomy, has formed stools, and has an ostomy that doesn't secrete much mucus, he may choose to wear only a pouch. In this case, make sure the pouch opening closely matches the stoma size.
- Between 6 weeks and 1 year after surgery, the stoma will shrink to its permanent size. At that point, pattern-making preparations will be unnecessary unless the patient gains weight, has additional surgery, or injures the stoma.

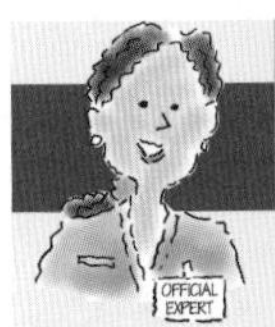

Advice from the experts

Applying a skin barrier and pouch

Fitting a skin barrier and ostomy pouch properly can be done in a few steps:

- Measure the stoma using a measuring guide.
- Trace the appropriate circle carefully on the back of the skin barrier.
- Cut the circular opening in the skin barrier. Bevel the edges to keep them from irritating the patient.

There are flat skin barriers and convex skin barriers depending on what the stoma looks like.

For stomas that stick out *at least an inch* from the body, the flat skin barrier usually provides the best seal for the pouching system to attach securely to the patient's body.

For flat stomas, or ones that do not protrude at least an inch from the patient's body, the convex skin barrier is the best choice. These are usually better for patients with soft abdomens or if there is any "denting" near the area around the stoma.

- Remove the backing from the skin barrier and moisten it or apply barrier paste as needed along the edge of the circular opening.
- Center the skin barrier over the stoma, adhesive side down, and gently press it to the skin.
- Gently press the pouch opening onto the ring until it snaps into place.

Applying or changing the pouch

- Collect all equipment.
- Perform hand hygiene and provide privacy.
- Explain the procedure to the patient *because the patient will eventually perform the procedure himself.*
- Put on gloves.

Out with the old

- Remove and discard the old pouch in a plastic bag. Wipe the stoma and peristomal skin gently with a facial tissue or gauze.
- Carefully wash the peristomal skin with mild soap and water and dry it by patting gently. Allow the skin to dry thoroughly. Inspect the peristomal skin and stoma. If necessary, shave surrounding hair (in a direction away from the stoma) *to promote a better seal and avoid skin irritation from hair pulling against the adhesive.*
- If applying a separate skin barrier, peel off the paper backing of the prepared skin barrier, center the barrier over the stoma, and press gently *to ensure adhesion.*
- You may want to outline the stoma on the back of the skin barrier (depending on the product) with a thin ring of stoma paste *to provide extra skin protection.* (Skip this step if the patient has a sigmoid or descending colostomy, formed stools, and little mucus.)

Peel and press

- Remove the paper backing from the adhesive side of the pouching system and center the pouch opening over the stoma. Press gently to secure.
- For a pouching system with flanges, align the lip of the pouch flange with the bottom edge of the skin barrier flange. Gently press around the circumference of the pouch flange, beginning at the bottom, until the pouch securely adheres to the barrier flange. (The pouch will click into its secured position.) Holding the barrier against the skin, gently pull on the pouch *to confirm the seal between flanges.*

Body warmth improves adherence and softens a rigid skin barrier.

Warm to the task

- Encourage the patient to stay quietly in position for about 5 minutes *to improve adherence. The patient's body warmth also helps improve adherence and soften a rigid skin barrier*
- Attach an ostomy belt to further secure the pouch, if desired. (Some pouches have belt loops, and others have plastic adapters for belts.)

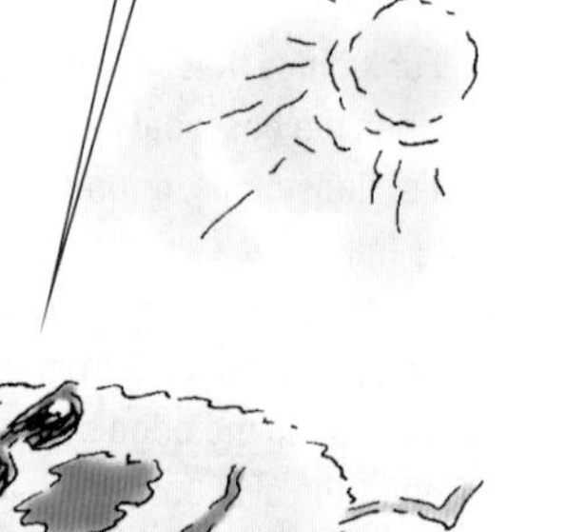

- Leave a bit of air in the pouch *to allow drainage to fall to the bottom.*
- Apply the closure clamp, if necessary. Some have a Lock 'n Roll closure; just roll the bottom end up onto itself three times and it snaps into place, like Velcro.
- If desired, apply paper tape in a picture-frame fashion to the pouch edges *for additional security.*

Documenting colostomy and ileostomy care

In your notes, record:
- date and time of the pouching system change
- character of drainage, including color, amount, type, and consistency
- appearance of the stoma and peristomal skin
- patient teaching
- patient's response to self-care and evaluation of his learning progress.

Emptying the pouch

- Perform hand hygiene. Don gloves.
- Tilt the bottom of the pouch upward and remove the closure clamp. Some pouches have the Lock 'n Roll closure. To open, just unfold the bottom three times.
- Turn up a cuff on the lower end of the pouch and allow it to drain into the toilet or bedpan.
- Wipe the bottom of the pouch and reapply the closure clamp.
- If desired, the bottom portion of the pouch can be rinsed with cool tap water. Don't aim water up near the top of the pouch *because this may loosen the seal on the skin.*
- A two-piece flanged system can also be emptied by unsnapping the pouch. Let the drainage flow into the toilet.

Gas release

- Release flatus through the gas release valve if the pouch has one. Otherwise, release flatus by tilting the pouch bottom upward, releasing the clamp, and expelling the flatus. To release flatus from a flanged system, loosen the seal between the flanges.

Practice pointers

- After explaining and performing the procedure to the patient, encourage the patient's increasing involvement in self-care.
- Use commercial pouch deodorants, if desired. However, most pouches are odor-free, and odor should only be evident when you empty the pouch or if it leaks. Before discharge, suggest that the patient avoid odor-causing foods. (See *Documenting colostomy and ileostomy care.*)

T-tube care

A T tube (or biliary drainage tube) may be placed in the common bile duct after cholecystectomy (removal of the gallbladder) or choledochostomy (removal of a portion of the bile duct). This tube helps drain bile while healing occurs.

The long and short of it

The surgeon inserts the short end (crossbar) of the T tube in the common bile duct and draws the long end through the incision. The tube then connects to a closed gravity drainage system. The tube remains in place for between 7 and 14 days after surgery. (See *Understanding T-tube placement.*)

Nursing responsibilities include emptying the drainage and caring for the T tube.

What you need

Graduated collection container ✱ small plastic bag ✱ sterile gloves and clean gloves ✱ clamp ✱ sterile 4″ × 4″ gauze pads ✱ transparent dressings ✱ rubber band ✱ normal saline solution ✱ sterile cleaning solution ✱ two sterile basins ✱ povidone-iodine pads ✱ sterile precut drain dressings ✱ hypoallergenic paper tape ✱ skin protectant, such as petroleum jelly, zinc oxide, or aluminum-based gel ✱ optional: Montgomery straps.

Getting ready

Assemble equipment at the bedside. Open all sterile equipment. Place one sterile 4″ × 4″ gauze pad in each sterile basin. Using sterile technique, pour 50 mL of cleaning solution into one basin and 50 mL of normal saline solution into the other basin.

Advice you can't refuse

Tape a small plastic bag on the table to use for refuse.

How you do it

- Provide privacy and explain the procedure to the patient. Perform hand hygiene.

Emptying drainage

- Don clean gloves.
- Place the graduated collection container under the outlet valve of the drainage bag. Without contaminating the clamp, valve, or outlet valve, empty the bag's contents completely into the container and reseal the outlet valve. Carefully measure and record the character, color, and amount of drainage. Discard your gloves.

Understanding T-tube placement

The T tube is placed in the common bile duct, anchored to the abdominal wall, and connected to a closed drainage system.

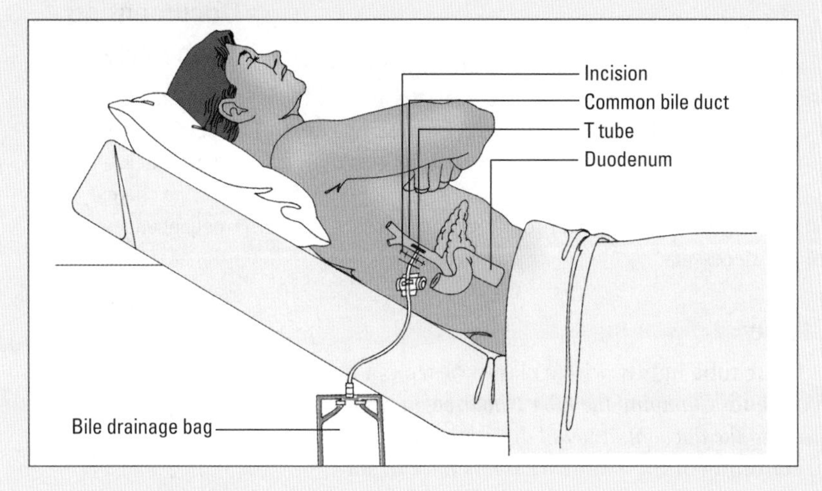

Redressing the T tube

- Perform hand hygiene *to prevent bacterial contamination of the incision*. Don clean gloves.
- Without dislodging the T tube, remove old dressings and dispose of them in the small plastic bag. Remove the clean gloves.

Now it's serious

- Perform hand hygiene again and put on sterile gloves. From this point on, follow strict aseptic technique *to prevent bacterial contamination of the incision*.
- Inspect the incision and tube site for signs or symptoms of infection, including redness, edema, warmth, tenderness, induration, or skin excoriation. Assess for wound dehiscence or evisceration.

Time for a wash

- Use sterile cleaning solution as prescribed to clean and remove dried matter or drainage from around the tube. Always start at the tube site and gently wipe outward in a continuous motion *to prevent recontamination of the incision*.
- Use normal saline solution to rinse off the prescribed cleaning solution. Dry the area with a sterile 4″ × 4″ gauze pad and discard all used materials.

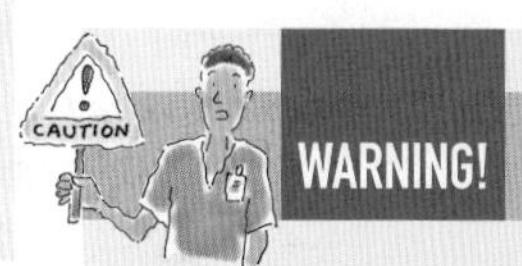

Managing T-tube obstruction

If your patient's T tube becomes blocked after cholecystectomy, notify the physician. Take these steps while you wait for the physician to arrive:

- Unclamp the T tube (if it was clamped before and after a meal) and connect it to a closed gravity drainage system.
- Inspect the tube for kinks and obstructions.
- Prepare the patient for possible T-tube irrigation or direct X-ray of the common bile duct. Describe these measures to reduce the patient's apprehension and promote cooperation.

- Using a povidone-iodine pad, wipe the incision site in a circular motion. Allow the area to dry thoroughly.
- Apply a sterile precut drain dressing on each side of the T tube *to absorb drainage.*

No kinks allowed

- Apply a sterile 4″ × 4″ gauze pad or transparent dressing over the T tube and the drain dressings. Be careful not to kink the tubing, *which might block the drainage.* Also avoid putting the dressing over the open end of the T tube *because this end connects to the closed drainage system.*
- Secure the dressings with the hypoallergenic paper tape or Montgomery straps if necessary.

Clamping the T tube

- As ordered, occlude the tube lightly with a clamp or wrap a rubber band around the end. *Clamping the tube 1 hour before and after meals diverts bile back to the duodenum to aid digestion.* Surgeons will usually order clamping of the T tube to assess patient status for a few days before deciding whether the T tube can be removed.
- Monitor the patient's response to clamping.
- *To ensure patient comfort and safety,* check bile drainage amounts regularly. Be alert for such signs of obstructed bile flow as chills, fever, tachycardia, nausea, right upper quadrant fullness and pain, jaundice, dark foamy urine, and clay-colored stools. **Report them immediately**. (See *Managing T-tube obstruction,* page 417.)

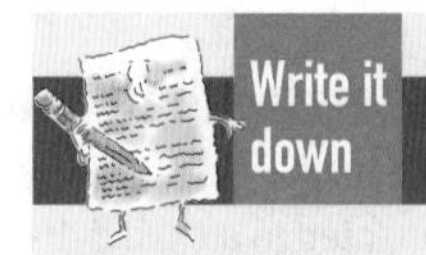

Documenting T-tube care

If your patient has a T tube, document:
- date and time of each dressing change
- patient education
- appearance of the wound and surrounding skin
- color, character, and volume of bile collected
- color of skin and mucous membranes around the T tube.

Also, be sure to keep a precise record of temperature trends as well as the amount and frequency of urination and bowel movements.

Practice pointers

- Normal daily bile drainage ranges from 500 to 1,000 mL of viscous, green-brown liquid. The T tube usually drains 300 to 500 mL of blood-tinged bile in the first 24 hours after surgery; report drainage exceeding 500 mL during this period. The amount typically declines to 200 mL or less after 4 days. Monitor the patient's fluid, electrolyte, liver function tests, and acid-base status carefully.
- Assess tube patency and site condition hourly for the first 8 hours and then every 4 hours until the physician removes the tube. (See *Documenting T-tube care.*)

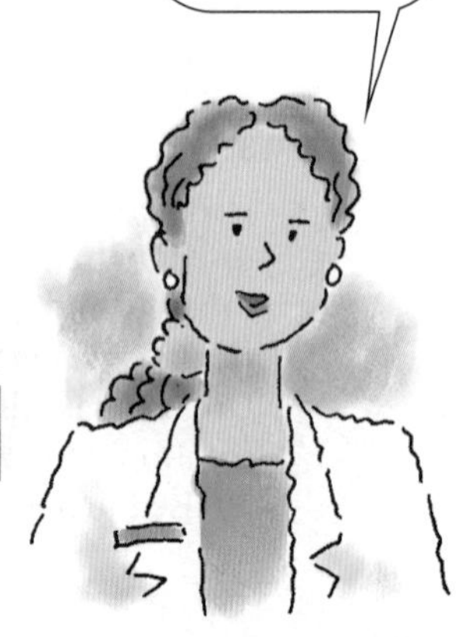
Bile drainage will ebb to 200 mL or less after 4 days.

Gastrostomy tube care and removal

Unless the patient has a PEG (see *Caring for a PEG or PEJ site,* page 402), a gastrostomy tube is usually placed during abdominal, especially pancreatic, resections. It is a large, typically rubber or silicone surgical drain. These types of gastrostomy or G tubes are mainly to provide drainage of stomach contents to prevent vomiting postoperatively and rest a new gastric or small bowel anastomosis. They are also placed palliatively in patients with a gastric outlet obstruction related to cancer or anastomotic stricture.

The G tube is place via a percutaneous incision during surgery and the tube is inserted into the stomach. There are two types, which is important to know for removal. One is anchored by a balloon filled with water, similar to a Foley catheter, whereas the other has a fenestrated end that opens up, anchoring the tube in place. A purse-string suture holds the tube in place on the skin to prevent it from being dislodged. As a nurse, the insertion site should be inspected for infection and be cleansed daily with normal saline and a fenestrated gauze should be placed over the insertion site with the cut/hole in the gauze for the tube to fit through.

In the hospital, the G tube is usually open and draining into a drainage bag. The amounts are recorded every shift. As the patient progresses, usually around postoperative day 3, the G tube is clamped (with a standard G-tube clamp or a rubber band) and an order is written to open the G tube every 6 hours unless the patient complains of nausea or vomiting (then it is left open to gravity drainage), during which time drainage amounts are measured and recorded. **Remember that about a liter of bile and a liter of saliva a day is produced by the human body**; therefore, if less than 500 mL per 6 hours are removed, then that is a good sign that there is no longer a postoperative ileus, and the patient can tolerate 24-hour clamping the next day, and subsequent progression to a clear liquid diet ordered by the surgeon. Usually, a G tube postoperatively is left in place for at least 10 days before removal. Think of it like an "escape valve" for the patient. As the patient's nurse, you may instruct the patient that she may open the G tube over a sink or toilet at home if she feels nauseated. This will empty the stomach contents in an effort to prevent vomiting. **A G tube does not require flushing, unless it is open and nothing is flowing out, and a patient is experiencing nausea.**

Keep in mind, however, that *the patient's surgeon would need to order the removal* of the G tube.

What you need

A suture removal kit: with scissors and tweezers or "pick-ups" ✳ a urinal—to open and drain the G tube before removal ✳ a 10-mL syringe ✳ linen-saver pad ✳ many pieces of gauze to soak up drainage after removal ✳ an ABD or extra absorbent dressing ✳ clear occlusive bandage (Tegaderm) or paper tape ✱ gown ✱ protective eye wear for splashes ✱ bedside procedure tray.

How you do it

- Provide privacy, perform hand hygiene, and put on gloves and gown.
- Change the patient into a gown, removing all of the clothing on the upper body, keeping the gown open to the front.
- It is best to remove the G tube after the patient has been fasting for about 4 hours.
- It is also best to have the patient take his prescribed pain medication about 1 hour before removal.

Removing a gastrostomy tube

- Explain the procedure to the patient. Tell him that he may experience a burning sensation and a feeling of "being wet" as the tube is removed but that it will only last a few seconds.
- Help the patient in a semi-Fowler's position because you need a little gravity to get all of the fluid out of the G tube when opened.
- Position your linen-saver pad under the left side of the patient (the side the G tube is placed) and tucked underneath the patient's clothing if wearing pants or a skirt.
- Stand on the left side of the patient and place the G tube into the opening in the urinal. Open the clamp. Be aware that gastric contents may flow out immediately into the urinal.
- Leave the G tube open and draining into the urinal until you are satisfied that the patient is done draining. Some patients may not drain until it is removed and then there could be a *lot* of drainage.

  The drainage is usually the same color as bile, ranging from green to yellow, and is mucousy and could reflect the qualities of the last meal that the patient ate.
- Remove the urinal and its contents.
- Bring your gauze pad, ABD pad, clear plastic occlusive dressing, 10-mL syringe, suture removal kit, and/or paper tape around to the left side of the bed or exam table.
- Open the suture kit and tell the patient that you are now removing the suture holding the G tube in place.
- Cut the loop of the purse-string and pull the entire suture out.
- If the G tube is of the silicone variety and has a port, attach the 10-mL syringe and pull back the fluid to deflate the balloon. If it is of the latex rubber variety, it is simply pulled out after the suture is removed and the fenestrated "balloon" end just "folds in" like an umbrella, when you close it, allowing for removal.
- Put on your protective eyewear.

- Tell the patient to take a deep breath, and as he let it out, you will pull the tube firmly but gently with one motion, dropping it onto the linen-saver pad, and pressing a handful of gauze on the now open and possibly draining wound.
- Continue to "mop up" the gastric contents, as they drain, and when drainage has stopped, help the patient to sit all the way up, again, using gravity to help assist any remaining fluid out.
- If nothing more drains, assist the patient back to semi-Fowler's and dress the wound. It is left open and unsutured to prevent infection. In the very rare occurrence that gastric contents continue to drain for at least 30 minutes after G-tube removal, a few sutures may need to be placed by the health care provider.
- Tell the patient that the open wound where the G tube was will close a little each day, and by a week's time, it will usually produce a scab.
- Dress the wound with an ABD extra absorbent pad and clear plastic occlusive dressing or paper tape. The clear plastic occlusive dressing is better in case of any further drainage.
- In the outpatient setting, tell the patient to leave the dressing on, unless it soaks through, until the next day and then he may remove this dressing and simply place a dry sterile gauze and paper tape over it.
- Instruct the patient to remain fasting, even with fluid, for about an hour to assist in the closure of the wound.
- Monitor the patient throughout for dizziness, nausea, and burning sensation on the skin. Remember that gastric secretions are acidic and that any gastric contents left on the skin can cause skin irritation. Just wipe the area clean with normal saline and dry it. (See *Documenting removal of the gastrostomy tube*.)

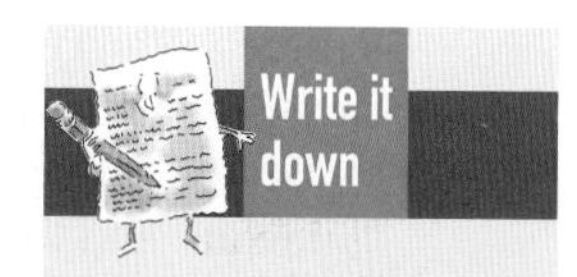

Documenting removal of the gastrostomy tube

In your notes, document:
- procedure
- patient and family education
- pain medication if given
- drainage from the site
- condition of the skin
- type of dressing applied
- patient's tolerance of the procedure.

Jackson-Pratt care and removal

A Jackson-Pratt (JP) drain is typically placed during abdominal, neck, breast surgery, and whenever drainage is likely to be produced after extensive tissue dissection. Here, we focus on JP care and removal after abdominal operations. The drain is a plastic bulb that typically is able to hold 100 mL of fluid. It contains a stopper (to be opened to empty the drainage in the bulb) and a catheter that is approximately 12″ (30.48 cm) in length. The catheter portion that hangs from the incision in which it was placed is thin and approximately 5 mm, and the end that is coiled into the abdominal cavity, near the area of the operation, is the same size as the outer portion at first and then it changes to a larger, approximately 1- to 1.5-cm portion to allow clots and fluid to pass through. The bulb of the drain should be compressed at all times except when emptying to create a vacuum in order to achieve gently suction and the removal of fluid around the area of the incision.

Fluid usually starts off as bloody, then progresses to serosanguineous, and then serous. If the patient has had a pancreatic resection and a pancreatic leak occurs, the fluid will look milky, cloudy, grayish, yellow-tinged to green. A biliary leak can be frankly bilious (green resembling bile).

A JP drain should be emptied before it is completely full, in the hospital or at home, so that suction and drainage can be maintained. Every time the bulb drain is emptied, the amount should be recorded and the color and character of the drainage should be noted. The drainage should **not** have an odor, unless there is a pancreatic leak following resection or there is drainage which contains frank enteric contents (stool). A JP drain that has been draining serosanguineous fluid, or serous fluid, that suddenly drains frank blood could indicate postoperative bleeding. **These situations require immediate reporting to the surgeon.**

What is my job in JP care?

As a nurse, you are required to provide care to the insertion site, milk the drain, empty and record amount and quality of drainage, reapply suction, and anchor the bulb to the patient's gown (with a safety pin, so that it does not hang and pull on the suture).

What you need

A container that is large enough to hold 100 mL of fluid (and has marked measurements on it every 5 or 10 mL) to empty the bulb, usually a urinary specimen container is used ✳ linen-saver pad ✳ normal saline ✳ gauze to help cleanse the insertion site and also to place at the insertion site, fenestrated if possible, after cleansing ✳ paper tape.

How you do it

- Wash and dry your hands and put on gloves.
- At the beginning of your shift or at the initial point of contact (in a home or outpatient setting), the JP drain should be inspected. The skin at the point of entry into the body should also be inspected for drainage, redness, pus, or swelling. It is normal for the skin to be red, right around the area where the drain/catheter enters the body, where a purse-string suture holds it in place. *If fluid is draining out of the insertion site, this could indicate that a clot has blocked drainage and that the tube may require milking, suction is lost, or the stopper on top is not completely closed.*

Milk the drain by holding the catheter in your fingers, at first closest to the insertion site, while gently pressing the tube between them with your nondominant hand, and then with the other, hold the tube between your thumb and second and third fingers while again applying gentle pressure and running your fingers along the length of the tube. Move your fingers of both hands down and repeat this procedure until the entire length of the drain is milked all the way to the bulb.

- Next, place the linen-saver pad near the patient, unpin the JP from the patient's gown, and place the bulb drain on the linen saver pad.
- Open your specimen or drainage container that contains measurement marks and place it next to the drain.
- Open the stopper, turn the drain upside down, and allow the drainage to fall into the container. When it has all drained out, close the measured container to avoid spills.
- *Next, be sure to squeeze the JP drain between your fingers until they meet at opposite sides of the bulb and close the stopper.* This ensures that suction has been reestablished.
- Next, cleanse the insertion site with normal saline and pat dry with dry sterile gauze. Dress the insertion site with a fenestrated dry sterile gauze and tape it into place.
- Pin the JP to the patient's gown.
- Clean up the linen saver and record the amount and quality of the drainage in the patient's chart as well as the condition of the insertion site. **Check to see if there is an order for fluid analysis from the health care provider before discarding the JP drainage.**
- If a patient is discharged from the hospital with a JP drain, explain these exact same steps to the patient and give him a sheet to record the drainage amounts and the quality of the drainage.
- Usually, when drainage has decreased to 30 mL/day, the JP drain is removed. *Remember, the surgeon or physician must order its removal.*

Removal of a JP drain

As a nurse, you may be required to remove a JP drain.

What you need

A suture removal kit ✳ a linen-saver pad ✳ dry sterile gauze ✳ paper tape ✳ gown.

How you do it

- First, explain the procedure to the patient. If possible, administer the patient's prescribed analgesic 1 hour before removal. If the patient is having the removal done in the outpatient setting, instruct the patient to take his prescribed pain medication 1 hour prior to his appointment.

- Explain that when the drain is removed, the patient will feel a burning sensation, but this will quickly subside. You may also tell him that he will have a sensation that "his stomach feels as if something is falling out." Tell the patient that slow deep breathing through the discomfort helps.
- Perform hand hygiene and don gloves and a gown.
- Help your patient to a completely supine position, unless contraindicated or the patient is unable because of discomfort or breathing difficulties. For this patient, you may place him in semi-Fowler's position. Being supine helps to relax the stomach musculature.
- Unpin the safety pin from the patient's gown and position the linen-saver pad near the area the JP is located and rest the bulb on top.
- Stand on the same side of the patient that the JP is placed.
- Grab your suture removal kit, open it, and cut the purse-string suture with the scissors, and remove the entire suture with the tweezers or pick-ups.

Documenting removal of a Jackson-Pratt drain

Upon removal of the JP drain, document:

- how much fluid remained in the bulb
- how the patient tolerated the procedure.

Prepare for removal

- Tell the patient to take a deep breath, and as she lets it out, pull on the JP drain at the site closest to the point of insertion. *At first, it is common to feel resistance. Remember that you are pulling a drain that is approximately a foot long, through the abdominal wall, from the abdominal cavity. Do not be deterred by the resistance, but continue to apply gentle pressure.*
- You will feel it "give way" and then slip out. Drop it onto the linen-saver pad and attend to your patient.
- Press a gauze pad to the insertion site and encourage your patient to breathe through the discomfort that is *temporary*; however, monitor for any signs of distress or bleeding.
- Usually, little drainage accompanies a JP removal, but it is very normal for the site to bleed a little. Hold gentle pressure until the bleeding stops and then place a dry sterile gauze on the area and hold it in place with paper tape.
- Make sure the entire length of the JP drain is removed as you examine it on the linen-saver pad and get ready to dispose of it in the medical waste container. *If for any reason the entire length of tubing is not present, notify the physician immediately.* This is exceedingly uncommon, as the JP system is typically removed in its entirety. (See *Documenting removal of a Jackson-Pratt drain.*)

Abdominal paracentesis

A bedside procedure, abdominal paracentesis involves using a needle, trocar, or cannula to aspirate fluid from the peritoneal space. It's used to diagnose and treat massive ascites (accumulation of fluid in abdominal cavity) that doesn't respond to other therapy.

The procedure also helps determine the cause of ascites and relieve pressure. It may also precede other procedures, including radiography, peritoneal dialysis, and surgery. Abdominal paracentesis can also detect intra-abdominal bleeding after traumatic injury and obtain a peritoneal fluid specimen for laboratory analysis.

Proceed with caution

The procedure must be performed cautiously in pregnant patients and in patients with bleeding tendencies or unstable vital signs.

What you need

Tape measure ✳ sterile gloves ✳ clean gloves ✳ gown ✳ goggles ✳ linen-saver pads ✳ four Vacutainer laboratory tubes ✳ blood culture bottles ✳ two large glass Vacutainer bottles (1,000 mL or larger) ✳ dry, sterile pressure dressing ✳ laboratory request forms ✳ povidone-iodine solution ✳ local anesthetic (multidose vial of 1% or 2% lidocaine with epinephrine) ✳ 4″ × 4″ sterile gauze pads ✳ sterile paracentesis tray (containing needle, trocar, cannula, three-way stopcock), usually disposable ✳ sterile drapes ✳ marking pen ✳ 5-mL syringe with 22G or 25G needle ✳ scalpel #10 ✳ optional: alcohol pad, 50-mL syringe, suture materials. Sometimes, the health care provider will do the procedure using ultrasound guidance to avoid intestinal perforation. The portable ultrasound machine can be used right at the bedside.

How you do it

- Identify the patient with two patient identifiers.
- Explain the procedure to the patient *to ease his anxiety and promote cooperation*. Reassure him that he should feel no pain but may feel a stinging sensation from the local anesthetic injection and pressure from the scalpel as a small incision is made to allow the trocar and cannula insertion.

First order of business

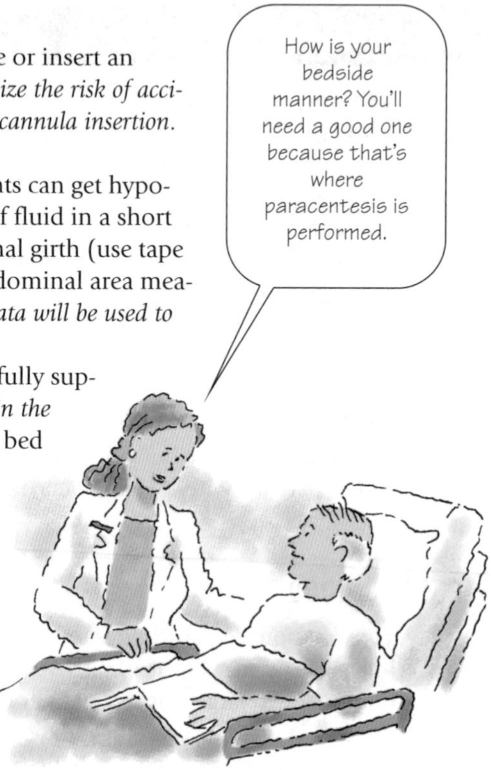

- Instruct the patient to void before the procedure or insert an indwelling urinary catheter, if ordered, *to minimize the risk of accidental bladder injury from the needle or trocar and cannula insertion.*
- Perform hand hygiene.
- Record baseline values especially because patients can get hypotensive after the procedure because of the loss of fluid in a short period of time: vital signs, weight, and abdominal girth (use tape measure) at the umbilical level. Indicate the abdominal area measured with a felt-tipped marking pen. *Baseline data will be used to monitor the patient's status.*
- Help the patient sit up in bed or in a chair that fully supports his arms and legs *so that fluid accumulates in the lower abdomen* or help him sit on the side of the bed and use pillows to support his back.

How is your bedside manner? You'll need a good one because that's where paracentesis is performed.

Southern exposure

- Expose the patient's abdomen from diaphragm to pubis. Keep the rest of the patient covered *to avoid chilling him.*
- Place a linen-saver pad under him *for protection from drainage.*
- Remind the patient to stay as still as possible during the procedure *to prevent injury from the scalpel, needle, or trocar and cannula.*
- Perform hand hygiene. Open the paracentesis tray using aseptic technique *to ensure a sterile field.* Next, put on gloves before assisting the health care provider as he prepares the patient's abdomen with 4″ × 4″ sterile gauze pads soaked in povidone-iodine solution, drapes the operative site with sterile drapes, and administers the local anesthetic.
- If the paracentesis tray doesn't contain a sterile ampule of anesthetic, wipe the top of a multidose vial of anesthetic solution with an alcohol pad and invert the vial at a 45-degree angle. *This will allow the health care provider to insert the sterile 5-mL syringe with the 22G or 25G needle and withdraw the anesthetic without touching the nonsterile vial.*
- Using the scalpel, the physician may make a small incision before inserting the needle or trocar and cannula (usually 1″ to 2″ [2.5 to 5 cm] below the umbilicus).

Collect call

- Assist the physician with specimen collection in the appropriate containers. Ensure the labels are verified with two patient identifiers that match the medical record as well as the lab requisition. Wear clean gloves, gown, and goggles *to protect you from possible body fluid contamination*. If the physician orders substantial drainage, connect the three-way stopcock and tubing to the cannula. Run the other end of the tubing to a large sterile Vacutainer or aspirate the fluid with a three-way stopcock and 50-mL syringe.

- Gently turn the patient from side to side *to enhance drainage* if necessary.

First, monitor . . .

- As the fluid drains, monitor the patient's vital signs every 15 minutes. Observe him closely for vertigo, faintness, diaphoresis, pallor, heightened anxiety, tachycardia, dyspnea, and hypotension—especially if more than 1,500 mL of peritoneal fluid was aspirated at one time. *This loss may induce a fluid shift and hypovolemic shock.*
- When the procedure ends and the physician removes the needle or trocar and cannula, he may suture the incision. Wearing sterile gloves, apply the dry, sterile pressure dressing to the site.

. . . and then monitor some more

- Monitor the patient's vital signs and check the dressing for drainage every 15 minutes for 1 hour, every 30 minutes for 2 hours, every hour for 4 hours, and then every 4 hours for 24 hours *to detect delayed reactions to the procedure*. Be sure to note drainage color, amount, and character.
- Send specimens to the laboratory with the appropriate laboratory request forms. If the patient is receiving antibiotics, note this on the request form.
- Remove and dispose of all equipment properly.

Practice pointers

- *To prevent fluid shifts and hypovolemia*, the physician should limit aspirated fluid to between 1,500 and 2,000 mL.
- After the procedure, observe for peritoneal fluid leakage, it is usually a clear yellow (straw) color but may be milky if it is chylous ascites. Chylous ascites is the presence of lymph fluid from thoracic or intestinal lymph in the abdominal cavity. This is very rare and usually occurs from the obstruction of lymph flow usually because of cancer. If this develops, notify the physician. Always maintain daily patient weight and abdominal girth records. Compare these values with the baseline figures *to detect recurrent ascites*. (See *Documenting abdominal paracentesis*.)

Documenting abdominal paracentesis

After abdominal paracentesis, document:

- date and time of the procedure
- patient education
- puncture site location
- whether the wound was sutured
- amount, color, viscosity, and odor of aspirated fluid (Note this in the patient's chart and in the fluid intake and output record.)
- number of specimens sent to the laboratory
- patient's vital signs, weight, and abdominal girth measurements before and after the procedure
- vital signs during the procedure
- complications
- patient's tolerance of the procedure.

Peritoneal lavage

Peritoneal lavage is used as a diagnostic procedure in a patient with blunt abdominal trauma and thoracic or abdominal stab wounds and helps detect bleeding and/or the presence of enteric contents in the peritoneal cavity.

The procedure involves several steps. Initially, the physician inserts a catheter through the abdominal wall into the peritoneal cavity and aspirates the peritoneal fluid with a syringe. If he can't see blood in the aspirated fluid, he then infuses a balanced saline solution and siphons the fluid from the cavity. He inspects the siphoned fluid for blood or enteric contents and also sends fluid samples to the laboratory for microscopic examination.

If you don't watch out, my next stop will be the peritoneum.

What's my job?

The medical team maintains strict aseptic technique throughout this procedure to avoid introducing microorganisms into the peritoneum and causing peritonitis. (See *Tapping the peritoneal cavity*.) It is also very important, if possible, to determine if

Tapping the peritoneal cavity

After administering a local anesthetic to numb the area near the patient's navel, the surgeon makes a smaller incision (about ¾″ [2 cm]) through the skin and subcutaneous tissues of the abdominal wall. He retracts the tissue, ligates several blood vessels, and uses 4″ × 4″ gauze pads to absorb and keep incisional blood from entering the wound and producing a false-positive test result.

Next, he directs the trocar through the incision into the pelvic midline until it enters the peritoneum. Then he advances the peritoneal catheter (through the trocar) 6″ to 8″ (15 to 20 cm) into the pelvis.

Using a syringe attached to the catheter, the surgeon aspirates fluid from the peritoneal cavity and looks for blood, enteric contents, and other abnormal findings.

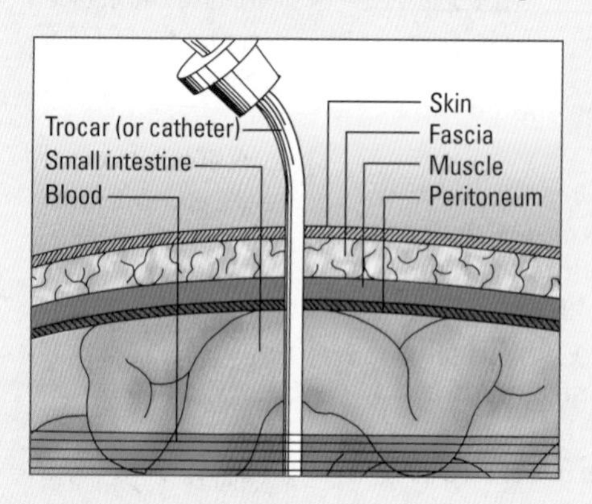

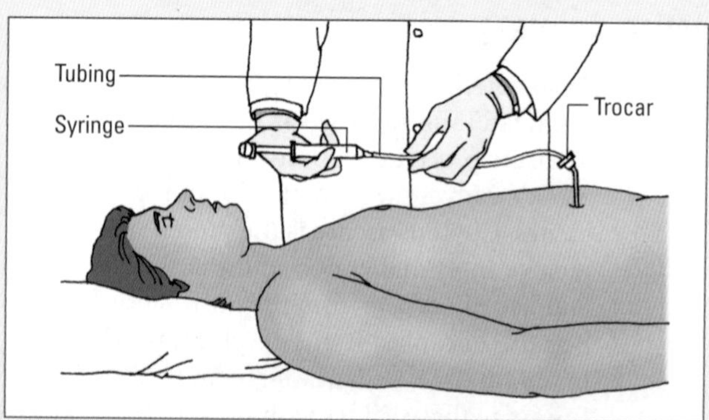

the patient is in the early stages of pregnancy. This would necessitate a supraumbilical rather than an incision inferior to the umbilicus. Pelvic fractures or a previous incision in that area may also necessitate a supraumbilical approach.

What you need

Indwelling urinary catheter, catheter insertion kit, and drainage bag ✳ NG tube ✳ gastric suction machine ✳ shaving kit ✳ I.V. pole ✳ macrodrip I.V. tubing ✳ I.V. solutions (1 L of warmed, balanced saline solution, usually lactated Ringer's solution or normal saline solution) ✳ peritoneal dialysis tray or peritoneal lavage kit ✳ sterile gloves ✳ gown ✳ goggles ✳ antiseptic solution (such as povidone-iodine) ✳ 3-mL syringe with 25G 1″ needle ✳ bottle of 1% lidocaine with epinephrine ✳ 8″ (20.3 cm) #14 intracatheter extension tubing and a small sterile hemostat (to clamp tubing) ✳ 30-mL syringe ✳ one 20G 1½″ needle ✳ #11 scalpel blade✳ sterile towels ✳ three containers for specimen collection, including one sterile tube for a culture and sensitivity specimen ✳ labels ✳ antiseptic ointment ✳ 4″ × 4″ gauze pads ✳ alcohol pads ✳ 1″ hypoallergenic tape ✳ 2-0 and 3-0 sutures.

We pause for this commercial announcement

If using a commercially prepared peritoneal dialysis kit (containing a #15 peritoneal dialysis catheter, trocar, and extension tubing with roller clamp), make sure the macrodrip I.V. tubing doesn't have a reverse flow (or back-check) valve that prevents infused fluid from draining out of the peritoneal cavity. A standard peritoneal lavage kit should have the correct tubing.

How you do it

- Identify the patient using two patient identifiers per facility policy.
- Provide privacy and perform hand hygiene. Reinforce the physician's explanation of the procedure.
- Don gown and goggles.

You'll feel a little full

- Before the procedure, advise the patient to expect a sensation of abdominal fullness. Also inform him that he may experience a chill if the lavage solution isn't warmed or doesn't reach his body temperature.
- Then catheterize the patient with the indwelling urinary catheter and connect this catheter to the drainage bag *to prevent laceration or puncture of the bladder.*

Totally tubular

- Insert the NG tube. Attach this tube to the gastric suction machine (set for low intermittent suction) to drain the patient's stomach contents. *Decompressing the stomach prevents vomiting and subsequent aspiration and minimizes the possibility of bowel perforation during trocar or catheter insertion.*
- Using the shaving kit, clip or shave the hair, as ordered, from the area between the patient's umbilicus and pubis.
- Set up the I.V. pole. Attach the macrodrip tubing to the lavage solution container and clear air from the tubing *to avoid introducing air into the peritoneal cavity during the lavage.*
- Using aseptic technique, open the peritoneal dialysis or peritoneal lavage tray.

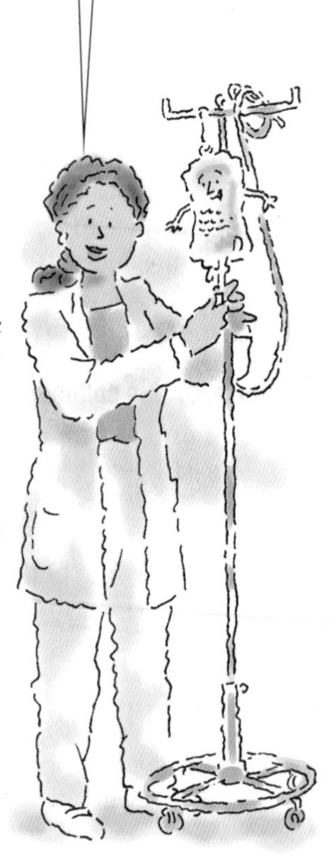
When you set up the I.V. pole for peritoneal lavage, make sure to clear air from the tubing—otherwise, air can enter the peritoneal cavity.

Cleaning duties

- The physician will wipe the patient's abdomen with the antiseptic solution and drape the area with sterile towels *to create a sterile field.*
- Using aseptic technique, hand the physician the 3-mL syringe and the 25G 1″ needle. If the peritoneal dialysis tray doesn't contain a sterile ampule of anesthetic, wipe the top of a multidose vial of 1% lidocaine with epinephrine with an alcohol pad and invert the vial at a 45-degree angle. *This allows the physician to insert the needle and withdraw the anesthetic without touching the nonsterile vial.*
- The physician will inject the anesthetic directly below the umbilicus (or at an adjacent site if the patient has a surgical scar). (See "What's my job?" for further contraindications of an incision below the umbilicus.) Then he'll make an incision, insert the catheter or trocar, withdraw fluid, and check the findings. If the findings are positive, the procedure ends and you'll prepare the patient for laparotomy and further measures. Even if retrieved fluid looks normal, lavage will continue.

Catheter connection

- Wearing gloves, connect the catheter extension tubing to the I.V. tubing, if ordered, and instill 500 to 1,000 mL (10 mL/kg body weight, especially in a pediatric patient) of the warmed I.V. solution into the peritoneal cavity over 5 to 10 minutes. Then clamp the tubing with the hemostat.
- Unless contraindicated by the patient's injuries (such as a spinal cord injury, fractured ribs, or an unstable pelvic fracture), gently tilt the patient from side to side *to distribute the fluid throughout the peritoneal cavity.* (If the patient's condition contraindicates tilting, the physician may gently palpate the sides of the abdomen *to distribute the fluid.*)

I.V. adjustment

- After 5 to 10 minutes, place the I.V. container below the level of the patient's body and open the clamp on the I.V. tubing. *Lowering the container helps excess fluid to drain.* Gently drain as much of the fluid as possible from the peritoneal cavity to the container. At least 75% of the fluid should be returned. Be careful not to disconnect the tubing from the catheter. The peritoneal cavity may take 20 to 30 minutes to drain completely.
- Although you don't need to vent a plastic bag container, be sure to vent glass I.V. containers with a needle *to promote flow.*

Fluid to go

- To obtain a fluid specimen, put on gloves and use a 30-mL syringe and 20G 1½″ needle to withdraw between 25 and 30 mL of fluid from a port in the I.V. tubing. Clean the top of each specimen container with an alcohol pad. Deposit fluid specimens in the labeled containers and send the specimens to the laboratory. *Note:* If you didn't obtain the culture and sensitivity specimen first, change the needle before drawing this fluid sample *to avoid contaminating the specimen.*
- With positive test results, the physician will usually perform a laparotomy. If test results are normal, the physician will close the incision.
- Wearing sterile gloves, apply antiseptic ointment to the site and dress the incision with a 4″ × 4″ gauze pad secured with hypoallergenic tape.
- Discard disposable equipment. Return reusable equipment to the appropriate department for cleaning and sterilization.

Practice pointers

- After lavage, monitor the patient's vital signs frequently. Report signs and symptoms of shock (tachycardia, decreased blood pressure, diaphoresis, dyspnea or shortness of breath, and vertigo) at once. Assess the incisional site frequently for bleeding.
- If the physician orders abdominal X-rays, they'll probably precede peritoneal lavage. *X-ray films made after lavage may be unreliable because of air introduced into the peritoneal cavity.* (See *Documenting peritoneal lavage.*) A CT scan may have been ordered before the procedure as well.

Documenting peritoneal lavage

After peritoneal lavage, record:

- patient education
- type and size of the peritoneal dialysis catheter used
- type and amount of solution instilled into and withdrawn from the peritoneal cavity
- amount and color of fluid returned
- whether the fluid flowed freely into and out of the abdomen
- specimens obtained and sent to the laboratory
- patient's tolerance of procedure
- complications and nursing interventions.

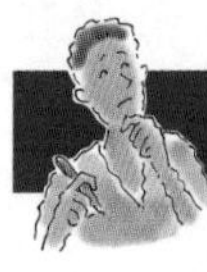

Quick quiz

1. What is the function of an NG tube?
   A. Prevention of postoperative vomiting
   B. Collection of duodenal contents for analysis
   C. Prepare the stomach for full liquid diet
   D. To provide fluid administration

Answer: A. An NG tube sits in the stomach and prevents postoperative vomiting.

2. An adhesive-backed opening should be how much larger than the stoma?
   A. 1/3″
   B. 1/4″
   C. 1/8″
   D. 1″

Answer: C. Because the stoma has no pain receptors, an opening that fits too tightly can injure the stoma. If the opening is too large, skin surrounding the stoma may come in contact with feces, causing skin breakdown. In general, the opening should be 1/8″ larger than the stoma itself.

3. During peritoneal lavage, why does the nurse gently tilt the patient from side to side after fluid instillation?
   A. To help excess fluid drain
   B. To distribute fluid throughout the peritoneal cavity
   C. To prevent bowel perforation
   D. To increase the flow of the fluids

Answer: B. Tilting the patient from side to side while the fluid dwells distributes the fluid throughout the peritoneal cavity.

4. What is not a way for the nurse to confirm NG tube placement?
   A. Aspirate stomach contents.
   B. Place the tube's end in a container of water.
   C. Inject 10 cc of air and auscultate for air sounds over the epigastric region.
   D. Have an X-ray taken to verify tube placement.

Answer: B. When confirming tube placement, avoid placing the tube's end in a container of water. If the tube isn't properly placed, the patient may aspirate water.

5. The nurse is preparing her patient for NG tube insertion. Which position should she place the patient?
   A. Semi-Fowler's
   B. Supine
   C. Dorsal recumbent
   D. Prone

Answer: A. A patient receiving a gastric feeding should be placed in semi-Fowler's or high Fowler's position to prevent aspiration.

6. A patient that has high nutritional requirements is receiving a hypertonic tube feed while simultaneously receiving continuous I.V. solution of normal saline. This patient is at risk for which electrolyte disturbance?

A. Hypokalemia
B. Hyponatremia
C. Hypernatremia
D. Hypomagnesemia

Answer: C. A hypertonic tube feed pulls water into the intestine and normal saline is adding salt to the patient's circulatory system, therefore potentially causing *hypernatremia*.

7. According to the American Association of Critical Care Nurses (AACN) practice guidelines, pH monitoring of NG tube fluid aspirates is **best** used to ascertain which assessment?

A. Placement in the esophagus
B. Migration from the stomach to small bowel (intestine)
C. Placement in the lungs
D. Correct placement in the stomach

Answer: B. The AACN guidelines state that serial pH monitoring of the NG tube fluid aspirate can eliminate the need for more than one X-ray to confirm migration into the correct small intestinal placement.

8. What is the **first action** the nurse should do when a physician orders a diagnostic peritoneal lavage?

A. Insert an NG tube and Foley catheter.
B. Assist the physician in administering lidocaine to the planned site.
C. Give the patient an enema.
D. Deposit fluid specimens in the labeled containers.

Answer: A. After explaining the procedure to the patient, the nurse should immediately place an indwelling urinary catheter and then insert an NG tube to prevent bladder or bowel laceration and to prevent vomiting and aspiration.

9. A patient with a clamped T tube placed during a cholecystectomy develops sudden chills, fever, and nausea. What should the nurse do **first**?

A. Unclamp the T tube and connect to a gravity drainage system.
B. Irrigate the T tube.
C. Administer an antipyretic.
D. Prepare the patient to return to the operating room.

Answer: A. The nurse should immediately unclamp the T tube and then call the patient's surgeon.

10. What type of skin barrier should a nurse use for a client that has a stoma that protrudes at least an inch from the body?

A. A convex skin barrier
B. An emollient skin barrier
C. A large skin barrier
D. A flat skin barrier

Answer: D. For stomas that protrude at least an inch from the body, a flat skin barrier works the best.

11. Which tube is **not** routinely flushed by a nurse?

A. A PEG feeding tube
B. A G tube
C. A PEJ feeding tube
D. An NG feeding tube

Answer: B. A G tube should almost never be flushed unless it is opened for nausea or postoperatively and no gastric contents are draining out.

12. After administering an oil-retention enema to a patient, what should the nurse do next? *Select all that apply.*

A. Encourage the patient to avoid defecation for at least 30 minutes.
B. Place an indwelling catheter to promote retention.
C. Immediately start a digital disimpaction.
D. Help the patient to the commode or bathroom in 15 minutes.
E. Follow with a soap and water enema 1 hour later.

Answer: A, B, E. An oil retention enema should be held by the patient for at least 30 minutes. An indwelling catheter can be used to promote retention especially in patients with poor sphincter tone, and a soap and water enema is usually administered after an oil-retention enema to help expel the softened feces completely.

13. When administering medications through a feeding tube, what should the nurse plan to do? *Select all that apply.*

A. Grind up sustained-release medications for better absorption.
B. Open and dilute capsules in water before administering them.
C. Flush the tubing afterward to ensure full instillation of medication.
D. Crush tablets and dilute them in water before administration.
E. Flush enteric-coated drugs, without crushing them, through the feeding tube.

Answer: B, C, D. Sustained-release and enteric-coated medications should **never** be crushed, opened, or placed/flushed through a feeding tube.

Scoring

☆☆☆ If you answered 12 or 13 items correctly, marvelous! Your retention level is simply GI-ant!

☆☆ If you answered 10 or 11 items correctly, wonderful! You're as efficient as a well-placed NG tube.

☆ If you answered fewer than 9 items correctly, stay mellow. Remember, GI procedures may take some time to digest.

Selected References

Araghizadeh, F. (2005). Fecal impaction. *Clinics in Colon and Rectal Surgery, 18*(2), 116–119.

Dandeles, L. (2010). *What products can be used to unclog feeding tubes.* Retrieved from http://dig.pharm.uic.edu/faq/Jul10/feedingtube.aspx

Durai, R., Venkatraman, R., & Ng, P. C. (2009). Nasogastric tubes. 1: Insertion techniques and confirming position. *Nursing Times, 105*(16), 12–13.

Hollister. (2009). *Colostomy: What's right for me?* Retrieved from http://www.hollister.com/us/files/pdfs/osted_pcb_colostomy.pdf

Kirby, D. F., Delegge, M. H., & Fleming, C. R. (1995). American Gastroenterological Association technical review on tube feeding for enteral nutrition. *Gastroenterology, 108*(4), 1282–1301.

Memorial Sloan Kettering Cancer Center. (2013). *Caring for your Jackson-Pratt drainage system.* Retrieved from http://www.mskcc.org/cancer-care/patient-education/resources/caring-your-jackson-pratt-drainage-system

Metheny, N. (2009). *Verification of feeding tube placement: Blindly inserted.* Retrieved from http://www.aacn.org/wd/practice/docs/practicealerts/verification-feeding-tube-placement.pdf?menu=aboutus

Perry, A., Potter, P., & Desmarais, P. L. (2015). *Mosby's pocket guide to nursing skills and procedures* (8th ed.). St. Louis, MO: Elsevier.

Physician's Desk Reference. (2014). *Lidocaine ointment.* Retrieved from http://www.pdr.net/drug-summary/lidocaine-ointment?druglabelid=753

Turgay, A., & Khorshid, L. (2010). Effectiveness of the auscultatory and pH methods in predicting feeding tube placement. *Journal of Clinical Nursing, 19*, 1553–1559.

VHA Pharmacy Benefits Management Strategic Healthcare Group and the Medical Advisory Panel and the National Center for Patient Safety. (2006). *A guidance on the use of topical anesthetics for naso/oropharyngeal and laryngotracheal procedures.* Retrieved from http://intranasal.net/documentstoload/topicalanestheticsreview.pdf

Chapter 9

Renal care

Just the facts

In this chapter, you'll learn:

- about renal and urologic care procedures and how to perform them
- what patient care is associated with each procedure
- how to manage complications associated with each procedure
- about essential documentation for each procedure.

Indwelling catheter insertion

An indwelling urinary catheter, also called a Foley or retention catheter, provides the patient with continuous urine drainage. It's inserted into the bladder and a balloon is inflated at the catheter's distal end to prevent it from slipping out. Insert the catheter with extreme care to prevent injury and infection.

Catheters should only be inserted for appropriate reasons and only leave in place as long as needed to prevent infection. Minimize urinary catheter use and duration of use in all patients, especially those at risk for catheter-associated urinary tract infection (CAUTI), elderly, women, and those with compromised immune systems. Avoid use in patients and nursing home patients for management of incontinence. Use urinary catheters only if necessary in operative patients and not routinely. For patients who need a urinary catheter for surgery, it should be removed as soon as possible postoperatively, preferably within 24 hours unless there is an appropriate indication for use. (See *Centers for Disease Control and Prevention*.)

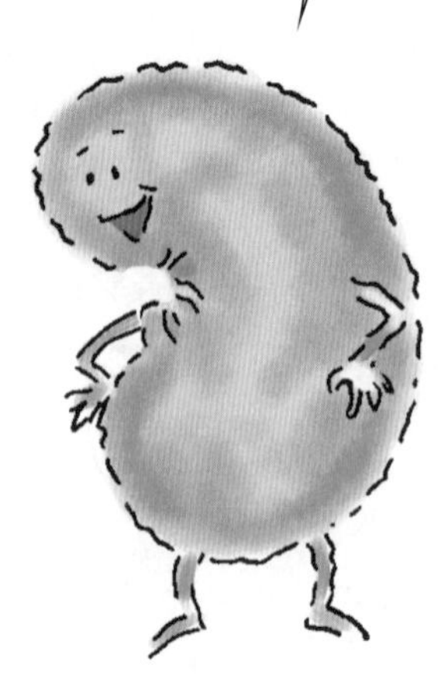
Here's everything you need to know about kidney procedures. Plus, you get the urinary system, too—no extra charge!

What you need

Sterile indwelling catheter (latex or silicone #10 to #22 French [average adult sizes are #16 to #18 French])—check for latex allergy ✱ syringe filled with 5 to 8 mL of normal saline solution

Centers for Disease Control and Prevention

A. Examples of appropriate indications for indwelling urethral catheter use
Patient has acute urinary retention or bladder outlet obstruction
Need for accurate measurements of urinary output in critically ill patients
Perioperative use for selected surgical procedures: • Patients undergoing urologic surgery or other surgery on contiguous structures of the genitourinary tract • Anticipated prolonged duration of surgery (catheters inserted for this reason should be removed in postanesthesia care unit [PACU]) • Patients anticipated to receive large-volume infusions or diuretics during surgery • Need for intraoperative monitoring of urinary output
To assist in healing of open sacral or perineal wounds in incontinent patients
Patient requires prolonged immobilization (e.g., potentially unstable thoracic or lumbar spine, multiple traumatic injuries such as pelvic fractures)
To improve comfort for end of life care if needed
B. Examples of inappropriate uses of indwelling catheters
As a substitute for nursing care of the patient or resident with incontinence
As a means of obtaining urine for culture or other diagnostic tests when the patient can voluntarily void
For prolonged postoperative duration without appropriate indications (e.g., structural repair of urethra or contiguous structures, prolonged effect of epidural anesthesia, etc.)

Note: These indications are based primarily on expert consensus.

✳ washcloth ✳ towel ✳ soap and water ✳ two linen-saver pads ✳ sterile gloves ✳ gloves ✳ sterile drape ✳ sterile fenestrated drape ✳ sterile cotton-tipped applicators (or cotton balls and plastic forceps) ✳ povidone-iodine or other antiseptic cleaning agent ✳ urine receptacle ✳ sterile water-soluble lubricant ✳ sterile drainage collection bag ✳ intake and output sheet ✳ optional: urine specimen container and laboratory request form, leg band with Velcro closure, gooseneck lamp or flashlight, pillows or rolled blankets or towels.

At your disposal

Prepackaged sterile disposable kits that usually contain all the necessary equipment are available. The syringes in these kits are prefilled with 10 mL of normal saline solution.

In case of contamination

In addition, gather an extra pair of sterile gloves and two catheters of an appropriate size to be readily available at the bedside in case of contamination during insertion.

Getting ready

Check the order on the patient's chart *to determine if a catheter size or type has been specified*. Then perform hand hygiene, select the appropriate equipment, and assemble it at the patient's bedside.

How you do it

- Identify the patient using two patient identifiers per facility policy. Explain the procedure to the patient and provide privacy. Check his chart and ask when he voided last. Percuss and palpate the bladder *to establish baseline data*. Ask if the patient feels the urge to void. Make sure he isn't allergic to iodine solution; if he *is* allergic, obtain another antiseptic cleaning agent. Raise the bed to appropriate working height. Stand on the left side of the bed if right-handed and on the right side of the bed if left-handed.
- Have a coworker hold a flashlight or place a gooseneck lamp next to the patient's bed *so that you can see the urinary meatus clearly in poor lighting*.

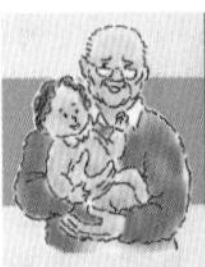

Ages and stages

Positioning the elderly female

The elderly female patient may need pillows or rolled towels or blankets for positioning support. If necessary, ask her to lie on her side with one knee drawn up to her chest during catheterization (as shown below). This position also may be helpful for disabled patients.

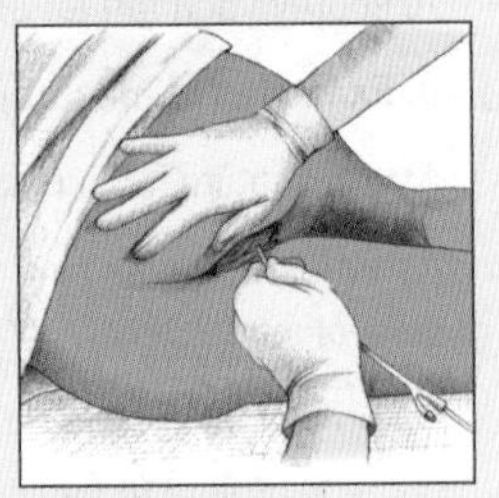

Assume the position

- Place the female patient in the supine position, with her knees flexed and separated and her feet flat on the bed, about 2′ (61 cm) apart. If she finds this position uncomfortable, have her flex one knee and keep the other leg flat on the bed. (See *Positioning the elderly female*.)
- Place the male patient in the supine position with his legs extended and flat on the bed. Ask the patient to hold the position *to give you a clear view of the urinary meatus and to prevent contamination of the sterile field*.

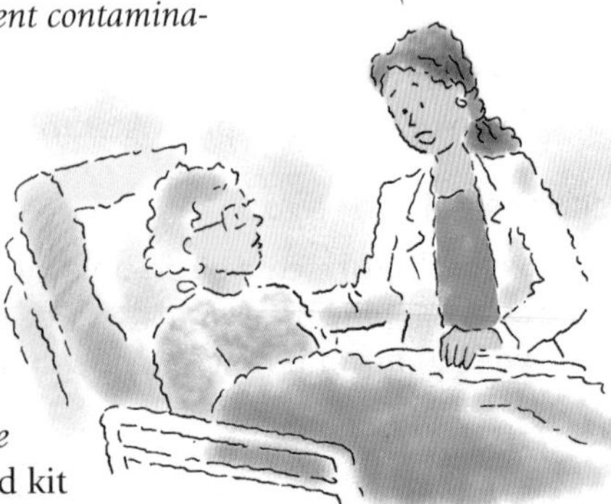
I'll need you to lie flat, with your knees flexed and separated.

Sterile fieldwork

- Don clean gloves. Clean the patient's genital area and perineum thoroughly with soap and water. Dry the area with the towel. Then remove the gloves and perform hand hygiene.
- Place the linen-saver pads on the bed between the patient's legs and under the hips. *To create the sterile field*, using aseptic technique, open the prepackaged kit

or equipment tray and place it between the female patient's legs or next to the male patient's hip. Place the sterile drape under the patient's hips. Then drape the patient's lower abdomen with the sterile fenestrated drape so that only the genital area remains exposed. Take care not to contaminate your gloves.

- Open the rest of the kit or tray. Don sterile gloves using strict sterile technique for Foley insertion.
- Tear open the packet of povidone-iodine or other antiseptic cleaning agent and use it to saturate the sterile cotton balls or applicators. Loosen lid of sterile specimen container if specimen needed.
- Open the packet of water-soluble lubricant and squeeze onto sterile field and place 2.5 to 5 cm of catheter tip into the lubricant; attach the drainage bag to the other end of the catheter. (If you're using a commercial kit, the drainage bag may be attached.) Check that all connections are secure. Make sure all tubing ends remain sterile and be sure the clamp at the emptying port of the drainage bag is closed *to prevent urine leakage from the bag.*
- Before inserting the catheter, inflate the balloon with normal saline solution *to inspect it for leaks.* To do this, attach the saline-filled syringe to the luer-lock, then push the plunger and check for seepage as the balloon expands. Aspirate the saline *to deflate the balloon.*

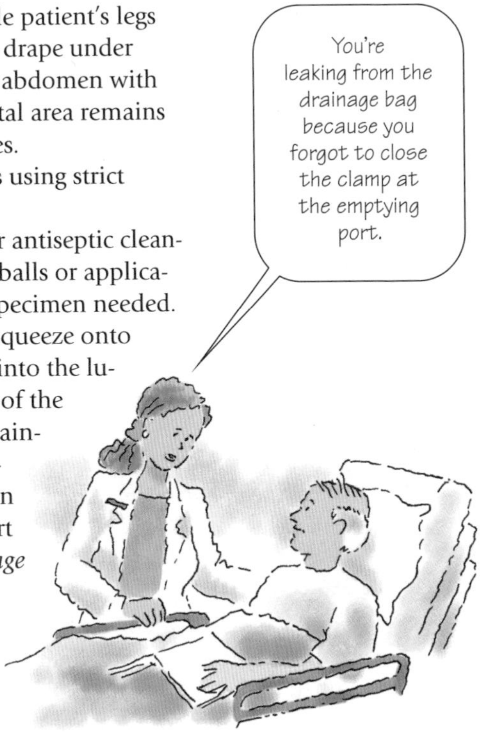

You're leaking from the drainage bag because you forgot to close the clamp at the emptying port.

Female facts

- For the female patient, separate the labia majora and labia minora as widely as possible with the thumb, middle, and index fingers of your nondominant hand *so you have a full view of the urinary meatus.* The nondominant hand is no longer considered sterile. Keep the labia well separated throughout the procedure *so they don't obscure the urinary meatus or contaminate the area when it's cleaned.*
- With your dominant hand, use a sterile, cotton-tipped applicator (or pick up a sterile cotton ball with the plastic forceps) and wipe one side of the urinary meatus with a single downward motion (as shown at right). Wipe the far side with another sterile applicator or cotton ball in the same way. Then wipe directly over the meatus with still another sterile applicator or cotton ball. Take care not to contaminate your sterile glove. If the labia closes during cleansing, the cleaning process must be repeated.

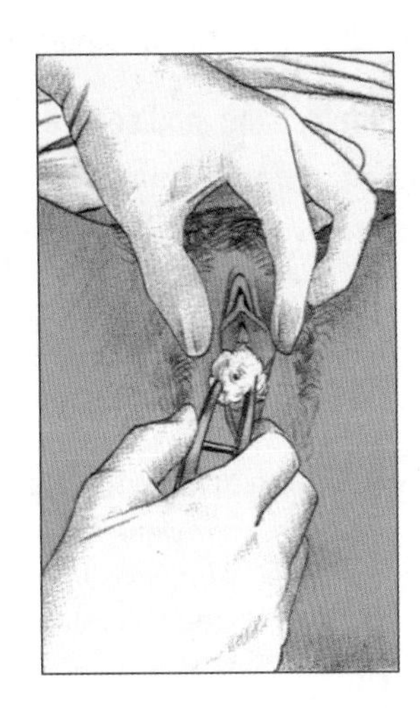

Male matters

- For the male patient, hold the penis at the shaft just below the glans with your nondominant hand; this hand is no longer sterile. If he's uncircumcised, retract the foreskin. Then gently lift the penis perpendicular to the patient's body and apply light traction. Hold the penis this way throughout the procedure *to straighten the urethra and maintain a sterile field.*

- Use your dominant hand to clean the glans with a sterile cotton-tipped applicator or a sterile cotton ball held in the forceps. Clean in a circular motion, starting at the urinary meatus and working outward down to the base of the glans.
- Repeat the procedure (three times) using another sterile applicator or cotton ball and taking care not to contaminate your sterile glove.
- Pick up the catheter with your dominant hand and prepare to insert the lubricated tip into the urinary meatus. *To facilitate insertion by relaxing the sphincter,* ask the patient to cough or bear down as you insert the catheter. Tell him to breathe deeply and slowly *to further relax the sphincter and spasms.* Hold the catheter close to its tip *to ease insertion and control its direction.* (See *Preventing indwelling catheter problems.*)

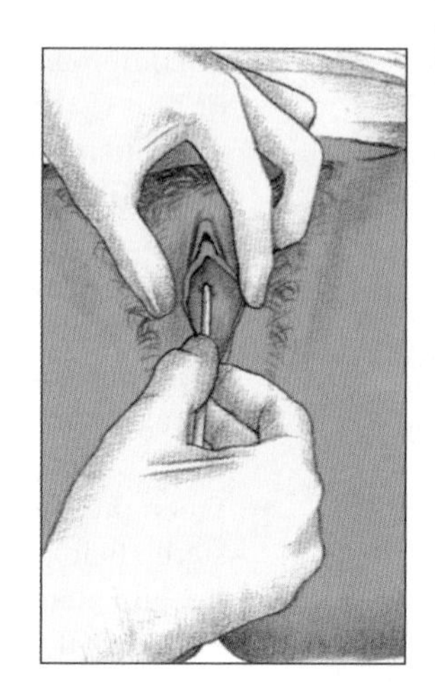

Advanced class

- For the female patient, with the sterile, dominant hand, pick up catheter and hold approximately 7.5 to 10 cm from tip loosely coiled in the palm of the hand; advance the catheter 2″ to 3″ (5 to 7.6 cm)—while continuing to hold the labia apart—until urine begins to flow (as shown in top illustration). Release labia and hold catheter securely. Collect urine specimen if needed.
  If the catheter is inadvertently inserted into the vagina, leave it there as a landmark. Then begin the procedure again using new supplies.
- For the male patient, advance the catheter to the bifurcation and check for urine flow (as shown in middle illustration). If the foreskin was retracted, replace it *to prevent compromised circulation and painful swelling.*

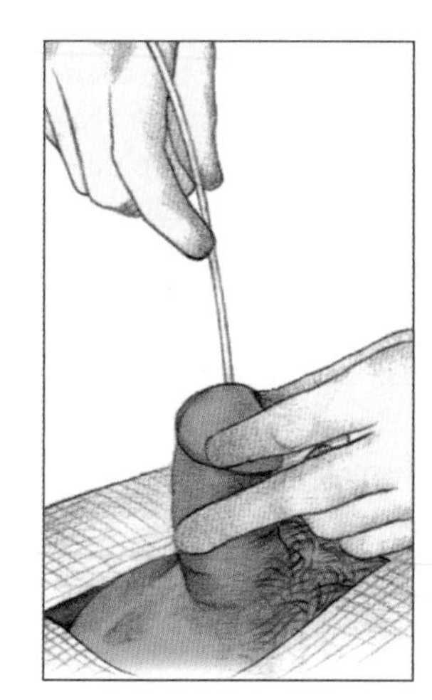

Inflate, hang, and secure

- Advance the catheter another inch. Push the plunger and slowly inflate the balloon *to keep the catheter in place in the bladder. Ask the patient to tell you if he feels any discomfort with balloon inflation. If he feels discomfort, the catheter is in the urethra. Deflate the balloon and advance the catheter into the bladder. Slowly inflate the balloon with 10 mL of saline and withdraw the catheter slowly until it meets resistance at the bladder neck.*
- Hang the collection bag below bladder level *to prevent urine reflux into the bladder, which can cause infection, and to promote gravity drainage of the bladder.* Make sure the tubing doesn't get tangled in the bed's side rails. Do not place bag on side rails.

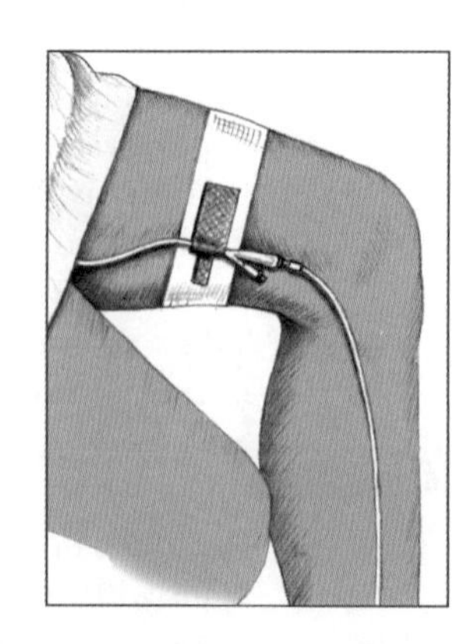

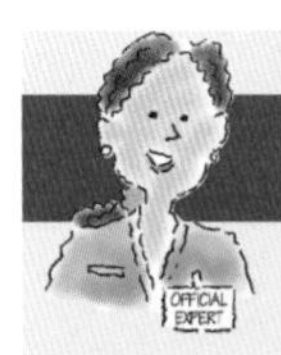

Advice from the experts

Preventing indwelling catheter problems

The following precautions can help prevent problems with an indwelling urinary catheter:

- Never force the catheter during insertion. Instead, maneuver it gently as the patient bears down or coughs. If you still meet resistance, stop and notify the doctor. Sphincter spasms, strictures, misplacement in the vagina (in females), or an enlarged prostate (in males) may cause resistance.
- Establish urine flow, and then inflate the balloon. This ensures that the catheter is in the bladder.

More helpful hints

Observe the patient carefully for hypovolemic shock and other adverse reactions caused by removing excessive volumes of residual urine. Check your facility's policy in advance to determine the maximum amount of urine that may be drained at one time; some facilities limit the amount to 700 to 1,000 mL. (Be aware, though, that controversy exists over the wisdom of limiting the amount of urine drainage.) Clamp the catheter at the first sign of an adverse reaction and notify the doctor.

- Secure the catheter to the patient's thigh using a leg band with a Velcro closure (as shown in lower illustration). *This reduces trauma and bleeding of the urethra and prevents bladder spasms caused by pressure and traction from movement of the catheter, prevents dislodgement and skin irritation, and may reduce risk of CAUTI.*
- Dispose of all used supplies properly.

Practice pointers

- The balloon size determines the amount of solution needed for inflation; the exact amount is usually printed on the distal extension of the catheter used for inflating the balloon.
- Unless otherwise clinically indicated, consider using the smallest bore catheter possible to minimize bladder neck and urethral trauma.
- If intermittent catheterization is used, perform it at regular intervals to prevent bladder overdistention.
- For monitoring purposes, empty the collection bag at least every 8 hours. Excessive fluid volume may require more frequent emptying *to prevent traction on the catheter wall.* (See *Documenting indwelling catheter insertion.*)

Write it down

Documenting indwelling catheter insertion

If your patient has an indwelling catheter, document:

- patient education
- date and time of catheter insertion
- size and type of catheter used
- amount, color, and other characteristics of urine drainage
- patient's tolerance of the procedure (if large volumes of urine were drained)
- whether a urine specimen was sent for laboratory analysis.

Be aware that your facility may require you to record fluid balance information only on the intake and output sheet.

Indwelling catheter care and removal

When performed, catheter care is completed after the patient's morning bath, immediately after perineal care. When the patient's condition warrants catheter removal, you'll also be required to remove the indwelling catheter.

Catheter care and maintenance

- Maintain a closed drainage system.
- Maintain unobstructed urine flow.
- Keep the tube free from kinking.
- Keep the drainage bag below the level of the bladder at all times.
- Empty the drainage bag frequently using a separate clean container. Do not let the drainage spigot make contact with the container.
- Use standard precautions, including using the gloves and gown as appropriate, during any manipulation of the catheter or the collecting system.
- Do not routinely change catheters or drainage bags. Only do it when clinically indicated.
- Routine bladder irrigation is not recommended per the Centers for Disease Control and Prevention.
- Do not clean the periurethral area with antiseptics to prevent CAUTI while the catheter is in place. Routine hygiene (e.g., cleansing of the meatal surface during daily bathing or showering) is appropriate.

What you need

For catheter removal

Absorbent cotton * gloves * alcohol pad * 10-mL syringe with a luer-lock * bedpan * linen-saver pad * optional: clamp for bladder retraining.

How you do it

- Identify the patient with two patient identifiers. Explain the procedure to the patient and provide privacy.

Catheter removal

Deflating the balloon

- Allow balloon to deflate by negative pressure and allow pressure within balloon to fill syringe with water. Use gentle aspiration if needed. The amount of fluid injected is usually indicated on the tip of the catheter's balloon lumen as well as on the Kardex and the patient's chart. Do not clamp the Foley before removing.

- Before removing the catheter, offer the patient a bedpan. Then grasp the catheter with the absorbent cotton and gently pull it from the urethra as patient exhales. Inspect the balloon to be sure that it's intact. If it isn't, report this to the doctor.
- Measure and record the amount of urine in the collection bag before discarding it.

Practice pointers

Stay low

- Avoid raising the drainage bag above bladder level. *This prevents reflux of urine, which may contain bacteria.*

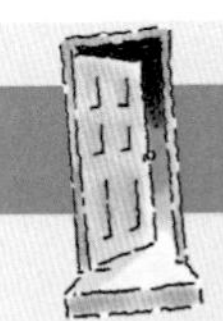

Home care connection

Teaching about leg bags

A urine drainage bag attached to the leg gives a catheterized patient greater mobility. Because the bag is hidden under clothing, it also may help him feel more comfortable about catheterization. Leg bags usually are worn during the day and replaced at night with a standard collection device.

If your patient will be discharged with an indwelling catheter, teach him how to attach and remove a leg bag. To demonstrate, gather a bag with a short drainage tube, two straps, an alcohol pad, adhesive tape, and a screw clamp or hemostat.

Attaching the leg bag

When teaching the patient how to attach the leg bag, follow these steps:

- Provide privacy and explain the procedure. Emphasize that a leg bag is smaller than a standard collection device and may have to be emptied more frequently.
- Remove the protective covering from the tip of the drainage tube. Then show the patient how to clean the tip with an alcohol pad, wiping away from the opening to avoid contaminating the tube. Show him how to attach the tube to the catheter.
- Place the drainage bag on the patient's calf or thigh. Have him fasten the straps securely (as shown) and show him how to tape the catheter to his leg.

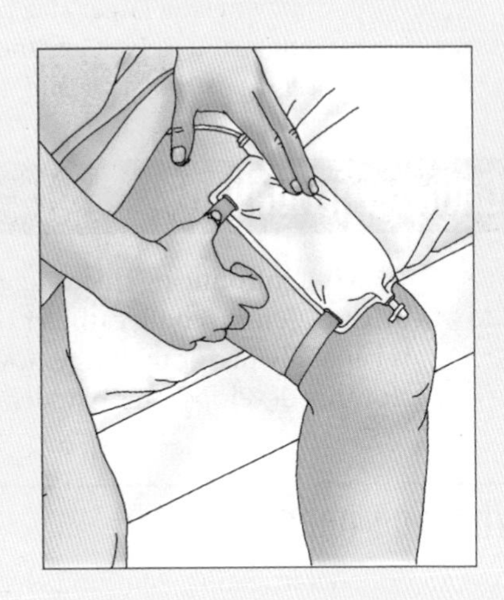

Let's not get complicated

To avoid complications, provide the following guidelines:

- To prevent a full leg bag from damaging the bladder wall and urethra, instruct the patient to empty the bag when it's only half full.
- To prevent infection, tell the patient to wash the leg bag with one part vinegar and three parts water. Soak bag for 20 minutes. Rinse bag with warm water and hang up to dry.

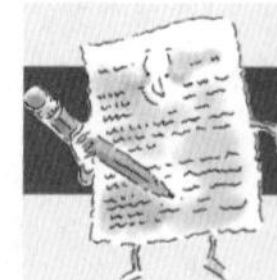

Write it down

Documenting indwelling catheter care and removal

When providing care for a patient with an indwelling catheter, document:
- care you performed
- care modifications required
- patient complaints
- condition of the perineum and urinary meatus
- characteristics of urine in the drainage bag
- whether a specimen was sent for laboratory analysis
- fluid intake and output. (Usually, an hourly record is required for critically ill patients and hemodynamically unstable patients with renal insufficiency.)

Catheter removal

Be sure to record:
- date and time of catheter removal
- patient's tolerance of the procedure
- when and how much the patient voided after removal (usually for first 24 hours)
- associated problems.

Bladder retraining

Document:
- date and time the catheter was clamped and released
- volume and appearance of urine.

- If the patient will be discharged with an indwelling catheter, teach him how to use a leg bag. (See *Teaching about leg bags*, page 443.)
- When changing catheters after long-term use (usually 30 days), you may need a larger size catheter because the meatus enlarges, causing urine to leak around the catheter. (See *Documenting indwelling catheter care and removal*.)

Catheter irrigation

To avoid introducing microorganisms into the bladder, you should irrigate an indwelling catheter only when necessary. The procedure is generally performed to remove an obstruction—such as a blood clot that develops after bladder, kidney, or prostate surgery.

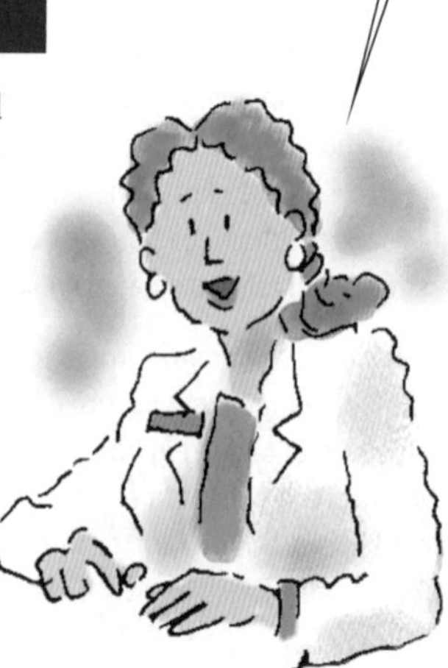
Perform catheter irrigation to remove an obstruction such as a blood clot.

What you need

Ordered irrigating solution (such as normal saline solution) ✳ sterile graduated receptacle or emesis basin ✳ sterile bulb syringe or 50-mL catheter-tip syringe ✳ two alcohol pads ✳ sterile gloves ✳ linen-saver pad ✳ intake-output sheet ✳ optional: basin of warm water.

We pause for this commercial message

Commercially packaged kits containing sterile irrigating solution, a graduated receptacle, and a bulb or 50-mL catheter-tip syringe are available. If the volume of irrigating solution instilled must be measured, use a graduated syringe instead of a noncalibrated bulb syringe.

Getting ready

Check the expiration date on the irrigating solution. *To prevent bladder spasms during instillation of solution,* warm it to room temperature. If necessary, place the container in a basin of warm water. Never heat the solution on a burner or in a microwave oven. *Hot irrigating solution can injure the patient's bladder.*

How you do it

- Identify the patient with two patient identifiers. Perform hand hygiene and assemble the equipment at the bedside. Explain the procedure to the patient and provide privacy.
- Place the linen-saver pad under the patient's buttocks *to protect the bed linens.*
- Create a sterile field at the patient's bedside by opening the sterile equipment tray or commercial kit. Using aseptic technique, clean the lip of the solution bottle by pouring a small amount into a sink or waste receptacle. Then pour the prescribed amount of solution into the graduated receptacle or sterile container.

Fill'er up

- Don sterile gloves and place the tip of the syringe into the solution. Squeeze the bulb or pull back the plunger (depending on the type of syringe) and fill the syringe with the appropriate amount of solution (usually 30 mL).
- Open the package of alcohol pads. Clean the juncture of the catheter and drainage tube with an alcohol pad *to remove as many bacterial contaminants as possible.*

Don't let go

- Disconnect the catheter and drainage tube by twisting them in opposite directions and carefully pulling them apart without creating tension on the catheter. Don't let go of the catheter—hold it in your nondominant hand. Then place the end of the drainage tube on the sterile field, making sure not to contaminate the tube.

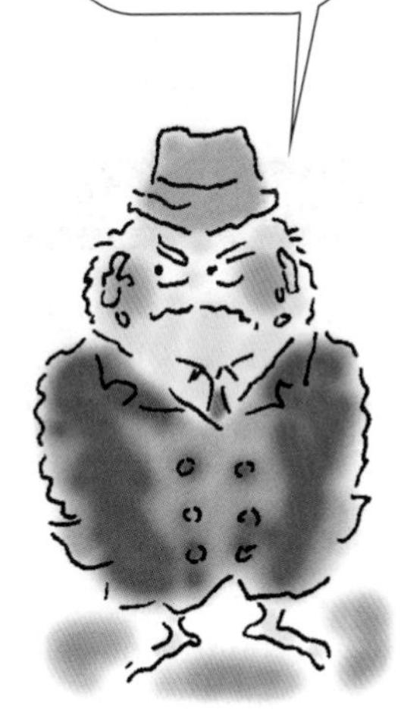
I'm always looking for new territory. Be careful when performing catheter irrigation or I'll take over.

- Twist the bulb syringe or catheter-tip syringe onto the catheter's distal end.

Flash flood

- Squeeze the bulb or slowly push the plunger of the syringe *to instill the irrigating solution through the catheter*. If necessary, refill the syringe and repeat this step until you've instilled the prescribed amount of irrigating solution.
- Remove the syringe and direct the return flow from the catheter into a graduated receptacle or emesis basis. Don't let the catheter end touch the drainage in the receptacle or become contaminated in any other way.
- Wipe the end of the drainage tube and catheter with the remaining alcohol pad.
- Wait a few seconds until the alcohol evaporates, then reattach the drainage tubing to the catheter.
- Dispose of all used supplies properly.

Documenting catheter irrigation

In your notes, record:
- patient education
- amount, color, and consistency of return urine flow
- patient's tolerance of the procedure
- any resistance met during instillation of the solution.

If the return flow volume measures less than the amount of solution instilled, note this on the fluid intake and output balance sheets as well as in your notes.

Practice pointers

- Catheter irrigation requires strict aseptic technique *to prevent bacteria from entering the bladder*. The ends of the catheter and drainage tube and the tip of the syringe must be kept sterile throughout the procedure.

In-stall-ation

- If you encounter resistance during instillation of the irrigating solution, don't try to force the solution into the bladder. Instead, stop the procedure and notify the doctor. If an indwelling catheter becomes totally obstructed, obtain an order to remove it and replace it with a new one *to prevent bladder distention, acute renal failure, urinary stasis, and subsequent infection*. (See *Documenting catheter irrigation*.)

Continuous bladder irrigation

Continuous bladder irrigation can help prevent urinary tract obstruction by flushing out small blood clots that form after prostate or bladder surgery. It may also be used to treat an irritated, inflamed, or infected bladder lining.

Triple threat

This procedure requires placement of a triple-lumen catheter. One lumen controls balloon inflation, one allows irrigant inflow, and one allows irrigant outflow. The continuous flow of irrigating solution through the bladder also creates a mild tamponade that may help prevent venous hemorrhage. (See *Setup for continuous bladder irrigation*.)

What you need

One 4-L container or two 2-L containers of irrigating solution (usually normal saline solution) or the prescribed amount of medicated solution ✱ Y-type tubing made specifically for bladder irrigation ✱ alcohol or povidone-iodine pad ✱ intravenous (I.V.) pole.

Getting ready

Before starting continuous bladder irrigation, double-check the irrigating solution against the doctor's order. If the solution contains an antibiotic, check the patient's chart *to make sure he isn't allergic to the drug.*

Setup for continuous bladder irrigation

In continuous bladder irrigation, a triple-lumen catheter allows irrigating solution to flow into the bladder through one lumen and flow out through another, as shown in the inset. The third lumen is used to inflate the balloon that holds the catheter in place.

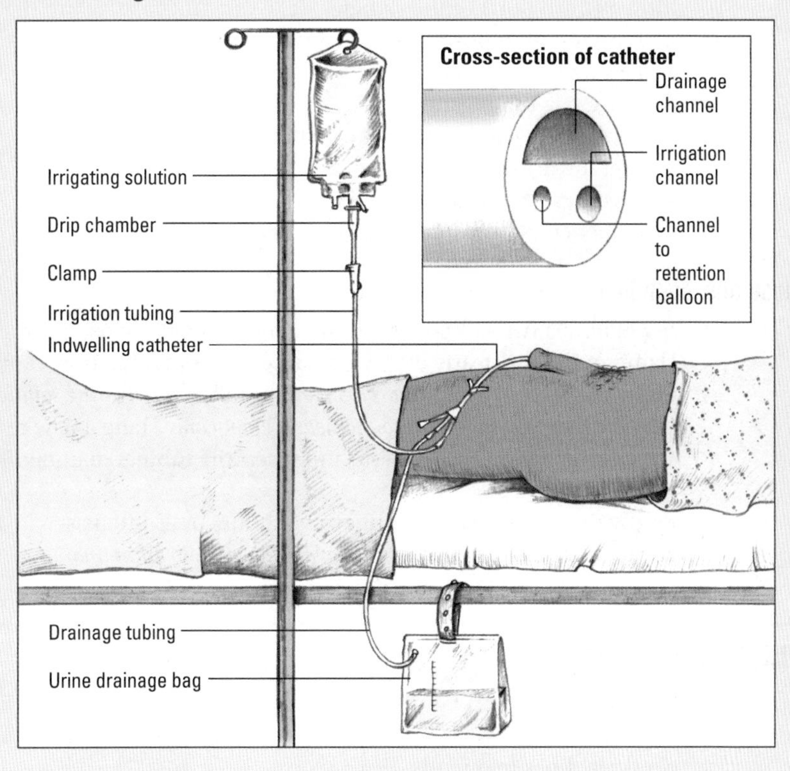

How you do it

- Identify the patient using two patient identifiers. Perform hand hygiene. Assemble all equipment at the patient's bedside. Explain the procedure to the patient and provide privacy.
- Hang the bag of irrigating solution on I.V. pole. Insert the spike of the Y-type tubing into the container of irrigating solution. (If you have a two-container system, insert one spike into each container.)
- Squeeze the drip chamber on the spike of the tubing until drip chamber is half full.
- Open the flow clamp and flush the tubing *to remove air, which could cause bladder distention*. Then close the clamp.

Hanging out

- Use standard precautions. To begin, hang the bag of irrigating solution on the I.V. pole.
- Clean the opening to the inflow lumen of the catheter with the alcohol or povidone-iodine pad.
- Insert the distal end of the Y-type tubing securely into the inflow lumen (third port) of the catheter. Take care not to attach to the balloon inflation port; this will cause balloon rupture.
- Make sure the catheter's outflow lumen is securely attached to the drainage bag tubing and is unclamped.
- Open the flow clamp under the container of irrigating solution and set the drip rate as ordered.
- *To prevent air from entering the system*, don't let the primary container empty completely before replacing it.

Close this, open that

- If you have a two-container system, simultaneously close the flow clamp under the nearly empty container and open the flow clamp under the reserve container. *This prevents reflux of irrigating solution from the reserve container into the nearly empty one.* Hang a new reserve container on the I.V. pole and insert the tubing, maintaining asepsis.
- Empty the drainage bag about every 4 hours or as often as needed. Use sterile technique *to avoid the risk of contamination*.

Practice pointers

- Check the inflow and outflow lines periodically for kinks *to make sure the solution is running freely*. If the solution flows rapidly, check the lines frequently.

Go all out—measure and assess

- Measure the outflow volume accurately. It should equal or, allowing for urine production, slightly exceed inflow volume. If inflow volume exceeds outflow volume postoperatively, suspect bladder rupture at the suture lines or renal damage and notify the doctor immediately.
- Also assess outflow for changes in appearance and for blood clots, especially if irrigation is being performed postoperatively to control bleeding. If drainage is bright red, irrigating solution should usually be infused rapidly *with the clamp wide open* until drainage clears. **Notify the doctor at once if you suspect hemorrhage.** If drainage is clear, the solution is usually given at a rate of 40 to 60 drops/minute. The doctor typically specifies the rate for antibiotic solutions. (See *Documenting continuous bladder irrigation*.)

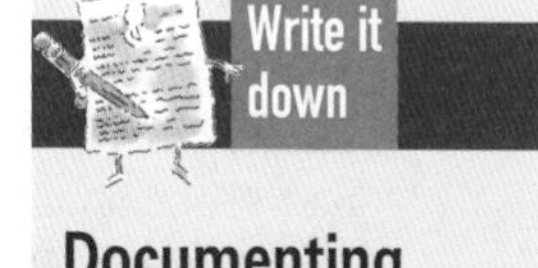

Documenting continuous bladder irrigation

Each time you finish a container of irrigating solution, record the date, time, and amount of fluid given on the patient's intake and output record.

Each time you empty the drainage bag, record the time and amount of drainage, appearance of the drainage, and any patient complaints.

Nephrostomy and cystostomy tube care

A nephrostomy tube drains urine directly from a kidney when a disorder inhibits the normal flow of urine. The tube is usually placed percutaneously, although sometimes, it's surgically inserted through the renal cortex and medulla into the renal pelvis from a lateral incision in the flank. Draining urine with a nephrostomy tube also allows kidney tissue damaged by obstructive disease to heal.

Creating a diversion

A cystostomy tube drains urine from the bladder, diverting it from the urethra. This type of tube is used after certain gynecologic procedures, bladder surgery, prostatectomy, and for severe urethral strictures or traumatic injury. Inserted about 2″ (5 cm) above the symphysis pubis, a cystostomy tube may be used alone or with an indwelling urethral catheter. Care involves changing the dressing daily (or more often if it becomes soiled) and irrigating the tube if necessary.

What you need

For dressing changes

Povidone-iodine solution or povidone-iodine pads ✱ 4″ × 4″ gauze pads ✱ sterile cup or emesis basin ✱ paper bag ✱ linen-saver pad ✱ clean gloves (for dressing removal) ✱ sterile gloves (for new dressing) ✱ forceps ✱ precut 4″ × 4″ drain dressings or transparent semipermeable dressings ✱ adhesive tape (preferably hypoallergenic).

For nephrostomy tube irrigation

3-mL syringe ✳ alcohol pad or povidone-iodine pad (some institutions use chlorhexidine) ✳ normal saline solution ✳ disposable linen-saver pad ✳ personal protective equipment (PPE) ✳ optional: hemostat.

Commercially prepared sterile dressing kits may be available.

Getting ready

- Confirm the order in the patient's medical record.
- Perform hand hygiene and assemble all equipment at the patient's bedside. Open several packages of gauze pads, place them in the sterile cup or emesis basin, and pour the povidone-iodine solution over them. Or, if available, open several packages of povidone-iodine pads. If you're using a commercially packaged dressing kit, open it using aseptic technique. Fill the cup with antiseptic solution. Check the patient for an allergy to iodine.

Cleanliness isn't next to the other equipment

Open the paper bag and place it away from the other equipment *to avoid contaminating the sterile field.*

How you do it

- Identify the patient using two patient identifiers per facility policy. Provide privacy and explain the procedure to the patient.

Changing a dressing

- Help the patient to lie on his back (for a cystostomy tube) or on the side opposite the tube (for a nephrostomy tube) *so that you can see the tube clearly and change the dressing more easily.*
- Place the linen-saver pad under the patient *to absorb excess drainage and keep him dry.*

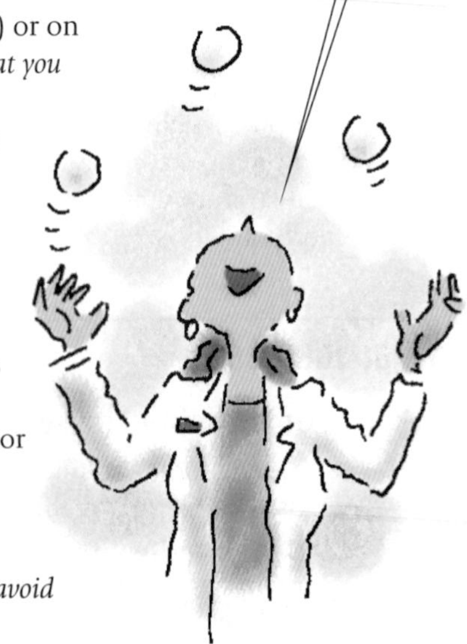
As a nurse, I sure could use four hands at times! For these tube changes, however, I need two sets of gloves.

Changing hands (just gloves really)

- Don clean gloves. Carefully remove the tape around the tube and then remove the wet or soiled dressing. Discard the tape and dressing in the paper bag. Remove the gloves and discard them in the bag.
- Don sterile gloves. Using forceps, pick up a saturated pad or dip a dry one into the cup of antiseptic solution.
- To clean the wound, wipe only once with each pad or pad, moving from the insertion site outward. Discard the used pad or pad in the paper bag. Don't touch the bag *to avoid contaminating your gloves.*

All dressed up

- Pick up a sterile 4″ × 4″ drain dressing and place it around the tube. If necessary, overlap two drain dressings *to provide maximum absorption*. Or, depending on your facility's policy, apply a transparent semipermeable dressing over the site and tubing *to allow observation of the site without removing the dressing*.
- Secure the dressing with hypoallergenic tape. Then tape the tube to the patient's lateral abdomen *to prevent tension on the tube*. (See *Taping a nephrostomy tube*.)
- Dispose of all equipment appropriately.

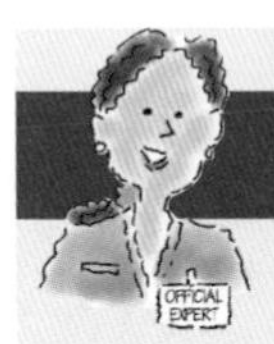

Advice from the experts

Taping a nephrostomy tube

To tape a nephrostomy tube directly to the patient's skin, follow these steps:

- Cut a wide piece of hypoallergenic adhesive tape twice lengthwise to its midpoint.

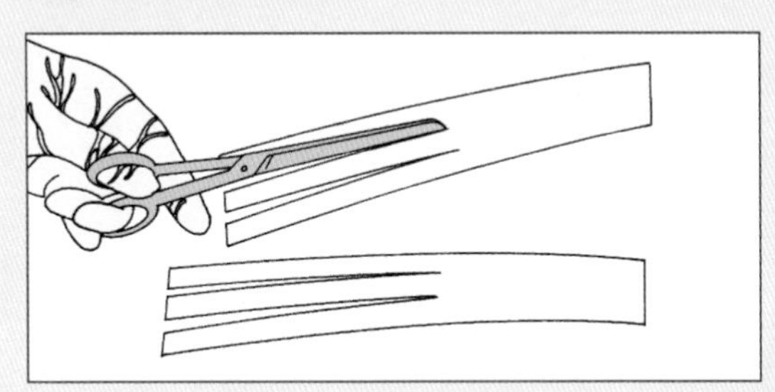

- Apply the uncut end of the tape to the skin so that the midpoint meets the tube.
- Wrap the middle strip around the tube in spiral fashion.

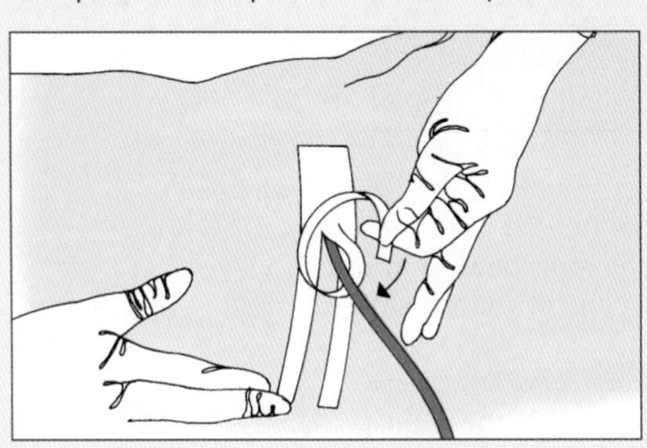

- Tape the other two strips to the patient's skin on both sides of the tube. For greater security, repeat this step with a second piece of tape, applying it in the reverse direction. You may also apply two more strips of tape perpendicular to and over the first two pieces.

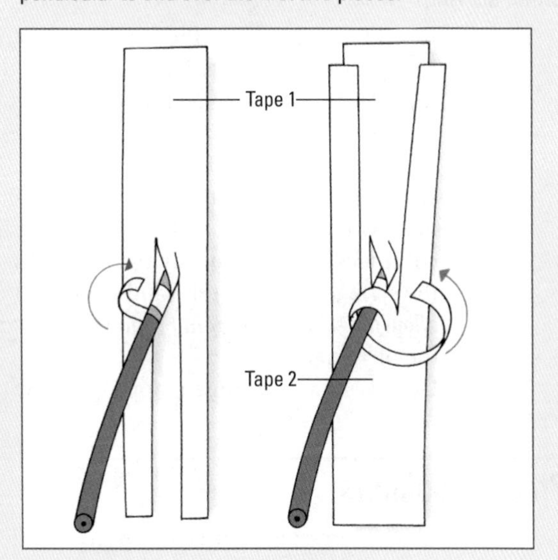

Dropping anchor

Always apply another strip of tape lower down on the tube in the direction of the drainage tube to further anchor the tube. Don't put tension on any sutures that prevent tube distention.

Irrigating a nephrostomy tube

This is required if there is absence of urine, if urine remains heavily blood stained, and if patient has persistent flank pain or suspected blockage.

This is a sterile procedure.

How you do it

- Confirm the order in the medical record. Identify the patient using two patient identifiers per facility policy.
- Explain the procedure to the patient.
- Assemble equipment at the bedside.
- Assist the patient to lie on the opposite side as the nephrostomy tube.
- Place the disposable sheet under the patient.
- Perform hand hygiene. Wear PPE.
- Fill the 3-mL syringe with the normal saline solution.
- Clean the junction of the nephrostomy tube and drainage tube with the alcohol pad or povidone-iodine pad and disconnect the tubes.

Small serving

- Insert the syringe into the nephrostomy tube opening (may have a stopcock) and gently instill 2 to 3 mL of saline solution into the tube. Never irrigate a nephrostomy tube with more than 10 mL of solution *because the capacity of the renal pelvis is usually between 4 and 8 mL.*
- Do not aspirate or force; if resistance occurs, ask the patient to lie down on his back and then again on his side. If resistance continues, stop and **notify the physician immediately**. Remove the syringe from the tube and reattach it to the drainage tubing *to allow the solution to drain by gravity*. If no drainage returns, notify the physician.
- Dispose of all equipment appropriately.

Practice pointers

- Change dressings once a day or more often if needed.
- When necessary, irrigate a cystostomy tube as you would an indwelling urinary catheter. Be sure to perform the irrigation gently *to avoid damaging any suture lines.*
- Check a nephrostomy tube frequently for kinks or obstructions. Suspect an obstruction when the amount of urine in the drainage bag decreases or the amount of urine around the insertion site

increases. Pressure created by urine backing up in the tube can damage nephrons. Gently curve a cystostomy tube *to prevent kinks.*

- Observe for continuous urine flow and signs of infection.
- **Notify the physician immediately** if the tube becomes dislodged or falls out. In a community setting, refer the patient to the emergency department.
- Observe for leakage at conjunction joints and seek advice from the physician if leakage seems evident.
- Typically, a cystostomy tube for a postoperative urologic patient should be checked hourly for 24 hours *to ensure adequate drainage and tube patency.* (See *Documenting nephrostomy and cystostomy care.*)

Documenting nephrostomy and cystostomy care

In your notes, record:

- patient education
- color and amount of drainage from the nephrostomy or cystostomy tube
- drainage color changes (as they occur)
- drainage color, amount, and characteristics from each tube if the patient has more than one tube
- amount and type of irrigant used (if irrigation is necessary)
- whether a complete return was obtained.

Urinary diversion stoma care

Urinary diversions provide an alternative route for urine flow when a disorder, such as an invasive bladder tumor, impedes normal drainage.

Temporary diversion

In conditions requiring temporary urinary drainage or diversion, a suprapubic or urethral catheter is usually inserted to divert the flow of urine temporarily. The catheter remains in place until the incision heals.

Permanent addition

A permanent urinary diversion is indicated in any condition that requires a total cystectomy (removal of the bladder). Ileal conduit (also known as ileal loop, Bricker's loop, or ileal bladder) and continent urinary diversion are the two types of permanent urinary diversions with stomas. These procedures usually require the patient to wear a urine collection appliance and to care for the stoma created during surgery. (See *Types of permanent urinary diversion,* page 454.)

What you need

Soap and warm water ✳ waste receptacle (such as an impervious or wax-coated bag) ✳ linen-saver pad ✳ hypoallergenic paper tape ✳ povidone-iodine pads ✳ urine collection container ✳ rubber catheter (usually #14 or #16 French) ✳ ruler ✳ scissors ✳ urine collection appliance (with or without antireflux valve) ✳ graduated cylinder ✳ cottonless gauze pads (some rolled, some flat) ✳ washcloth ✳ skin barrier in liquid, paste, wafer, or sheet form ✳ appliance belt ✳ two pairs of gloves ✳ optional: adhesive solvent, irrigating syringe, tampon, hair dryer, electric razor, regular gauze pads.

Types of permanent urinary diversion

The two main types of permanent urinary diversions are the ileal conduit and the continent urinary diversion. The steps involved in creating each are described here.

Ileal conduit

A segment of the ileum is excised and the two ends of the ileum that result from this excision are sutured closed. Then the ureters are dissected from the bladder and anastomosed to the ileal segment. One end of the ileal segment is closed with sutures; the opposite end is brought through the abdominal wall, forming a stoma.

Continent urinary diversion

A tube is formed from part of the ascending colon and ileum. One end of the tube is brought to the skin to form the stoma. At the internal end of this tube, a nipple valve is constructed so urine won't drain out unless a catheter is inserted through the stoma into the newly formed bladder pouch. The urethral neck is sutured closed.

Another recently developed type of continent urinary diversion is "hooked" back to the urethra, obviating the need for a stoma.

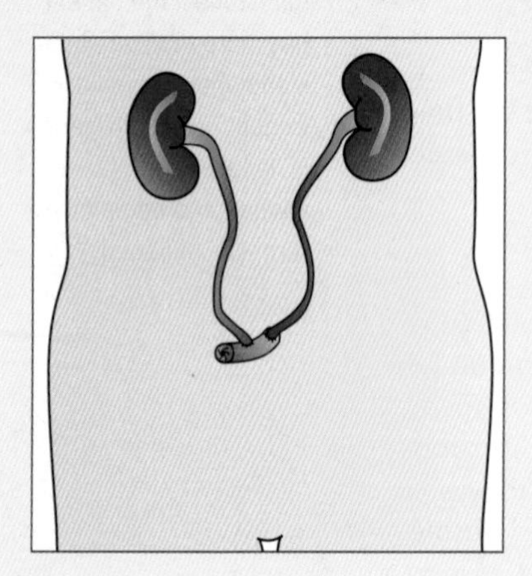

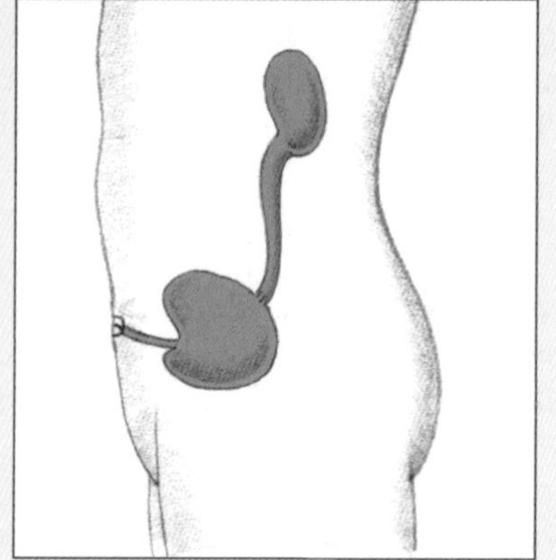

Commercial break

Commercially packaged stoma care kits are available. In place of soap and water, you can use adhesive remover pads, if available, or cotton gauze saturated with adhesive solvent.

Getting ready

- Confirm the order on the patient's medical record.
- Identify the patient using two patient identifiers per facility policy.
- Assemble all the equipment on the patient's overbed table. Tape the waste receptacle to the table for ready access. Provide privacy for the

patient and wash your hands. Measure the diameter of the stoma with a ruler. Cut the opening of the appliance with the scissors—it shouldn't be more than ⅛″ to ⅙″ (0.3 to 0.4 cm) larger than the diameter of the stoma. Moisten the faceplate of the appliance with a small amount of solvent or water *to prepare it for adhesion.*

Performance art

Performing these preliminary steps at the bedside *allows you to demonstrate the procedure and show the patient that it isn't difficult, which will help him relax.*

Let's take it from the beginning. Places! Nurse, I want you at the patient's bedside . . .
and...
action

How you do it

- Perform hand hygiene. Explain the procedure to the patient as you go along and offer constant reinforcement and reassurance *to counteract negative reactions that may be elicited by stoma care.*
- Place the bed in low Fowler's position so the patient's abdomen is flat. *This position eliminates skin folds that could cause the appliance to slip or irritate the skin and allows the patient to observe or participate.*
- Don gloves and place the linen-saver pad under the patient's side, near the stoma. Open the drain valve of the appliance being replaced *to empty the urine into the graduated cylinder.* Then, *to remove the appliance,* apply soap and water or adhesive solvent as you gently push the skin back from the pouch. If stents are present, pull appliance gently around stents. If the appliance is disposable, discard it into the waste receptacle. If it's reusable, clean it with soap and lukewarm water and let it air-dry.

Adhere to this: avoid adhesive

- *To avoid irritating the patient's stoma,* avoid touching it with adhesive solvent. If adhesive remains on the skin, gently rub it off with a dry gauze pad.
- *To prevent a constant flow of urine onto the skin while you're changing the appliance,* wick the urine with an absorbent, lint-free material. (See *Wicking urine from a stoma.*)

Wash and dry

- Use a washcloth and water to carefully wash off any crystal deposits that may have formed around the stoma. If urine has stagnated and has a strong odor, use soap to wash it off. Be sure to rinse thoroughly *to remove any oily residue that could cause the appliance to slip.*
- Follow your facility's skin care protocol to treat any minor skin problems.

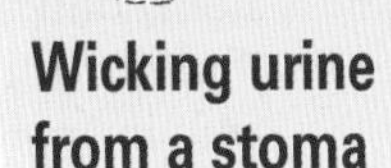

Wicking urine from a stoma

Use a piece of rolled, cottonless gauze or a tampon to wick urine from a stoma. Working by capillary action, wicking absorbs urine while you prepare the patient's skin to hold a urine collection appliance.

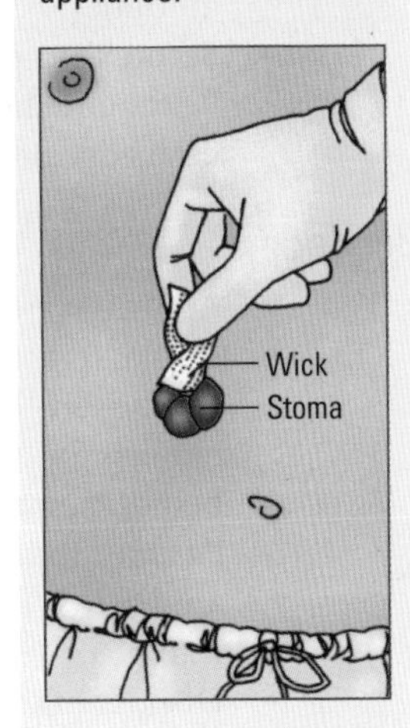

- Dry the peristomal area thoroughly with a gauze pad *because moisture will keep the appliance from sticking.* Remove any hair from the area with scissors or an electric razor *to prevent hair follicles from becoming irritated when the pouch is removed, which can cause folliculitis.*
- Inspect the stoma *to see if it's healing properly and to detect complications.* Inspect the peristomal skin for redness, irritation, and intactness.

Skin sense

- Apply the skin barrier. If you apply a wafer or sheet, cut it to fit over the stoma. Remove any protective backing and set the barrier aside with the adhesive side up. If you apply a liquid barrier (such as Skin-Prep), saturate a gauze pad with it and coat the peristomal skin. Move in concentric circles outward from the stoma until you've covered an area 2″ (5 cm) larger than the wafer. Let the skin dry for several minutes—it should feel tacky. Gently press the wafer around the stoma, sticky side down, smoothing from the stoma outward.
- If you're using a barrier paste, open the tube, squeeze out a small amount, and then discard it. Then squeeze a ribbon of paste directly onto the peristomal skin about ½″ (1.3 cm) from the stoma, making a complete circle. Make several more concentric circles outward. Dip your fingers into lukewarm water and smooth the paste until the skin is completely covered from the edge of the stoma to 3″ to 4″ (7.6 to 10.2 cm) outward. The paste should be ¼″ to ½″ (0.6 to 1.3 cm) thick. Then discard the gloves, wash your hands, and put on new gloves.
- Remove and discard the material used for wicking urine.
- Now place the appliance over the stoma, leaving only a small amount (⅜″ to ¾″ [1 to 2 cm]) of skin exposed.
- Secure the faceplate of the appliance to the skin with paper tape, if recommended. To do this, place a piece of tape lengthwise on each edge of the faceplate so that the tape overlaps onto the skin.

Buckle up

- Apply the appliance belt, making sure that it's on a level with the stoma. *If the belt is applied above or below the stoma, it could break the bag's seal or rub or injure the stoma.* The belt should be loose enough for you to insert two fingers between the skin and the belt. *If the belt is too tight, it could irritate the skin or cause internal damage.* Some devices don't require a belt. Instead, the pouch has a ridge that fits over the rim of barrier adhesive and snaps securely into place.
- Dispose of the used materials appropriately.

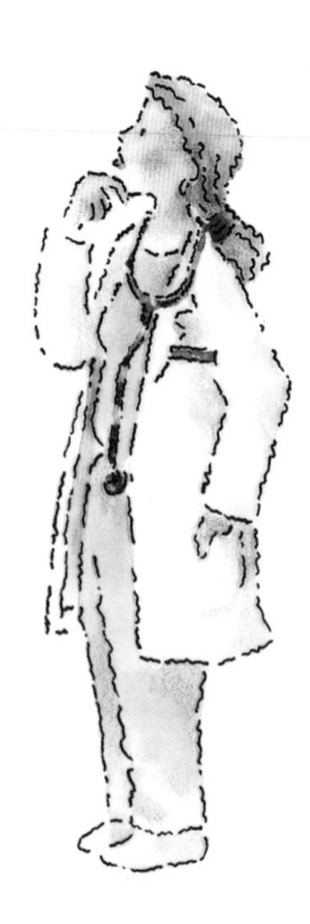

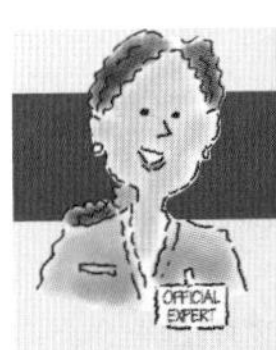

Advice from the experts

Caring for the patient with a continent urinary diversion

In a continent urinary diversion (an alternative to the traditional ileal conduit), a pouch created from the ascending colon and terminal ileum serves as a new bladder, which empties through a stoma. To drain urine continuously, several drains are inserted into this reconstructed bladder and left in place for 3 to 6 weeks until the new stoma heals. The patient will be discharged from the hospital with the drains in place. He'll return to have them removed and to learn how to catheterize his stoma.

First hospitalization

After the patient undergoes the procedure, follow these steps:

- Immediately after surgery, monitor intake and output from each drain. Stay alert for decreased output, which may indicate that urine flow is obstructed.
- Watch for common postoperative complications, such as infection and bleeding. Also watch for signs of urinary leakage, which include increased abdominal distention and urine appearing around the drains or midline incision.
- Using an irrigating syringe, irrigate the drains as ordered.
- Clean the area around the drains daily—first with povidone-iodine solution and then with sterile water. Apply a dry, sterile dressing to the area. Use precut 4″ × 4″ drain dressings around the drain to absorb leakage.
- To increase the patient's mobility and comfort, connect the drains to a leg bag.

Second hospitalization or outpatient visit

When the patient requires care after the initial hospitalization, follow these steps:

- After the patient's drains are removed, teach the patient how to catheterize the stoma. Gather the following equipment on a clean towel: rubber catheter (usually #14 or #16 French), water-soluble lubricant, washcloth, stoma covering (nonadherent gauze pad or panty liner), hypoallergenic adhesive tape, and an irrigating solution (optional).
- Apply water-soluble lubricant to the catheter tip to ease insertion.
- Remove and discard the stoma cover. Using the washcloth, clean the stoma and the area around it, starting at the stoma and working outward in a circular motion.
- Hold the urine collection container under the catheter, then slowly insert the catheter into the stoma. Urine should begin to flow into the container. If it doesn't, gently rotate the catheter or redirect its angle. If the catheter drains slowly, it may be plugged with mucus. Irrigate it with sterile saline solution or sterile water to clear it. When the flow stops, pinch the catheter closed and remove it.

Home care

When the patient goes home, provide these instructions:

- Teach the patient how to care for the drains and their insertion sites during the 3 to 6 weeks he'll be at home before their removal and teach him how to attach them to a leg bag. Also teach him how to recognize signs and symptoms of infection and obstruction.
- After the drains are removed, teach the patient how to empty the pouch and how to establish a schedule. Initially, he should catheterize the stoma and empty the pouch every 2 to 3 hours. Later, he should catheterize every 4 hours while awake and also irrigate the pouch each morning and evening, if ordered. Instruct him to empty the pouch whenever he feels a sensation of fullness.
- Tell the patient that the catheters are reusable but only after they've been cleaned. Advise him to clean the catheters inside and out every 2 days with distilled white vinegar to prevent crystal formation and hang it to dry over a clean towel. Tell him to store cleaned and dried catheters in plastic bags and change bag daily. Mention that he can reuse catheters for up to 1 month before discarding them. However, he should immediately discard any catheter that becomes discolored or cracked.

Practice pointers

- Tell the patient to empty the appliance through the drain valve when it's one-third to one-half full *to prevent the weight of the urine from loosening the seal around the stoma.*

Night collection

- Instruct the patient to connect his appliance to a urine collection container before he goes to sleep. *The continuous flow of urine into the container during the night prevents the urine from accumulating and stagnating in the appliance.*
- If the patient has a continent urinary diversion, make sure you know how to meet his special needs. (See *Caring for the patient with a continent urinary diversion,* page 457.)
- Inform the patient about support services provided by ostomy clubs and the American Cancer Society. (See *Documenting urinary diversion stoma care.*)

Write it down

Documenting urinary diversion stoma care

Record the appearance and color of the stoma and whether it's inverted, flush with the skin, or protruding. If it protrudes, note by how much it protrudes above the skin. (The normal range is ½" to ¾" [1.3 to 2 cm].) Record the appearance and condition of the peristomal skin, noting any redness or irritation or complaints of itching or burning.

Continuous ambulatory peritoneal dialysis

Continuous ambulatory peritoneal dialysis (CAPD) requires insertion of a permanent peritoneal catheter (such as a Tenckhoff catheter) to circulate dialysate in the peritoneal cavity. Inserted under local anesthetic, the catheter is sutured in place and its distal portion tunneled subcutaneously to the skin surface. There it serves as a port for the dialysate, which flows in and out of the peritoneal cavity by gravity. (See *Three major steps of continuous ambulatory peritoneal dialysis.*)

Three cheers for CAPD!

CAPD can be a welcome alternative to hemodialysis because the patient can perform the dialysis at home. It also provides more stable fluid and electrolyte levels than conventional hemodialysis.

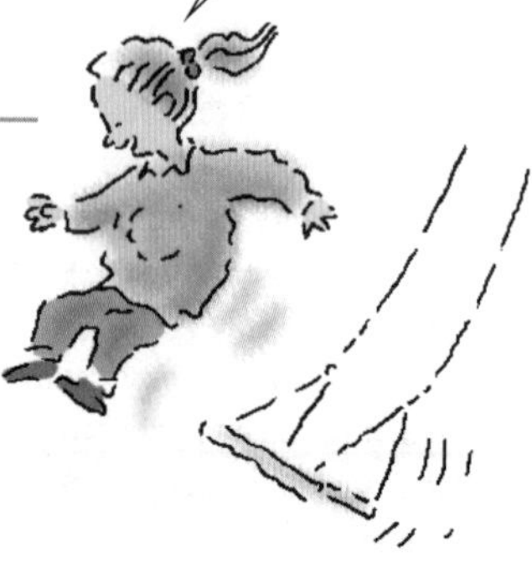
Totally awesome! CAPD gives dialysis patients more freedom.

What you need

To infuse dialysate

Prescribed amount of dialysate (usually in 2-L bags) ✱ heating pad or commercial warmer ✱ three face masks ✱ 42″ (106.7 cm) connective tubing with drain clamp ✱ six to eight packages of sterile 4″ × 4″ gauze pads ✱ medication, if ordered ✱ povidone-iodine pads ✱ hypoallergenic tape ✱ plastic snap-top container ✱ povidone-iodine solution ✱ sterile basin ✱ container of alcohol ✱ sterile gloves ✱ belt or fabric pouch ✱ two sterile waterproof

Three major steps of continuous ambulatory peritoneal dialysis

These illustrations show the patient setting up a CAPD system.

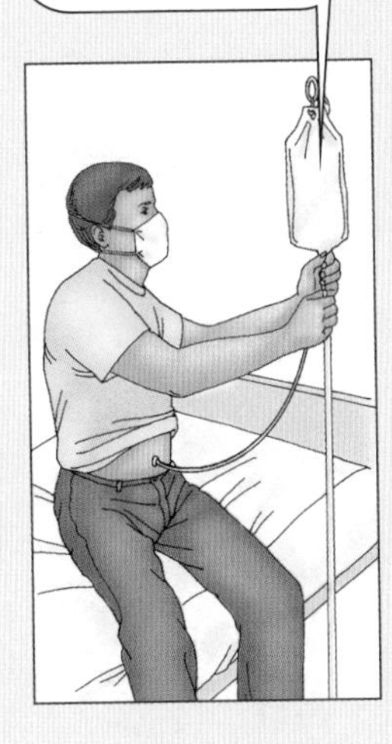
A bag of dialysate is attached to the tube entering the patient's abdominal area so the fluid flows into the peritoneal cavity.

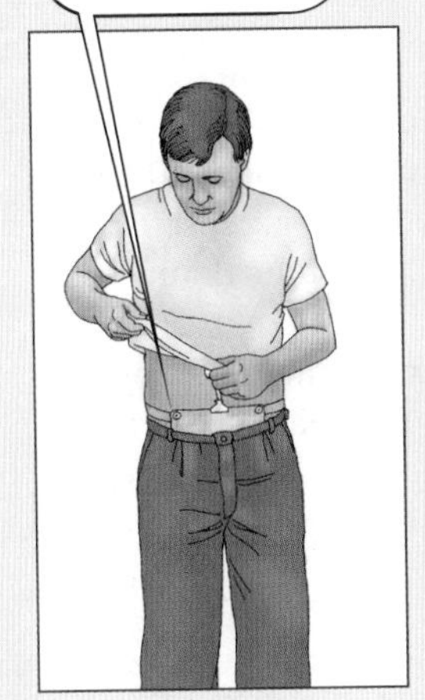
While the dialysate remains in the peritoneal cavity, the patient can roll up the bag, place it under his shirt, and go about his normal activities.

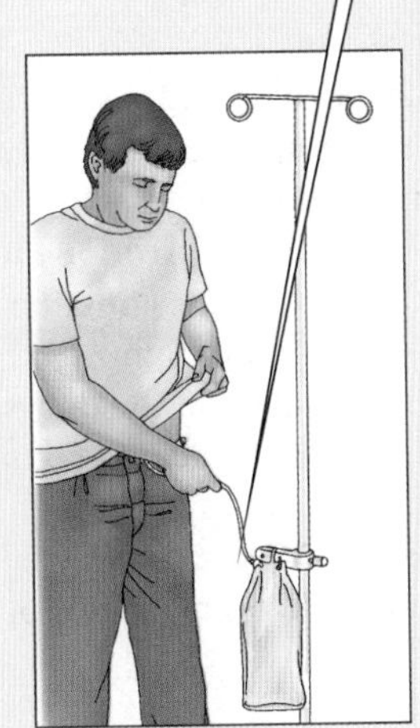
Unrolling the bag and suspending it below the pelvis allows the dialysate to drain from the peritoneal cavity back into the bag.

paper drapes (one fenestrated) ✳ optional: syringes, labeled specimen container.

To discontinue dialysis temporarily

Three sterile waterproof paper barriers (two fenestrated) ✳ 4″ × 4″ gauze pads (for cleaning and dressing the catheter) ✳ two face masks ✳ sterile basin ✳ hypoallergenic tape ✳ povidone-iodine solution ✳ sterile gloves ✳ sterile rubber catheter cap.

Sterility is a must

All equipment for infusing the dialysate and discontinuing the procedure must be sterile. Commercially prepared sterile CAPD kits are available.

Getting ready

Check the concentration of the dialysate against the doctor's order. Also check the expiration date and appearance of the solution—it should be clear, not cloudy. Warm the solution to body temperature with a heating pad or a commercial warmer if one is available. Don't warm the solution in a microwave oven *because the temperature is unpredictable.*

To minimize the risk of contaminating the bag's port, leave the dialysate container's wrapper in place. This also keeps the bag dry, which makes examining it for leakage easier after you remove the wrapper.

Perform hand hygiene and put on a surgical mask. Remove the dialysate container from the warming setup and remove its protective wrapper. Squeeze the bag firmly to check for leaks.

Anything to add?

If ordered, use a syringe to add any prescribed medication to the dialysate, using sterile technique *to avoid contamination.* (The ideal approach is to add medication under a laminar flow hood.) Disinfect multiple-dose vials in a 5-minute povidone-iodine soak. Insert the connective tubing into the dialysate container. Open the drain clamp to prime the tube. Then close the clamp.

Place a povidone-iodine pad on the dialysate container's port. Cover the port with a dry gauze pad and secure the pad with tape. Remove and discard the surgical mask. Tear the tape so it will be ready to secure the new dressing. Commercial devices with povidone-iodine pads are available for covering the dialysate container and tubing connection.

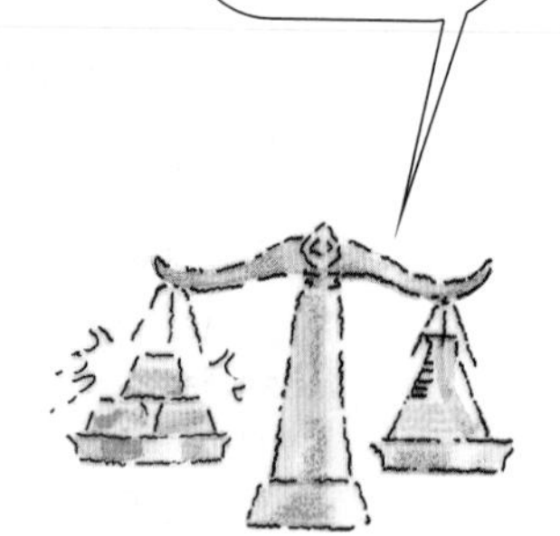
Weigh the patient daily to help monitor fluid balance.

How you do it

- Identify the patient using two patient identifiers per the facility policy.
- Weigh the patient *to establish a baseline level.* Weigh him at the same time and on the same scale every day *to help monitor fluid balance.*

Infusing dialysate

- Assemble all equipment at the patient's bedside and explain the procedure to him. Perform hand hygiene. Prepare the sterile field by placing a waterproof, sterile paper drape on a dry surface near the patient. Take care to maintain the drape's sterility.
- Fill the snap-top container with povidone-iodine solution and place it on the sterile field. Place the basin on the sterile field. Then place four pairs of sterile gauze pads in the sterile basin and saturate them with the povidone-iodine solution. Drop the remaining gauze pads on the sterile field. Loosen the cap on the alcohol container and place it next to the sterile field.

- Put on a clean surgical mask and provide one for the patient.
- Carefully remove the dressing covering the peritoneal catheter and discard it. Be careful not to touch the catheter or skin. Check skin integrity at the catheter site and look for signs of infection. If drainage is present, obtain a swab specimen and notify the doctor.
- Don sterile gloves and palpate the insertion site and subcutaneous tunnel route for tenderness or pain. If present, notify the doctor.

Catheter cleaning

- Wrap one gauze pad saturated with povidone-iodine solution around the distal end of the catheter and leave it in place for 5 minutes. Clean the catheter and insertion site with the rest of the gauze pads, moving in concentric circles away from the insertion site. Use straight strokes to clean the catheter, beginning at the insertion site and moving outward. Use a clean area of the pad for each stroke. Loosen the catheter cap one notch and clean the exposed area. Place each used pad at the base of the catheter *to help support it*. After using the third pair of pads, place the fenestrated paper drape around the base of the catheter. Continue cleaning the catheter for another minute with one of the remaining pads soaked with povidone-iodine.
- Remove the povidone-iodine pad on the catheter cap, remove the cap, and use the remaining povidone-iodine pad to clean the end of the catheter hub. Attach the connective tubing from the dialysate container to the catheter. Be sure to secure the luer-lock connector tightly.

What goes up must come down. Gravity allows the solution to enter the peritoneal cavity.

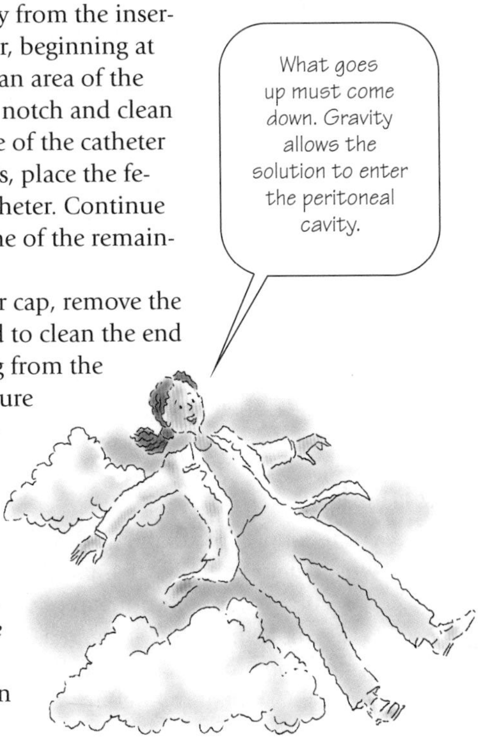

Open and fold

- Open the drain clamp on the dialysate container *to allow the solution to enter the peritoneal cavity by gravity* over a period of 5 to 10 minutes. Leave a small amount of fluid in the bag *to make folding it easier*. Close the drain clamp.
- Fold the bag and secure it with a belt or tuck it in the patient's clothing or a small fabric pouch.
- After the prescribed dwell time (usually 4 to 6 hours), unfold the bag, open the clamp, and allow peritoneal fluid to drain back into the bag by gravity.
- When drainage is complete, attach a new bag of dialysate and repeat the infusion.
- Discard used supplies appropriately.

Discontinuing dialysis temporarily

- Perform hand hygiene, put on a surgical mask, and provide one for the patient. Explain the procedure to him.

Sterile setup

- Using sterile gloves, remove and discard the dressing over the peritoneal catheter.
- Set up a sterile field next to the patient by covering a clean, dry surface with a waterproof drape. Be sure to maintain the drape's sterility. Place all equipment on the sterile field and place the 4″ × 4″ gauze pads in the basin. Saturate them with the povidone-iodine solution. Open the 4″ × 4″ gauze pads to be used as the dressing and drop them onto the sterile field. Tear pieces of tape as needed.
- Tape the dialysate tubing to the side rail of the bed *to keep the catheter and tubing off the patient's abdomen.*

Get more gloves

- Change to another pair of sterile gloves. Then place one of the fenestrated drapes around the base of the catheter.
- Use a pair of povidone-iodine pads to clean about 6″ (15.2 cm) of the dialysis tubing. Clean for 1 minute, moving in one direction only, away from the catheter. Then clean the catheter, moving from the insertion site to the junction of the catheter and dialysis tubing. Place used pads at the base of the catheter *to prop it up*. Use two more pairs of pads to clean the junction for a total of 3 minutes.
- Place the second fenestrated paper drape over the first at the base of the catheter. With the fourth pair of pads, clean the junction of the catheter and 6″ of the dialysate tubing for another minute.

Break in the line

- Disconnect the dialysate tubing from the catheter. Pick up the catheter cap and fasten it to the catheter, making sure it fits securely over both notches of the hard plastic catheter tip.
- Clean the insertion site and a 2″ (5 cm) radius around it with povidone-iodine pads, working from the insertion site outward. Let the skin air-dry before applying the dressing.
- Discard used supplies appropriately.

Practice pointers

- If inflow and outflow are slow or absent, check the tubing for kinks. You can also try raising the solution or repositioning the patient *to increase the inflow rate*. Repositioning the patient or applying manual pressure to the lateral aspects of the patient's abdomen may also help increase drainage.

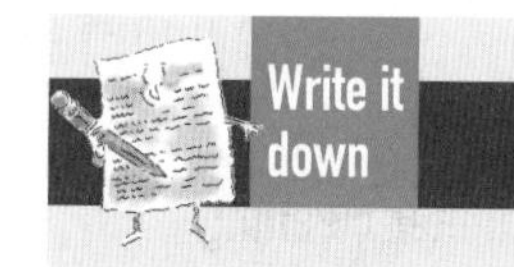

Documenting continuous ambulatory peritoneal dialysis

In your notes, record:

- patient education
- type and amount of fluid instilled and returned for each exchange
- time and duration of the exchange
- medications added to the dialysate
- color and clarity of the returned exchange fluid
- whether the returned fluid contains presence of mucus, pus, or blood
- fluid intake and output balance
- signs of fluid imbalance, such as weight change, decreased breath sounds, peripheral edema, ascites, or skin turgor change
- patient's weight, blood pressure, and pulse rate after the day's last fluid exchange.

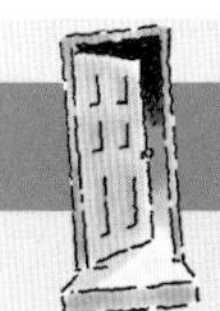

Home care connection

Using continuous-cycle peritoneal dialysis

CAPD is easier for the patient who uses an automated continuous cycler system. When set up, this system runs the dialysis treatment automatically until all the dialysate is infused. The system remains closed throughout the treatment, which cuts the risk of contamination. Continuous-cycle peritoneal dialysis (CCPD) can be performed while the patient is awake or asleep. The system's alarms warn about general system, dialysate, and patient problems.

Cycling through the day

The cycler can be set to an intermittent or continuous dialysate schedule at home or in a health care facility. The patient typically initiates CCPD at bedtime and undergoes three to seven exchanges, depending on individual prescriptions. On awakening, the patient infuses the prescribed dialysis volume, disconnects himself from the unit, and carries the dialysate in his peritoneal cavity during the day.

The continuous cycler follows the same aseptic care and maintenance procedures as the manual method.

- Keep a close watch for signs of infection.
- Inform the patient about the advantages of an automated continuous-cycle system for home use. (See *Using continuous-cycle peritoneal dialysis* and *Documenting continuous ambulatory peritoneal dialysis*.)
- Patient education materials can be found at the National Kidney and Urologic Diseases Information Clearing House at http://kidney.niddk.nih.gov/KUDiseases/pubs/peritoneal/index.aspx

An AV shunt site requires regular cleaning and dressing—more frequently if it gets wet.

Arteriovenous shunt care

An arteriovenous (AV) shunt consists of two segments of tubing joined (in a U shape) to divert blood from an artery to a vein. Inserted surgically, usually in a forearm or (rarely) an ankle, the AV shunt provides access to the circulatory system for hemodialysis.

An AV avocation

After insertion, the shunt requires regular assessment for patency and examination of the surrounding skin for signs of infection. AV shunt care also includes aseptically cleaning the arterial and venous exit sites, applying antiseptic ointment, and dressing the sites with sterile bandages. When performed just before hemodialysis, this procedure prolongs the life of the shunt, helps prevent infection, and allows early detection of clotting. Shunt site care is done more often if the dressing becomes wet or nonocclusive.

What you need

Drape ✱ stethoscope ✱ sterile gloves ✱ sterile 4″ × 4″ gauze pads ✱ sterile cotton-tipped applicators ✱ antiseptic (usually povidone-iodine solution) ✱ bulldog clamps ✱ plasticized or hypoallergenic tape ✱ optional: swab specimen kit, prescribed antimicrobial ointment (usually povidone-iodine), sterile elastic gauze bandage, 2″ × 2″ gauze pads.

Kits containing all the necessary equipment can be prepackaged and stored for use.

How you do it

- Identify the patient using two patient identifiers per facility policy.
- Explain the procedure to the patient. Provide privacy and perform hand hygiene.
- Place the drape on a stable surface, such as a bedside table, *to reduce the risk of traumatic injury to the shunt site.* Then place the shunted extremity on the draped surface.

Beware of dogs

- Remove the two bulldog clamps from the elastic gauze bandage and unwrap the bandage from the shunt area.
- Carefully remove the gauze dressing covering the shunt and the 4″ × 4″ gauze pad under the shunt.
- Assess the arterial and venous exit sites for signs of infection, such as erythema, swelling, excessive tenderness, or drainage. Obtain a swab specimen of any purulent drainage and notify the doctor immediately of any signs of infection.

The red and the black

- Check blood flow through the shunt by inspecting the color of the blood and comparing the warmth of the shunt with that of the surrounding skin. The blood should be bright red; the shunt should feel as warn as the skin. If the blood is dark purple or black and the temperature of the shunt is lower than the surrounding skin, clotting has occurred. **Notify the doctor immediately.**

Feel the vibe

- Use the stethoscope to auscultate the shunt between the arterial and venous exit sites. A bruit confirms normal blood flow. Palpate the shunt for a thrill (by lightly placing fingertips over the access site and feeling for vibration), which also indicates normal blood flow. Don't use a Doppler device to auscultate because it will detect peripheral blood flow as well as shunt-related sounds.
- Open a few packages of 4″ × 4″ gauze pads and cotton-tipped applicators and soak them with the antiseptic. Put on the sterile gloves.
- Using a soaked 4″ × 4″ gauze pad, start cleaning the skin at one of the exit sites. Wipe away from the site *to remove bacteria and reduce the chance of contaminating the shunt*. Use each 4″ × 4″ gauze pad only once to minimize the contamination risk.

They love crust

- Use the soaked cotton-tipped applicators to remove any crusted material from the exit site *because the encrustations provide a medium for bacterial growth*.
- Clean the other exit site using fresh, soaked 4″ × 4″ gauze pads and cotton-tipped applicators.
- Clean the rest of the skin that was covered by the gauze dressing with fresh, soaked 4″ × 4″ gauze pads.
- If ordered, apply antimicrobial ointment to the exit sites *to help prevent infection*.
- Place a dry, sterile 4″ × 4″ gauze pad under the shunt. This prevents the shunt from contacting the skin, which could cause skin irritation and breakdown.

Close the exits

- Cover the exit sites with a dry, sterile 4″ × 4″ gauze pad and tape the pad securely *to keep the exit sites clean and protected*. Make sure the tape doesn't kink or occlude the shunt.
- For routine daily care, wrap the shunt with an elastic gauze bandage. Leave a small portion of the shunt cannula exposed *so the patient can check for patency without removing the dressing*.
- Place the bulldog clamps on the edge of the elastic gauze bandage *so that the patient can use them quickly to stop hemorrhage in case the shunt separates*.
- For care before hemodialysis, don't redress the shunt, but keep the bulldog clamps readily accessible.

Practice pointers

- Make sure the AV junction of the shunt is secured with plasticized or hypoallergenic tape. *This prevents separation of the two halves of the shunt, minimizing the risk of hemorrhage.*

Don't measure, don't puncture

- Blood pressure measurement and venipuncture should be avoided in the affected arm to *prevent shunt occlusion.*
- Never remove the tape securing the AV junction during dressing changes.
- Make sure the patient isn't allergic to iodine before using povidone-iodine solution or ointment. (See *Documenting shunt care.*)

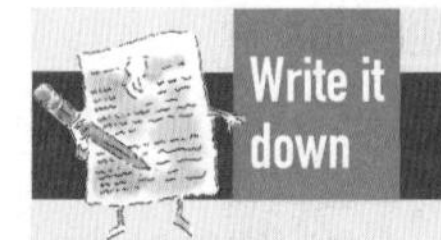

Documenting shunt care

In your notes, record:
- patient education
- that shunt care was performed
- condition of the shunt and surrounding skin, + bruit and thrill
- ointment used
- instructions given to the patient.

Continuous arteriovenous hemofiltration

When patients have fluid overload but don't require dialysis, continuous arteriovenous hemofiltration (CAVH) is used for treatment. CAVH filters fluid, solutes, and electrolytes from the patient's blood and infuses a replacement solution.

The hemofilter, composed of about 5,000 hollow fiber capillaries, filters blood at a rate of about 100 to 250 mL/minute and is driven by the patient's arterial blood pressure (a systolic blood pressure of 60 mm Hg is adequate for the procedure). Some of the ultrafiltrate collected during CAVH is replaced with a replacement fluid, which can be lactated Ringer's solution or any solution that resembles plasma. Because the amount of fluid removed exceeds the amount replaced, the patient gradually loses fluid (12 to 15 L daily).

Slow drain

CAVH carries a much lower risk of hypotension than conventional hemodialysis because it withdraws fluid more slowly—at about 200 mL/hour. CAVH is commonly used to treat patients in acute renal failure. It's also used for treating fluid overload that doesn't respond to diuretics and for some electrolyte and acid-base disturbances. Possible complications include bleeding, hemorrhage, hemofilter occlusion, infection, and thrombosis.

What you need

CAVH equipment ✳ heparin flush solution ✳ occlusive dressings for catheter insertion sites ✳ sterile gloves ✳ sterile mask ✳ povidone-iodine solution ✳ sterile 4″ × 4″ gauze pads ✳ tape ✳ filtration replacement fluid (FRF), as ordered ✳ infusion pump.

How you do it

- Perform hand hygiene. Assemble your equipment at the patient's bedside and explain the procedure to him.
- If necessary, assist with inserting the catheters into the femoral artery and vein using strict aseptic technique. (In some cases, an internal AV fistula or external AV shunt may be used instead of the femoral route.) If ordered, flush both catheters with the heparin flush solution *to prevent clotting.*
- Apply occlusive dressings to the insertion sites and mark the dressings with the date and time. Secure the tubing and connections with tape.
- Assess all pulses in the affected leg every hour for the first 4 hours, then every 2 hours afterward.

Weights and measures

- Weigh the patient, take baseline vital signs, and make sure that all necessary laboratory studies have been done. Monitor the patient's weight and vital signs hourly.
- Don sterile gloves and mask. Prepare the connection sites by cleaning them with gauze pads soaked in povidone-iodine solution; then connect them to the exit port of each catheter.
- Connect the arterial and venous lines to the hemofilter. Use aseptic technique.

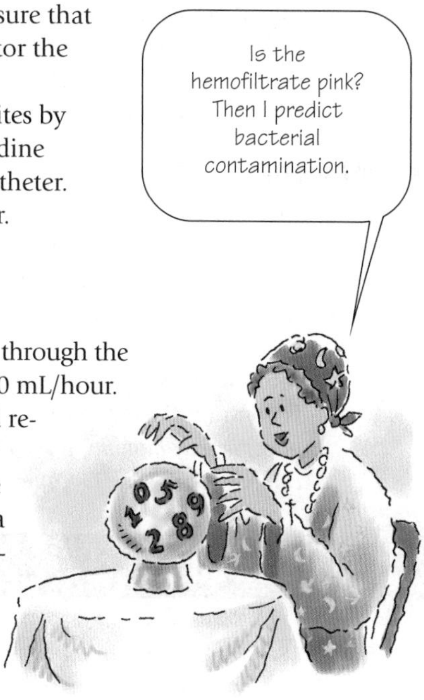

Let the flow go

- Turn on the hemofilter and monitor the blood flow rate through the circuit. The flow rate is usually kept between 500 and 900 mL/hour.
- Inspect the ultrafiltrate during the procedure. It should remain clear yellow, with no gross blood. Pink-tinged or bloody ultrafiltrate may signal a membrane leak in the hemofilter, which permits bacterial contamination. If a leak occurs, notify the doctor so he can have the hemofilter replaced.

When cool isn't cool

- Assess the affected leg for signs of obstructed blood flow, such as coolness, pallor, and weak pulse.
  Check the groin area on the affected side for signs of hematoma. Also ask the patient if he has pain at the insertion sites.
- Calculate the amount of FRF every hour, or as ordered, according to policy. Then infuse the prescribed amount and type of FRF through the infusion pump into the arterial side of the circuit.
- Stay alert for decreased blood pressure, which may indicate hypovolemia, from removal of ultrafiltrate too rapidly.

Practice pointers

- *Because blood flows through an extracorporeal circuit during CAVH,* the blood in the hemofilter may need to be anticoagulated. To do this, infuse heparin in low doses (usually starting at 500 units/hour) into an infusion port on the arterial side of the setup. Then measure thrombin clotting time or the activated clotting time (ACT). *This ensures that the circuit, not the patient, is anticoagulated.* A normal ACT is 100 seconds; during CAVH, keep it between 100 and 300 seconds, depending on the patient's clotting times. If the ACT is too high or too low, the doctor will adjust the heparin dose accordingly.

Rerouted

- Another way to prevent clotting in the hemofilter is to infuse medications or blood through a line other than the venous line, if possible.
- A third way to help prevent clots in the hemofilter, and also to prevent kinks in the catheter, is to make sure the patient doesn't bend the affected leg more than 30 degrees at the hip for femoral lines.

Beating bacteria

- *To prevent infection,* perform skin care at the catheter insertion sites every 48 hours (some institutions use 72 hours) using aseptic technique. Cover the sites with an occlusive dressing.
- If the ultrafiltrate flow rate decreases, raise the bed *to increase the distance between the collection device and the hemofilter.* Lower the bed *to decrease the flow rate.* Clamping the ultrafiltrate line is contraindicated with some types of hemofilters *because pressure may buildup in the filter, clotting it and collapsing the blood compartment.* (See *Documenting CAVH.*)

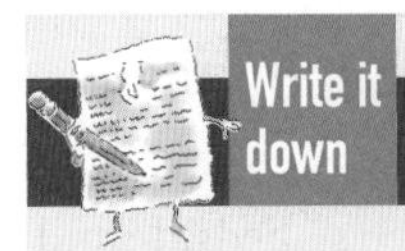

Documenting CAVH

In your notes, record:
- patient education
- time the treatment began and ended
- fluid balance information
- times of dressing changes
- any complications
- medications given
- patient's vital signs and tolerance of the procedure.

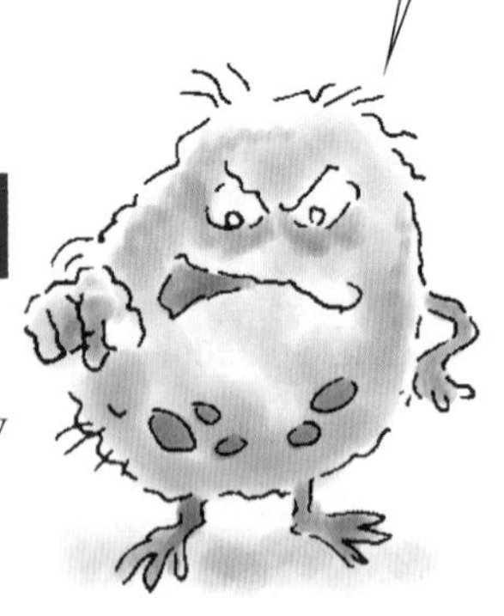
Wanna keep me out? Perform skin care at the CAVH site every 2 days.

Quick quiz

1. Securing the catheter to the patient's thigh using a leg band with a Velcro closure prevents several issues. Which issue is not affected by securing the catheter?
   A. Prevention of bladder spasms
   B. Balloon rupture
   C. Reduction in trauma and bleeding
   D. Decreases unintended catheter removal

Answer: B. Leg securement reduces trauma and bleeding and bladder spasms, which result from traction and pressure on the urethra from unsecured catheters. Leg securement does not prevent balloon rupture.

2. If drainage from continuous bladder irrigation is bright red, at what rate should the nurse infuse the irrigating solution?

A. 40 to 60 drops/minute
B. 20 to 60 drops/minute
C. A rapid rate with the clamp wide open
D. Intermittent rate depending on the patient's age

Answer: C. If drainage is bright red, run the irrigating solution rapidly until drainage clears. Continuous flow of irrigating solution through the bladder helps create a mild tamponade that may help prevent hemorrhage. Notify the doctor if you suspect hemorrhage.

3. What's the total volume of solution that can be safely used to irrigate a nephrostomy tube?

A. 2 to 3 mL
B. 5 to 10 mL
C. 10 to 20 mL
D. 30 mL

Answer: A. Never irrigate a nephrostomy tube with more than 5 mL of solution because renal pelvis capacity usually is between 4 and 8 mL.

4. When assessing an AV shunt for normal blood flow, what should the nurse detect?

A. Dark purple or black blood in the shunt
B. A shunt temperature that is lower than the surrounding skin
C. A positive bruit and thrill
D. No audible sounds at the shunt

Answer: C. A positive bruit and thrill confirms normal blood flow. The blood in the shunt should be bright red and the shunt should feel as warm as the skin. If the blood is dark purple or black and the temperature of the shunt is lower than the surrounding skin, clotting has occurred.

5. If inflow or outflow during CAPD is slow or absent, which step is contraindicated in trying to increase blood flow?

A. Checking the tubing for kinks
B. Repositioning the patient
C. Lowering the solution
D. Increasing the solution height

Answer: C. Raising, not lowering, the solution may increase the flow rate of the solution by increasing the pressure of gravity.

Scoring

☆☆☆ If you answered all five items correctly, super! You're as smooth as a perfect catheter insertion.

☆☆ If you answered three or four items correctly, cool! You've got a ken for kidney procedures.

☆ If you answered fewer than three items correctly, that's okay. Just read the chapter again, and you'll begin to filter all the important facts.

Selected References

Agency for Clinical Innovation. (2012). *Nursing management of patient's with nephrostomy tubes: Guidelines and patient information*. Retrieved from http://www.aci.health.nsw.gov.au/__data/assets/pdf_file/0011//165917/Nephrostomy-Tubes-Toolkit.pdf

National Institute of Diabetes and Digestive and Kidney Diseases, National Institutes of Health. (2014a). *Treatment methods for kidney failure: Peritoneal dialysis*. Retrieved from http://kidney.niddk.nih.gov/KUDiseases/pubs/peritoneal/index.aspx

National Institute of Diabetes and Digestive and Kidney Diseases, National Institutes of Health. (2014b). *Urinary diversion*. Retrieved from http://kidney.niddk.nih.gov/kudiseases/pubs/urostomy/#diversion

Northwestern Memorial Hospital. (2007). *A patient guide to urinary diversions*. Retrieved from https://www.nm.org/sites/default/files/urinary-diversion-guide-08-07.pdf

Chapter 10

Orthopedic care

Just the facts

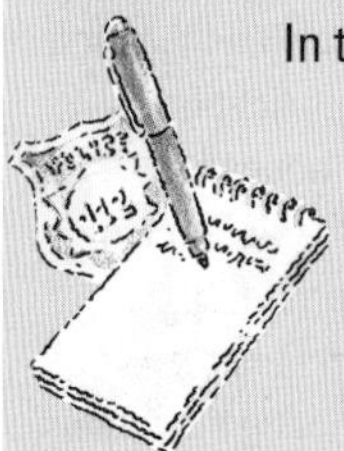

In this chapter, you'll learn:

- about orthopedic procedures and how to perform them
- what patient care is associated with each procedure
- how to manage complications associated with each procedure
- about patient teaching and documentation for each procedure.

Arm sling application

Slings have traditionally been made from a triangular piece of muslin, canvas, or cotton. Modern slings are commercially manufactured and come in several sizes. Slings promote healing by supporting and immobilizing an injured arm, wrist, shoulder, or hand. A sling may be applied to restrict movement of a fracture or dislocation or to support a muscle sprain. It also can support the weight of a splint and help secure a dressing.

What you need

Commercially manufactured sling in the appropriate size (pediatric or adult size small, medium, or large).

How you do it

- Identify the patient using two patient identifiers per facility policy.
- Perform hand hygiene and explain the procedure to the patient.
- Have the patient remove any hand or wrist jewelry.
- Position the affected arm across the patient's chest with the elbow flexed to 90 degrees. To help prevent dependent edema and possible neurovascular compromise, keep the patient's fingers slightly higher than the hand and the hand slightly higher than the elbow.

- Slide the patient's arm into the sling placing the elbow snugly into the corner of the sling sleeve. *Note:* The forearm should rest across the chest with the wrist supported by the sling. The fingers should be visible with the thumb pointing up or toward the body.
- Place the neck strap *outside of the shirt* to reduce irritation and fasten strap to the back of the sling.
- Assess the capillary bed refill of the patient's fingers and radial and ulnar pulses. Instruct patient to report any numbness or tingling that might indicate a too-tight sling or the development of compartment syndrome.

Documenting sling application

In your notes, record:
- date, time, and location of sling application
- patient education
- patient's tolerance of the procedure
- circulation to the fingers, noting their color and temperature.

Practice pointers

- Teach the patient signs and symptoms of skin irritation and breakdown and the proper care of the sling while at home. (See *Documenting sling application*.)

Clavicle strap application

Also called a figure-eight strap, a clavicle strap reduces and immobilizes a fracture of the clavicle by gently pulling the shoulders back and putting the clavicle in a healing position. A commercially available figure-eight strap is most commonly used.

What you need

Figure-eight clavicle strap ✳ marking pen ✳ analgesics as ordered.

How you do it

- Identify the patient using two patient identifiers per facility policy.
- Perform hand hygiene and explain the procedure to the patient. The strap can be worn over an undershirt or t-shirt for patient comfort.
- Assess neurovascular integrity by palpating skin temperature; noting the color of the hand and fingers; palpating the radial, ulnar, and brachial pulses bilaterally; and then comparing the affected side with the unaffected side. Ask the patient about any numbness or tingling distal to the injury and assess motor function.
- Perform a pain assessment and administer analgesics as ordered.
- Ask the patient to sit or stand up with his arms loosely at his sides.

Applying a figure-eight strap

- Place the apex of the triangle between the scapulae and drape the straps over the shoulders. Bring the strap with the Velcro or buckle end under one axilla and through the loop. Pull the other strap under the other axilla and through the loop. (See *Types of clavicle straps.*)
- Gently tighten each strap so that the shoulders are gently pulled back and the patient is comfortable with the amount of support.

Completing a figure-eight strap

- Secure the ends using Velcro pads, or a buckle, depending on the equipment. Make sure a buckle or any sharp edges face away from the skin. Tape the secured ends to the underlying strap or bandage.

You've got a pen pal

- Use a pen to mark the strap at the site of the loop of the figure-eight strap. *If the strap loosens, this mark helps you tighten it to the original position.*
- Assess neurovascular integrity, *which may be impaired by a strap that's too tight.* If neurovascular integrity is compromised when the strap is correctly applied, notify the physician. The physician may order another treatment.

Practice pointers

- If patient cannot tolerate the figure-eight strap, you can immobilize the clavicle by applying a sling alone. (See "Arm sling application," page 471, and *Clavicle immobilization.*)

Types of clavicle straps

Clavicle straps provide support to the shoulder by gently pulling the shoulders back and creating a proper alignment to promote healing.

Commercially available clavicle straps have a short back panel and long straps that extend around the patient's shoulders and axillae. Velcro pads or buckles on the ends allow for easy fastening.

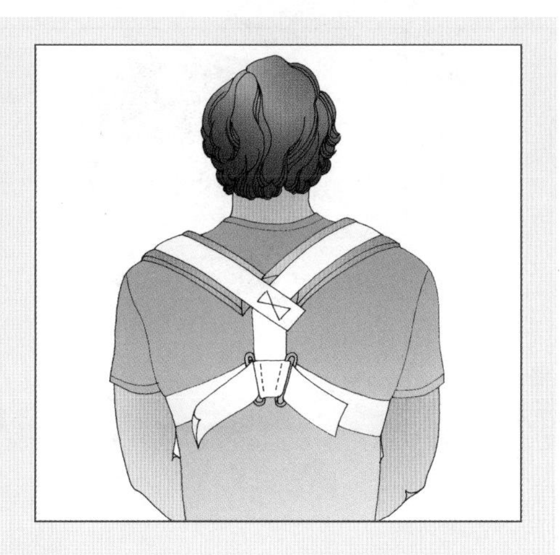

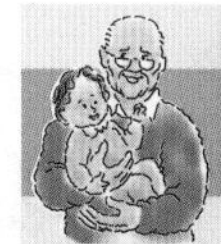

Ages and stages

Clavicle immobilization

For a small child or a confused adult, a clavicle strap may be restrictive and cause discomfort. Using a simple sling instead to support the arm and limit movement is an acceptable alternative.

Permanent addition

- Instruct the patient to wear the clavicle strap for the time instructed by the physician or until patient is pain-free, typically 1 to 3 weeks. The strap can be removed for bathing and removed when sleeping. (See *Documenting clavicle strap application*.)

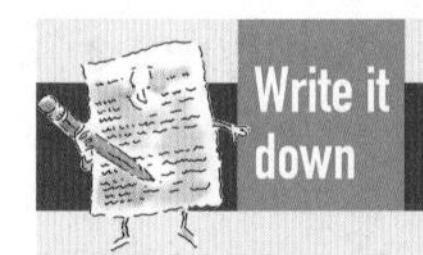

Documenting clavicle strap application

In your notes, record:
- date and time of strap application
- type of clavicle strap applied
- pain assessment and any medications given
- bilateral neurovascular integrity before and after the procedure
- patient teaching provided.

Cervical collar application

A cervical collar holds the neck straight in a neutral position. It immobilizes the cervical spine, decreases muscle spasms, and helps relieve pain. The collar also prevents further injury and promotes healing.

Off it comes, slowly

A cervical collar may be used for an acute injury (such as a strained cervical muscle) or a chronic condition (such as arthritis or cervical metastasis). It can be used after cervical surgery. It can also be used with a splinting device, such as a spine board, to prevent potential spinal cord damage.

Types of cervical collars

Cervical collars can be molded from hard plastic or soft.

Hard and firm

Made of rigid plastic, the *molded* cervical collar holds the patient's neck firmly, keeping it straight in a neutral position.

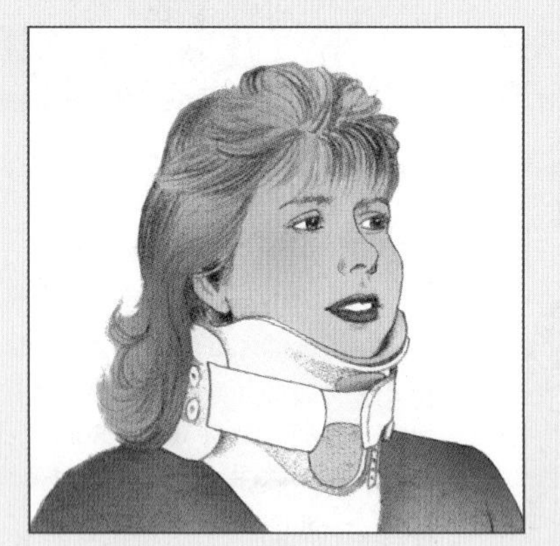

Soft and gentle

The *soft* cervical collar, made of spongy foam, provides gentler support and reminds the patient to avoid cervical spine motion.

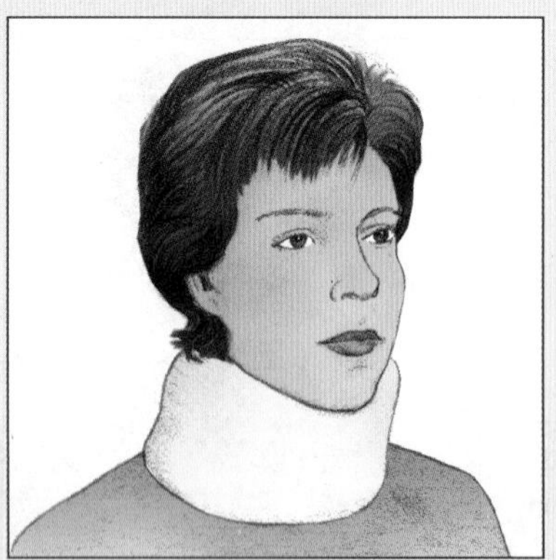

As acute injury symptoms subside, the patient may discontinue wearing the collar gradually, alternating periods of wear with increasing periods of removal until he no longer needs the collar.

What you need

Cervical collar in the appropriate size ✱ optional: cotton (for padding). (See *Types of cervical collars*.)

How you do it

- Identify the patient with two patient identifiers per facility policy.
- Perform hand hygiene.
- Explain the procedure to the patient.
- Check the patient's neurovascular status before application.
- Instruct the patient to position his head slowly to face directly forward in a *neutral* position.
- Measure the distance between the underside of the tip of the chin (not the jawline) and the top of the shoulder where the cervical collar will rest. You can do this by holding your hand in a "karate chop" parallel to the side of the neck at those landmarks.

Fit and fasten

- Slide the front of the collar up the front of the neck until the "chin ledge" rests under the tip of the chin. Fit the collar snugly around the neck and attach the Velcro fasteners at the back of the neck.
- Check the patient's airway and neurovascular status *to ensure that the collar isn't too tight.*

Practice pointers

- For a sprain, make sure the collar isn't too high in front *because this may hyperextend the neck.* In a neck sprain, such hyperextension may cause ligaments to heal in a shortened position.

A little padding, please

- If the patient complains of pressure, the collar may be too tight. Remove and reapply it. If the patient complains of skin irritation or friction, the collar itself may be irritating him. Apply protective cotton padding between the irritated skin and the collar.

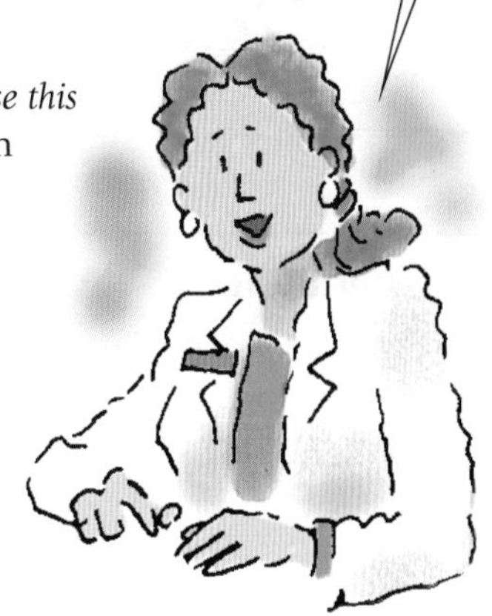
Here's a hint. If the cervical collar is too high in the front, it may hyperextend the neck.

- Before discharge, teach the patient how to apply the cervical collar and how to do a neurovascular check. Some collars are complex and the patient (or a caregiver) may need to practice if he'll be responsible for application. After showing him how to apply the collar, have him perform a return demonstration. If indicated, advise the patient to sleep without a pillow. (See *Documenting cervical collar application*.)

Documenting cervical collar application

In your notes, record:
- type and size of the cervical collar
- time and date of application
- results of neurovascular checks
- pain assessment and any medications given
- collar's snugness
- all patient instructions.

Splint application

By immobilizing the injury site, a splint relieves pain and allows the injury to heal in proper alignment. It also minimizes possible complications, such as excessive bleeding into tissues, restricted blood flow caused by bone pressing against vessels, and possible paralysis from an unstable spinal cord injury.

Moving insurance

In cases of multiple serious injuries, a splint or spine board allows caregivers to move the patient without risking further damage to bones, muscles, nerves, blood vessels, and skin.

A splint can be applied to immobilize a simple or compound fracture, a dislocation, or a subluxation. During an emergency, apply a splint to a suspected fracture, dislocation, or subluxation. Be aware that traction splints are contraindicated for upper extremity injuries and open fractures. (See *Three types of splints*.)

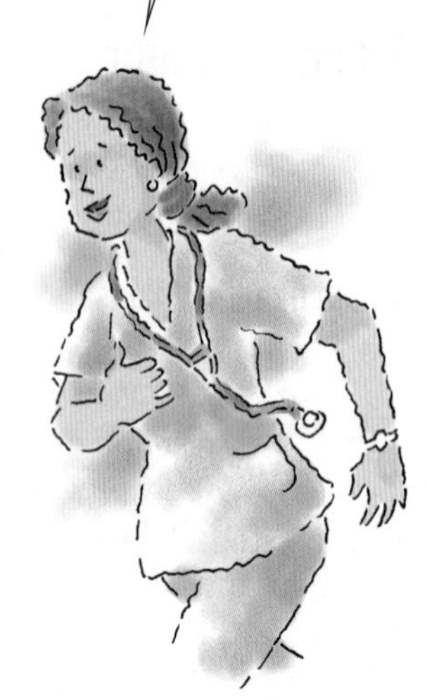
In an emergency, splint an injury if you suspect it's a fracture, dislocation, or subluxation.

What you need

Rigid splint, Velcro support splint, spine board, or traction splint ✻ bindings ✻ padding ✻ sandbags or rolled towels or clothing ✻ optional: roller gauze, cloth strips, ice bag.

Several commercial splints are widely available. An inflatable semirigid splint, called an air splint, can often be used to secure an injured extremity. (See *Using an air splint*, page 478.) Velcro straps, 2″ roller gauze, or 2″ cloth strips can be used as bindings.

How you do it

- Identify the patient using two patient identifiers per facility policy.
- Obtain a complete history of the injury.
- Perform hand hygiene. Follow standard precautions.
- Begin a thorough head-to-toe assessment, checking for obvious deformities, swelling, or bleeding.

Three types of splints

Three types of splints commonly are used to help support injured or weakened limbs or to help correct deformities.

Rigid splint

A rigid splint is used to immobilize a fracture or dislocation in an extremity, as shown. Ideally, two people should apply a rigid splint to an extremity.

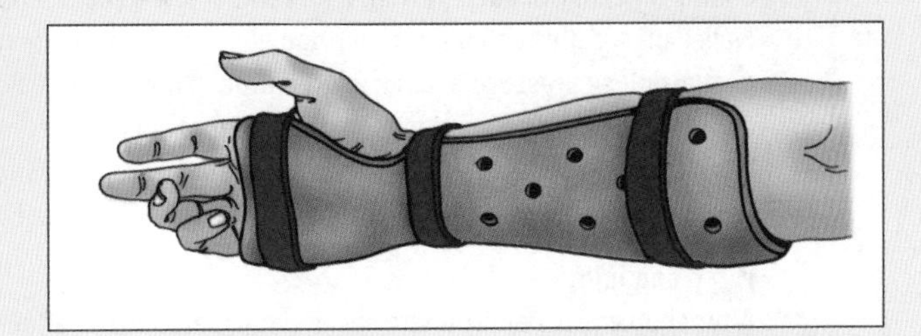

Traction splint

A traction splint immobilizes a fracture and exerts a longitudinal pull that reduces muscle spasms, pain, and arterial and neural damage. Used primarily for femoral fractures, a traction splint also may be applied for a fractured hip or tibia. Two trained people should apply a traction splint.

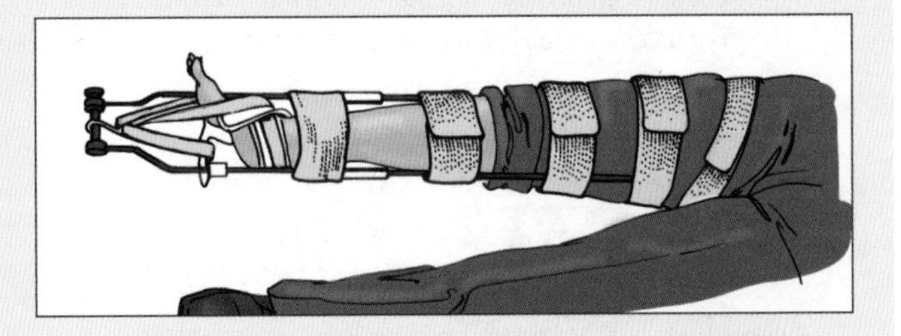

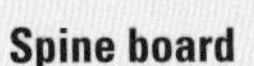

Spine board

Used for a suspected spinal fracture, a spine board is a rigid splint that supports the injured person's entire body. Three people should apply a spine board.

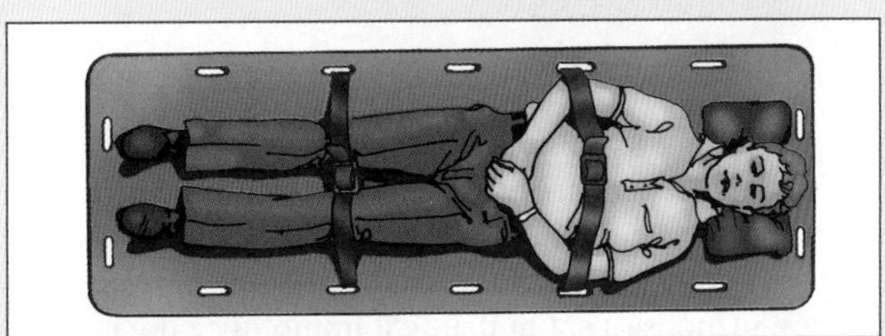

- Ask the patient if he can move the injured area (typically an extremity). Compare the injured extremity with the uninjured extremity, where applicable. Gently palpate the injured area, inspecting for swelling, obvious deformities, bleeding, discoloration, and evidence of fracture or dislocation.
- Remove or cut away clothing from the injury site, if necessary. Check neurovascular integrity distal to the site. Explain the procedure to the patient *to allay his fears.*

Everything in its place

- If an obvious bone misalignment causes the patient acute distress or severe neurovascular problems, align the extremity in its normal anatomic position, if possible. Stop, however, if this causes further neurovascular deterioration.

Using an air splint

In an emergency, an air splint can be used to immobilize a fracture or control bleeding, especially from a forearm or lower leg. Made of double-walled plastic, this compact, comfortable splint (shown below) provides gentle, diffuse pressure over an injured area. It may control bleeding better than a local pressure bandage. Also, its clear plastic construction simplifies inspection of the affected site for bleeding, pallor, or cyanosis and allows the patient to be moved without further damage to the injured limb.

Wrap and inflate

After choosing the appropriate splint, wrap it around the affected extremity, secure it with Velcro or other strips, and then inflate. The fit should be snug enough to immobilize the extremity without impairing circulation.

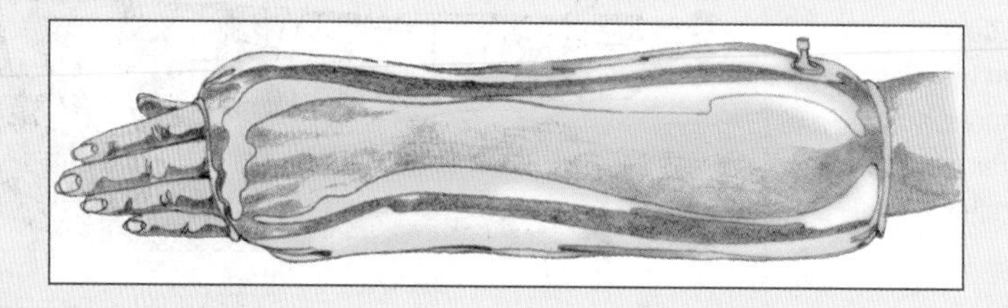

- Don't try to straighten a dislocation; *doing so could damage displaced vessels and nerves.* Also, don't attempt reduction of a contaminated bone end *because this may cause additional laceration of soft tissues, vessels, and nerves as well as gross contamination of deep tissues.*
- Choose a splint that will immobilize the joints above and below the fracture. Pad the splint as necessary *to protect bony prominences.*

Applying a rigid splint

- Support the injured extremity and apply firm, gentle traction.
- Have an assistant place the splint under, beside, or on top of the extremity, as ordered.
- Tell the assistant to apply the bindings *to secure the splint.* Don't let them obstruct circulation.

Applying a spine board

Pad the spine board carefully, especially the areas that will support the lumbar region and knees, *to prevent uneven pressure and discomfort.*

A job for three

- If the patient is lying on his back, place one hand on each side of his head and keep the head aligned with the body. Have one

Assessing an injured extremity

When assessing an injured extremity, take the following steps. Be sure to compare your findings to the unaffected limb.

- Inspect the color of the patient's fingers or toes.
- Assess for edema by noting the size of the area and/or distal digits.
- Simultaneously touch the digits of the affected and unaffected extremities and compare temperature.
- Check capillary refill by pressing on the distal tip of one digit until it's white. Then release the pressure and note how soon normal color returns. It should return quickly (less than 2 seconds) in both the affected and unaffected extremities.
- Check sensation by touching the fingers or toes and asking the patient how they feel. Note reports of numbness or tingling.
- To test movement, tell the patient to wiggle his toes or move his fingers.
- Palpate the distal pulses to assess vascular patency.

Record your findings for both the affected and unaffected extremities using standard terms to avoid ambiguity. Warmth, free movement, rapid capillary refill, normal color, and sensation indicate good neurovascular status.

assistant logroll the patient onto his side while another slides the spine board under him. Then instruct the assistants to roll the patient onto the board while you maintain alignment.

- If the patient is prone, logroll him onto the board so he ends up in a supine position.
- *To maintain body alignment,* use straps to secure the patient on the spine board. *To keep head and neck aligned,* use commercial cervical spine immobilizer equipment or rolled towels or clothing on both sides of his head.

Applying a traction splint

- Place the splint beside the injured leg. (Never use a traction splint on an arm *because the major axillary plexus of nerves and blood vessels can't tolerate countertraction.*) Adjust the splint to the correct length and open and adjust the Velcro straps.
- Have an assistant keep the leg motionless while you pad the ankle and foot and fasten the ankle hitch around them. (You may leave the shoe on.)
- Tell the assistant to lift and support the leg at the injury site as you apply firm, gentle traction.

Documenting splint application

In your notes, record:

- circumstances and cause of the injury
- patient education
- patient's complaints (including whether symptoms are localized)
- neurovascular status before and after applying the splint
- type of wound
- amount and type of any drainage
- time of splint application
- slippage of the bone end into surrounding tissue
- pain assessment and any medications given
- change in degree of dislocation resulting from transportation.

Slide, pad, and strap

- While you maintain traction, tell the assistant to slide the splint under the leg, pad the groin *to avoid excessive pressure on external genitalia,* and gently apply the ischial strap.
- Have the assistant connect the loops of the ankle hitch to the end of the splint.
- Adjust the splint to apply enough traction *to secure the leg comfortably in the corrected position.*
- After applying traction, fasten the Velcro support splints *to secure the leg closely to the splint.*
- Don't use a traction splint for a severely angulated femur or knee fracture.

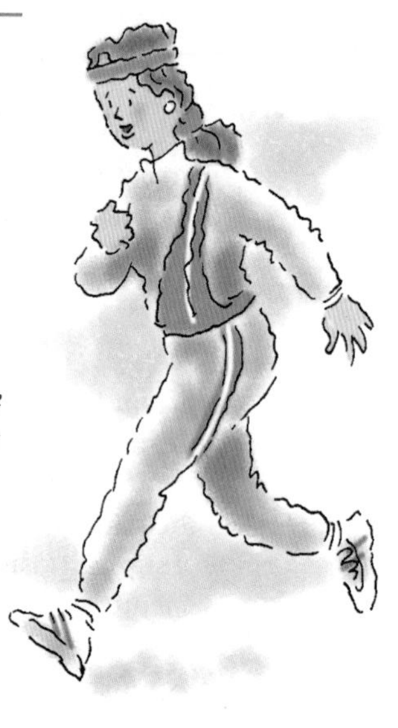
If you encounter an unconscious patient, assume he could have a cervical injury. Apply a splint before moving him.

Practice pointers

- At the accident scene, always examine the patient completely for other injuries. Avoid unnecessary movement or manipulation, *which might cause additional pain or injury.*
- Always consider the possibility of cervical injury in an unconscious patient. If possible, apply the splint before repositioning the patient.
- After applying any type of splint, monitor vital signs frequently *because bleeding in fractured bones and surrounding tissues may cause shock.* Also monitor neurovascular status of the fractured limb by assessing skin color and checking for numbness in the fingers or toes. *Numbness or paralysis distal to the injury indicates pressure on nerves.* (See *Assessing an injured extremity,* page 479.)

Don't stop for snacks

- Transport the patient to a hospital as soon as possible. Apply ice to the injury. (See *From fracture to fat embolism* and *Documenting splint application,* page 479.)

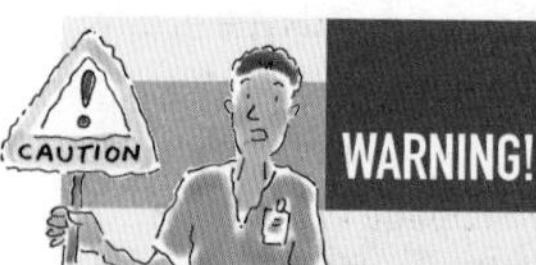

WARNING!

From fracture to fat embolism

Multiple patient transfers and repeated manipulation of a fracture may lead to fat embolism. Signs and symptoms of this complication include shortness of breath; agitation; confusion; and petechiae on the skin, buccal membranes, and conjunctival sacs. Fat embolism usually occurs 24 to 72 hours after injury or manipulation.

Cast preparation

A cast is a hard mold that encases a body part—usually an extremity—to provide immobilization without discomfort. It can be used to treat injuries (including fractures), correct orthopedic conditions (such as deformities), or promote healing after general or plastic surgery, amputation, or nerve and vascular repair.

Casting call

Casts may be made of plaster, fiberglass, or other synthetic materials. Fiberglass, the most commonly used material, is lighter, stronger, and more resilient than plaster. Because fiberglass dries rapidly, it's more difficult to mold. However, it can bear body weight immediately if needed.

No definite no-no's

Contraindications for casting may include skin diseases, peripheral vascular disease, diabetes mellitus, open or draining wounds, and susceptibility to skin irritations. However, these aren't strict contraindications; the physician must weigh potential risks and benefits for each patient. (See *Casts and compartment syndrome.*)

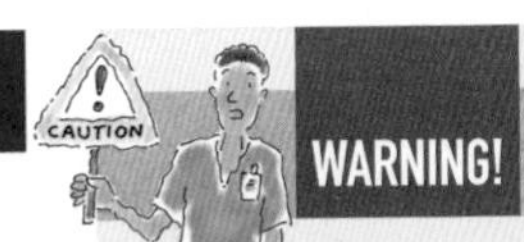
CAUTION
WARNING!

Casts and compartment syndrome

Improper cast application can lead to compartment syndrome, palsy, paresthesia, ischemia, ischemic myositis, pressure necrosis, and, eventually, misalignment or nonunion of fractured bones.

What you need

Tubular stockinette ✱ casting material ✱ plaster splints (if necessary) ✱ bucket of water ✱ sink equipped with plaster trap ✱ linen-saver pad ✱ sheet wadding ✱ sponge or felt padding (if necessary) ✱ cast scissors, cast saw, and cast spreader (if necessary) ✱ pillows or bath blankets ✱ optional: rubber gloves, cast stand, moleskin or adhesive tape.

Gather the tubular stockinette, cast material, and plaster splints in the appropriate sizes. Tubular stockinettes range from 2″ to 12″ (5 to 30.5 cm) wide; plaster rolls, from 2″ to 6″ (5 to 15 cm) wide; and plaster splints, from 3″ to 6″ (7.5 to 15 cm) wide. Wear rubber gloves, especially if applying a fiberglass cast.

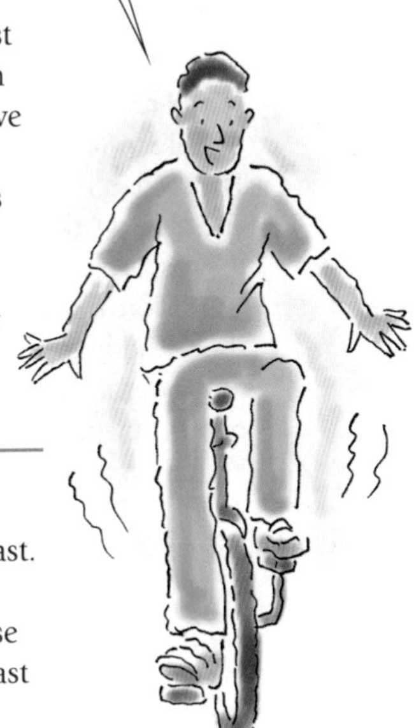
Hmmm. After I crash, I think I'd like a fiberglass cast.

Getting ready

Follow the manufacturer's directions for preparing the fiberglass cast. Place all equipment within reach.

Cast application is often a two-person procedure, with the nurse typically supporting the heath care professional who applies the cast as well as supporting the patient.

How you do it

- Identify the patient using two patient identifiers per facility policy.
- Perform hand hygiene.
- *To allay the patient's fears,* explain the procedure. Also begin explaining some aspects of proper cast care *to prepare him for patient teaching and to assess his knowledge level.*
- Assess pain status and administer adequate analgesia before the cast is applied.
- Cover appropriate parts of the patient's bedding and gown with a linen-saver pad.
- Remove any jewelry from the affected extremity before casting. Finger rings and toe rings can later interfere with circulation and neurologic status because of extremity swelling.

Skin survey

- Assess skin condition in the affected area, noting any redness, contusions, or open wounds. *This will aid evaluation of complaints the patient may have after the cast is applied.*
- If the patient has severe contusions or open wounds, prepare the patient for treatment of these *before* casting.
- *To establish baseline measurements,* assess neurovascular status. Palpate distal pulses; assess color, temperature, and capillary refill of the appropriate fingers or toes; and check neurologic function, including sensation and motion in the affected and unaffected extremities.

Assume the position

- Help the patient to hold the limb in the medically desired position. (Most extremities are placed in either a neutral position or in the case of an arm fracture, a 90-degree angle). If the patient is unable to maintain the ordered position, maintain it for him.
- The second health care professional applies the tubular stockinette and sheet wadding. The stockinette should extend beyond the ends of the cast *to pad the edges.* (If the patient has an open wound or a severe contusion, other material may be used.) The limb is then wrapped in sheet wadding, starting at the distal end, and extra wadding is applied to the distal and proximal ends of the cast area as well as any points of prominence. As the sheet wadding is applied, check for wrinkles.
- Prepare cast materials as directed.

Chemistry class

- Put on rubber gloves.
- If you're using water-activated fiberglass, immerse the tape rolls in tepid water for 10 to 15 minutes *to initiate the chemical reaction that causes the cast to harden.* Open one roll at a time. Avoid squeezing out excess water before application.

- If you're using light-cured fiberglass, you can unroll the material more slowly. This casting remains soft and malleable until it's exposed to ultraviolet light, which sets it.

Completing the cast

- Use a cast stand or your palm to support the cast in the therapeutic position until it becomes firm to the touch (usually 6 to 8 minutes).

This little piggy . . .

To check circulation in the casted limb, palpate the distal pulse and assess color, temperature, and capillary refill of the fingers or toes. Assess neurologic status by asking the patient if he's experiencing paresthesia in the extremity or decreased motion of the extremity's uncovered joints. Evaluate the unaffected extremity the same way and compare findings.

Raise the bar

- Elevate the injured limb above heart level with pillows or bath blankets, as ordered, *to promote venous return and reduce edema. To prevent molding,* make sure pressure is evenly distributed under the cast.
- The patient may have additional X-rays *to ensure proper positioning.*
- Instruct the patient to report pain, foul odor, drainage, or burning sensation under the cast. (After the cast hardens, a window may be cut into the cast to inspect the painful or burning area.)

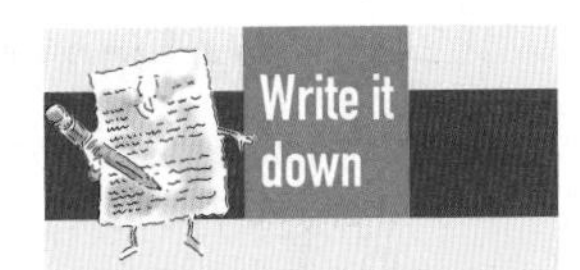

Documenting cast application

In your notes, record:
- date and time of cast application
- pain assessment and any medications given
- skin condition of the extremity before the cast was applied
- contusions, redness, or open wounds
- neurovascular findings before and after application (for both the affected and unaffected extremities)
- location of special devices, such as felt pads or plaster splints
- patient teaching provided.

Practice pointers

- A fiberglass cast dries immediately after application. During this drying period, the cast must be properly positioned *to prevent a surface depression that could cause pressure areas or dependent edema.* Neurovascular status must be assessed, drainage monitored, and the condition of the cast checked periodically.
- After the cast dries completely, it looks shiny and no longer feels damp or soft. Care consists of monitoring for drainage pattern changes, preventing skin breakdown near the cast, and averting complications of immobility.

School starts

- Patient teaching must begin immediately after the cast is applied and should continue until the patient or a family member can care for the cast.
- Never use the bed or a table to support the cast as it sets *because molding can result, causing pressure necrosis of underlying tissue.* Also, don't use rubber- or plastic-covered pillows before the cast hardens *because they can trap heat under the cast.*

- If a cast is applied after surgery or traumatic injury, remember that the most accurate way to assess for bleeding is to monitor vital signs. A visible blood spot on the cast can be misleading: One drop of blood can produce a circle 3″ (7.5 cm) in diameter.

Ugh! That's my leg?

- Tell the patient that when the cast is removed, his casted limb will appear thinner and flabbier than the uncasted limb and the skin will appear yellowish or gray from accumulated dead skin and oils from glands near the skin surface. Reassure him that with exercise and good skin care, his limb will return to normal. (See *Teaching your patient about cast care* and *Documenting cast application*, page 483.)

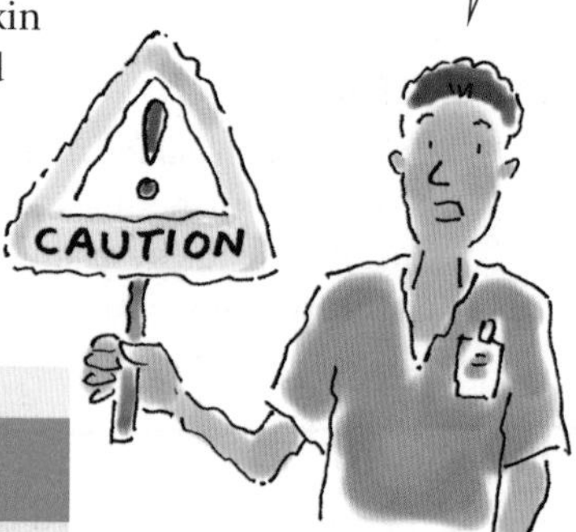
Don't be fooled by a drop of blood on the cast. To check for bleeding, monitor vital signs.
CAUTION

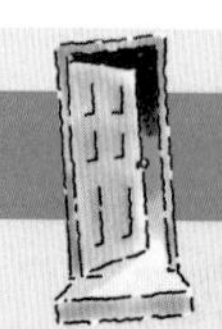

Home care connection

Teaching your patient about cast care

Before the patient goes home, teach him how to care for his cast. Tell him to keep the casted limb elevated above heart level to minimize swelling. Explain that he should raise a casted leg by lying in a supine position with his leg on top of pillows and that he should prop a casted arm so that his hand and elbow are higher than his shoulder.

Warning signs

Instruct the patient to call the physician if he can't move his fingers or toes, if he has numbness or tingling in the affected limb, or if he has signs or symptoms of infection, such as fever, unusual pain, or a foul odor from the cast. Advise him to maintain muscle strength by continuing recommended exercises.

A few more cast caveats

- If the cast needs repair (if it loosens and slips) or if the patient has questions about cast care, advise him to contact his physician.
- Warn the patient not to get the cast wet. Moisture will weaken or destroy it.
- Urge the patient not to insert anything (such as a back scratcher or powder) into the cast to relieve itching. Foreign matter can damage the skin and cause an infection. Tell him, however, that he can apply alcohol on the skin at the cast edges.
- Caution the patient not to chip, crush, cut, or otherwise break any area of the cast and not to bear weight on it unless the physician instructs him to do so.
- If the patient must use crutches, instruct him to remove throw rugs from the floor and to rearrange furniture to reduce the risk of tripping and falling.
- If the patient has a cast on his dominant arm, determine if he needs help with bathing, toileting, eating, and dressing.

Mechanical traction

Mechanical traction exerts a pulling force on a part of the body—usually the spine, pelvis, or long bones of the arms and legs. It can be used to reduce fractures, treat dislocations, correct or prevent deformities, improve or correct contractures, or decrease muscle spasms. It is not used as frequently as it was in the past because of improved surgical interventions and decreases in length of hospital stays.

Pressure? Or pins?

Depending on the injury or condition, an orthopedist may order either skin or skeletal traction. *Skin traction*, applied directly to the skin and thus indirectly to the bone, is ordered when a light, temporary, or noncontinuous pulling force is required and is more commonly used in pediatrics. Contraindications include a severe injury with open wounds, an allergy to tape or other skin traction equipment, circulatory disturbances, dermatitis, and varicose veins.

In *skeletal traction*, an orthopedist inserts a pin or wire through the bone and attaches the traction equipment to the pin or wire to exert a direct, constant, longitudinal pulling force. Indications include fractures of the tibia, femur, and humerus *where surgery is either delayed or contraindicated*. Infections, such as osteomyelitis, contraindicate skeletal traction. (See *Complications of traction*.)

Your concerns: immobility, inspection, infection

An orthopedic assistant usually is responsible for setting up the traction frame. After the patient is placed in the ordered type of traction, the nurse is responsible for preventing complications from immobility; for routinely inspecting the equipment; for adding traction weights as ordered; and, in patients with skeletal traction, for monitoring pin insertion sites for signs of infection. (See *Comparing types of traction*, page 486.)

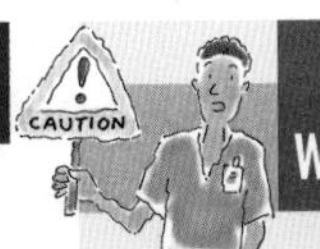

WARNING!

Complications of traction

Immobility during traction may result in pressure ulcers, muscle atrophy, weakness, contractures, and osteoporosis.

The list goes on

Immobility can also cause:

- gastrointestinal (GI) disturbances such as constipation
- urinary problems, including stasis and calculi
- respiratory problems, such as stasis of secretions and hypostatic pneumonia
- circulatory disturbances, including stasis and thrombophlebitis.

Long-term troubles

Prolonged immobility, especially after traumatic injury, may promote depression or other emotional disturbances. Skeletal traction may cause osteomyelitis originating at the pin or wire sites.

What you need

Overhead frame: There are three basic frames: the claw-type frame, the intravenous (I.V.)-type frame, and the Balkan frame. All frames consist of bars and clamps to form an overhead frame. The physician will order the type of frame desired, and either the physician or the orthopedic assistant will assemble.

Comparing types of traction

Traction restricts movement of a patient's affected limb or body part. The limb is immobilized by pulling with equal force on each end of the injured area—an equal mix of traction and countertraction. Weights provide the pulling force. Use of other weights or positioning the patient's body weight against the traction pull provides countertraction.

Skin traction

Skin traction immobilizes a body part intermittently over an extended period through direct application of a pulling force on the skin. The force may be applied using adhesive or nonadhesive traction tape or other skin traction devices, such as a boot, belt, or halter.

Adhesive attachment permits more continuous traction, whereas nonadhesive attachment allows easier removal for daily skin care.

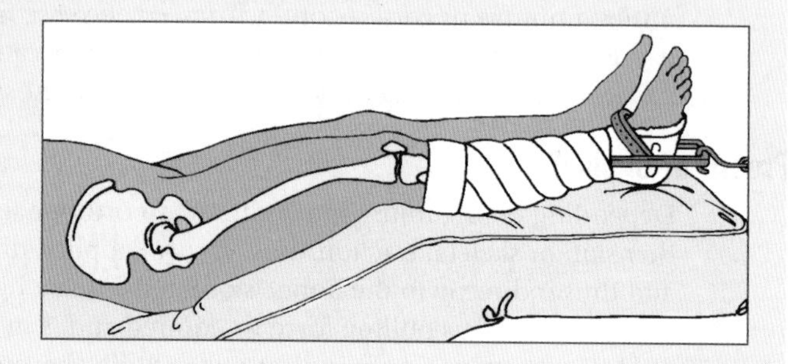

Skeletal traction

Skeletal traction immobilizes a body part for prolonged periods by attaching weighted equipment directly to the bones. This may be accomplished with pins, screws, wires, or tongs.

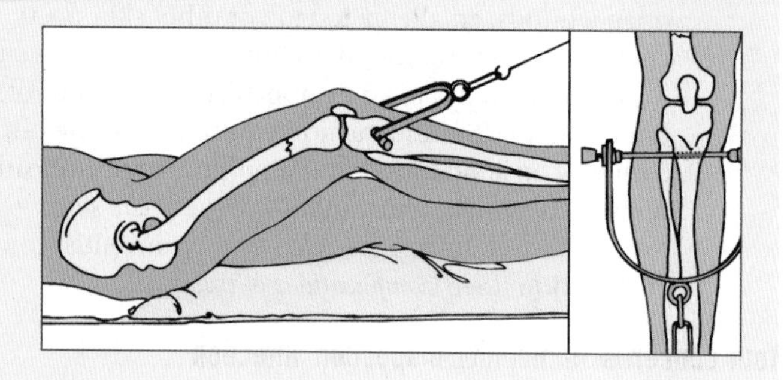

For all frame types: trapeze with clamp ✻ wall bumper or roller.

For skeletal traction care: sterile cotton-tipped applicators ✻ prescribed antiseptic solution ✻ sterile gauze pads ✻ povidone-iodine solution * optional: antimicrobial ointment.

Getting ready

Arrange with central supply or the appropriate department to have traction equipment transported to the patient's room on a traction cart. If appropriate, gather equipment for pin site care at the patient's bedside. Pin site care protocols may vary with each hospital or physician.

How you do it

- Explain the purpose of traction to the patient. Emphasize the importance of maintaining proper body alignment after the traction equipment is set up.

Caring for the traction patient

- After traction is set up, show the patient how much movement he's allowed and instruct him not to readjust the equipment. Also tell him to report pain or pressure from the traction equipment.
- At least once per shift, make sure traction equipment connections are tight and that no parts touch the bedding, the patient, or inappropriate portions of the apparatus. Check for impingements such as ropes rubbing on the footboard or getting caught between pulleys. *Friction and impingement reduce the effectiveness of traction.*

> Make sure the traction weights stay in the air. Touching the floor or bed reduces the amount of traction.

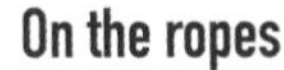

On the ropes

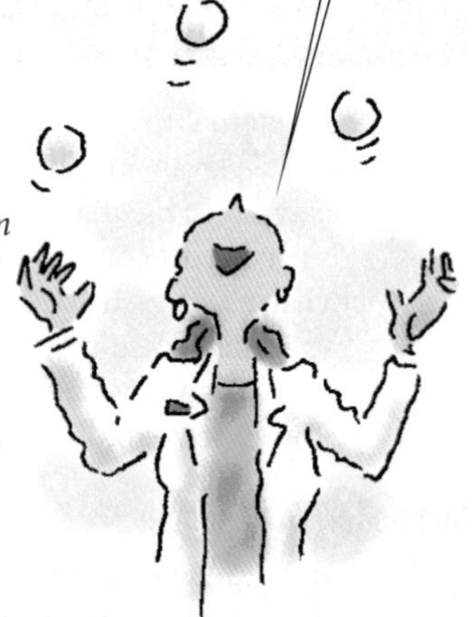

- Inspect traction equipment *to ensure correct alignment.*
- Inspect ropes for fraying, *which eventually can cause a rope to break.*
- Make sure ropes are positioned properly in the pulley track. *An improperly positioned rope changes the degree of traction.*
- *To prevent tampering and aid stability and security,* make sure all rope ends are taped above the knot.
- Inspect equipment regularly to make sure traction weights hang freely. *Weights that touch the floor, bed, or each other reduce the amount of traction.*

Check alignment—every 2 hours or 3,000 miles

- About every 2 hours, check the patient for proper body alignment and reposition him as necessary. *Misalignment causes ineffective traction and may keep the fracture from healing properly.*
- *To prevent complications from immobility,* assess neurovascular integrity routinely. The patient's condition, hospital routine, and physician's orders determine the frequency of neurovascular assessments.
- Provide skin care, encourage coughing and deep-breathing exercises, and assist with ordered range-of-motion (ROM) exercises for unaffected extremities. Typically, the physician will order a sequential compression device for the unaffected leg(s). Check elimination patterns and provide laxatives as ordered.

- Check the pin site and surrounding skin regularly for signs of infection.
- If ordered, clean the pin site and surrounding skin with a cotton-tipped applicator dipped in the ordered antiseptic. If ordered, apply antimicrobial ointment to the pin sites. Apply a loose sterile dressing or dress with sterile gauze pads soaked in povidone-iodine solution.

Practice pointers

- When using skin traction, apply ordered weights slowly and carefully *to avoid jerking the affected extremity.*
- When applying Buck's traction, make sure the line of pull is always parallel to the bed and not angled downward *to prevent pressure on the heel.* (See *Documenting mechanical traction.*)

Documenting mechanical traction

In your notes, record:
- amount of traction weight used daily
- application of additional weights and the patient's tolerance
- equipment inspections
- patient care, including routine checks of neurovascular integrity, skin condition, respiratory status, pain assessment, and elimination patterns
- condition of the pin site and pin site care given, if applicable.

External fixation

In external fixation, the physician inserts metal pins through skin and muscle layers into broken bones and affixes the pins to an adjustable external frame that maintains their proper alignment. This procedure is used most commonly to treat open, unstable fractures with extensive soft tissue damage; comminuted closed fractures; and septic, nonunion fractures and to promote surgical joint immobilization. Specialized types of external fixators may be used to lengthen leg bones or immobilize the cervical spine.

See better, walk sooner

An advantage of external fixation over other immobilization techniques is that it stabilizes the fracture while allowing full visualization and access to open wounds. It also promotes early ambulation, thus reducing the risk of complications from immobilization.

Hi-tech helper

The Ilizarov fixator, a special type of external fixation device, is a combination of rings and tensioned transosseous wires. It's used primarily in limb lengthening, bone transport, and limb salvage. This highly complex device provides gradual distraction (separation of bone surfaces by extension), resulting in good-quality bone formation with minimal complications.

What you need

Sterile cotton-tipped applicators ✱ prescribed antiseptic cleaning solution ✱ sterile gauze pads ✱ povidone-iodine solution ✱ ice bag ✱ optional: antimicrobial ointment, analgesic.

Equipment varies with the type of fixator and the fracture type and location. Typically, sets of pins, stabilizing rods, and clips are available from manufacturers. Don't reuse pins.

Getting ready

Make sure the external fixation set includes all the equipment it's supposed to include and that the equipment has been sterilized according to your facility's policy.

How you do it

- Explain the procedure to the patient *to reduce his anxiety*. Assure him that he'll feel little pain after the fixation device is in place and that he'll be able to adjust to the apparatus.
- Tell the patient he'll be able to move about with the apparatus in place, which may help him resume normal activities more quickly.
- After the fixation device is in place, perform neurovascular checks according to your facility's protocol *to assess for possible neurologic damage*. Evaluate color, motion, sensation, digital movement, edema, capillary refill, and pulses of the affected extremity. Compare with the unaffected side.

You're swell

- Apply an ice bag to the surgical site as ordered *to reduce swelling, relieve pain, and lessen bleeding*.
- Administer analgesics, as ordered, before exercising or mobilizing the affected extremity *to promote comfort*.
- Monitor the patient for pain unrelieved by analgesics and for burning, tingling, or numbness, *which may indicate nerve damage or circulatory impairment*.
- Elevate the affected extremity, if appropriate, *to minimize edema*.

Pin pointers

- Perform pin site care, as ordered, *to prevent infection*. Use sterile technique. If ordered, clean the pin site and surrounding skin with a cotton-tipped applicator dipped in ordered antiseptic solution. If ordered, apply an antimicrobial ointment to the pin sites. Apply a loose sterile dressing or dress with sterile gauze pads soaked in povidone-iodine solution.

- Also check for redness, skin tenting, prolonged or purulent drainage from the pin site, swelling, elevated body or pin site temperature, and bowing or bending of pins, which may stress the skin.

Documenting external fixation

In your notes, record:
- condition of the pin sites and patient's skin
- patient's reaction to the apparatus and to ambulation
- patient's understanding of teaching.

For the patient with an Ilizarov fixator

After the device has been placed and preliminary calluses have begun to form at the insertion sites (in 5 to 7 days), gentle distraction is initiated by turning the appropriate screws one-quarter turn (1 mm) every 4 to 6 hours as ordered.

Turning of the screw

Tell the patient he must be consistent in turning the screws every 4 to 6 hours around the clock. Make sure he understands he must be strongly committed to compliance for the procedure to succeed. Because the treatment period may be prolonged (4 to 10 months), discuss the psychological effects of long-term care with the patient and family members.

No to NSAIDs

Don't administer nonsteroidal anti-inflammatory drugs (NSAIDs) to a patient who's being treated with the Ilizarov fixator. *NSAIDs may decrease necessary inflammation caused by the distraction, resulting in delayed bone formation.*

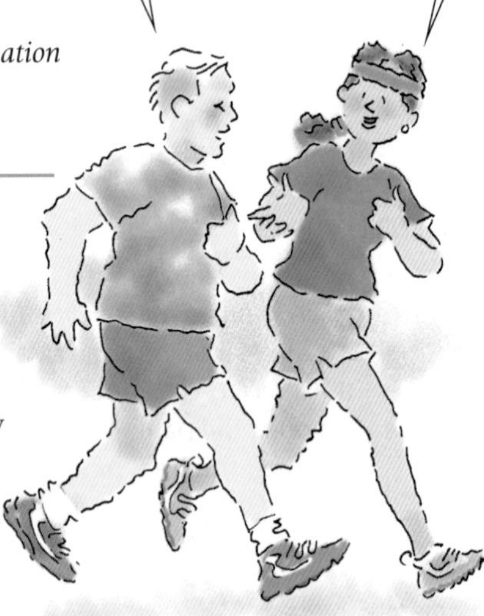
Thanks for encouraging me to adjust the screws on the fixator.
That's the only way the Ilizarov device will be effective.

Practice pointers

- Before discharge, teach the patient and family members how to provide pin site care. Clean technique can be used at home. Teach them how to recognize signs and symptoms of pin site infection. Have the patient and family do a return demonstration to verify understanding.
- Tell the patient to keep the affected limb elevated when sitting or lying down.
- Complications of external fixation include loosening of pins and loss of fracture stabilization, pin tract or wound infection, skin breakdown, nerve damage, and muscle impingement. (See *Documenting external fixation*.)

Internal fixation

In internal fixation (also called surgical reduction or open reduction), the physician implants fixation devices—using no external framework—to stabilize the fracture. Internal fixation devices include nails, screws, pins, wires, and rods, all of which may be used in combination with metal plates.

Internal fixation is typically used to treat fractures of the face and jaw, spine, and arm or leg bones as well as fractures involving a joint (most commonly the hip). Internal fixation permits earlier mobilization than other treatment options and can shorten hospitalization—particularly in elderly patients with hip fractures.

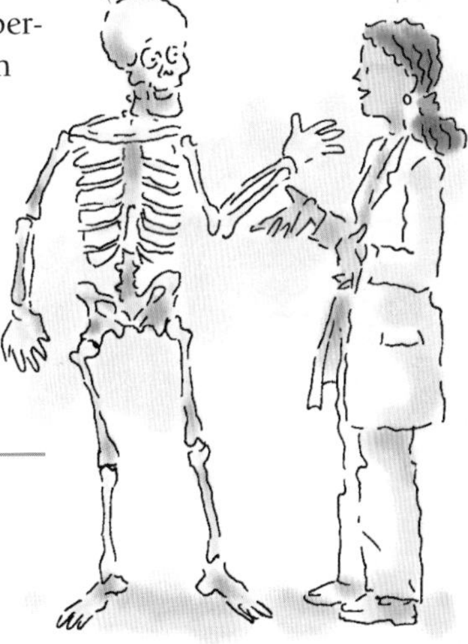

What's with the hardware?
Internal fixation devices, such as screws, are implanted permanently— unless a problem develops.

Bionic man

Internal fixation devices stay in the body indefinitely unless the patient has adverse reactions after healing is complete. (See *Reviewing internal fixation devices,* page 492.)

What you need

Ice bag ✳ pain medication (analgesic or narcotic) ✳ incentive spirometer or intermittent positive-pressure breathing (IPPB) device ✳ sequential compression device for unaffected leg(s).

Patients with leg fractures may also need the following: overhead frame with trapeze ✳ pressure-relief mattress ✳ crutches or walker ✳ pillow (hip fractures may require abductor pillows).

Getting ready

Equipment is collected and prepared in the operating room.

How you do it

- Explain the procedure to the patient *to allay his fears.* Encourage the patient to ask the physician any questions that he may have.

Reviewing internal fixation devices

Choice of a specific internal fixation device depends on the location, type, and configuration of the fracture.

In trochanteric or subtrochanteric fractures, the surgeon may use a hip pin or nail, with or without a screw plate. A pin or plate with extra nails stabilizes the fracture by impacting the bone ends at the fracture site.

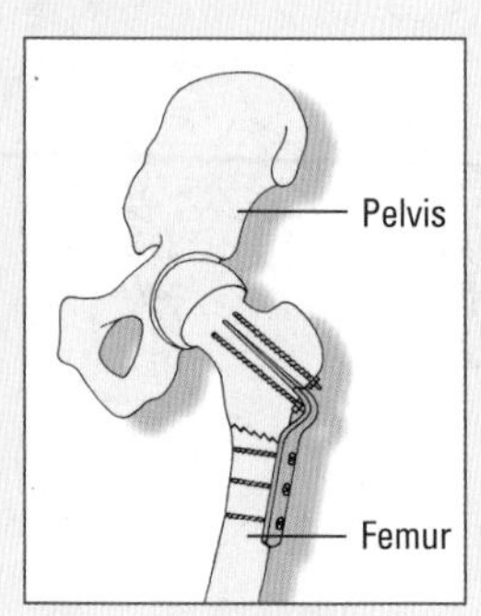

In an uncomplicated fracture of the femoral shaft, the surgeon may use an intramedullary rod. This device permits early ambulation with partial weight.

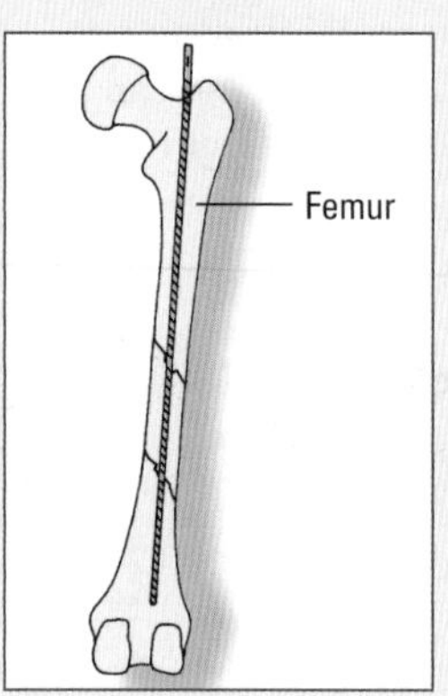

Another choice for fixation of a long-bone fracture is a screw plate, shown here on the tibia.

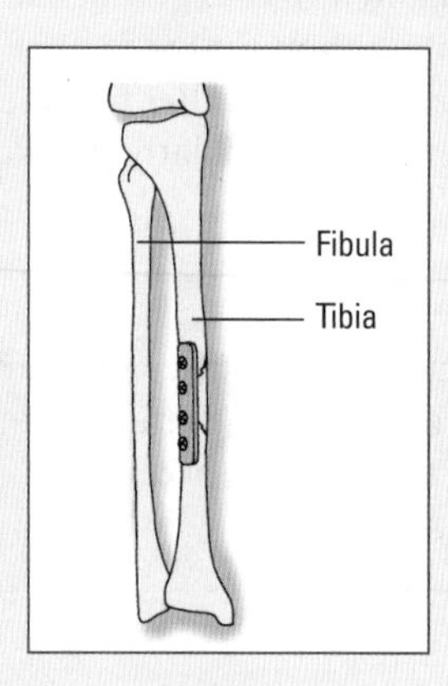

In an arm fracture, the surgeon may fix the involved bones with a plate, rod, or nail. Most radial and ulnar fractures may be fixed with plates, whereas humeral fractures commonly are fixed with rods.

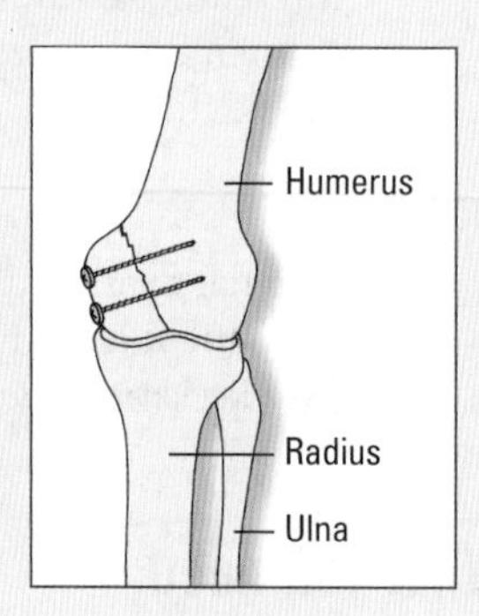

Checkout line

- After the procedure, monitor the patient's vital signs according to your facility's protocol. *Changes in vital signs may indicate hemorrhage or infection.*
- Monitor fluid intake and output every 4 to 8 hours.
- Perform neurovascular checks following your facility's protocol. Assess color, motion, sensation, digital movement, edema, capillary refill, and pulses of the affected area. Compare findings with the unaffected side.

Comfort care

- Apply an ice bag to the operative site as ordered *to reduce swelling, relieve pain, and lessen bleeding.*
- Administer analgesics, as ordered, before exercising or mobilizing the affected area *to promote comfort.*
- Monitor the patient for pain unrelieved by analgesics and for burning, tingling, or numbness, *which may indicate infection or impaired circulation.*

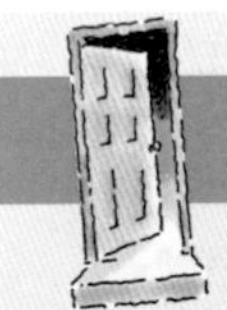

Home care connection

Recovering from internal fixation

Before discharge, teach the patient and family members how to care for the incision site and recognize signs and symptoms of wound infection. Also teach them about administering pain medication, practicing an exercise regimen (if ordered), and using assistive ambulation devices (such as crutches or a walker), if appropriate.

Write it down

Documenting internal fixation

In your notes, record:

- patient's perioperative cardiovascular, respiratory, and neurovascular status
- pain assessment
- pain management techniques used
- wound appearance
- alignment of the affected bone
- patient's response to teaching about appropriate exercise, infection site care, use of assistive devices (if appropriate), and symptoms to report.

- Elevate the affected limb on a pillow, if appropriate, *to minimize edema.*
- Check surgical dressings for excessive drainage or bleeding. Check the incision site for signs and symptoms of infection, such as erythema, drainage, edema, and unusual pain.

Time to stretch

- Assist and encourage the patient to perform ROM and other muscle-strengthening exercises as ordered *to promote circulation, improve muscle tone, and maintain joint function.*
- Teach the patient to perform progressive ambulation and mobilization using an overhead frame with trapeze, or crutches or a walker, as appropriate.

Practice pointers

- *To avoid complications of immobility after surgery,* have the patient use an incentive spirometer. Apply sequential compression devices to both legs as appropriate. The patient also may require a pressure-relief mattress. (See *Recovering from internal fixation* and *Documenting internal fixation.*)

Stump and prosthesis care

Patient care immediately after limb amputation includes monitoring drainage from the stump, positioning the affected limb, assisting with prescribed exercises, wrapping and conditioning the stump, and assessing psychological support to the patient.

Postoperative stump care will vary slightly, depending on the amputation site (arm or leg). After the stump heals, it requires only routine daily care, such as proper hygiene and continued muscle-strengthening exercises.

Clean and lube

The prosthesis, when in use, also requires daily care. Typically, a plastic prosthesis must be cleaned, lubricated, and checked for proper fit. As the patient recovers from the physical and psychological trauma of amputation, he will need to learn correct procedures for routine daily care of the stump and the prosthesis.

What you need

For postoperative stump care: pressure dressing ✳ abdominal (ABD) pad ✳ suction equipment, if ordered ✳ overhead trapeze ✳ 1″ adhesive tape ✳ sandbags or trochanter roll (for a leg) ✳ elastic stump shrinker or 4″ elastic bandage with Velcro closures.

For stump and prosthesis care: mild soap or alcohol pads ✳ stump socks or athletic tube socks ✳ two washcloths ✳ two towels ✳ appropriate lubricating oil.

How you do it

- Perform routine postoperative care. Frequently assess the patient's respiratory status and level of consciousness, monitor vital signs and I.V. infusions, check tube patency, and promote patient comfort and safety.

Monitoring stump drainage

- *Because gravity causes fluid to accumulate at the stump,* frequently check the amount of blood and drainage on the dressing. Notify the physician if drainage or blood accumulations increase rapidly. If excessive bleeding occurs, notify the physician immediately and apply a pressure dressing or compress the appropriate pressure points. If this doesn't control bleeding, use a tourniquet only **as a last resort**. Keep a tourniquet available, if needed.
- Tape the ABD pad over the moist part of the dressing as needed. *Providing a dry area helps prevent bacterial infection.*
- Monitor the suction drainage equipment and note the amount and type of drainage.

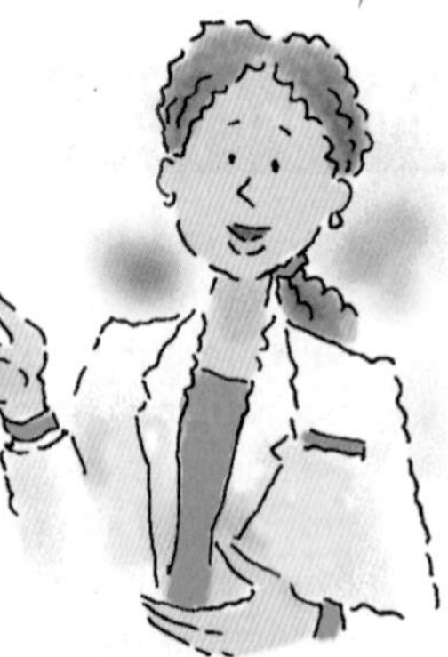
Phantom pain isn't a fantasy. It can be a real complication of an amputation.

Positioning the extremity

- *To prevent contractures,* position an arm with the patient's elbow extended and the shoulder abducted.
- *To correctly position a leg,* elevate the foot of the bed slightly and place sandbags or a trochanter roll against the patient's hip *to*

prevent external rotation. Don't place a pillow under the thigh to flex the hip; *this can cause hip flexion contracture.* For the same reason, tell the patient to avoid prolonged sitting.

- After a below-the-knee amputation, maintain knee extension *to prevent hamstring muscle contractures.*

Firm basis for care

After leg amputation, place the patient on a firm surface in the prone position for at least 4 hours per day, with his legs close together and without pillows under his stomach, hips, knees, or stump (unless this position is contraindicated). *This position helps prevent hip flexion, contractures, and abduction; it also stretches the flexor muscles.*

Assisting with prescribed exercises

- After arm amputation, encourage the patient to exercise the remaining arm *to prevent muscle contractures.* Help him perform isometric and ROM exercises for both shoulders as prescribed *because prosthesis use requires both shoulders.*
- After leg amputation, stand behind the patient and, if necessary, support him with your hands at his waist during balancing exercises.
- Instruct the patient to exercise the affected and unaffected limbs *to maintain muscle tone and increase muscle strength.* A patient with a leg amputation may perform push-ups, as ordered (in the sitting position, arms at his sides), or pull-ups on the overhead trapeze *to strengthen his arms, shoulders, and back in preparation for using crutches.*

Wrapping and conditioning the stump

- Wrapping the stump properly is important to provide equal, firm compression and to ready the stump for a prosthesis. Using a 4" elastic bandage, stretch the bandage to about two-thirds its maximum length as you wrap it diagonally around the stump, with the greatest pressure distally. (Depending on the size of the patient's leg, you may need to use two 4" bandages.) Secure the bandage with the Velcro closures or use tape. Make sure the bandage covers all portions of the stump smoothly *because wrinkles or exposed areas encourage skin breakdown.* (See *Wrapping a stump,* page 496.)
- If the patient experiences throbbing after the stump is wrapped, remove the bandage immediately and reapply it less tightly. *Throbbing indicates impaired circulation.*
- Check the bandage regularly. Rewrap it when it begins to bunch up at the end (usually about every 12 hours for a moderately active patient) or every 24 hours.

Wrapping a stump

Proper stump care helps protect the limb, reduces swelling, and prepares the limb for a prosthesis. As you perform the procedure, teach it to the patient.

- Obtain two 4″ elastic bandages with Velcro closures or use tape.
- Center the end of the first 4″ bandage at the top of the patient's thigh.
- Unroll the bandage downward over the stump and to the back of the leg.
- Make three figure-eight turns to adequately cover the ends of the stump. As you wrap, be sure to include the roll of flesh in the groin area. Use enough pressure to ensure that the stump narrows toward the end so that it fits comfortably into the prosthesis.
- Use the second 4″ bandage to anchor the first bandage around the waist. For a below-the-knee amputation, use the knee to anchor the bandage in place.
- Secure the bandage with the Velcro closures or tape.
- Check the stump bandage regularly and rewrap it if it bunches at the end.

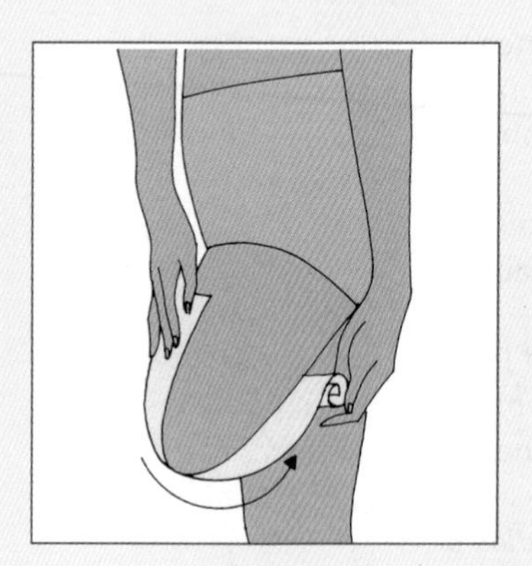

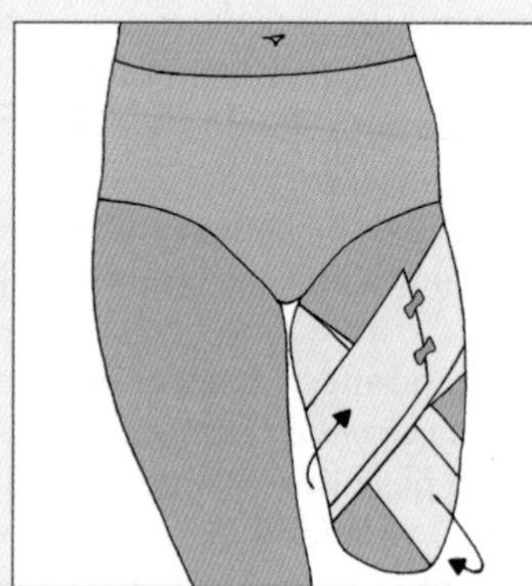

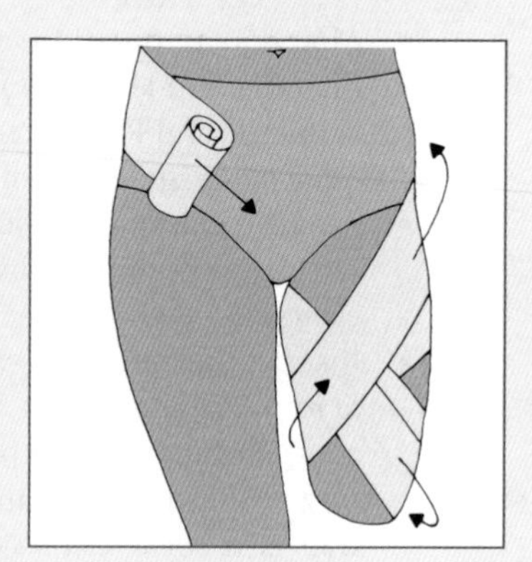

- After removing the bandage to rewrap it, massage the stump gently, always pushing *toward* the suture line rather than away from it. *This stimulates circulation and prevents scar tissue from adhering to the bone.*

Conditioning the stump

- When healing begins, instruct the patient to push the stump against a pillow. Then have him progress gradually to pushing against harder surfaces, such as a padded chair, then a hard chair. *These conditioning exercises help the patient adjust to experiencing pressure and sensation in the stump.*

Note: An elastic stump shrinker may be used after the wound has healed. The shrinker is used to control swelling and to help ready the stump for a prosthesis.

Caring for the healed stump

- *To prevent a rash,* bathe the stump but never shave it. If possible, bathe the stump at the end of the day *because warm water may cause swelling, making reapplication of the prosthesis difficult.*

Inspection report

- Inspect the stump for redness, swelling, irritation, and calluses. Report these findings to the physician. Tell the patient to avoid putting weight on the stump. (The skin should be firm but not taut over the bony end of the limb.)
- Continue muscle-strengthening exercises *so the patient can build the strength he'll need to control the prosthesis.*
- Change the patient's stump socks as necessary *to avoid exposing the skin to excessive perspiration, which can be irritating.* Wash the socks in warm water and gentle nondetergent soap; lay them flat on a towel to dry. *Machine washing or drying may shrink the socks.*

Caring for the plastic prosthesis

- Wipe the plastic socket of the prosthesis with a damp cloth and mild alcohol *to prevent bacterial accumulation.*
- Wipe the insert (if the prosthesis has one) with a dry cloth.
- Dry the prosthesis thoroughly; if possible, allow it to dry overnight.
- Maintain and lubricate the prosthesis, as instructed by the manufacturer.
- Check for malfunctions and adjust or repair the prosthesis as necessary *to prevent further damage.*
- Check the condition of the shoe on a foot prosthesis frequently and change it as necessary.

Applying the prosthesis

- Apply a stump sock. Keep the seams away from bony prominences.
- If the prosthesis has an insert, remove it from the socket, place it over the stump, and insert the stump into the prosthesis.
- If it has no insert, merely slide the prosthesis over the stump. Secure the prosthesis onto the stump according to the manufacturer's directions.

Practice pointers

- If a patient arrives at the hospital with a traumatic amputation, the amputated part may be saved for possible reimplantation. (See *Caring for an amputated body part,* page 498.)

Documenting stump and prosthesis care

In your notes, record:
- date, time, and specific procedures performed for all postoperative care
- amount and type of drainage
- condition of the dressing
- need for dressing reinforcement
- appearance of the suture line and surrounding tissue
- signs and symptoms of skin irritation or infection
- complications and nursing actions taken
- patient's tolerance of exercise
- patient's psychological reaction to the amputation.

During routine daily care, document:
- date, time, type of care given
- condition of the skin and suture line, including signs and symptoms of irritation (such as redness or tenderness)
- patient education
- patient's progress in caring for the stump or prosthesis.

Caring for an amputated body part

After traumatic amputation, a surgeon may be able to reimplant the severed body part through microsurgery. The chance of successful reimplantation is much greater if the amputated part has received proper care.

If a patient arrives at the hospital with a severed body part, first make sure the bleeding at the amputation site has been controlled. Then follow these guidelines for preserving the body part.

- Put on sterile gloves. Carefully remove any clothing, dirt, or debris from the body part. It may be gently irrigated with sterile saline to aid in this process. Wrap the body part in several saline-soaked gauze pads, combine pads, or roller gauze. *Cover completely with saline-soaked material.* Place in a watertight bag and either wrap with another ice-filled bag or immerse in a sterile container filled with ice and water.
- Always protect the part from direct contact with ice—and *never* use dry ice. Otherwise, irreversible tissue damage may occur, making the part unsuitable for reimplantation.) Keep this bag ice-cold until the patient is readied for reimplantation surgery.
- Label the bag with the patient's name, name of body part, hospital identification number, and date and time when cooling began. Verify if the label matches the information in the patient's medical record.

Note: The body part must be wrapped and cooled quickly.

Irreversible tissue damage occurs after only 6 hours at ambient temperature. However, hypothermic management seldom preserves tissues for more than 24 hours.

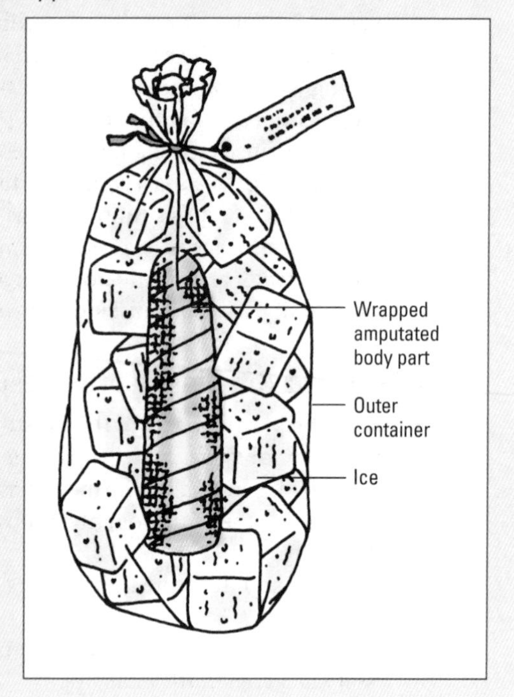

- Teach the patient how to care for his stump and prosthesis properly. Make sure he knows what signs and symptoms indicate problems in the stump. Explain that a 10-lb (4.5 kg) change in body weight will alter his stump size and require a new prosthesis socket *to ensure a correct fit.* (See *Caring for a stump at home.*)
- Exercise of the remaining muscles in an amputated limb must begin the day after surgery. A physical therapist will direct these exercises. For example, arm exercises progress from isometrics to assisted ROM to active ROM. Leg exercises include rising from a chair, balancing on one leg, and ROM exercises of the knees and hips. (See *Documenting stump and prosthesis care,* page 497.)

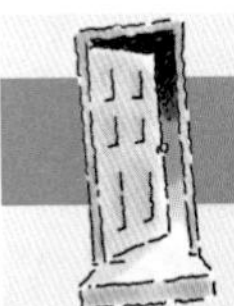

Home care connection

Caring for a stump at home

Before your patient returns home after a limb amputation, emphasize that proper care of his stump can speed healing. Tell him to inspect the stump carefully every day, using a mirror, and to continue proper daily stump care. Instruct him to call his physician if the incision appears to be opening, looks red or swollen, feels warm, is painful to touch, or is seeping drainage.

Tell the patient to massage the stump toward the suture line to mobilize the scar and prevent its adherence to bone. Advise him to avoid exposing the skin around the stump to excessive perspiration, which can be irritating. Tell him to change his elastic bandages or stump socks during the day to avoid this.

Ease the pain

Tell the patient that he may experience twitching, spasms, or phantom limb pain, as his stump muscles are adjusting to amputation. Advise him that he can ease these symptoms with heat, massage, or gentle pressure. If his stump is sensitive to touch, tell him to rub it with a dry washcloth for 4 minutes three times per day.

Stress the importance of performing prescribed exercises to help minimize complications, maintain muscle strength and tone, prevent contractures, and promote independence. Also, urge him to maintain proper positioning to prevent contractures and edema.

Electrical bone growth stimulation

Bone growth stimulation is the technique of promoting bone growth in difficult-to-heal fractures by applying a low electrical current or ultrasound to the fracture. By imitating the body's natural electrical forces, electrical bone growth stimulation initiates or accelerates the healing process in a fractured bone that has failed to heal.

Three styles of stimulation

Three basic electrical bone stimulation techniques are available: fully implantable direct current stimulation, semi-invasive percutaneous stimulation, and noninvasive electromagnetic coil stimulation. The first two techniques can lead to complications. (See *Bone stimulation and complications*.) Choice of technique depends on the fracture type and location, the physician's preference, and the patient's ability and willingness to comply. The invasive device requires little or no patient involvement. With the other two methods, however, the patient must manage his own treatment schedule and maintain the equipment. Treatment time averages 3 to 6 months.

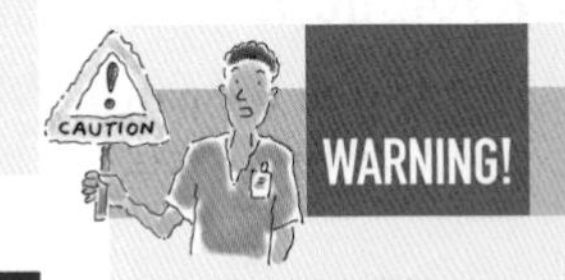

WARNING!

Bone stimulation and complications

Direct current electrical bone stimulation equipment may cause any of the complications associated with any surgical procedure, including increased infection risk. Local irritation or skin ulceration may arise around cathode pin sites with percutaneous devices. No complications are associated with electromagnetic coils.

What you need

For direct current stimulation: The equipment set consists of a small generator and leadwires that connect to a titanium cathode wire that's surgically implanted into the nonunited bone site.

For percutaneous stimulation: The set consists of an external anode skin pad with a leadwire, lithium battery pack, and one to four Teflon-coated stainless steel cathode wires that are surgically implanted.

For electromagnetic stimulation: The set consists of a generator that plugs into a standard 110-volt outlet and two strong electromagnetic coils placed on either side of the injured area. The coils can be incorporated into a cast, cuff, or orthotic device.

Getting ready

All equipment comes in sets with instructions provided by the manufacturer. Follow the instructions carefully. Make sure all parts are included and are sterilized according to hospital policy and procedure.

How you do it

- Tell the patient whether he'll have an anesthetic and, if possible, which kind.

Direct current stimulation

- Implantation is performed with the patient under general anesthesia. Afterward, the physician may apply a cast or external fixator to immobilize the limb. The patient may be hospitalized for observation after implantation. Weight bearing may be ordered, but most patients must remain *non-weight-bearing until the fracture has healed.*
- After the bone fragments join, the generator and leadwire can be removed under local anesthesia. The titanium cathode remains implanted.

Percutaneous stimulation

Remove excessive body hair from the injured site before applying the anode pad. Avoid stressing or pulling on the anode wire. Instruct the patient to change the anode pad every 48 hours. Tell him to report local pain to his physician and not to bear weight for the duration of treatment.

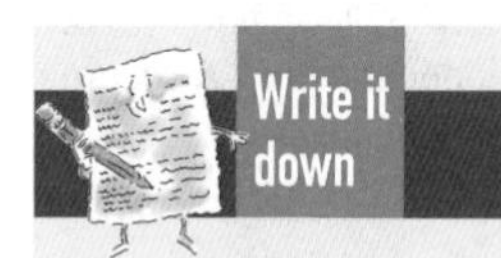

Documenting electrical bone growth stimulation

In your notes, record:
- type of electrical bone stimulation equipment provided (including date, time, and location, as appropriate)
- skin condition
- patient's tolerance of the procedure
- instructions given to the patient and family members and their ability to understand and act on instructions.

Electromagnetic stimulation

- Show the patient where to place the coils and tell him to apply them for 3 to 10 hours each day, as ordered by his physician. Many patients find it most convenient to perform the procedure at night.
- Urge the patient not to interrupt treatments for more than 10 minutes at a time.
- Teach the patient how to use and care for the generator.
- Weight bearing may be ordered, but most patients must remain *non-weight-bearing until the fracture has healed.*

Practice pointers

- A patient with a direct current electrical bone stimulation shouldn't undergo electrocauterization, diathermy, or magnetic resonance imaging (MRI). *Electrocautery may "short" the system; diathermy may potentiate the electrical current, possibly causing tissue damage; and MRI will interfere with or stop the current.*
- Percutaneous electrical bone stimulation is contraindicated in patients with any inflammatory process. Ask the patient if he's sensitive to nickel or chromium; *both are present in the electrical bone stimulation system.* (See *Documenting electrical bone growth stimulation.*)

No-no's: pregnancy, pacemaker

Electromagnetic coils are contraindicated for a pregnant patient, a patient with a tumor, or a patient with an arm fracture and a pacemaker.

Continuous passive motion

Continuous passive motion (CPM) devices are used to control postoperative pain, reduce inflammation, provide passive motion in a specific plane of movement, and protect the healing repair of tissue. A CPM device constantly moves the joint through a controlled ROM. The device is applied to the affected extremity using pads and straps that are connected to the device. The physician will prescribe usage instructions, including the speed of the machine, the duration of usage, amount of motion, and the rate of the motion increase.

These devices are indicated for treatment of joint stiffness and limited ROM resulting from fractures, dislocations, ligament and tendon repairs, joint arthroplasty, burns, total knee replacement, spinal cord injuries, rheumatoid arthritis, tendon release, cerebral palsy, multiple sclerosis, and other traumatic and nontraumatic disorders.

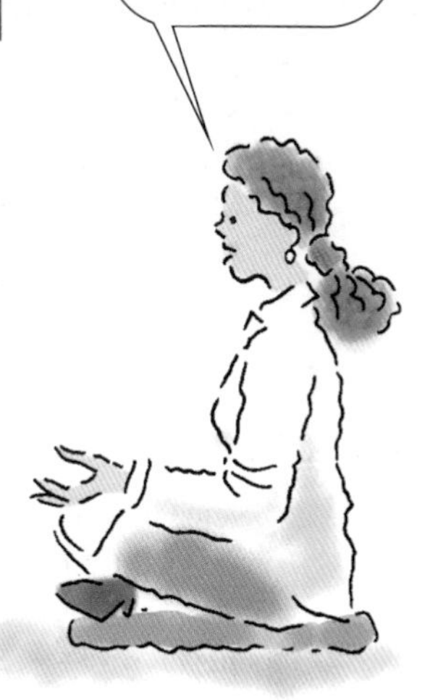
Meditate on this: Knee extension systems can help restore range-of-motion to stiff joints.

What you need

CPM device.

The device is typically applied by the representative from the device maker or the orthopedic assistant, but nursing should be aware of the application, how to change settings, and general operation procedures.

How you do it

- Check the order on the patient's chart.
- Identify the patient using two patient identifiers per facility policy.
- Explain the procedure to the patient.
- Secure the appropriate soft goods to the device as directed. (Written instructions accompany each new device.)
- Fit the patient according to the written instructions by first measuring the length of the patient's femur from the greater trochanter (hip joint) to the center or joint line of the knee.
- Transfer this measurement to the thigh cradle.
- Loosen the calf cradle adjustment knobs and extend the foot assembly. Position the patient's leg in the unit with the soft goods in place.
- Tighten and adjust the calf cradle and foot assembly as appropriate.

Remember: The goal is to align the knee axis of the patient with the pivot axis of the CPM.

- Stabilize the device by extending the base rods against a solid barrier such as the footboard.

Setting splint tension

- Locate ON/OFF switch. Turn unit ON.
- Set flexion range, extension range, speed, and pause according to the physician's order.
- Make sure the patient has the ability to turn the unit ON and OFF at any time desired.
- Make sure the patient practices applying and removing the splint.

Practice pointers

- The CPM device is contraindicated if passive ROM treatments are inappropriate, as in unhealed or unstable fractures. It should be used cautiously in patients with thrombophlebitis, osteoporosis, spasticity, edema, gross ligament instability, and circulatory impairment. (See *Documenting CPM device use*.)

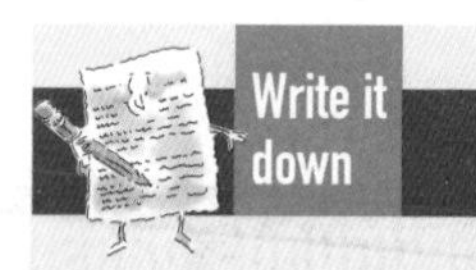

Documenting CPM device use

In your notes, record:
- time and date of the procedure
- settings ordered by the physician
- length of time the patient can tolerate the ordered settings
- setting changes
- reason for the change in settings.

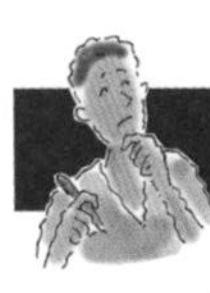

Quick quiz

1. Which type of splint immobilizes a fracture with a longitudinal pull that reduces muscle spasms?
   A. Rigid splint
   B. Traction splint
   C. Spine board splint
   D. Circular splint

Answer: B. A traction splint immobilizes a fracture with a longitudinal pull that reduces muscle spasms, pain, and arterial and neural damage.

2. Which finding indicates pressure on the nerves?
   A. Numbness or paralysis distal to the injury site
   B. Pain localized at the injury site
   C. Cyanosis of the extremity
   D. Blanching of the fingernails

Answer: A. Numbness or paralysis distal to the injury site indicates pressure on nerves.

3. Which procedure is used most commonly to treat open, unstable fractures with extensive soft tissue damage?
   A. External fixation
   B. Mechanical traction
   C. Skin traction
   D. Buck's traction

Answer: A. External fixation is used most commonly to treat open, unstable fractures with extensive soft tissue damage.

4. What is the best way for the nurse to care for an amputated body part?
   A. Clean the amputated part thoroughly with alcohol and saline solution.
   B. Pour dextrose and water over the part and seal in a bag.
   C. Place in saline-soaked gauze pads in a watertight container and then put the container on ice.
   D. Immediately pack the extremity in a cooler with ice and alcohol.

Answer: C. Place the amputated part in saline-soaked gauze pads in a watertight container and then put the container on ice.

Scoring

☆☆☆ If you answered all four items correctly, fabulous! You've demonstrated a fixation for fine answers.

☆☆ If you answered three items correctly, terrific. You've certainly found some traction in this chapter.

☆ If you answered fewer than two items correctly, don't get bent out of shape. A quick chapter review will give you all the support you need.

Selected References

Behrens, S. B., Deren, M. E., & Monchik, K. O. (2013). A review of bone growth stimulation for fracture treatment. *Current Orthopaedic Practice, 24*(1), 84–91.

Drozd, M., Miles, S., & Davies, J. (2009a). Casting: Complications and after care. *Emergency Nurse, 17*(3), 26–27.

Drozd, M., Miles, S., & Davies, J. (2009b). Essential practice in casting. *Emergency Nurse, 17*(2), 18–19.

Liu, F., Williams, R. M., Liu, H.E., et al. (2010). The lived experience of persons with lower extremity amputation. *Journal of Clinical Nursing, 19*, 2152–2161.

Malik, S., Chiampas, G., & Leonard, H. (2010). Emergent evaluation of injuries to the shoulder, clavicle and humerus. *Emergency Medicine Clinics of North America, 28*(4), 739–763.

McConnell, E. A. (1991). Correctly positioning an arm sling. *Nursing, 21*, 70.

Osmond, T. (1999). Principles of traction. *Australian Nursing Journal, 6*(7 Suppl.), 1–4.

Salter, R. B., Hamilton, H. W., Wedge, J. H., et al. (1984). Clinical application of basic research on continuous passive motion for disorders and injuries of synovial joints: A preliminary report of a feasibility study. *Journal of Orthopaedic Research, 1*(3), 325–342.

Springhouse. (2003). *Best practices: A guide to excellence in nursing care*. Philadelphia, PA: Lippincott Williams & Wilkins.

Williams, H., & Griffiths, P. (2004). The effectiveness of pin site care for patients with external fixators. *British Journal of Community Nursing, 9*(5), 206–210.

Chapter 11

Skin care

Just the facts

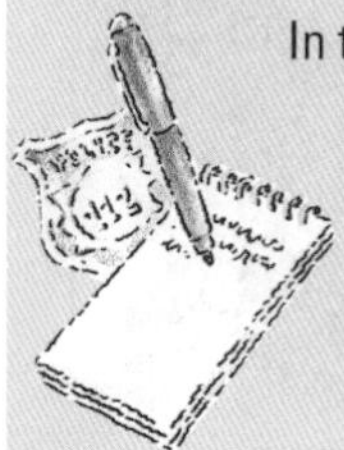

In this chapter, you'll learn:

- about skin care procedures and how to perform them
- what patient care is associated with each procedure
- how to manage complications associated with each procedure
- about patient teaching and documentation for each procedure.

Burn care

Goals of burn care are to maintain the patient's physiologic stability, repair skin integrity, prevent infection, and promote maximal functioning and psychosocial health. Reintegration of the patient into the home/school/work/community environment is important. A particular focus is care immediately after a burn occurs. Competent care at that time can dramatically improve the success of overall treatment.

Burn severity and percent of total body surface area affects the type of care you'll provide. Burn severity is determined by the burn's depth and extent and other factors, such as age, complications, and coexisting illnesses. (See *Evaluating burn severity*, page 506.) Effective pain management during procedures is imperative.

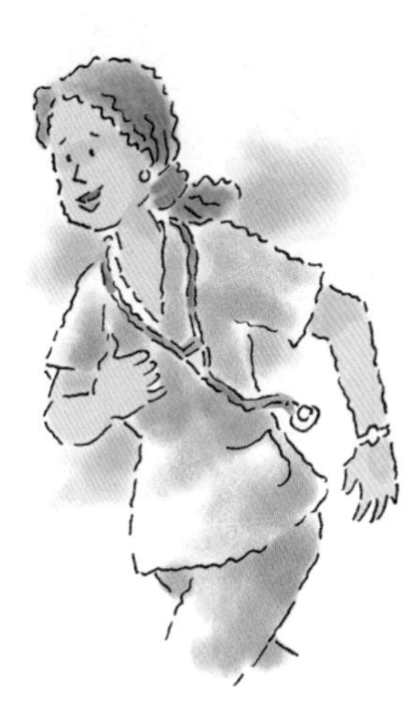
Competent care immediately after a burn makes recovery more likely.

Dress for success

Infection of a burn can increase wound depth, cause skin graft rejection, slow healing, increase pain, and prolong hospitalization. It can even lead to death. To help prevent infection, use strict aseptic technique during care; dress the burn site as ordered; monitor and rotate intravenous (I.V.) lines regularly; and carefully assess the burn extent, body system functions, and the patient's emotional status. Other interventions—such as careful positioning and regular exercise for burned extremities—help maintain joint function, prevent contractures, and minimize deformity. (See *Positioning the patient to prevent deformity*, page 507.)

Evaluating burn severity

To judge a burn's severity, assess its depth and extent as well as the presence of other factors.

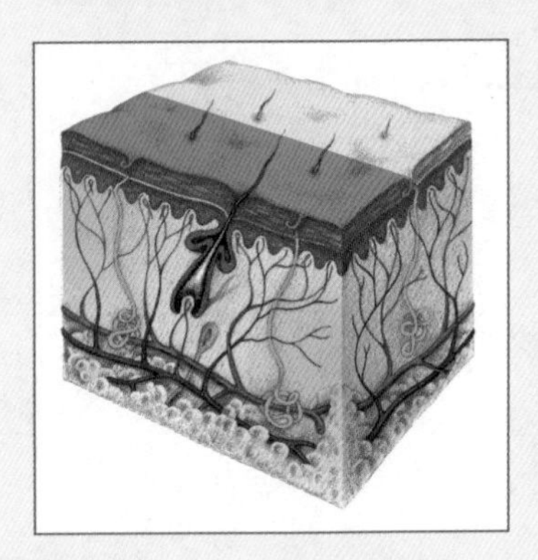

Superficial partial-thickness (first-degree) burn
The burned area appears pink or red with minimal edema.

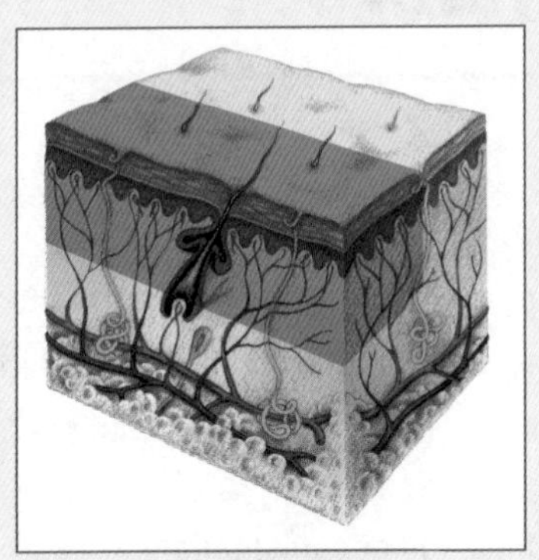

Deep partial-thickness (second-degree) burn
The burned area is pink or red with a mottled appearance.

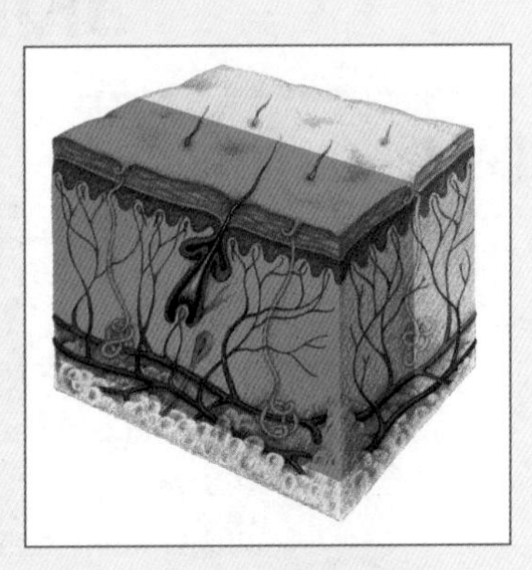

Full-thickness (third-degree) burn
The burned area appears red, waxy, white, brown, or black.

Therapeutic Guidelines

Lund and Browder chart for calculating the percentage of total body surface area burnt

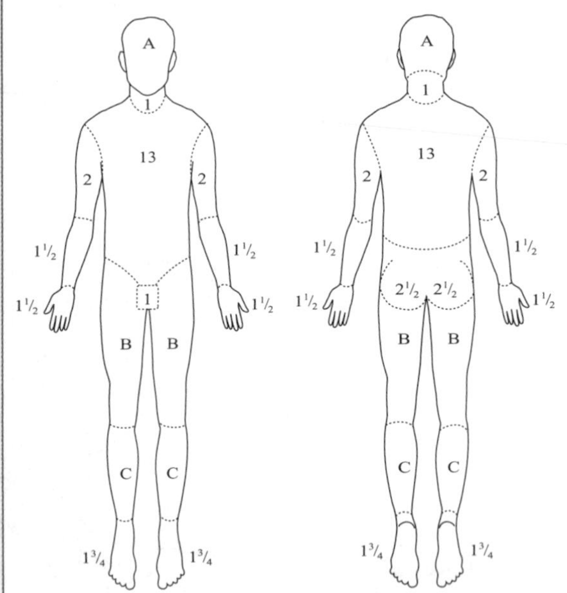

Region	Partial thickness (%) [NB1]	Full thickness (%)
head		
neck		
anterior trunk		
posterior trunk		
right arm		
left arm		
buttocks		
genitalia		
right leg		
left leg		
Total burn		

NB1: Do not include erythema

Area	Age 0	1	5	10	15	Adult
A = half of head	9½	8½	6½	5½	4½	3½
B = half of one thigh	2¾	3¼	4	4½	4½	4¾
C = half of one lower leg	2½	2½	2¾	3	3¼	3½

Therapeutic Guidelines Limited is an independent not-for-profit organisation dedicated to deriving guidelines for therapy from the latest world literature, interpreted and distilled by Australia's most eminent and respected experts.

Positioning the patient to prevent deformity

For each potential deformity listed below, you can use the corresponding positioning and interventions to help prevent the deformity.

Burned area	Potential deformity	Preventive positioning	Nursing interventions
Neck	• Flexion contraction • Extensor contraction	• Extension • Prone with head slightly raised	• Remove pillow from bed. • Place pillow under upper chest to flex cervical spine or apply cervical collar.
Elbow	• Flexion and pronation	• Arm extended and supinated	• Use an elbow splint.
Wrist	• Flexion	• Splint in 15-degree extension	• Apply a hand splint.
Fingers	• Extension	• Splint in 15-degree flexion	• Apply a hand splint.
Hand	• Adhesions of the extensor tendons; loss of palmar grip	• Metacarpophalangeal joints in maximum flexion; interphalangeal joints in slight flexion; thumb in abduction	• Apply a hand splint; wrap fingers separately.
Hip	• Internal rotation, flexion, and adduction	• Neutral rotation and abduction; maintain extension with prone position	• Trochanter rolls • Long leg splints • Pillow under buttocks • Foam wedge
Knee	• Internal rotation, flexion, and adduction	• Neutral rotation and abduction; maintain extension	• Knee splint
Ankle	• Flexion • Plantar flexion	• 90-degree dorsiflexion	• Use a footboard or ankle splint.

The next step

Repair of skin integrity requires aggressive wound debridement followed by maintenance of a clean wound bed until the wound heals or is covered with a skin graft.

What you need

A sterile field is required, and all equipment and supplies used in the dressing should be sterile. Sterile towels to set up the sterile field ✳ ordered pain medication ✳ normal saline solution ✳ fluffed gauze pads ✳ sterile bowl ✳ blunt scissors ✳ tissue forceps ✳ ordered topical medication ✳ burn gauze ✳ roller gauze ✳ fine-mesh gauze ✳ elastic gauze ✳ elastic netting or tape ✳ cotton-tipped applicators ✳ three pairs of sterile gloves ✳ two sterile gowns ✳ two masks ✳ surgical cap ✳ shoe covers ✳ heat lamps ✳ bath blanket ✳ impervious plastic trash bag.

Getting ready

Warm normal saline solution by immersing unopened bottles in warm water. Check expiration dates on packaging. Assemble equipment on the dressing table. Make sure the treatment area has adequate light *to allow accurate wound assessment*. Open equipment packages using aseptic technique. Arrange supplies on a sterile field in order of use.

Low exposure

To prevent cross-contamination, plan to dress the cleanest areas first and the dirtiest or most contaminated areas last. *To help prevent excessive pain or cross-contamination*, you may need to perform the dressing in stages to avoid exposing all wounds at the same time.

How you do it

- Verify the physician/clinician orders.
- Identify the patient with at least two patient identifiers, according to facility policy.
- Assess the patient's level of pain per facility policy.
- Administer ordered oral pain analgesic about 20 minutes before beginning wound care and/or I.V. analgesic immediately before the procedure *to maximize patient comfort and cooperation*.
- Explain the procedure to the patient and provide privacy.
- Turn on overhead heat lamps *to keep the patient warm*. Make sure they don't overheat the patient.
- Pour warmed normal saline solution into the sterile bowl in the sterile field.
- Perform hand hygiene.

Removing a dressing without hydrotherapy

- Put on a gown, a mask, and sterile gloves.
- Remove dressing layers down to the innermost layer by cutting the outer dressings with sterile blunt scissors.
- If the inner layer appears dry, soak it with warm normal saline solution *to ease removal*.
- Remove the inner dressing with sterile tissue forceps or your sterile gloved hand.

Take out the trash

- *Because soiled dressings harbor infectious microorganisms*, dispose of dressings carefully in the impervious plastic trash bag according to facility policy. Dispose of your gloves and perform hand hygiene.

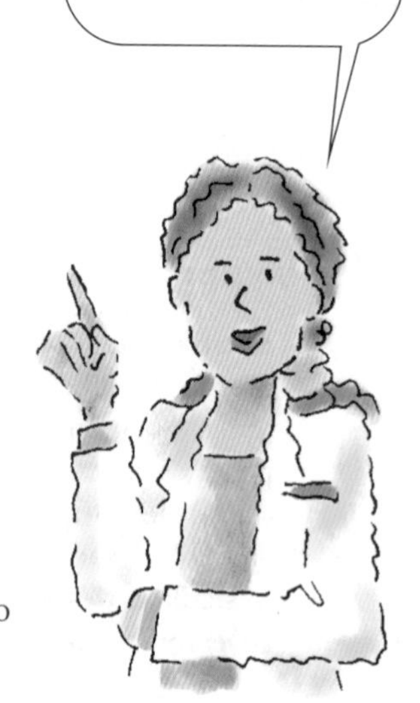
Be sure to dump soiled dressings where they won't spread infection. Afterward, change your gloves.

- Put on a new pair of sterile gloves. Using gauze pads moistened with normal saline solution, gently remove exudate and old topical medication. Move from the center of the wound outward.
- Carefully remove all loose eschar with sterile forceps and scissors if ordered. (See "Mechanical and chemical debridement," page 515.)

What's in the margin?

Wound assessment

- Assess wound condition. Note the location, size of wound, and tissue description. The wound should appear clean, with no debris, loose tissue, purulence, inflammation, or darkened margins.
- Before applying a new dressing, remove your gown and gloves. Discard them according to your facility policy, perform hand hygiene, and put on new barrier attire with sterile gloves.

Applying a wet dressing

- Soak fine-mesh gauze and the elastic gauze dressing in a large sterile basin containing the ordered solution (for example, saline or silver nitrate).
- Wring out the fine-mesh gauze until it's moist but not dripping and apply it to the wound. Warn the patient that he may feel transient pain when you apply the dressing.
- Wring out the elastic gauze dressing and position it to hold the fine-mesh gauze in place.
- Roll an elastic gauze dressing over these two dressings *to keep them intact.*

Warm and cozy—but not wet

- Cover the patient with a warm cotton bath blanket *to prevent chills.* Change the blanket if it becomes damp. Use an overhead heat lamp if necessary.
- Change dressings as ordered, *to keep the wound moist,* especially if you're using silver nitrate. *Silver nitrate becomes ineffective and the silver ions may damage tissue if dressings become dry.* (To maintain moisture, some protocols call for irrigating the dressing with solution at least every 4 hours through small slits cut into the outer dressing.)

Applying a dry dressing with a topical medication

- Remove old dressings, dispose of properly, and clean the wound (as described previously).
- Apply ordered medication to the wound in a thin layer (about 2 to 4 mm thick) with your sterile gloved hand. If the area is large

and painful, the medication may be applied to the gauze first, then laid onto the burn surface. Place several layers of burn gauze on top *to contain the medication but allow exudate to escape.*

Cut to fit

- Don't cover unburned areas.
- Cover the entire dressing with roller gauze and secure it with elastic netting or tape.

Providing arm and leg care

- Apply dressings from the distal to the proximal area *to stimulate circulation and prevent constriction.* Wrap the burn gauze once around the patient's arm or leg so the edges overlap slightly. Continue wrapping in this way until the gauze covers the wound.
- Apply a dry roller gauze dressing *to hold the bottom layers in place.* Secure with elastic netting or tape. Elastic/ace bandages may be ordered for the lower extremities to help maintain venous blood return.

Providing hand and foot care

- Wrap each finger separately with a single layer of a 4″ × 4″ gauze pad *to allow the patient to use his hands and to prevent webbing contractures.*
- Put gauze between each toe as appropriate *to prevent webbing contractures.*
- Place the hand/foot in a functional position and secure this position using a dressing. Apply splints if ordered.

Providing chest, abdomen, and back care

- Apply the ordered medication to the wound in a thin layer. Then cover the entire burned area with sheets of burn gauze.
- Wrap the area with roller gauze or apply a specialty vest dressing *to hold the burn gauze in place.*

Netting a good result

Secure the dressing with elastic netting or tape. Make sure the dressing doesn't restrict respiratory motion, especially in very young or elderly patients and in those with circumferential injuries (injuries to the body's periphery).

Providing facial care

- If the patient has scalp burns, clip or shave the hair around the burn as ordered. Clip other hair until it's about 2″ (5 cm) long *to prevent contamination of burned scalp areas.*

- Shave facial hair if it comes in contact with burned areas.
- Typically, facial burns are managed with milder topical agents (such as triple antibiotic ointment) and are left open to air. If dressings are required, make sure they don't cover the patient's eyes, nostrils, or mouth.

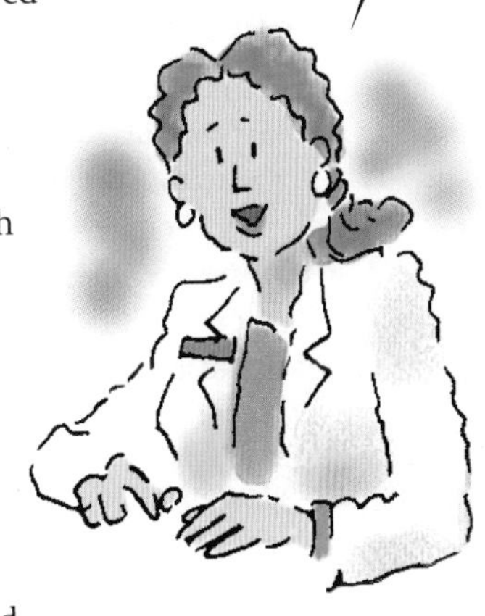
With facial burns, use a milder topical agent and leave the burn open to air.

Providing ear care

- Clip hair around the affected ear.
- Remove exudate and crusts with cotton-tipped applicators dipped in normal saline solution.
- Place a 4″ × 4″ layer of gauze behind the auricle *to prevent webbing*.
- Apply the ordered medication to 4″ × 4″ gauze pads and place the pads over the burned area. Before securing the dressing with a roller bandage, position the patient's ears normally *to avoid damaging the auricular cartilage. The ears may be left open after topical medication is applied.*
- Examine the ear canals for patency.
- Assess the patient's hearing ability.

Providing eye care

- Clean the area around the eyes and eyelids with a cotton-tipped applicator and normal saline solution every 4 to 6 hours, or as needed, *to remove crusts and drainage.*
- Administer ordered eye ointments or drops.
- If the eyes can't be closed, apply lubricating ointments or drops as ordered.
- Be sure to close the patient's eyes before applying eye pads *to prevent corneal abrasion*. Don't apply topical ointments near the eyes without a doctor's order.

Providing nasal care

Check the nostrils for signs of inhalation injury, including inflamed mucosa, singed hairs inside the nostrils, and soot.

Up the chimney

- Clean the nostrils with cotton-tipped applicators dipped in normal saline solution. Remove crusts.
- Apply ordered ointments.
- If the patient has a nasogastric tube, use tracheostomy ties to secure the tube or bridle type device that doesn't require external ties/tape. Be sure to check the ties frequently for tightness resulting from swelling of facial tissue. Clean the area around the tube every 4 to 6 hours.

Practice pointers

- Assess/document level of pain again after dressing wounds to determine effectiveness of pain medications and tolerance of the procedure.
- Perform dressing changes in stages to prevent cross-contamination and excessive exposure, which increases pain. Change sterile gloves for each stage.

Wound condition

- Thorough assessment and documentation of the wound's appearance are essential *to detect infection and other complications.* A purulent wound or green-gray exudate indicates infection; an overly dry wound suggests dehydration; and a wound with a swollen, red edge suggests cellulitis. Suspect a fungal infection if the wound is white and powdery. Healthy granulation tissue appears clean, pinkish, faintly shiny, free of exudate, and bleeds easily.

No popping allowed

- *Because blisters protect underlying tissue,* leave them intact unless they impede joint motion, become infected, or cause patient discomfort.

Super-size that order

- Keep in mind that the patient with healing burns has increased nutritional needs. He'll require extra protein and carbohydrates *to accommodate an almost doubled basal metabolism.*
- Begin discharge planning as soon as the patient enters the facility *to help him (and his family) make a smooth transition from facility to home.* (See *Documenting burn care.*)

Documenting burn care

In your notes, record:
- date and time of all care provided
- wound condition
- special dressing-change techniques
- topical medications administered
- positioning of the burned area
- patient's tolerance of care procedures.

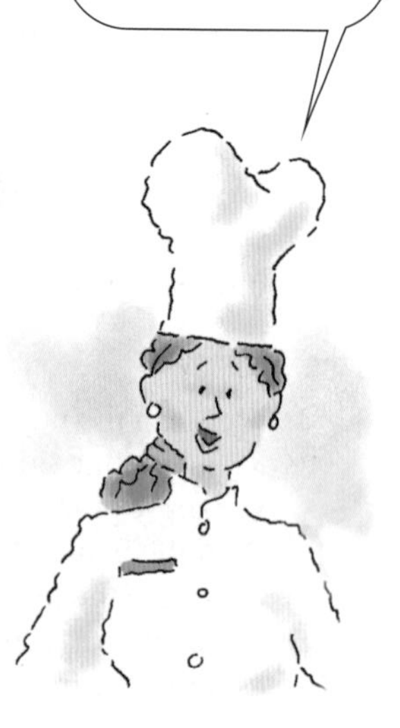
A burn patient needs extra calories. That's because his basal metabolism nearly doubles to help healing.

Biologic burn dressings

Biologic burn dressings provide a temporary protective covering for burn wounds and clean granulation tissue. They also temporarily secure fresh skin grafts and protect graft donor sites.

This little piggy provides burn dressings

Three organic materials are commonly used as burn dressings: pigskin, cadaver skin, and amniotic membrane. One biocomposite material, Biobrane, is also used. (See *Comparing biologic dressings.*) Besides stimulating new skin growth, these dressings act like normal skin: They reduce heat loss; block infection; and minimize fluid, electrolyte, and protein losses.

Comparing biologic dressings

Type	Description and uses	Nursing considerations
Cadaver (homograft)	• Obtained at autopsy up to 24 hours after death • Available as fresh cryopreserved homografts in tissue banks • Provides protection to granulation tissue after escharotomy • May be used in some patients as a test graft for autografting • Covers excised wounds immediately • Applied by clinician in the operating room (OR) or at bedside	• Observe for exudate. • Watch for signs of rejection. • Keep in mind that the gauze dressing may be removed every 8 hours to observe the graft.
Pigskin (heterograft or xenograft)	• Comes fresh or frozen in rolls or sheets • Can cover and protect debrided, untidy wounds, mesh autografts, clean (eschar-free) partial-thickness burns, and exposed tendons • Applied by the clinician in the OR or at bedside	• Reconstitute frozen form with normal saline solution 30 minutes before use. • Watch for signs of rejection. • Dressing is typically changed every 2 to 5 days.
Amniotic membrane (homograft)	• Bacteriostatic condition doesn't require antimicrobials • May be used to protect partial-thickness burns or (temporarily) granulation tissue before autografting • Applied by the clinician	• Change the membrane every 48 hours. • Cover the membrane with a gauze dressing or leave it exposed as ordered. • If you apply a gauze dressing, change it every 48 hours.
Biobrane (biocomposite dressing)	• Comes in sterile, prepackaged sheets in various sizes • Used to cover donor sites, superficial partial-thickness burns, debrided wounds awaiting autograft, and meshed autografts • Provides significant pain relief • Applied by clinician or nurse	• Leave the membrane in place for 3 to 14 days, possibly longer. • Don't use dressing for preparing a granulation bed for subsequent autografting.

Amniotic membrane or fresh cadaver skin usually is applied to the patient in the operating room. Pigskin or Biobrane may be applied in either the operating room or a treatment room. Before applying a biologic dressing, the wound must be clean and free of eschar. The frequency of dressing changes will vary, depending on wound type and the specific function of the dressing.

What you need

Ordered analgesic ✱ cap ✱ mask ✱ two pairs of sterile gloves ✱ sterile or clean gown ✱ shoe covers ✱ biologic dressing ✱ tape ✱ roller gauze ✱ normal saline solution ✱ sterile basin ✱ Xeroflo gauze ✱ elastic netting ✱ sterile forceps ✱ sterile scissors ✱ sterile hemostat.

Getting ready

Place the biologic dressing in the sterile basin containing sterile normal saline solution (or open the Biobrane package). Using aseptic technique, open the sterile dressing packages. Arrange the equipment on the dressing cart and keep the cart readily accessible. Make sure the treatment area has adequate light to allow accurate wound assessment and dressing placement.

How you do it

- Verify the orders for specific dressings to be used.
- Verify the patient's identity using at least two patient identifiers according to facility policy.
- If this is the patient's first treatment, explain the procedure *to allay his fears and promote cooperation*. Provide privacy.
- Assess the patient's level of pain using the facility's established pain scale. If ordered, administer an analgesic to the patient 20 minutes before beginning the procedure and/or give an I.V. analgesic immediately before the procedure *to increase the patient's comfort and tolerance levels.*
- Perform hand hygiene and put on a cap, mask, gown, shoe covers, and sterile gloves.
- Clean and debride the wound *to reduce bacteria*. Remove and dispose of gloves. Wash your hands and put on a fresh pair of sterile gloves.

Shiny is down—unless it's up

- Place the dressing directly on the wound surface.
- Pigskin is shiny side **down**.
- Biobrane is shiny side **up**; follow manufacturer's instructions for other products ordered.
- Roll the dressing directly onto the skin if applicable. Place the dressing strips so that the edges touch but don't overlap. Use sterile forceps if necessary. Smooth the dressing. Eliminate folds, wrinkles, and air pockets by rolling out the dressing with the hemostat/forceps handle or your sterile-gloved hand *to cover the wound completely and ensure adherence.*
- Use scissors to trim the dressing around the wound so it fits the wound without overlapping adjacent areas.

Over organics

- Place ordered dressing (such as Xeroform gauze) directly over a cadaver skin graft, a pigskin graft, or an amniotic membrane. Place a few layers of gauze on top *to absorb exudate* and wrap with a roller gauze dressing. Secure the dressing with tape or elastic netting. During daily dressing changes, the dressing will be removed down to the original covering, and the gauze will be replaced after inspecting for drainage, adherence, and signs of infection.

Over synthetics/biocomposites

- Place a nonadhesive dressing as ordered (such as Exu-Dry) over the Biobrane *to absorb drainage and provide stability*. Wrap the dressing with a roller gauze dressing and secure it with tape or elastic netting. During daily dressing changes, the dressing will be removed down to the Biobrane and the site inspected for signs of infection. After the Biobrane adheres (usually in 2 to 3 days), it doesn't need to be covered with a dressing.
- Position the patient comfortably, elevating the area if possible. *This reduces edema, which may prevent the biologic dressing from adhering.*

Documenting biologic burn dressings

In your notes, record:

- time and date of dressing changes
- types of dressings applied
- areas of dressing application
- quality of dressing adherence
- purulent drainage or other infection signs
- patient's tolerance of the dressing procedure
- level of pain pre- and postprocedure.

Practice pointers

- Reassess the patient's level of pain after the mentioned procedures.
- Be aware that infection may develop under a biologic dressing. Observe the wound carefully during dressing changes for signs of infection. If wound drainage appears purulent, remove the dressing, clean the area with normal saline solution or another prescribed cleaning solution as ordered, and apply a fresh biologic dressing. (See *Documenting biologic burn dressings*.)

Mechanical and chemical debridement

Debridement involves removing necrotic (dead) tissue to allow underlying healthy tissue to regenerate. Mechanical debridement procedures include irrigation, hydrotherapy, and dead tissue excision with forceps and scissors. The procedure may be done at the bedside, in a procedure room, or tub room. Chemical debridement attacks the collagen in tissue and helps remove dead tissue.

Eschar-go

Burn wound debridement removes eschar (hardened, dead tissue). This prevents or controls infection, promotes healing, and prepares the wound surface to receive a graft. Ideally, the wound should be debrided daily during the dressing change. Frequent, regular debridement guards against hemorrhage resulting from more extensive and forceful debridement. It also reduces the need to conduct extensive debridement under anesthesia.

Escharotomy

If thick eschar is present in a third-degree burn that is circumferential, an escharotomy may be performed. The thick eschar does not allow for expansion when fluid resuscitation is given and may directly impact circulation to an extremity. Electrical burns are at greater risk. When Doppler pulses and oximetry decrease or cease, this procedure becomes imminent. Ventilating the lungs may become difficult for a patient with thick eschar in a circumferential burn of the trunk/chest. Physicians perform this procedure. The eschar is opened longitudinally and sometimes laterally down to the subcutaneous tissue to relieve the pressure. The area is dressed just as the burn is thereafter and will fill in over time.

Combo order

Mechanical debridement may be combined with other debridement techniques, such as chemical/enzymatic debridement (with topical agents that dissolve dead tissue) or surgical excision and skin grafting (usually reserved for deep burns or ulcers). Typically, the patient receives a local or general anesthetic.

What you need

Ordered pain medication ✳ two pairs of sterile gloves ✳ two gowns ✳ shoe covers ✳ mask ✳ cap ✳ sterile scissors ✳ sterile forceps ✳ 4″ × 4″ sterile gauze pads ✳ sterile solutions and medications as ordered ✳ hemostatic agent as ordered.

Be sure to have the following equipment immediately available to control hemorrhage: needle holder ✳ gut suture with needle.

How you do it

- Identify the patient using two patient identifiers, per facility policy.
- Explain the procedure to the patient *to allay his fears and promote cooperation*. Teach him distraction and relaxation techniques, if possible, *to minimize his discomfort*.
- Assess level of pain.

Early start

- Provide privacy. Administer an analgesic 20 minutes before debridement begins and/or give an I.V. analgesic immediately before the procedure.
- Keep the patient warm. Expose only the area to be debrided *to prevent chilling and fluid and electrolyte loss*.

- Perform hand hygiene and put on a cap, mask, gown, shoe covers, and sterile gloves.

Flip back a few pages

- Remove the burn dressings and clean the wound. (For detailed instructions, see "Burn care," page 505.)
- Remove your gown and dirty gloves and change to another gown and sterile gloves.
- Lift loosened edges of eschar with forceps. Use the blunt edge of scissors or forceps to probe the eschar. Cut the dead tissue from the wound with the scissors. *To avoid cutting into viable tissue,* leave a ¼″ (0.6 cm) edge on the remaining eschar.

If bleeding occurs

- Because debridement removes only dead tissue, bleeding should be minimal. If bleeding occurs, apply gentle pressure on the wound with sterile 4″ × 4″ gauze pads. Apply the hemostatic agent if needed. If bleeding persists, notify the doctor and maintain pressure on the wound until arrival. Excessive bleeding or spurting vessels may warrant ligation.
- Perform additional procedures, such as application of topical medications and dressing replacements, as ordered.

Documenting mechanical debridement

In your notes, record:
- date and time of wound debridement
- area debrided
- solutions and medications used
- wound condition, including signs of infection or skin breakdown
- patient's tolerance of and reaction to the procedure
- pain assessment
- indications for additional therapy.

Practice pointers

- Work quickly, with an assistant if possible, to complete this painful procedure as soon as possible. Limit procedure time to 20 minutes if possible. (See *Documenting mechanical debridement.*)
- Debride no more than a 4″ (10-cm) square area at one time.

Note to self: Debridement is a painful procedure, so limit it to 20 minutes at most.

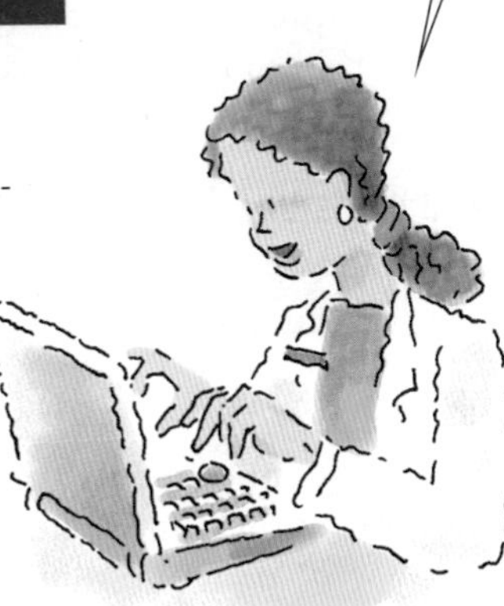

Skin graft care

A skin graft consists of healthy skin taken either from the patient (autograft) or a donor (allograft) and applied to a prepared burn surface. There, the graft resurfaces an area damaged by burns, traumatic injury, or surgery.

Split, full, or pedicle

The graft itself may be one of several types: split-thickness, full-thickness, or pedicle-flap. (See *Understanding types of grafts,* page 518.)

If and when

The size and depth of the patient's burns determine whether grafting is required. Grafting usually occurs at the completion of wound debridement. The goal is to cover all wounds with an autograft or allograft within 2 weeks. With enzymatic debridement, grafting may be performed 5 to 7 days after debridement is complete; with surgical debridement, grafting can occur the same day as the surgery.

Depending on your facility's policy, a doctor or a specially trained nurse may change graft dressings. The dressings usually stay in place for 3 to 5 days after surgery *to avoid disturbing the graft site.*

Double duty

Care procedures for an autograft or an allograft are essentially the same. However, an autograft requires care for two sites: the graft site and the donor site. (See *How to care for a donor graft site.*)

What you need

Ordered analgesic * clean and sterile gloves * sterile gown * cap * mask * sterile forceps * sterile scissors * sterile scalpel * burn gauze * Xeroform gauze * warm saline solution * moisturizing cream * roller bandage * optional: sterile cotton-tipped applicators.

Getting ready

Assemble the equipment on the dressing cart.

How you do it

- Identify the patient via two patient identifiers, according to facility policy.
- Assess the patient's level of pain.
- Explain the procedure to the patient and provide privacy.
- Administer an analgesic as ordered, 20 to 30 minutes before beginning the procedure and/or give an I.V. analgesic immediately before the procedure.

Even if they aren't dirty

- Perform hand hygiene.
- Put on the sterile gown and the clean mask, cap, and gloves.

Soak always

- Gently lift off all outer dressings. Soak the middle dressings with warm saline solution. Remove these carefully and slowly *to avoid disturbing the graft site.* Leave the primary dressing layer intact *to avoid dislodging the graft.*

Understanding types of grafts

A burn patient may receive one or more graft types.

Split-thickness
Most commonly used to cover open burns, a split-thickness graft includes the epidermis and part of the dermis. It may be applied as a sheet or a mesh. Mesh grafts prevent fluids from collecting under the graft and typically are used over extensive full-thickness burns.

Full-thickness
A full-thickness graft includes the epidermis and the entire dermis. It contains hair follicles, sweat glands, and sebaceous glands. These grafts usually are used for small burns that cause deep wounds, especially of the face.

Pedicle-flap
A pedicle-flap graft—a type of full-thickness graft—include skin and subcutaneous tissue and blood vessels to provide continued blood supply. It may be used in reconstructive surgery to cover defects.

How to care for a donor graft site

Autografts usually are taken from another area of the patient's body with a dermatome, an instrument that cuts uniform, split-thickness skin portions—typically about 0.013 to 0.05 cm thick. Autografting makes the donor site a partial-thickness wound, which may bleed, drain, and cause pain.

This site needs scrupulous care to prevent infection, which could convert the site to a full-thickness wound. Depending on the graft's thickness, tissue may be obtained from the donor site again as soon as 10 days later.

Usually, Biobrane or ordered covering is applied postoperatively. The outer gauze dressing can be removed after 24 hours; the Biobrane will protect the new epithelial proliferation.

Dressing the wound

Care for the donor site as you care for the autograft, using dressing changes at the initial stages to prevent infection and promote healing. Follow these guidelines:

- Identify the patient using two patient identifiers per facility policy.
- Perform hand hygiene and put on sterile gloves.
- Remove the outer gauze dressings within 24 hours. Inspect the Biobrane/primary covering for signs of infection, then leave it open to the air to speed drying and healing.
- Leave small amounts of fluid accumulation alone. Using aseptic technique, aspirate larger amounts through the dressing with a small gauge needle and syringe. Trim Biobrane as it curls.
- Apply ordered moisturizer daily to healed donor sites to keep skin tissue pliable and to remove crusts.

- Remove and discard the clean gloves, wash your hands, and put on the sterile gloves.
- Assess the condition of the graft. If you see purulent drainage, notify the doctor.

Soak if necessary

- Remove the primary layer only when there is an order to remove the dressings down to the graft. Use sterile forceps, and then clean the area gently. If necessary, soak with warm saline solution *to ease removal.*
- Inspect an allograft for signs of rejection or infection.
- Inspect a sheet graft for blebs. If ordered, evacuate them carefully with a sterile scalpel. (See *Removing fluid from a sheet graft,* page 520.)
- Place fresh Xeroform or ordered covering over the site *to promote wound healing and prevent infection.* Cover this with burn gauze and a roller bandage. Using sterile scissors, cut the roller bandage to the desired length.
- Clean any completely healed areas and apply a moisturizing cream to them *to keep the skin pliable and to retard scarring.*

Removing fluid from a sheet graft

When small pockets of fluid (called blebs) accumulate beneath a sheet graft, you'll need to remove the fluid using a sterile scalpel and sterile cotton-tipped applicators.

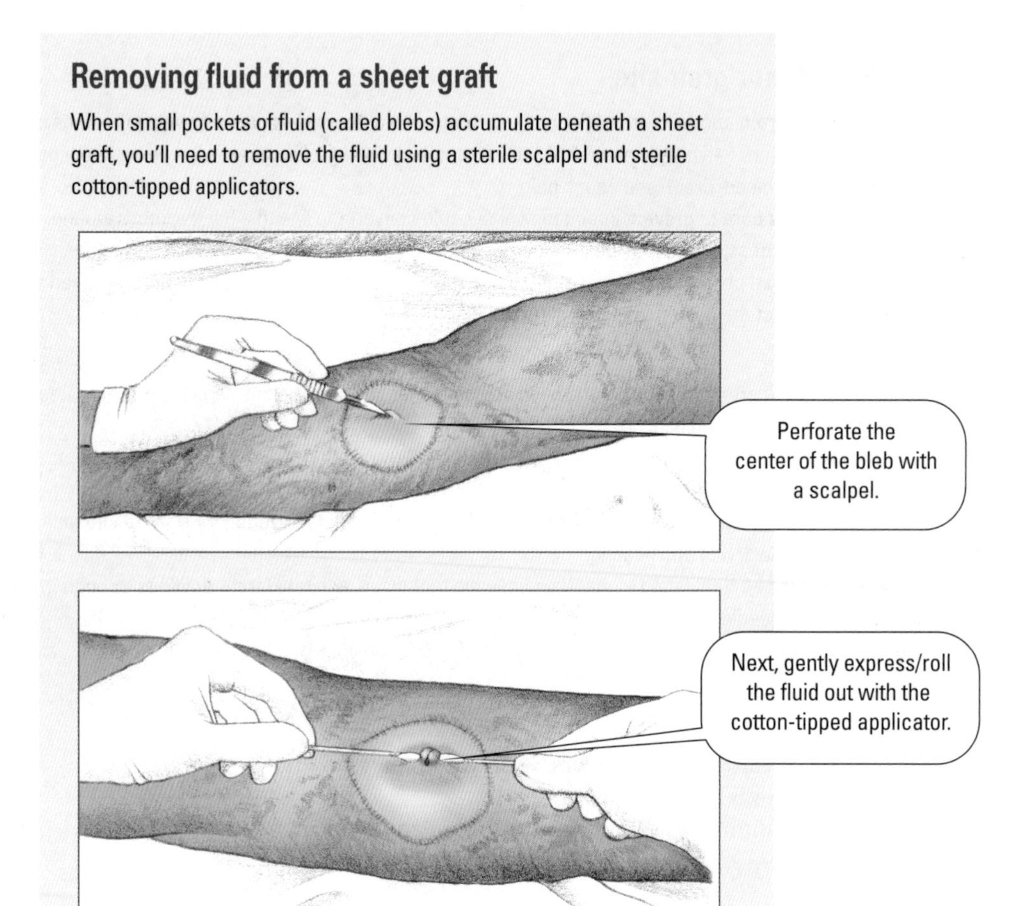
Perforate the center of the bleb with a scalpel.
Next, gently express/roll the fluid out with the cotton-tipped applicator.

Practice pointers

- *To avoid dislodging the graft,* hydrotherapy usually is discontinued, as ordered, for 3 to 4 days after grafting. Avoid using a blood pressure cuff over the graft. Don't tug or pull dressings during dressing changes. Keep the patient from lying on the graft. Hydrotherapy then will proceed with gentle cleansing/spray suspended over the tub without the whirlpool action.

Steps for slippage

- If the graft dislodges, apply sterile skin compresses *to keep the area moist until the surgeon reapplies the graft.* If the graft affects an arm or a leg, elevate the affected extremity *to reduce postoperative edema.* Check for bleeding and signs of neurovascular impairment, such as increasing pain, numbness or tingling, coolness, and pallor.

- Graft failure may result from traumatic injury, hematoma or seroma formation, infection, an inadequate graft bed, rejection, or compromised nutritional status. (See *Documenting skin graft care.*)

Documenting skin graft care

In your notes, record:
- time and date of all dressing changes
- medications used
- patient's response to medications
- condition of the skin graft
- signs and symptoms of infection or rejection
- additional treatments
- patient's reaction to the graft dressing change.

Hypertrophic scars or keloids

Some patients develop hypertrophic scars after deep burns. These scars are pink, raised, and firm to the touch. Keloids are raised and purplish in color, and the firmness is more delineated than hypertrophic scars. These types of scars are of concern in treatment options and contribute to poor body image postburn in a dramatic fashion.

Scarring is a subject for research the cause of hypertrophic scars, how to minimize the formation, determine the timing of the intervention, and measuring the success of an intervention. Several scar assessment scales have been developed, and their reliability and validity is being studied.

Wound healing is initiated by an injury phase, followed by a proliferative phase where fibroblasts and keratinocytes migrate to reepithelialize, and finally by remodeling, which involves collagen formation and degradation. There is some dysfunction in this process that causes hypertrophic scarring.

Pressure garments have been the mainstay in prevention since the early 1970s and are still used regularly. We know that when pressure is applied to developing scar tissue, it helps limit scar formation. When pressure garments fail, plastic surgery to remove the scar is sometimes successful.

We are now looking at scar formation at a cellular level postburn to try and determine the correct timing of treatment to avoid scar hypertrophy. Here are some of the treatments that have been studied:

- Iontophoresis—a method of applying a medication or substance to the skin directly, then applying an electrical charge (electric stimulation) to open up the cells and assist with transport. Corticosteroids and local anesthesia are two items that may use this delivery method.
- Massage—multiple times a day
- Injections of corticosteroids and interferon
- Topicals such as:
  - paraffin, beeswax, and plant-based ointments
  - Silicone gel sheeting along with pressure garments has shown improvement in scar thickness and decrease in itch and pain.
  - topicals with hyaluronic acid
  - over-the-counter creams and ointments
- Laser treatment (See "Laser surgery" section, page 523.)

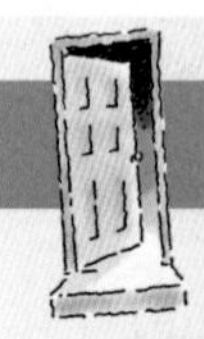

Home care connection

Discharge instructions for burn patients

Educate patient/caregivers
- Hand hygiene
- Dressing changes—clean or sterile technique
- Adequate diet/nutrition/fluid intake
- Avoidance of caffeine, alcohol, tobacco, and driving while on pain medications.

Skin care
- Itch control
- Protection from sun, frostbite, insects
- Moisturizers to use daily
- New skin fragility.

Hypertrophic scars
- Pressure garments—application, laundering, hours per day to wear signs of constriction—cool skin, numbness, discoloration, red marks lasting longer than 10 minutes
- Massage frequency—vertical, horizontal, and circular massage.

Socialization
- Family, friends, community, support groups, burn victim's camping events
- Work reintegration
- Advocacy.

Controlling the itch

The itch of a healing burn is as uncomfortable for many patients as the pain was. (See *Discharge instructions for burn patients*.) Skin grafts are lost to itching as a result of scratching or writhing. Controlling itch continues to be investigated to determine what medications systemically as well as topically are beneficial. Antihistamines are the mainstay but fall short of the comfort goal. Here is what is being researched.

- Antihistamines
- Corticosteroid injection
- Verapamil injections
- Naltrexone
- Gabapentin
- Doxepin
- Ondansetron
- TENS machine/unit
- Guided imagery

- Topical creams, gels
- Ice/cooling

Laser surgery—the Jedi force

Lasers became useful for skin treatments in the early 1980s. Think Star Wars, 1977. Laser surgery is used to treat various skin lesions. This type of surgery has several advantages. The laser offers precise control, spares normal tissue, speeds healing, and deters infection by sterilizing the operative site. In addition, the laser beam leaves a nearly bloodless operative field by sealing tiny blood vessels as it vaporizes tissue. The procedure can be performed on an outpatient basis.

Lasers most commonly used to treat skin lesions include vascular, pigment, and carbon dioxide (CO_2) lasers. (See *Understanding types of laser therapy*.)

Job hazard—initiate Jedi tricks

In general, laser surgery is safe, although bleeding and scarring can result. One pronounced hazard—to the patient and treatment staff alike—is eye damage or other injury caused by unintended laser beam reflection. For this reason, everyone in the surgical suite, including the patient, must wear special goggles to filter laser light. Also, the surgeon must use special nonreflective instruments. Room access must be strictly controlled, and all windows must be covered. Vaporized tissue has low potential for spreading infection, but there

Understanding types of laser therapy

Laser therapy is an essential tool for treating many types of skin lesions. The term *laser* is an acronym for Light Amplification by Stimulated Emission of Radiation.

The number of lasers used in dermatology is ever growing. Each type of laser emits its own wavelength within the color spectrum, making it effective against specific lesions.

The *argon* laser produces a blue-green light that's absorbed by vascular tissue. This makes it useful for treating vascular lesions, such as port-wine stains, hemangiomas, venous lake, rosacea, telangiectasia, and Kaposi's sarcoma.

The *pulsed dye* laser contains various wavelengths. It's most useful in treating cutaneous vascular lesions, such as port-wine stains, telangiectasis, and hypertrophic scars.

The *carbon dioxide* laser emits infrared light. It's used to treat such lesions as actinic cheilitis, rhinophyma, warts, and hypertrophic scars/keloids.

The *Nd:YAG* laser is used for dark hair removal as well as tattoo removal and some vascular lesions.

are reports of viral transmission linked back to the patient. Most facilities have a laser safety committee to ensure strict adherence to the safety protocols specific to the type of laser.

What you need

Laser ✳ filtration face masks ✳ specific protective eyewear ✳ smoke evacuator (vacuum) ✳ extra vacuum filters ✳ prescribed cleaning solution ✳ antibiotic ointment ✳ surgical drape ✳ sterile gauze ✳ nonadherent dressings ✳ surgical tape ✳ cotton-tipped applicators ✳ nonreflective surgical instruments ✳ gowns ✳ masks ✳ gloves ✳ shoe covers.

Getting ready

Before the procedure begins, prepare the tray. It should include a local anesthetic, as ordered, as well as dry and wet gauze. The gauze will be used *to control bleeding, protect healthy tissue,* and *abrade and remove any eschar*, which would otherwise inhibit laser absorption. Prepare surgical instruments as needed. Cover all windows in the operating suite and have water, saline, and fire extinguisher readily available.

How you do it

- Identify the patient using two patient identifier per facility policy. Call a time out to verify the correct procedure on the correct body part and correct patient per facility policy.
- Tell the patient how the laser works and explain its benefits. Point out the equipment and outline the procedure *to help allay the patient's concerns.*
- Position the patient comfortably.
- Perform hand hygiene; put on shoe covers, a gown, a mask, and gloves.
- Perform a time out before beginning the procedure to ensure that the correct patient, site, procedure, and equipment are identified.
- Place gauze moistened with saline around areas close to the operative site. Moisten all surgical drapes on the operative area.

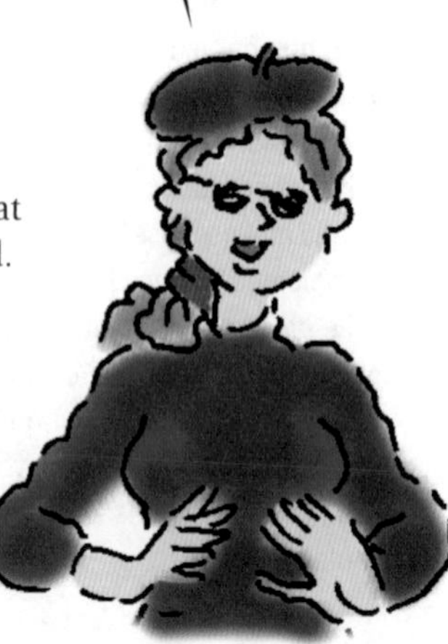
My shades are hip—but to assist with laser surgery, you'll need extra special specs.

I wear eye wear

- Confirm that everyone in the room—including the patient—has safety goggles specific to the type of laser being used.
- Keep doors that enter the surgical suite closed and be sure that warning signs are posted on the doors per the facility protocol.

Off limits

- After the surgeon administers the anesthetic and it takes effect, activate the laser vacuum. Many lasers now have the vacuum attached to the laser handle, but it may be separate and needs to be near the surgical site. The vacuum has a filter that traps and collects the vaporized tissue. Change the filter whenever suction decreases, and follow facility guidelines for filter disposal.

Full-court press

- When the surgeon finishes the procedure, put on sterile gloves and apply direct pressure with a sterile gauze pad to a bleeding wound for 20 minutes. If the wound continues to bleed, notify the doctor.
- Once the bleeding is controlled, clean the area with a cotton-tipped applicator dipped in the prescribed cleaning solution. Then size and cut a nonadherent dressing. Spread a thin layer of antibiotic ointment on one side of the dressing. Place the ointment side over the wound and secure the dressing with surgical tape.
- Discard disposable equipment and materials according to your facility policy.
- Perform hand hygiene.

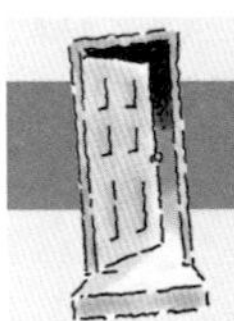

Home care connection

Caring for a laser surgery site

Teach the patient how to dress his wound or care for his skin daily, as ordered by the surgeon. To promote wound healing and prevent infection, tell him he can take showers but shouldn't immerse the wound site in water or take a tub bath.

Press here
If the wound bleeds at home, show how to apply direct pressure on the site with clean gauze or a washcloth for 20 minutes. If bleeding persists, tell the patient to call his doctor.

Elevate here
If the patient's foot or leg was operated on, urge him to keep the extremity elevated and to use it as little as possible because pressure can inhibit healing.

Cover here
Warn the patient to shield the treated area from sun exposure to avoid changes in pigmentation. Tell him to call the doctor if a fever of 100° F (37.8° C) or higher lasts more than 1 day.

Practice pointers

- Vascular and pigment lasers won't result in a wound; only superficial skin changes will occur.
- Warn the patient to expect a burning odor during the procedure. Tell him that a machine called a smoke evacuator, which sounds like a vacuum cleaner, will clear away any smoke. Explain that he may sense heat from the laser. Urge him to tell the doctor at once if pain develops.
- Know that bleeding, scarring, and infection are rare complications of laser surgery. (See *Caring for a laser surgery site*, page 525, and *Documenting laser surgery care*.)

Documenting laser surgery care

Most patients who have laser surgery for skin lesions are treated as outpatients. Record:
- patient's skin condition before and after the procedure
- any bleeding
- type of dressing applied
- patient complaints of pain
- patient's understanding of home care instructions.

Pressure ulcer care

Most pressure ulcers develop over bony prominences, where friction and shearing force combine with pressure to break down skin and underlying tissues. Common sites include the sacrum, coccyx, ischial tuberosities, and greater trochanters. Other common sites include the skin over the vertebrae, scapulae, elbows, knees, and heels in bedridden and relatively immobile patients. (See *Assessing pressure ulcers*, page 528.)

An ounce of . . . Prevention city

Prevention is the key to avoiding extensive tissue damage. Preventive measures include ensuring adequate nourishment and mobility to relieve pressure and promote circulation. It is important to evaluate each patient's risk of developing pressure ulcers. The Braden Scale is a good tool to use in calculating risk.

Preventative measures

The Braden Scale will identify the majority of patients at risk for pressure ulcers. Those with preexisting conditions that have partial paralysis or changes in sensation are a special consideration in your initial assessment, especially if the patient moves well. Patients with neural tube defects such as spina bifida who have low-level lesions are at greater risk to score lower on the Braden Scale. If the patient uses a wheelchair, teach how to do push-ups and shift position.

Specialty beds provide some assistance for the patient with decreased sensation, obesity, or preexisting pressure ulcers. Special low air-loss beds should never negate the need to have frequent position changes. Patients undergoing a surgery that will render them immobile or greatly decrease mobility will benefit from specialty beds and

BRADEN SCALE – For Predicting Pressure Sore Risk

SEVERE RISK: Total score ≤ 9 **HIGH RISK:** Total score 10-12
MODERATE RISK: Total score 13-14 **MILD RISK:** Total score 15-18

RISK FACTOR	SCORE/DESCRIPTION				DATE OF ASSESS ➡ 1	2	3	4
SENSORY PERCEPTION Ability to respond meaningfully to pressure-related discomfort	1. **COMPLETELY LIMITED** – Unresponsive (does not moan, flinch, or grasp) to painful stimuli, due to diminished level of consciousness or sedation, **OR** limited ability to feel pain over most of body surface.	2. **VERY LIMITED** – Responds only to painful stimuli. Cannot communicate discomfort except by moaning or restlessness, **OR** has a sensory impairment which limits the ability to feel pain or discomfort over ½ of body.	3. **SLIGHTLY LIMITED** – Responds to verbal commands but cannot always communicate discomfort or need to be turned, **OR** has some sensory impairment which limits ability to feel pain or discomfort in 1 or 2 extremities.	4. **NO IMPAIRMENT** – Responds to verbal commands. Has no sensory deficit which would limit ability to feel or voice pain or discomfort.				
MOISTURE Degree to which skin is exposed to moisture	1. **CONSTANTLY MOIST**– Skin is kept moist almost constantly by perspiration, urine, etc. Dampness is detected every time patient is moved or turned.	2. **OFTEN MOIST** – Skin is often but not always moist. Linen must be changed at least once a shift.	3. **OCCASIONALLY MOIST** – Skin is occasionally moist, requiring an extra linen change approximately once a day.	4. **RARELY MOIST** – Skin is usually dry; linen only requires changing at routine intervals.				
ACTIVITY Degree of physical activity	1. **BEDFAST** – Confined to bed.	2. **CHAIRFAST** – Ability to walk severely limited or nonexistent. Cannot bear own weight and/or must be assisted into chair or wheelchair.	3. **WALKS OCCASIONALLY** – Walks occasionally during day, but for very short distances, with or without assistance. Spends majority of each shift in bed or chair.	4. **WALKS FREQUENTLY**– Walks outside the room at least twice a day and inside room at least once every 2 hours during waking hours.				
MOBILITY Ability to change and control body position	1. **COMPLETELY IMMOBILE** – Does not make even slight changes in body or extremity position without assistance.	2. **VERY LIMITED** – Makes occasional slight changes in body or extremity position but unable to make frequent or significant changes independently.	3. **SLIGHTLY LIMITED** – Makes frequent though slight changes in body or extremity position independently.	4. **NO LIMITATIONS** – Makes major and frequent changes in position without assistance.				
NUTRITION Usual food intake pattern [1]NPO: Nothing by mouth. [2]IV: Intravenously. [3]TPN: Total parenteral nutrition.	1. **VERY POOR** – Never eats a complete meal. Rarely eats more than 1/3 of any food offered. Eats 2 servings or less of protein (meat or dairy products) per day. Takes fluids poorly. Does not take a liquid dietary supplement, **OR** is NPO[1] and/or maintained on clear liquids or IV[2] for more than 5 days.	2. **PROBABLY INADEQUATE** – Rarely eats a complete meal and generally eats only about ½ of any food offered. Protein intake includes only 3 servings of meat or dairy products per day. Occasionally will take a dietary supplement **OR** receives less than optimum amount of liquid diet or tube feeding.	3. **ADEQUATE** – Eats over half of most meals. Eats a total of 4 servings of protein (meat, dairy products) each day. Occasionally refuses a meal, but will usually take a supplement if offered, **OR** is on a tube feeding or TPN[3] regimen, which probably meets most of nutritional needs.	4. **EXCELLENT** – Eats most of every meal. Never refuses a meal. Usually eats a total of 4 or more servings of meat and dairy products. Occasionally eats between meals. Does not require supplementation.				
FRICTION AND SHEAR	1. **PROBLEM**- Requires moderate to maximum assistance in moving. Complete lifting without sliding against sheets is impossible. Frequently slides down in bed or chair, requiring frequent repositioning with maximum assistance. Spasticity, contractures, or agitation leads to almost constant friction.	2. **POTENTIAL PROBLEM**– Moves feebly or requires minimum assistance. During a move, skin probably slides to some extent against sheets, chair, restraints, or other devices. Maintains relatively good position in chair or bed most of the time but occasionally slides down.	3. **NO APPARENT PROBLEM** – Moves in bed and in chair independently and has sufficient muscle strength to lift up completely during move. Maintains good position in bed or chair at all times.					
TOTAL SCORE	Total score of 12 or less represents HIGH RISK							

ASSESS	DATE	EVALUATOR SIGNATURE/TITLE	ASSESS.	DATE	EVALUATOR SIGNATURE/TITLE
1	/ /		3	/ /	
2	/ /		4	/ /	

NAME-Last	First	Middle	Attending Physician	Record No.	Room/Bed

Form 3166P BRIGGS, Des Moines, IA 50306 (800) 247-2343 www.BriggsCorp.com
R304 PRINTED IN U.S.A

BRADEN SCALE

Assessing pressure ulcers

To choose the most effective treatment for a pressure ulcer, you must first assess its characteristics. The pressure ulcer staging system described below, used by the National Pressure Ulcer Advisory Panel and the Agency for Healthcare Research and Quality, reflects the anatomic depth of exposed tissue (http://www.npuap.org/resources/educational-and-clinical-resources/pressure-ulcer-categorystaging-illustrations/).

Keep in mind that if the wound contains necrotic tissue, you won't be able to determine the stage until you can see the wound base.

Stage 1

In stage 1, the heralding lesion of a pressure ulcer is persistent redness in lightly pigmented skin and persistent red, blue, or purple hues on darker skin. Other indicators include changes in temperature, consistency, or sensation.

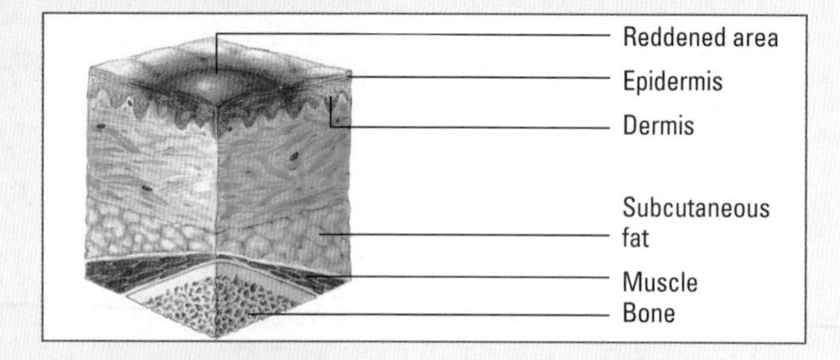

Stage 2

Stage 2 is marked by partial-thickness skin loss involving the epidermis, dermis, or both. The ulcer is superficial and appears as an abrasion, a blister, or a shallow crater.

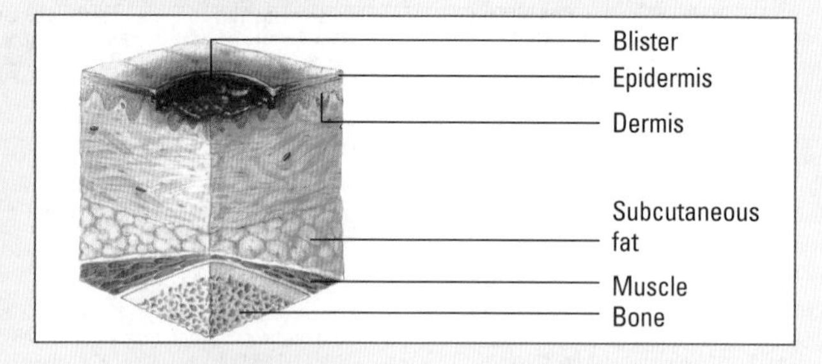

Stage 3

In stage 3, the ulcer constitutes a full-thickness wound penetrating the subcutaneous tissue, which may extend to—but not through—underlying fascia. The ulcer resembles a deep crater and may undermine adjacent tissue.

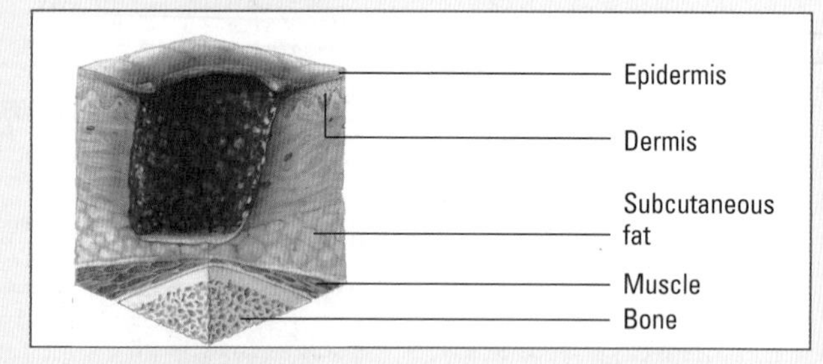

Stage 4

In stage 4, the ulcer extends through the skin, accompanied by extensive destruction; tissue necrosis; or damage to muscle, bone, or supporting structures (such as tendons and joint capsules).

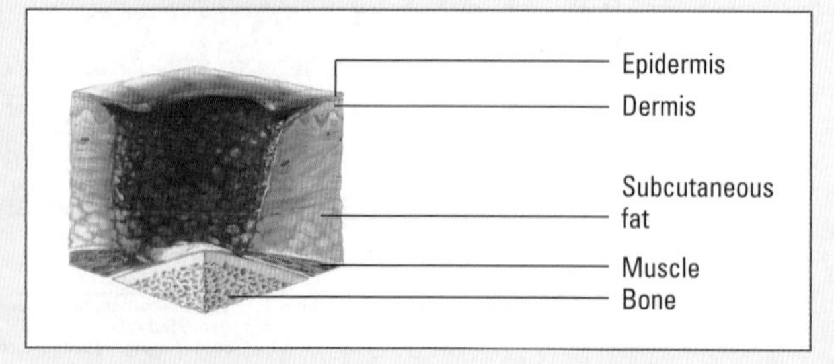

Assessing pressure ulcers *(continued)*

Unstageable/Unclassified: Full-thickness skin or tissue loss—depth unknown

Full-thickness tissue loss in which actual depth of the ulcer is completely obscured by slough (yellow, tan, gray, green, or brown) and/or eschar (tan, brown, or black) in the wound bed. Until enough slough and/or eschar are removed to expose the base of the wound, the true depth cannot be determined, but it will be either a category/stage III or IV. Stable (dry, adherent, intact without erythema or fluctuance) eschar on the heels serves as "the body's natural [biological] cover" and should not be removed.

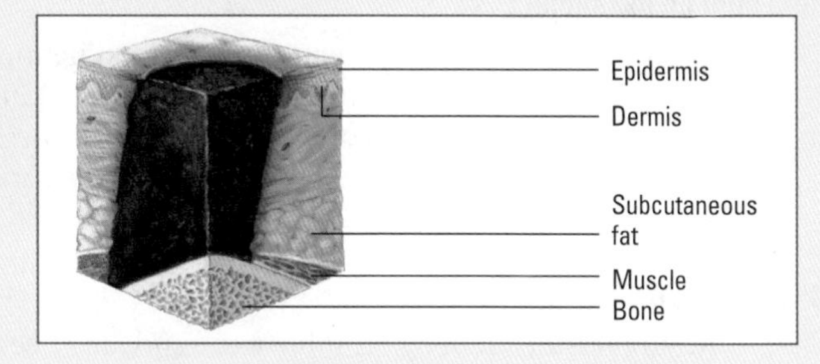

Suspected deep tissue injury—depth unknown

Purple or maroon localized area of discolored intact skin or blood-filled blister because of damage of underlying soft tissue from pressure and/or ***shear***. The area may be preceded by tissue that is painful, firm, mushy, boggy, warmer, or cooler as compared to adjacent tissue. Deep tissue injury may be difficult to detect in individuals with dark skin tones. Evolution may include a thin blister over a dark wound bed. The wound may further evolve and become covered by thin eschar. Evolution may be rapid exposing additional layers of tissue even with optimal treatment.

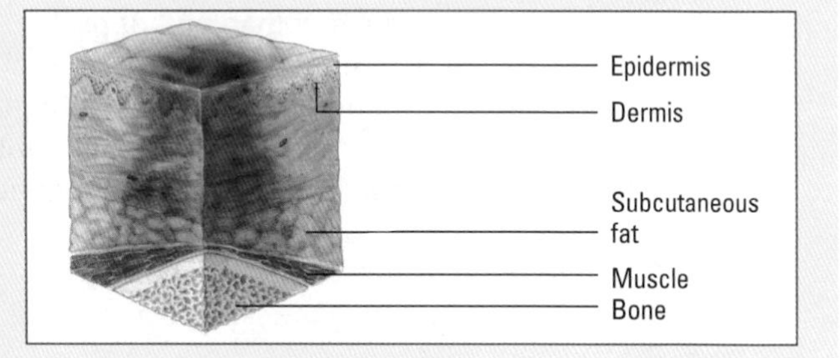

support surfaces for sitting. Place as few layers of linens between the patient and the support surface to ensure the optimal benefit.

Use turning sheets to help prevent shear and to assist with transfers. Never turn or transfer a bedfast, at-risk patient without assistance, this provides the least risk of damaging the skin. Many larger facilities employ a lift team to assist nurses in transfers and position changes, especially for the large patient.

If nutritional issues are identified as a problem, monitor prealbumin levels as an indicator of nutritional status. Encourage healthy food choices. If incontinence is an issue, encourage frequent voiding and evaluate the need for stool containment interventions.

Family engagement

Encourage family members/caregivers to assist the patient in remembering to change positions. You may ask them to alert the patient each time a TV commercial comes on. Small changes in position by shifting his weight are helpful and something family members may be able to assist with.

Put a light on the subject

Be sure to evaluate your patient's skin in good lighting and to palpate the skin as well. Patients with deeply pigmented skin are more difficult to assess skin changes of discoloration or redness.

Always assess the skin more frequently in the patient who scored any risk on the Braden Scale.

Take a new position

Avoid pressure on bony prominences, especially heels, trochanters and coccyx. Educate the patient at their level of understanding. When lying, the head of the bed should not be more than 30 degrees, and if sitting up in a chair, try to keep position at 90 degrees. Lubricate or powder bedpans and roll the patient onto the pan rather than pull or push. Apply transparent film or hydrocolloid dressings to bony areas that start to show any sign of irritation or redness. This may keep them from developing further skin breakdown. Reassess the skin daily or more often and chart your findings.

Keep intact skin hydrated by using topical moisturizers and avoid scrubbing the skin when bathing.

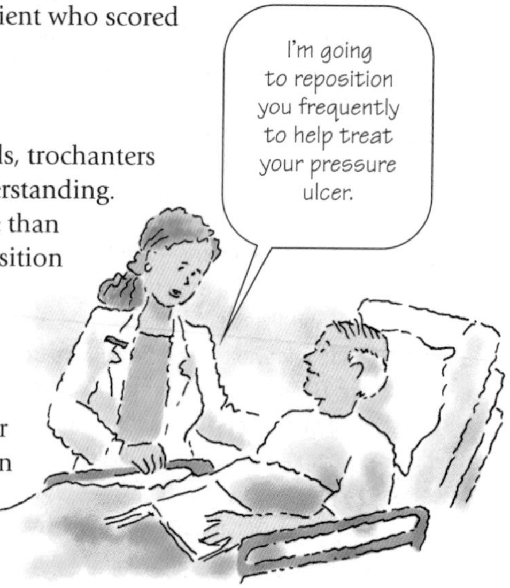

I'm going to reposition you frequently to help treat your pressure ulcer.

What you need

Hypoallergenic tape or elastic netting ✱ overbed table ✱ piston-type irrigating system ✱ two pairs of gloves ✱ normal saline solution, or antimicrobic or pH-balanced wound cleanser as ordered ✱ sterile 4″ × 4″ gauze pads ✱ sterile cotton-tipped applicators ✱ selected topical dressing ✱ linen-saver pads ✱ impervious plastic trash bag ✱ disposable wound-measuring device ✱ optional: alcohol pad ✱ 21G needle and syringe ✱ 19G angiocatheter ✱ 35-mL syringe.

Getting ready

Assemble the equipment at the patient's bedside as you check the expiration date of each item to ensure sterility. Cut tape into strips for securing dressings if necessary. Loosen lids on cleaning solutions and medications for easy removal. Loosen existing dressing edges and tapes before putting on gloves. Attach an impervious plastic trash bag to the overbed table to hold used dressings and refuse. Saline is only good for 24 hours, if outdated or unlabeled, discard.

How you do it—dress for success

- Identify the patient using two patient identifiers per facility policy.
- Perform hand hygiene.
- Assess level of pain.
- Provide privacy and explain the procedure to the patient *to allay his fears and promote cooperation.*
- Open the normal saline solution container and the piston syringe. Pour normal saline solution into an irrigation container.
- Put the piston syringe into the opening provided in the irrigation container.
- Open the packages of supplies.
- Position the patient in a way that maximizes his comfort while allowing access to the pressure ulcer site.
- Cover bed linens with a linen-saver pad *to prevent soiling.*

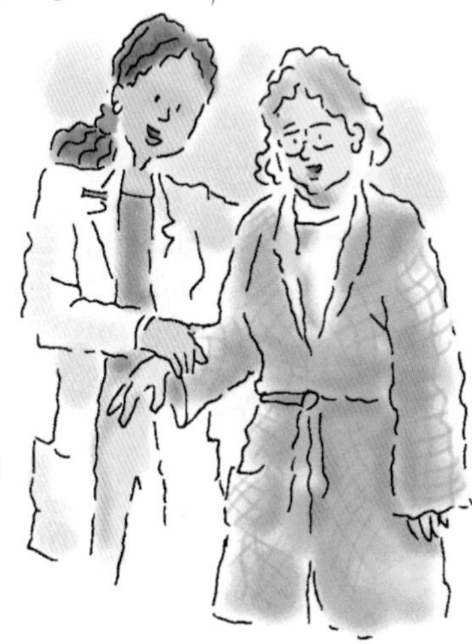
Keeping you mobile is key to preventing pressure ulcers.

Cleaning the pressure ulcer

- Put on gloves to remove the old dressing and expose the pressure ulcer. Discard the soiled dressing in the impervious plastic trash bag *to avoid contaminating the sterile field and spreading infection. Follow facility policy for body fluid disposal.*

Tale of the tape measure

- Inspect the wound. Note the color, amount, and odor of drainage and necrotic debris. Measure the wound perimeter with the disposable tape measure.
- Using the piston syringe, apply full force to irrigate the pressure ulcer *to remove necrotic debris and help decrease bacteria in the wound.* If debris remain, use the 35-mL syringe with 19G angiocatheter for increased pressure (8 psi stream).
- Use gauze pads to gently wash the area to remove tissue debris. Start in the center of the wound and rotate the gauze toward the outside.
- Dry the skin surrounding the wound.
- Remove and discard your soiled gloves and put on a fresh pair.

Tunnel test/Exit stage right

- Insert a gloved finger or sterile cotton-tipped applicator into the wound to assess wound tunneling or undermining. *Tunneling usually signals wound extension along fascial planes.* Gauge tunnel depth by inserting the cotton swab, marking the depth with your finger then measuring the length with the tape measure. Measure the perimeter of the wound in centimeters (length × width) at the widest points.

- Next, reassess the condition of the skin and ulcer. Note the character of the clean wound bed and the surrounding skin.
- If you observe adherent necrotic material, notify a wound care specialist or a doctor *to ensure appropriate debridement.*
- Prepare to apply the appropriate topical dressing. Instructions for applying typical moist saline gauze, hydrocolloid, transparent, alginate, foam, and hydrogel dressings follow. For other dressings or topical agents, follow your facility's protocol or the supplier's instructions.

Applying a moist saline gauze dressing

- Irrigate the pressure ulcer with normal saline solution. Blot the surrounding skin dry.
- Moisten the gauze dressing with normal saline solution.
- Gently place the dressing over the ulcer surface. *To separate surfaces within the wound that has tunnelling,* gently place a dressing between opposing wound surfaces. *To avoid damage to tissues, don't pack the gauze tightly.*
- Change the dressing often enough to keep the wound moist. (See *Choosing a pressure ulcer dressing.*)

Applying a hydrocolloid dressing

- Irrigate the pressure ulcer with normal saline solution. Blot the surrounding skin dry.

Smooth operator

- Choose a clean, dry, presized dressing or cut one to overlap the pressure ulcer by about 1" (2.5 cm). Remove the dressing from its package, pull the release paper from the adherent side of the dressing, and apply the dressing to the wound. *To minimize irritation,* carefully smooth out wrinkles as you apply the dressing.
- If the dressing's edges need to be secured with tape, apply a skin sealant to the intact skin around the ulcer. After the area dries, tape the dressing to the skin. *The sealant protects the skin and promotes tape adherence.* Avoid using tension or pressure when applying the tape.
- Remove your gloves and discard them in the impervious plastic trash bag. Dispose of refuse according to facility policy and perform hand hygiene.
- Change a hydrocolloid dressing every 2 to 7 days as necessary—for example, if the patient complains of pain, the dressing no longer adheres, or leakage occurs.

Applying a transparent dressing

- Select a dressing to overlap the ulcer by 2" (5 cm).

Choosing a pressure ulcer dressing

The patient's needs and ulcer characteristics determine which type of dressing to use on a pressure ulcer.

Gauze dressings

Made of absorptive cotton or synthetic fabric, gauze dressings are permeable to water, water vapor, and oxygen. Gauze may also be impregnated with petroleum jelly or another agent. When uncertain about which dressing to use, you should apply a gauze dressing moistened in saline solution until a wound specialist recommends definitive treatment. This type of dressing is commonly used to assist with debriding sloughed tissue and is called a *wet-to-dry dressing*.

Hydrocolloid dressings

Hydrocolloid dressings are adhesive, moldable wafers made of a carbohydrate-based material and usually have waterproof backings. They are impermeable to oxygen, water, and water vapor, and most have some absorptive properties. These may also be used preventatively to bony prominences that are showing signs of mild erythema. They are indicated as primary dressings for minimally to moderately exudative partial- and full-thickness wounds. They are also recommended for clean stage II and noninfected shallow stage III pressure ulcers for parts of the body where dressings won't melt or roll.

Transparent film dressings

Transparent film dressings are clear, adherent, and nonabsorptive. These polymer-based dressings are permeable to oxygen and water vapor but not to water. Their transparency allows visual inspection. Because they can't absorb drainage, they're used on partial-thickness wounds with minimal exudate. These are used on very fragile skin areas at times to help prevent shearing effects of movement against harsh hospital linens.

Alginate dressings

Made from seaweed, alginate dressings are nonwoven, absorptive dressings available as soft white sterile pads or ropes. They absorb excessive exudate and may be used on infected wounds. As these dressings absorb exudate, they turn into a gel that keeps the wound bed moist and promotes healing. When exudate is no longer excessive, switch to another type of dressing. They can be safely packed in deep tracking wounds and allow for easy removal without leaving pieces in the wound.

Foam dressings

Foam dressings are spongelike polymer dressings that may be impregnated or coated with other materials. Somewhat absorptive, they may be adherent. These dressings promote moist wound healing and are useful when a nonadherent surface is desired. Uses as a primary or secondary dressing to absorb heavy exudate. Their cooling properties also make them ideal for radiation burns.

Hydrogel dressings

Water-based and nonadherent, hydrogel dressings are polymer-based dressings that have some absorptive properties. They're available as a gel in a tube, as flexible sheets, and as saturated gauze packing strips. They may have a cooling effect, which eases pain. They are recommended for dry to minimally exudative pressure ulcers that are noninfected and granulating in areas of the body where the dressing won't slip.

Enzymatic biologic debridement dressing

Enzymatic debridement of necrotic tissue from wounds is used widely for pressure ulcer wounds. Collagenase Santyl is commonly used debriding biological. It contains *Clostridium histolyticum*, or collagenase I and collagenase II. Together they attack the collagen present in the eschar. It can be combined with other topicals that contain metal salts such as sodium and magnesium. Products that contain silver inhibit the enzymatic effect of collagenase. Ionic silver inhibits more than water-insoluble silver. Silvadene 10% is the most inhibiting. Many wound cleansers and other antibiotic dressings also decrease the effect of collagenase. Be sure to check manufacturer enclosure.

Negative pressure dressings

Negative pressure dressings have been found to enhance healing of chronic wounds by continually removing drainage in a closed system under suction. The usual setting is 125 mm Hg. (See chapter 3, "Vacuum-assisted closure therapy" section.)

Straighten the curls

- Gently lay the dressing over the ulcer. *To prevent shearing force,* don't stretch the dressing. Press firmly on the edges of the dressing to promote adherence. Although this type of dressing is self-adhesive, you may have to tape the edges *to prevent them from curling.*
- If necessary, aspirate accumulated fluid with a 21G needle and syringe. After aspirating the pocket of fluid, clean the aspiration site with an alcohol pad and cover it with another strip of transparent dressing.
- Change the dressing every 3 to 7 days, depending on the amount of drainage.

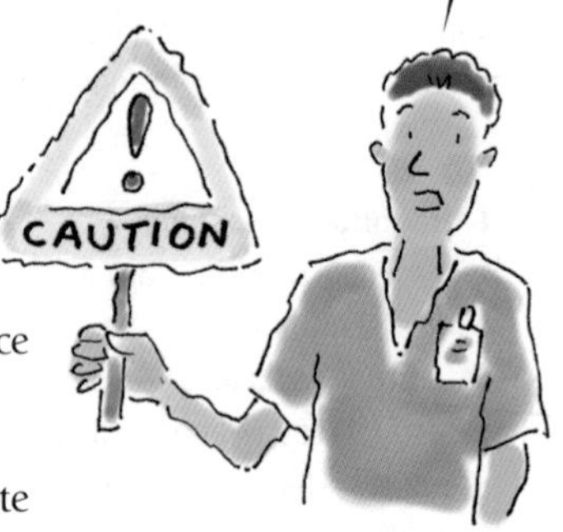
Never stretch a transparent dressing. If you do, you could cause shearing force.
CAUTION

Applying an alginate dressing

- Apply the alginate dressing to the ulcer surface. Cover the area with a secondary dressing (such as gauze pads) as ordered. Secure the dressing with tape or elastic netting.
- If the wound is draining heavily, change the dressing once or twice daily for the first 3 to 5 days. As drainage decreases, change the dressing less frequently—every 2 to 4 days or as ordered. When the drainage stops or the wound bed looks dry, stop using alginate dressing.

Applying a foam dressing

- Gently lay the foam dressing over the ulcer.
- Use tape, elastic netting, or gauze to hold the dressing in place.
- Change the dressing when the foam no longer absorbs the exudate.

Applying a hydrogel dressing

- Apply gel to the wound bed.
- Cover the area with a secondary dressing.
- Change the dressing daily or as needed *to keep the wound bed moist.*
- If the dressing you select comes in sheet form, cut the dressing to match the wound base; *otherwise, the intact surrounding skin can become macerated.*
- Hydrogel dressings also come in a prepackaged, saturated gauze for wounds that require "dead space" to be filled. Follow the manufacturer's directions.

Practice pointers

Remain tapeless

- Tape denudes the skin and can create new wounds in fragile skin. Limit using it as much as possible.

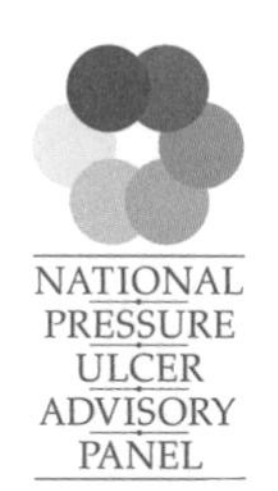

Pressure Ulcer Scale for Healing (PUSH)
PUSH Tool 3.0

Patient Name______________________ Patient ID# __________

Ulcer Location ______________________ Date __________

Directions:

Observe and measure the pressure ulcer. Categorize the ulcer with respect to surface area, exudate, and type of wound tissue. Record a sub-score for each of these ulcer characteristics. Add the sub-scores to obtain the total score. A comparison of total scores measured over time provides an indication of the improvement or deterioration in pressure ulcer healing.

LENGTH X WIDTH (in cm^2)	**0** 0	**1** < 0.3	**2** 0.3 – 0.6	**3** 0.7 – 1.0	**4** 1.1 – 2.0	**5** 2.1 – 3.0	**Sub-score**
		6 3.1 – 4.0	**7** 4.1 – 8.0	**8** 8.1 – 12.0	**9** 12.1 – 24.0	**10** > 24.0	
EXUDATE AMOUNT	**0** None	**1** Light	**2** Moderate	**3** Heavy			**Sub-score**
TISSUE TYPE	**0** Closed	**1** Epithelial Tissue	**2** Granulation Tissue	**3** Slough	**4** Necrotic Tissue		**Sub-score**
							TOTAL SCORE

Length x Width: Measure the greatest length (head to toe) and the greatest width (side to side) using a centimeter ruler. Multiply these two measurements (length x width) to obtain an estimate of surface area in square centimeters (cm^2). Caveat: Do not guess! Always use a centimeter ruler and always use the same method each time the ulcer is measured.

Exudate Amount: Estimate the amount of exudate (drainage) present after removal of the dressing and before applying any topical agent to the ulcer. Estimate the exudate (drainage) as none, light, moderate, or heavy.

Tissue Type: This refers to the types of tissue that are present in the wound (ulcer) bed. Score as a "4" if there is any necrotic tissue present. Score as a "3" if there is any amount of slough present and necrotic tissue is absent. Score as a "2" if the wound is clean and contains granulation tissue. A superficial wound that is reepithelializing is scored as a "1". When the wound is closed, score as a "0".

- **4** – **Necrotic Tissue (Eschar):** black, brown, or tan tissue that adheres firmly to the wound bed or ulcer edges and may be either firmer or softer than surrounding skin.
- **3** – **Slough:** yellow or white tissue that adheres to the ulcer bed in strings or thick clumps, or is mucinous.
- **2** – **Granulation Tissue:** pink or beefy red tissue with a shiny, moist, granular appearance.
- **1** – **Epithelial Tissue:** for superficial ulcers, new pink or shiny tissue (skin) that grows in from the edges or as islands on the ulcer surface.
- **0** – **Closed/Resurfaced:** the wound is completely covered with epithelium (new skin).

www.npuap.org
11F

PUSH Tool Version 3.0: 9/15/98

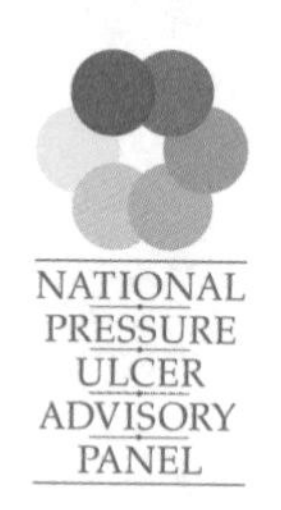

Pressure Ulcer Healing Chart

To monitor trends in PUSH Scores over time

(Use a separate page for each pressure ulcer)

Patient Name______________________ Patient ID# ____________

Ulcer Location ______________________ Date ____________

Directions:

Observe and measure pressure ulcers at regular intervals using the PUSH Tool.
Date and record PUSH Sub-scores and Total Scores on the Pressure Ulcer Healing Record below.

Pressure Ulcer Healing **Record**														
Date														
Length x Width														
Exudate Amount														
Tissue Type														
PUSH Total Score														

Graph the PUSH Total Scores on the Pressure Ulcer Healing Graph below.

PUSH Total Score	Pressure Ulcer Healing **Graph**													
17														
16														
15														
14														
13														
12														
11														
10														
9														
8														
7														
6														
5														
4														
3														
2														
1														
Healed = 0														
Date														

www.npuap.org
11F

PUSH Tool Version 3.0: 9/15/98

- Try to use the stretchy netting over dressings to hold in place. They can be cut creatively to cross over the hips and shoulders thereby helping to anchor the dressing.

Infection

- Be aware that infection may cause foul-smelling drainage, persistent pain, severe erythema, induration, and elevated skin and body temperatures. Advancing infection or cellulitis can lead to septicemia. Severe erythema may signal worsening cellulitis, which means the offending organisms have invaded the tissue and are no longer localized. (See *Documenting pressure ulcer care.*)

Documenting pressure ulcer care

In your notes, record:

- date and time of initial and subsequent treatments
- specific treatment given
- preventive strategies performed.

Use the PUSH tool to monitor the wound's progress.

- pressure ulcer location and size (length, width, and depth)
- color and appearance of the wound bed
- amount, odor, color, and consistency of drainage
- condition of the surrounding skin.

Reassess pressure ulcers with each dressing change and daily for exudate. Update the plan of care as required, noting changes in ulcer condition or size and skin temperature elevation on the clinical record. Record when the doctor was notified of abnormal observations. Record daily temperatures on the graphic sheet to allow easy assessment of body temperature patterns.

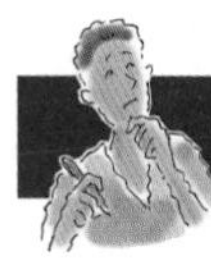

Quick quiz

1. An 83-year-old woman with 20% scald burns was admitted to the burn center last evening. The nurse who is assigned on tub team informs the patient's nurse that she is first on the list and to give her pain medication immediately. Her nurse will explain the procedure to her. What additional information is important to know about this patient?

A. Labs
B. Pulse
C. Blood pressure
D. Marital status

Answer: C. Because of the patient's age and the use of pain medications, she may have a drop in blood pressure that would decrease perfusion to her wounds as well as a safety risk for transferring onto and off the tub cart.

2. The nurse is discharging a 55-year-old male from the burn center and he states that he cannot wait to get home and have a beer and smoke a cigarette. He has had smoking cessation instructions previously. What should the nurse do?

A. Do nothing, as this is the patient's decision.
B. Provide smoking cessation information again.
C. Explain the effects cigarettes and alcohols have on circulation.
D. Tell him he should call his physician for approval.

Answer: C. If he restarts and continues these habits, his burns will be less likely to heal because of decreased circulation to the extremities as well as the pulmonary effects.

3. A patient with third-degree burns to her right hand and arm is complaining of numbness in her fingers. She has a hand splint in place. What should the nurse do first?

   A. Perform Doppler readings of pulses in her fingers.
   B. Inspect the dressings for any restrictions.
   C. Elevate the hand and arm.
   D. Call the clinician to perform an escharotomy.

Answer: B. The dressings may be the sole cause of her symptoms, especially if there is an ace wrap as well. The nurse can then assess Doppler pulses.

4. A 39-year-old female had autographs to her burned extremities 12 hours ago. Which assessment by the nurse is not to be performed on this patient?

   A. Remove the dressing down to the graft to check for adherence.
   B. Check the donor sites for drainage.
   C. Position the patient so there is no pressure on the graft sites.
   D. Elevate the grafted areas.

Answer: A. The dressings are left untouched for at least 24 hours and only removed if there is undue bleeding and only by the clinician at that point.

5. The nurse is caring for a 62-year-old male who has diabetes and a severe leg ulcer with thick black eschar present within the wound. The nurse prepares to cleanse the wound and replace the dressing. Which combination of topical agents is not appropriate for this patient?

   A. Saline-soaked gauze, dry gauze, and an ace wrap
   B. Maggots and a moist occlusive dressing
   C. Silver sulfadiazine and collagenase
   D. Papain and urea-based agents

Answer: C. The silver-based topical with heavy metal ions will make the collagenase ineffective.

6. The nurse is taking a health history of a patient from a nursing home facility who is being treated for dehydration and blood glucose control. Which assessment finding is not expected for this patient?

   A. Weight
   B. Pressure ulcer risk (Braden Score)
   C. Mental status
   D. Melena

Answer: D. You would not expect melena in a patient with dehydration and elevated blood sugar.

7. A 33-year-old female patient is being prepped in the OR for laser therapy to her face to treat severe acne scarring. Which action is contraindicated?

A. Lock the access doors to the OR so no one can enter.
B. Ensure all in the OR suite have the appropriate eye protection including the patient.
C. Ensure that the instrument set up is nonreflective.
D. Moisten all draping materials and gauze close to the operative site.

Answer: A. Rather than locking the OR doors, post large signs warning that no one enter because of laser in use.

8. A 45-year-old male patient has a large burn that is in the healing stages post graft. The patient is complaining of severe itching and was given diphenhydramine an hour ago, which is not providing any relief. Which adjunct therapy is not to be used with this patient?

A. Opiate antagonist
B. H_2 receptor blocker
C. Tacrolimus
D. Propranolol

Answer: C. Tacrolimus has not been studied for use in pruritus in burn patients.

9. A 28-year-old male returns to the outpatient burn area to evaluate the healing burns. He relates that he cannot stand to wear the pressure garments because of the heat (summer) and intense itching. Skin assessment shows increased hypertrophy of the scars. What would be the next step for his care?

A. Aloe gel and pressure garments
B. Laser therapy to the hypertrophic scars
C. Excision of the scars and W plasty
D. Silicone gel and hydroxyzine

Answer: D. Studies show that wearing the pressure garments with the addition of silicone gel aids the level of comfort and assists in decreasing hypertrophic scarring than either alone. The addition of hydroxyzine will help ensure greater comfort and reduce scratching.

10. The nurse is caring for a 13-year-old female with sacral level spina bifida who presents to the hospital for creation of an ileal conduit so she can more easily self-catheterize. She wears long leg braces at home and is able to do self-transfers with ease preoperatively. Which postoperative nursing diagnosis is not needed with this patient?

A. Increased risk on the Braden scale
B. Decreased mobility because of postsurgical pain
C. Knowledge deficit because of a new self-catheterization technique
D. Potential skin breakdown over her heels

Answer: A. Even though her mobility is decreased because of surgical pain, she would not score any higher on the Braden Scale.

Scoring

☆☆☆ If you answered all ten items correctly, awesome—you've got skin in the game!

☆☆ If you answered seven or eight items correctly, super! You've done a nice job.

☆ If you answered fewer than five items correctly, keep cool. A quick review should deliver you to success.

Selected References

Al-Mousawi, A., Suman, O., & Herndon, D. (2012). Teamwork for total burn care: Burn centers and multidisciplinary burn teams. In D. Herndon (Ed.), *Total burn care* (pp. 9–15). Beijing, China: Saunders Elsevier.

Castelluccio, D. (2012). Implementing AORN Recommended Practices for Laser Safety. *AORN Journal, 95*(5), 612–627. doi:10.1016/j.aorn.2012.03.001

Centers for Disease Control and Prevention. (2002). Guideline for hand hygiene in health-care settings: Recommendations of the Healthcare Infection Control Practices Advisory Committee HICPAC/SHEA/APIC/IDSA Hand Hygiene Task Force. *Morbidity and Mortality Weekly Report, 51*(RR-16), 1–45.

Curran, T., & Ghahary, A. (2013). Evidence of a role for fibrocyte and keratinocyte-like cells in formation of hypertrophic scars. *Journal of Burn Care and Research, 34*(2), 227–231. doi:10.1097/BCR.0b013e318254d1f9

Hassan, S., Reynold, G., & Clarkson, J. (2014). Challenging the dogma: Relationship between time to healing and formation of hypertrophic scars after burn injury. *Journal of Burn Care & Research, 35*(2), e118–e124. doi:10.1097/BCR.0b013e31829b330a

Jovanovic, A., Ermis, R., Mewaldt, R., et al. (2012). The influence of metal salts, surfactants, and wound care products on enzymatic activity of collagenase, the wound debriding enzyme. *Wounds, 24*(9), 242–253.

Kagan, R. J., Peck M. D., Ahrenholz, D. H., et al. (2009). *American Burn Association White Paper: Surgical management of the burn wound and use of skin substitutes.*

Retrieved from http://www.ucdenver.edu/academics/colleges/medicalschool/departments/surgery/divisions/GITES/burn/Documents/American%20Burn%20Association%20White%20Paper.pdf

Kirby, M. (2007). Negative pressure wound therapy. *British Journal of Diabetes & Vascular Disease, 7*(5), 230–234.

Kishner, S., Ioffe, J., & Sung, R. C. (2014). *Pain assessment.* Retrieved from http://emedicine.medscape.com/article/1948069

Li-Tsang, C. W., Zheng, Y. P., & Lau, J. C. (2010). A randomized clinical trial to study the effect of silicone gel dressing and pressure therapy on posttraumatic hypertrophic scars. *Journal of Burn Care & Research, 31*(3), 448–457. doi:10.1097/BCR.0b013e318db52a7

National Institute on Disability, Independent Living, and Rehabilitation Research. (1995). *An easy guide to outpatient burn rehabilitation* (Project No. H133A031402). Retrieved from http://www.google.com/url?sa=t&rct=j&q=&esrc=s&frm=1&source=web&cd=2&ved=0CCYQFjABahUKEwitzdmJ15TGAhVK0oAKHb0pANs&url=http%3A%2F%2Fsearch.naric.com%2Fresearch%2Frehab%2Fdownload.cfm%3FID%3D108848&ei=A1WAVe2_JcqkgwS904DYDQ&usg=AFQjCNET6aqt6wDVKz2gr_t7mvKb78cV2g&sig2=5pVThfdsBgYNePGTAzOzSQ

National Pressure Ulcer Advisory Panel & European Pressure Ulcer Advisory Panel. (2009). Pressure ulcer treatment recommendations. In *Prevention and treatment of pressure ulcers: Clinical practice guideline* (pp. 51–120). Washington, DC: National Pressure Ulcer Advisory Panel.

Nedelec, B., Correa, J., Rachelska, G., et al. (2008). Quantitative measurement of hypertrophic scar: Intrarater reliability, sensitivity, and specificity. *Journal of Burn Care & Research, 29*(3), 489–500. doi:10.1097/BCR.0b013e3181710869

Pallija, G., Mondozzi, M., & Webb, A. (1999). Skin care of the pediatric patient. *Journal of Pediatric Nursing, 14*(2), 80–87.

Serghiou, M., Ott, S., Whitehead, C., et al. (2012). Comprehensive rehabilitation of the burn patient. In D. Herndon (Ed.), *Total burn care* (pp. 517–527). Beijing, China: Saunders, Elsevier.

The Joint Commission. (2012). Standard NPSG.01.01.01. In *Comprehensive accreditation manual for hospitals: The official handbook.* Oakbrook Terrace, IL: Author.

The Joint Commission. (2012). Standard NPSG.07.01.01. In *Comprehensive accreditation manual for hospitals: The official handbook.* Oakbrook Terrace, IL: Author.

World Health Organization. (2009). *WHO guidelines on hand hygiene in health care: First global patient safety challenge. Clean care is safer care.* Geneva, Switzerland: Author.

Chapter 12

Maternal–neonatal care

Just the facts

In this chapter, you'll learn:

- about maternal-neonatal procedures
- what patient care and teaching are associated with each procedure
- how to manage complications associated with each procedure
- the essential documentation for each procedure.

Fetal heart rate monitoring

Fetal heart rate (FHR) is an important source of information about fetal well-being during gestation and labor. There are two main FHR monitoring methods. A lesser used method is manual auscultation with a fetoscope or a handheld Doppler device placed on the maternal abdomen. The more commonly used method is electronic fetal monitoring (EFM), which detects the FHR, the length of the uterine contractions, and the time between them. EFM allows nurses and physicians to measure the response of the FHR to uterine contractions. The normal FHR is 110 to 160 beats/minute. If the FHR does not vary or is outside of the normal parameters, it can signal a potential problem with the fetus.

Not for everyone

In a high-risk pregnancy, external (indirect) or internal (direct) EFM provides more accurate information on fetal status than auscultation can.

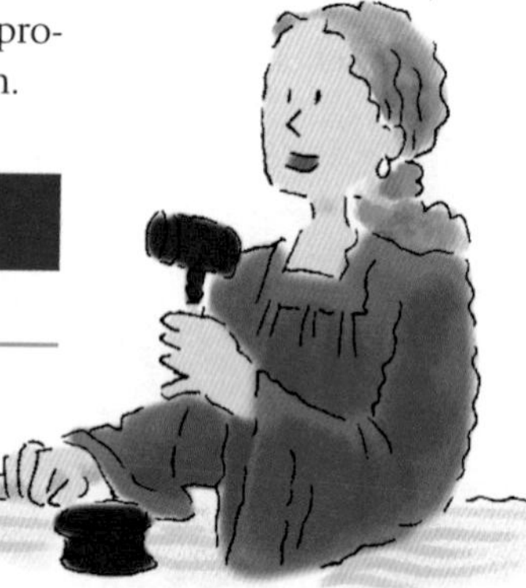
Now hear this! You can learn a lot about fetal health by listening to the heart rate.

Manual auscultation method

What you need

Fetoscope or Doppler stethoscope ✱ water-soluble lubricant (for ultrasound instrument) ✱ watch with second hand ✱ bath blanket.

Getting ready

Explain the procedure to the patient, wash your hands, and provide privacy. Reassure the patient that you may reposition the listening instrument frequently *to hear the loudest fetal heart tones*.

How you do it

- Assist the patient to a supine position with a wedge under her right hip, drape her with a bath blanket to minimize exposure, then apply the water-soluble lubricant to her abdomen or the monitoring device.

Calculating FHR during gestation

- To assess FHR in a fetus age 20 weeks or older, position the Doppler stethoscope or ultrasound on the abdominal midline above the pubic hairline. After 20 weeks' gestation, when you can palpate fetal position, use Leopold's maneuvers and position the listening instrument over the fetal back, *the ideal position to hear the heart*. (See *Performing Leopold's maneuvers*, page 544.)
- Using a Doppler stethoscope, place the earpieces in your ears, or if using a handheld Doppler device, turn it on and adjust the volume. Press the bell gently on the patient's abdomen. Start listening at the midline, midway between the umbilicus and the symphysis pubis.

Side to side

- Move the instrument slightly from side to side *to locate the loudest heart tones* then palpate the maternal pulse.
- Monitor the maternal pulse rate while counting the fetal heartbeats for at least 15 seconds. If the maternal radial pulse and FHR are the same, try to locate the fetal thorax or back by using Leopold's maneuvers; then reassess FHR. Record FHR.

Counting FHR during labor

- Allow the mother and her support person to listen to the fetal heart if they wish and document their participation.

Baseline beats

- After placing the device and locating the fetal heart tones, monitor maternal and fetal heartbeats for 60 seconds during the relaxation period between contractions *to determine baseline*.
- In a low-risk labor, assess FHR every 60 minutes during the latent phase, every 30 minutes during the active phase, and every

Performing Leopold's maneuvers

You can determine fetal position, presentation, and attitude by performing Leopold's maneuvers. Ask the patient to empty her bladder, assist her to a supine position with a wedge under her right hip, and expose her abdomen. Then perform the four maneuvers in order.

First maneuver

Face the patient and curl your fingers around the fundus. With the fetus in vertex position, the buttocks feel irregularly shaped and firm. With the fetus in breech position, the head feels hard, round, and movable.

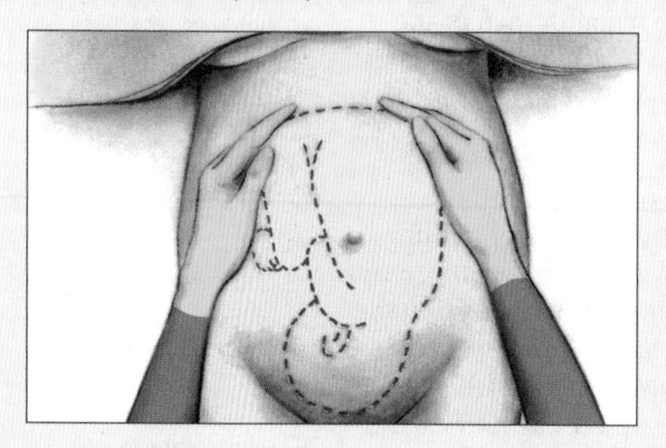

Second maneuver

Move your hands down the sides of the abdomen and apply gentle pressure. If the fetus lies in vertex position, you'll feel a smooth, hard surface on one side—the fetal back. Opposite, you'll feel lumps and knobs—the knees, hands, feet, and elbows. If the fetus lies in breech position, you may not feel the back at all.

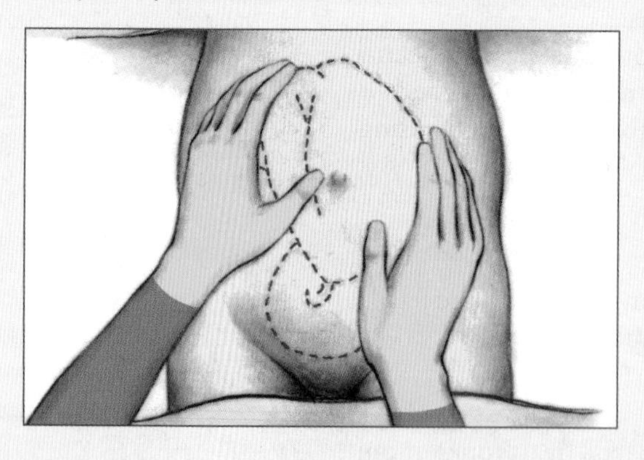

Third maneuver

Spread apart the thumb and fingers of one hand. Place them just above the patient's symphysis pubis. Bring your fingers together. If the fetus lies in vertex position (and hasn't descended), you'll feel the head. If the fetus lies in vertex position (and has descended), you'll feel a less distinct mass.

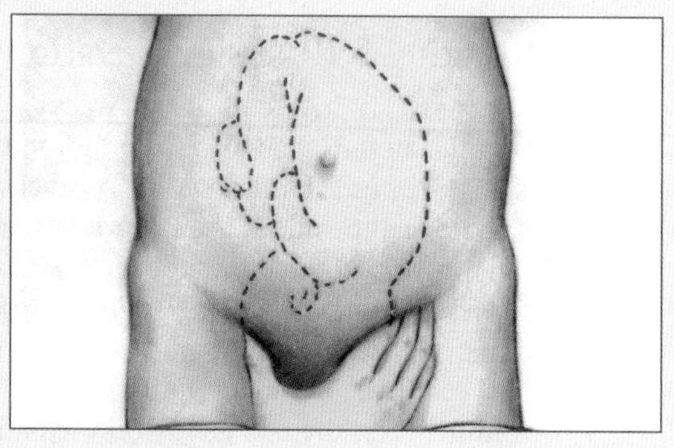

Fourth maneuver

Use this maneuver in late pregnancy. To determine flexion or extension of the fetal head and neck, place your hands on both sides of the lower abdomen. Apply gentle pressure with your fingers as you slide your hands downward, toward the symphysis pubis. If the head presents, one hand's descent will be stopped by the cephalic prominence. The other hand will be unobstructed. If the cephalic prominence is on the same side as the back, the head is extended; if it is opposite the back, the head is flexed.

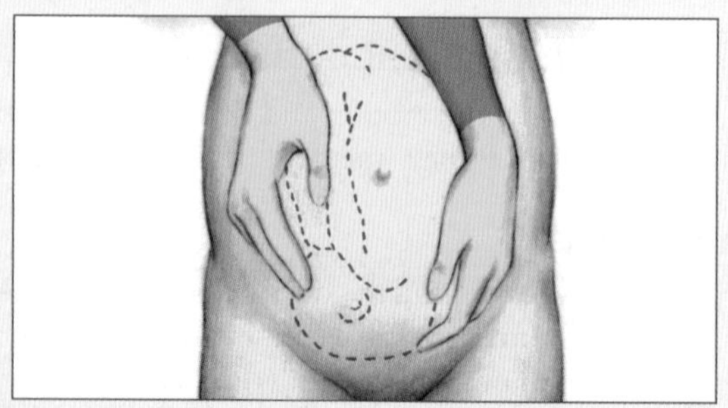

15 minutes during the second stage of labor. In a high-risk labor, assess FHR every 30 minutes during the latent phase, every 15 minutes during the active phase, and every 5 minutes during the second stage of labor.

Before and after

- Auscultate FHR during a contraction and for 30 seconds afterward *to identify the response to the contraction.*

Practice pointers

- Auscultate FHR before administration of medications, ambulation, and artificial rupture of membranes. Auscultate FHR after rupture of membranes, changes in the characteristics of the contractions, vaginal examinations, and medications. (See *Documenting FHR monitoring.*)

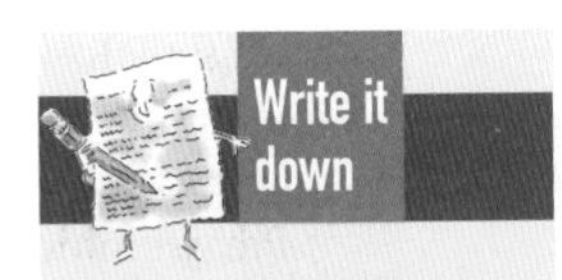

Documenting FHR monitoring

On the flowchart, record both the FHR and maternal pulse rate. Also record each auscultation.

Notify the doctor or nurse-midwife immediately if you observe marked changes in FHR from baseline values (especially during or immediately after a contraction, when signs of fetal distress typically occur). If fetal distress develops, begin indirect or direct EFM.

Amniocentesis

Amniocentesis, a needle aspiration of amniotic fluid for laboratory analysis, is usually performed between 14 and 20 weeks' gestation. This procedure can detect chromosomal and neural tube defects, metabolic and other disorders, and the sex of the fetus. It also helps assess overall fetal health. When performed in the final trimester, amniocentesis helps to evaluate fetal lung maturity and detect Rh hemolytic disease.

Older moms and others

Amniocentesis is indicated when maternal age is over 35 and in patients with a family history of chromosomal or neural tube defects or inborn errors of metabolism. Another test, chorionic villi sampling, can also be used to detect fetal disorders.

Amniocentesis is contraindicated when the anterior uterine wall is completely covered by the placenta or when amniotic fluid is insufficient.

What you need

Hospital gown ✳ two sets of sterile gloves, sterile gowns, and masks ✳ stethoscope ✳ Doppler stethoscope and other appropriate ultrasound equipment or electronic fetal monitor ✳ antiseptic solution with sterile container ✳ local anesthetic ✳ alcohol ✳ 10-mL syringe ✳ sterile 20G or 22G 4″ spinal needle with stylet ✳ 22G or 25G needle ✳ sterile 20-mL glass syringe ✳ clean amber glass specimen container for Rh sensitization and lecithin-sphingomyelin (L/S) ratio tests * three sterile glass specimen tubes (for genetic tests) * laboratory request forms * adhesive bandage.

Preassembled amniocentesis trays are available.

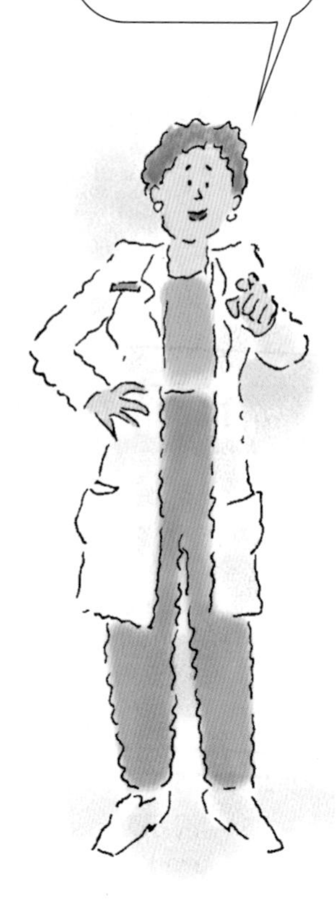
Amniocentesis is part of the standard care menu for expectant mothers over age 35.

Getting ready

If you don't have an amber specimen container, cover the outside of a clean test tube or glass container with adhesive tape or aluminum foil *to prevent the breakdown of bilirubin*. Properly label all specimen containers or tubes.

How you do it

- Identify the patient using two patient identifiers per the facility policy.
- Make sure that the consent form is signed.
- *To reduce the risk of bladder puncture*, ensure that the patient voids before the procedure if the pregnancy exceeds 20 weeks (before 20 weeks, a full bladder may help to hold the uterus steady).

Hip helper

- Provide privacy and explain the procedure to the patient. Have the patient put on a hospital gown and assist him to a supine position. Obtain baseline maternal vital signs. Next, determine the baseline FHR with a Doppler handheld device, Doppler stethoscope, or the fetoscope.
- Instruct the patient to fold her hands on her chest or rest her hands behind her head and tell her to remain still. Provide reassurance to the patient.
- The doctor will use ultrasonography to locate the fetus, placenta, and amniotic fluid pocket to determine the appropriate needle-insertion depth. Next, he'll put on the sterile gown, sterile gloves, and mask and clean the skin with an antiseptic solution.

Pain relief prep

- If the patient is receiving a local anesthetic, clean the diaphragm of the multidose vial of anesthetic solution with alcohol. Provide a 10-mL syringe and a 22G or 25G needle. Then invert the bottle *to allow the doctor to withdraw the anesthetic.*

Scrub in

- Perform hand hygiene and put on a sterile gown, sterile gloves, and mask.
- After the anesthetic takes effect, the doctor, guided by ultrasonographic imaging, advances the 20G needle with a stylet through the abdomen and uterine wall into the amniotic sac, removes the stylet, attaches the 20-mL glass syringe to the needle, and aspirates the amniotic fluid.

Sure, I could predict the sex of the fetus. But amniocentesis takes away the guesswork.

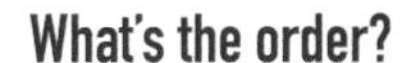

What's the order?

- If the patient is having genetic studies, open the sterile glass specimen tubes for the physician to transfer the amniotic fluid, then promptly close the tubes avoiding contamination.
- If the patient is having Rh sensitization or L/S ratio tests, open the amber or covered specimen container for the amniotic fluid and close the container promptly.
- After the needle is withdrawn, place an adhesive bandage over the insertion site.

Let's go to the lab

- Label the specimens and verify the information from the medical record matches the labels and the requisition. Send the specimens to the laboratory immediately.
- If the patient is in the final trimester of pregnancy, direct her to lie on her side.

Irritation inspection

- Assess maternal vital signs and FHR every 15 minutes for 30 minutes for tachycardia or bradycardia. Notify the doctor and continue to monitor FHR if these signs appear. In addition, electronically monitor the patient for uterine irritability and the fetus for changes in heart rate pattern for a few hours after the procedure.
- Instruct the patient to report signs and symptoms of complications, including a vaginal discharge (fluid or blood), decreased fetal movement, contractions, or fever and chills. (See *Complications of amniocentesis*, page 548.)
- Help the patient dress in preparation for discharge.

Practice pointers

- Inform the patient, her family, and her support person, as appropriate, that test results should be available in 2 to 4 weeks. Provide emotional support as needed. (See *Documenting amniocentesis*.)

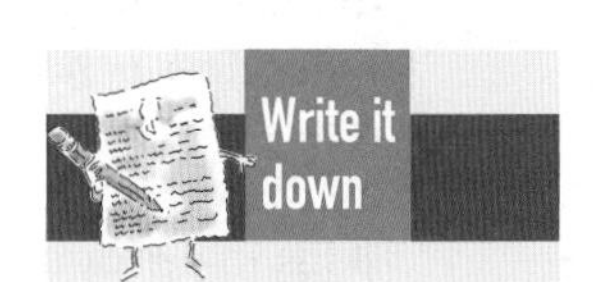

Documenting amniocentesis

In your notes, record:
- doctor's name
- patient education
- date and time of the procedure
- amount and appearance of the specimen and time of transport to the laboratory
- ordered laboratory tests
- baseline maternal vital signs and FHR and any changes
- patient's tolerance of the procedure
- discharge instructions.

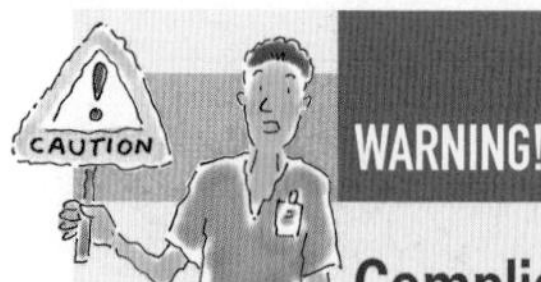

WARNING!

Complications of amniocentesis

Amniocentesis causes complications for the mother in less than 1% of patients. Possible complications include amniotic fluid embolism, hemorrhage, infection, premature labor, abruptio placentae, placenta or umbilical cord trauma, bladder or intestinal puncture, and Rh isoimmunization.

Fetal complications also are rare. They include intrauterine fetal death, amnionitis, injury from needle puncture, amniotic fluid leakage, bleeding, spontaneous abortion, and premature birth.

Biophysical profile

The nurse does not typically participate in assisting with the biophysical profile (BPP) but is responsible for explaining the procedure to the patient. Part of the BPP consists of a nonstress test, which the nurse does perform in the labor and delivery unit. After the nonstress test is completed, the patient receives an ultrasound, performed either in the nuclear medicine unit or at bedside. Some nurses have skills in performing ultrasounds. The BPP assesses fetal breathing movements, fetal movement, fetal tone, and amniotic fluid volume.

What you need

The nurse will attach the patient to an external monitor as described in the "External fetal monitoring" section. The external fetal monitor and the ultrasound machine are the only equipment that is needed.

How you do it

Help the patient sit in a semi-Fowler's position of supine with a wedge under her right hip.

Apply the external monitor tocotransducer and Doppler ultrasound. Locate the fetal heart tones and apply the Doppler in that location. Perform the nonstress test for at least 20 minutes. If the patient will have the rest of the BPP performed in the nuclear medicine unit, transport the patient to the unit. If it will be at bedside, the patient will have an ultrasound of the uterus, which usually takes at least 30 to 45 minutes to complete.

External fetal monitoring

External fetal monitoring is an indirect, noninvasive procedure. It uses two devices strapped to the mother's abdomen to evaluate fetal well-being during labor.

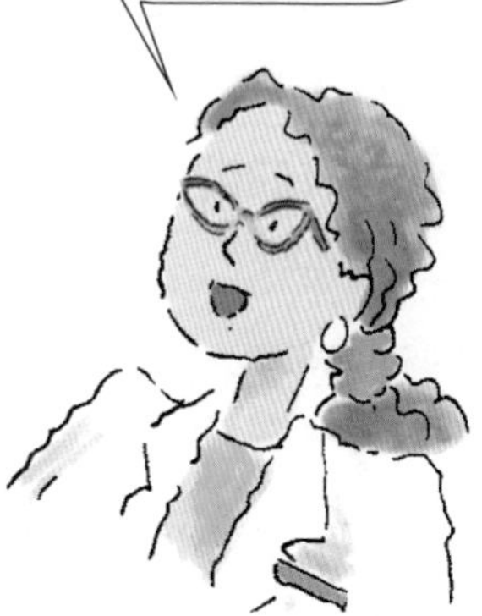
External fetal monitoring is a noninvasive way to assess contractions and fetal heart rate.

Two readings, one printout

The ultrasound transducer transmits high-frequency sound waves to the fetal heart. The tocotransducer, in turn, responds to the pressure exerted by uterine contractions and simultaneously records their duration and frequency. (See *Applying external fetal monitoring devices.*) The monitoring apparatus traces FHR and uterine contraction data onto the same printout paper.

External fetal monitoring may be used for high-risk pregnancy, oxytocin-induced labor, and antepartal nonstress—delete contraction stress tests, as they are not performed.

Applying external fetal monitoring devices

To ensure clear tracings that define fetal status and labor progress, be sure to precisely position external monitoring devices. These devices include an ultrasound transducer and a tocotransducer.

Fetal heart monitor

Palpate the uterus to locate the fetal back and place the ultrasound transducer over this site where the fetal heartbeat sounds the loudest. Then tighten the belt. Use the fetal heart tracing on the monitor strip to confirm the transducer's position.

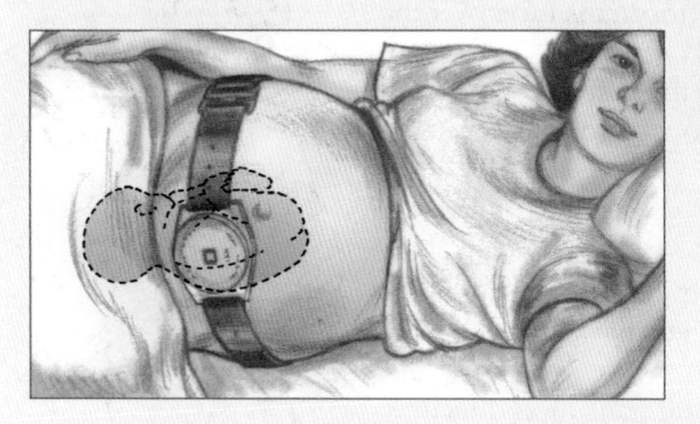

Labor monitor

A tocotransducer records uterine motion during contractions. Place the tocotransducer over the uterine fundus where it contracts, either midline or slightly to one side. Place your hand on the fundus and palpate a contraction to verify proper placement. Secure the tocotransducer's belt, then adjust the pen set so that the baseline values read between 5 and 15 mm Hg on the monitor strip.

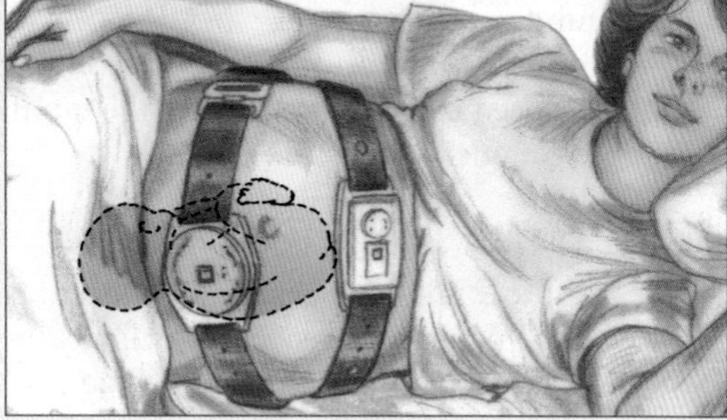

What you need

Electronic fetal monitor ✳ operator's manual ✳ ultrasound transducer ✳ tocotransducer ✳ conduction gel ✳ transducer straps ✳ damp cloth ✳ printout paper. Monitoring devices, such as phonotransducers and abdominal electrocardiogram (ECG) transducers, are commercially available.

Getting ready

After reviewing the operator's manual, prepare the machine for use.

Who and when

Label the printout paper with the patient's identification number or birth date and her name, the date, maternal vital signs and position, the paper speed, and the number of the strip paper.

How you do it

- Identify the patient using two patient identifiers per the facility policy.
- Explain the procedure to the patient.
- Make sure the patient has signed a consent form if required.
- Perform hand hygiene and provide privacy.

Beginning the procedure

- Assist the patient to the semi-Fowler's or left-lateral position with her abdomen exposed and palpate the abdomen to locate the fundus—the area of greatest muscle density in the uterus. Then, using transducer straps, secure the tocotransducer over the fundus.
- Adjust the pen set tracer controls so that the baseline values read between 5 and 15 mm Hg on the monitor strip or as indicated by the model.

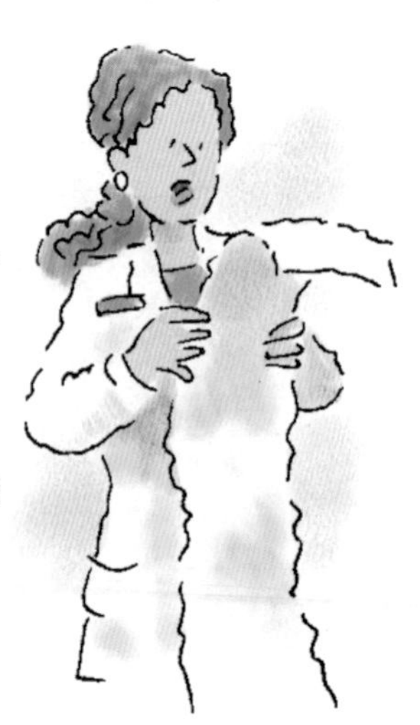

Goo for good contact

- Apply conduction gel to the ultrasound transducer crystals and use Leopold's maneuvers to palpate the fetal back, through which fetal heart tones resound most audibly.
- Start the monitor and apply the ultrasound transducer directly over the site having the strongest heart tones.
- Activate the control that begins the printout.

Monitoring the patient

- Observe the tracings *to identify the frequency and duration of uterine contractions* but palpate the uterus *to determine intensity of contractions. Using the external monitor does not allow measurement of the strength of the contractions. Palpation of the contraction as mild can be compared to the tip of one's nose, moderate strength to one's chin, and strong to the feeling of one's forehead. This provides the nurse with a reference point as the nurse compares the assessment of strength with another experienced nurse.*

Compare and contract

- Note the baseline FHR and assess periodic accelerations or decelerations from the baseline. Compare the FHR patterns with those of the uterine contractions.
- Move the tocotransducer and the ultrasound transducer *to accommodate changes in maternal or fetal position.* Readjust both transducers every hour and assess the patient's skin for reddened areas caused by the strap pressure.
- Clean the ultrasound transducer periodically with a damp cloth *to remove dried conduction gel* and apply fresh gel as necessary. After using the ultrasound transducer, place the cover over it.

Practice pointers

- If the patient reports discomfort in the position that provides the clearest signal, try to obtain a satisfactory 5- or 10-minute tracing with the patient in this position before assisting her to a more comfortable position. (See *Documenting external fetal monitoring.*)

Documenting external fetal monitoring

Number each fetal monitoring strip in sequence and label each printout sheet with the patient's identification number or birth date, her name, the date and time, and paper speed.

In your notes, record:

- time of vaginal examinations, membrane rupture, drug administration, and maternal or fetal movements
- patient education
- maternal vital signs
- intensity of uterine contractions
- each movement or readjustment of the tocotransducer and ultrasound transducer
- assessments and interventions (in correlation with monitor printout strips).

Internal fetal monitoring

Internal fetal monitoring, also called direct fetal monitoring, is an invasive procedure that uses a spiral electrode attached to the presenting fetal part (usually the scalp). This electrode detects the fetal heartbeat and transmits it to the monitor, which converts the signals to a fetal ECG waveform. This helps assess fetal response to uterine contraction, measures intrauterine pressure, tracks labor progress, and allows evaluation of short- and long-term FHR variability.

Only when the train has reached the station

Internal fetal monitoring is indicated for high-risk pregnancies. It's performed only if the amniotic sac has ruptured, the cervix is dilated at least 2 cm, and the presenting part of the fetus is at least at the −1 station. (See *Complications of internal fetal monitoring,* page 552.)

What you need

Electronic fetal monitor * spiral electrode and a drive tube * disposable leg plate pad or reusable leg plate with Velcro belt * conduction gel * antiseptic solution * hypoallergenic tape * sterile gloves * sterile drapes * intrauterine catheter connection cable and pressure-sensitive catheter * graph paper * operator's manual.

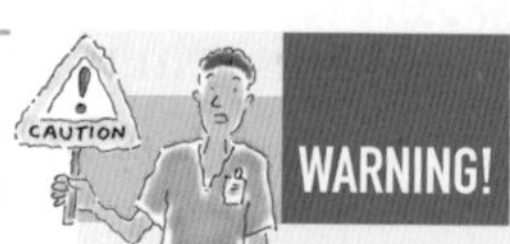

Complications of internal fetal monitoring

Maternal complications of internal fetal monitoring may include uterine perforation and intrauterine infection. Fetal complications may include abscess, hematoma, and infection.

Getting ready

Be sure to review the operator's manual before using the equipment. Perform hand hygiene and open the sterile equipment, maintaining aseptic technique.

How you do it

- Identify the patient using two patient identifiers per facility policy.
- Describe the procedure and make sure a consent form is signed.
- Label the printout paper with the patient's identification number or name and birth date, the date, the paper speed, and the number on the monitor strip.

Monitoring contractions

Assist the patient into the lithotomy position for a vaginal examination while the doctor puts on sterile gloves.

Lots of cable, no free movies

- Attach the connection cable to the outlet on the monitor marked uterine activity (UA), connect the cable to the intrauterine catheter, and then zero the catheter with a gauge on the distal end of the catheter.
- Cover the patient's perineum with a sterile drape and clean the perineum with antiseptic solution, according to facility policy. The physician performs a vaginal examination, inserts the catheter into the uterine cavity until it's advanced to the black line, and secures it with hypoallergenic tape to the inner thigh.

Strip tips

- Observe the monitoring strip *to verify proper placement and a clear tracing*. Periodically evaluate the strip to determine amount of pressure exerted with each contraction. Note all such data on the strip and the patient's medical record.

- The intrauterine catheter is usually removed during the second stage of labor. Dispose of the catheter and clean and store the cable according to facility policy. (See *Applying an internal electronic fetal monitor.*)

Monitoring FHR

- Apply conduction gel to the leg plate and secure to the patient's inner thigh with Velcro straps or 2" tape. Connect the leg plate cable to the ECG outlet on the monitor.
- After a vaginal examination to identify the fetal presenting part and level of descent, the spiral electrode will be placed in a drive tube and advanced through the vagina to the fetal presenting part. *To secure the electrode,* mild pressure will be applied and the drive tube will be turned clockwise 360 degrees.

Applying an internal electronic fetal monitor

During internal EFM, a spiral electrode monitors the FHR and an internal catheter monitors uterine contractions.

Monitoring FHR

The spiral electrode is inserted after a vaginal examination that determines the position of the fetus. As shown at right, the electrode is attached to the presenting fetal part, usually the scalp or buttocks.

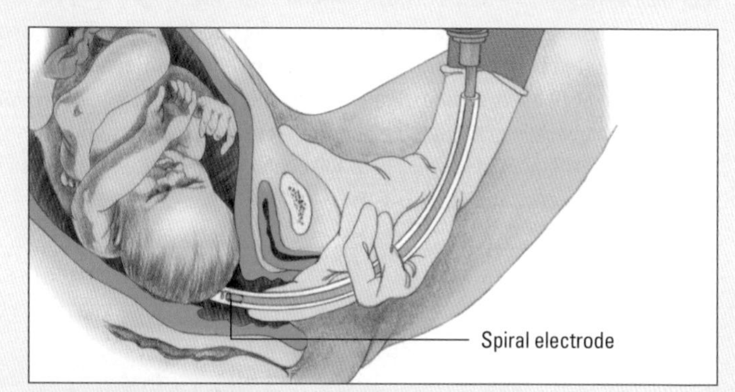

Monitoring uterine contractions

The intrauterine catheter is inserted up to a premarked level on the tubing and then connected to a monitor that interprets uterine contraction pressures.

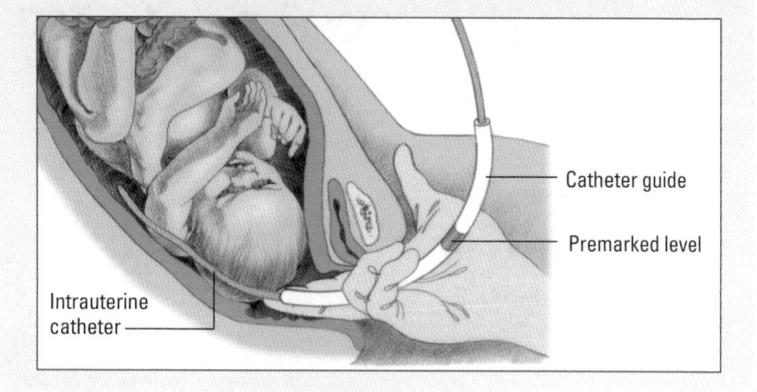

Connect the dots

- After the electrode is in place and the drive tube has been removed, connect the color-coded electrode wires to the corresponding color-coded leg plate posts.
- Turn on the recorder and note the time on the printout paper.
- Help the patient to a comfortable position and evaluate the strip *to verify proper placement and a clear FHR tracing.*

Monitoring the patient

Begin by noting the frequency, duration, and intensity of uterine contractions. Normal intrauterine pressure ranges from 8 to 12 mm Hg. (See *Reading a fetal monitor strip*.)

Reading a fetal monitor strip

Presented in two parallel recordings, the fetal monitor strip records the FHR in beats per minute in the top recording and UA in millimeters of mercury (mm Hg) in the bottom recording. You can obtain information on fetal status and labor progress by reading the strips horizontally and vertically.

Reading horizontally on the FHR or the UA strip, each small block represents 10 seconds. Six consecutive small blocks, separated by a dark vertical line, represent 1 minute. Reading vertically on the FHR strip, each block represents an amplitude of 10 beats/minute. Reading vertically on the UA strip, each block represents 5 mm Hg of pressure.

Assess the baseline FHR (the "resting" heart rate) between uterine contractions when fetal movement diminishes. This baseline FHR (normal range: 110 to 160 beats/minute) pattern serves as a reference for subsequent FHR tracings produced during contractions.

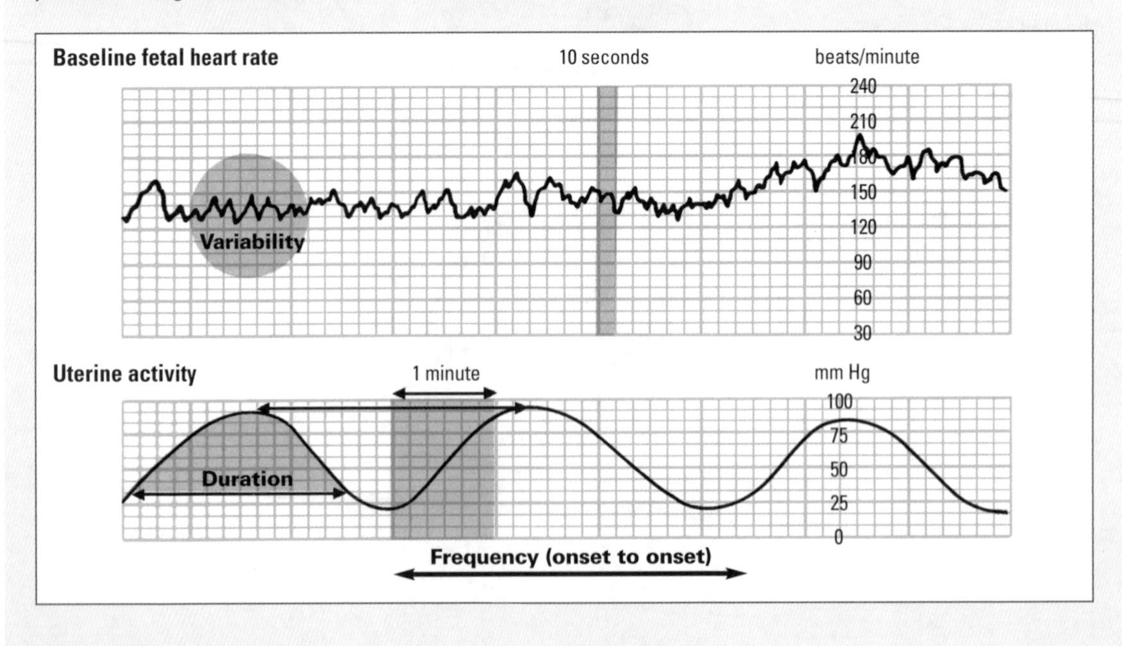

Check and compare

- Next, check the baseline FHR and assess periodic accelerations or decelerations from the baseline. (See *Identifying baseline FHR irregularities*, page 556.)
- Compare the FHR uterine contraction pattern. Note the interval between onset of deceleration and uterine contractions, the interval between the lowest level of an FHR deceleration and a uterine contraction peak, and the FHR deceleration range.
- Check for FHR variability, which is a measure of fetal oxygen reserve and neurologic integrity and stability.

Practice pointers

- Interpret FHR and uterine contractions at regular intervals. Guidelines of the Association of Women's Health, Obstetric, and Neonatal Nurses specify that high-risk patients need continuous FHR monitoring, whereas low-risk patients should have FHR auscultated every 30 minutes after a contraction during the first stage and every 15 minutes after a contraction during the second stage.
- First, determine the baseline FHR within 10 beats/minute; then assess the degree of baseline variability. Identify changes such as decelerations (early late, variable, or mixed) and nonperiodic changes such as a sinusoidal pattern.
- If vaginal delivery isn't imminent (within 30 minutes) and fetal distress patterns don't improve, cesarean delivery will be necessary. (See *Documenting internal fetal monitoring.*)

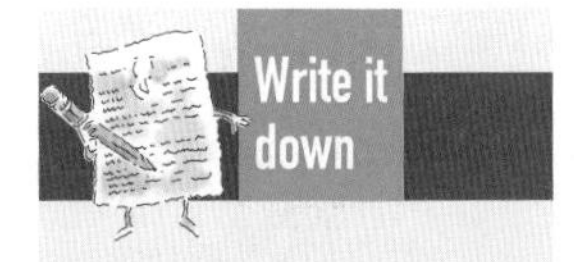

Documenting internal fetal monitoring

- Patient education
- Document all activity related to monitoring.
- Identify the monitoring strip with the patient's name, her doctor's name, your name, and the date and time. Record the paper speed and electrode placement.
- Document the patient's vital signs at regular intervals according to standards of care. Note her pushing efforts and record any change in her position. Document I.V. line insertion and changes in the I.V. solution or infusion rate. Note the use of oxytocin, regional anesthetics, or other medications.
- After a vaginal examination, document cervical dilation and effacement as well as fetal station, presentation, and position. Also document membrane rupture, including the time it occurred and whether it was spontaneous or artificial. Note the fluid amount, color, and odor.

Consistency in interpreting and communicating FHR patterns

The National Institute of Child Health and Human Development (NICHD) Workshop Report on Electronic Fetal Monitoring: Update on Definitions, Interpretations, and Research Guidelines has developed a three-tier FHR interpretation system. Nurses are part of the health care team and are responsible for accurately interpreting and communicating findings to the primary health care provider.

There are three NICHD categories.

Category I: considered normal

- Baseline rate between 110 and 160 beats/minute
- The baseline variability is moderate.
- Late or variable decelerations are absent.
- Early decelerations may be present or absent.
- Accelerations may be present or absent.

Identifying baseline FHR irregularities

When monitoring the FHR, you need to be familiar with irregularities that may occur, the possible causes, and nursing interventions to take. Here is a guide to these irregularities.

Irregularity	Possible causes	Clinical significance	Nursing interventions
Baseline tachycardia beats/minute 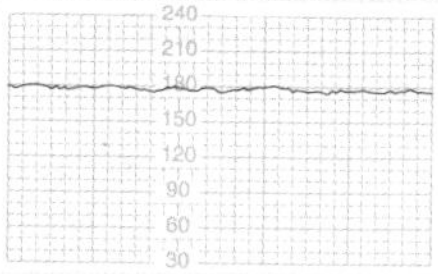	• Early fetal hypoxia • Maternal fever • Parasympathetic agents, such as atropine and scopolamine • Beta-adrenergics, such as ritodrine and terbutaline • Amnionitis (inflammation of inner layer of fetal membrane or amnion) • Maternal hyperthyroidism • Fetal anemia • Fetal heart failure • Fetal arrhythmias	Persistent tachycardia without periodic changes doesn't usually adversely affect fetal well-being, especially when associated with maternal fever. However, tachycardia is an ominous sign when associated with late decelerations, severe variable decelerations, or lack of variability.	• Intervene to alleviate the cause of fetal distress and provide supplemental oxygen as ordered. Also administer intravenous (I.V.) fluids as prescribed. • Discontinue oxytocin infusion to reduce uterine activity. • Turn the patient onto her left side and elevate her legs. • Continue to observe FHR. • Document interventions and outcomes. • Notify the doctor; further medical intervention may be necessary.
Baseline bradycardia beats/minute 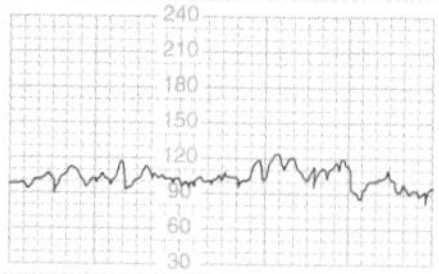	• Late fetal hypoxia • Beta-adrenergic blocking agents, such as propranolol, and anesthetics • Maternal hypotension • Prolonged umbilical cord compression • Fetal congenital heart block	Bradycardia with good variability and no periodic changes doesn't signal fetal distress if FHR remains higher than 80 beats/minute. However, bradycardia caused by hypoxia and acidosis is an ominous sign when associated with loss of variability and late decelerations.	• Intervene to correct the cause of fetal distress. Administer supplemental oxygen as ordered. Start an I.V. line and administer fluids as prescribed. • Discontinue oxytocin infusion to reduce uterine activity. • Turn the patient onto her left side and elevate her legs. • Continue observing FHR. • Document interventions and outcomes. • Notify the doctor; further medical intervention may be necessary.
Early decelerations beats/minute 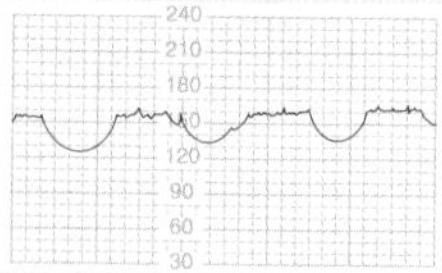 mm Hg 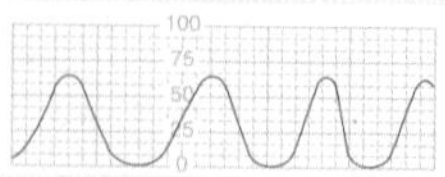	• Fetal head compression	Early decelerations are benign, indicating fetal head compression at dilation of 4 to 7 cm.	• Reassure the patient that the fetus isn't at risk. • Observe FHR. • Document the frequency of decelerations.

Identifying baseline FHR irregularities *(continued)*

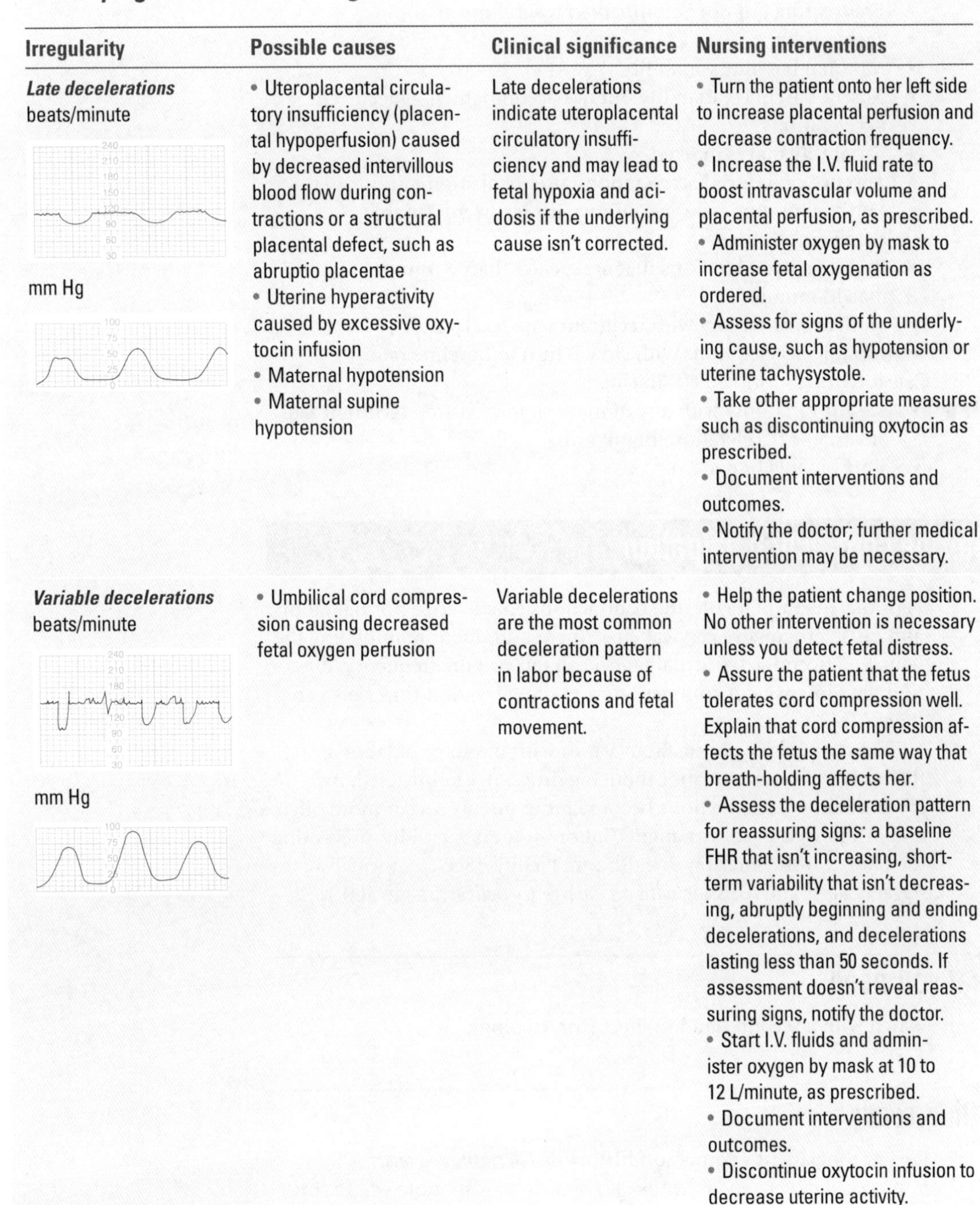

Irregularity	Possible causes	Clinical significance	Nursing interventions
Late decelerations beats/minute; mm Hg	• Uteroplacental circulatory insufficiency (placental hypoperfusion) caused by decreased intervillous blood flow during contractions or a structural placental defect, such as abruptio placentae • Uterine hyperactivity caused by excessive oxytocin infusion • Maternal hypotension • Maternal supine hypotension	Late decelerations indicate uteroplacental circulatory insufficiency and may lead to fetal hypoxia and acidosis if the underlying cause isn't corrected.	• Turn the patient onto her left side to increase placental perfusion and decrease contraction frequency. • Increase the I.V. fluid rate to boost intravascular volume and placental perfusion, as prescribed. • Administer oxygen by mask to increase fetal oxygenation as ordered. • Assess for signs of the underlying cause, such as hypotension or uterine tachysystole. • Take other appropriate measures such as discontinuing oxytocin as prescribed. • Document interventions and outcomes. • Notify the doctor; further medical intervention may be necessary.
Variable decelerations beats/minute; mm Hg	• Umbilical cord compression causing decreased fetal oxygen perfusion	Variable decelerations are the most common deceleration pattern in labor because of contractions and fetal movement.	• Help the patient change position. No other intervention is necessary unless you detect fetal distress. • Assure the patient that the fetus tolerates cord compression well. Explain that cord compression affects the fetus the same way that breath-holding affects her. • Assess the deceleration pattern for reassuring signs: a baseline FHR that isn't increasing, short-term variability that isn't decreasing, abruptly beginning and ending decelerations, and decelerations lasting less than 50 seconds. If assessment doesn't reveal reassuring signs, notify the doctor. • Start I.V. fluids and administer oxygen by mask at 10 to 12 L/minute, as prescribed. • Document interventions and outcomes. • Discontinue oxytocin infusion to decrease uterine activity.

Category II: evaluated as indeterminate; are not predictive of abnormal fetal acid-base status

- Bradycardia but not accompanied by absent variability
- Tachycardia
- Minimal baseline variability
- Absent baseline variability but not accompanied by recurrent decelerations
- Variability that is marked
- Absence of induced accelerations after fetal stimulation
- Minimal or moderate variability with recurrent variable decelerations
- Prolonged decelerations that are greater than 2 minutes and less that 10 minutes
- Moderate variability with recurrent late decelerations
- Variable decelerations with slow return to baseline rate.

Category III: abnormal FHR tracing

- Absent variability with any of these characteristics: recurrent late or variable deceleration, bradycardia.
- Sinusoidal FHR pattern.

Uterine contraction palpation

Periodic, involuntary uterine contractions characterize normal labor and cause progressive cervical effacement and dilation, impelling the fetus to descend. Uterine palpation can tell you the frequency, duration, and intensity of contractions and the relaxation time between them.

The character of contractions varies with the stage of labor and the body's response to labor-inducing drugs, if administered. As labor advances, contractions become more intense, occur more often, and last longer. In some patients, labor progresses rapidly, preventing the patient from entering a health care facility. (See *Quick guide to stages of labor* and *Assisting with an emergency delivery*, page 560.)

What you need

Watch with a second hand ✱ sheet (for draping).

Getting ready

Review the patient's admission history *to determine the onset, frequency, duration, and intensity of contractions*. Also, note where contractions feel strongest or exert the most pressure.

Quick guide to stages of labor

Normal labor advances through the four stages summarized here. Offer your patient encouragement and progress reports throughout the stages.

First stage

Regular contractions, which repeat at 15- to 20-minute intervals and last between 10 and 30 seconds, signal the onset of labor's first stage. This stage has three phases: latent, active, and transitional. In primiparous patients, the first stage of labor ranges from 3.3 to 19.7 hours; in multiparous patients, it ranges from 0.1 to 14.3 hours.

In the *latent phase* (characterized by irregular, brief, and mild contractions), the cervix dilates to 3 or 4 cm. Other signs and symptoms include abdominal cramping and backache. The patient may expel the mucus plug during this phase. This phase averages 8.6 hours in primiparous patients and 5.3 hours in multiparous patients.

During the *active phase*, cervical dilation increases to between 5 and 7 cm. Contractions occur every 3 to 5 minutes, last 30 to 45 seconds, and become moderately intense. In primiparous patients, this phase averages 5.8 hours; in multiparous patients, 2.5 hours.

In the *transitional phase*, the cervix dilates completely (8 to 10 cm). Uterine contractions grow intense, last between 45 and 60 seconds, and repeat at least every 2 minutes. The patient may thrash about, lose control of breathing techniques, and experience nausea and vomiting. This phase typically lasts less than 3 hours in primiparous patients and less than 1 hour in multiparous patients.

Second stage

In the second stage of labor, contractions occur every 1½ to 2 minutes and last up to 90 seconds. This stage commonly ends within 1 hour for a primiparous patient and possibly 15 minutes for a multiparous patient.

Signs and symptoms signaling onset of the second stage include increased bloody show, rupture of membranes (if they're still intact), severe rectal pressure and flaring, and reflexive bearing down with each contraction. The fetal head approaches the perineal floor and emerges at the vaginal opening. The second labor stage concludes with birth.

Third stage

Strong but less painful contractions expel the placenta, which normally emerges within 30 minutes after the neonate emerges. Signs indicating normal separation of the placenta from the uterine wall include lengthening of the umbilical cord, a sudden gush of dark blood from the vagina, and a palpable change in uterine shape from disklike to globular.

Fourth stage

This stage begins with placental expulsion and extends through the next 4 hours, while the patient's body rests and begins adjusting to the postpartum state.

Wash your hands and provide privacy. Describe the procedure to the patient, assist her to a comfortable side-lying position, and drape her with a sheet.

How you do it

- Plant the palmar surface of your fingers on the uterine fundus and palpate lightly *to assess contractions*. Each contraction has three phases: increment (rising), acme (peak), and decrement (letting down or ebbing). Palpate the contractions and determine the strength at the peak of the contractions.

Assisting with an emergency delivery

Emergency delivery—an unplanned birth outside of a health care facility—may occur when labor progresses quickly or when circumstances prevent the mother from entering a health care facility. Whether you're assisting at an emergency delivery or instructing the person who is, your goals include:

- establishing a clean, safe, private birth area
- promoting a controlled delivery
- preventing injury, infection, and hemorrhage.

What to gather

Gather the following items:

- large, clean cloth
- bath towel, blanket, or coat
- gloves
- clean, sharp object, such as a knife or scissors. (Boil at least 5 minutes, if possible.)

Prep steps

To promote a safe delivery, follow these steps:

- Provide privacy, wash your hands, and put on the gloves.
- Position the patient comfortably and place the open cloth under her buttocks.
- Elevate her buttocks slightly with the towel, blanket, or coat.
- Encourage her to pant during contractions.

Countdown to the birth

As delivery progresses, follow these guidelines:

- Place one hand gently on the patient's perineum.
- As the neonate's head emerges, break the amniotic sac, if it's intact.
- Support the neonate's head as it emerges.
- Locate the umbilical cord. If it's wrapped loosely around the neonate's neck, slip it over the neonate's head. If it's wrapped tightly around the neck, ligate the cord in two places. Then, using the sharp object, carefully cut between the two ligatures.
- Gently wipe mucus and amniotic fluid from the neonate's nose and mouth.
- Instruct the mother to bear down with the next contraction.
- Position your hands on either side of the neonate's head and support the neck.
- Exert gentle, downward pressure to deliver the posterior shoulder.
- Support the neonate's body in a slightly head-down position and wipe mucus from the face. If the neonate doesn't breathe spontaneously, gently pat the soles of the feet.
- Dry and cover the neonate with the blanket or towel.
- Ligate the umbilical cord.
- Cradle the neonate at uterus level or place on the mother's lower abdomen until the umbilical cord stops pulsating.

Wrapping things up

After delivery, take the following actions to ensure the mother's and neonate's welfare:

- Watch for signs of placental separation (a slight gush of dark blood from the vagina, cord lengthening, and a firm fundus). When you see these signs, apply gentle, downward pressure on the mother's abdomen while encouraging her to bear down.
- Gently massage the uterus.
- Encourage the mother to breastfeed.
- Check her for excessive bleeding. Apply a perineal pad, if available, and instruct her to press her thighs together.
- Arrange transportation to the hospital for the mother and neonate.

How fast?

- *To assess frequency,* time the interval between the beginning of one contraction and the beginning of the next.

How long?

- *To assess duration,* time the period from when the uterus begins tightening until it begins relaxing.

How hard?

- *To assess intensity*, press your fingertips into the uterine fundus when the uterus tightens. During mild contractions, the fundus indents easily; during moderate contractions, the fundus indents less easily; during strong contractions, the fundus resists indenting.
- Determine how the patient copes with discomfort by assessing her breathing and relaxation techniques.
- Assess contractions in low-risk patients every 30 to 60 minutes in the latent phase, every 15 to 30 minutes in the active phase, and every 10 to 15 minutes in the transition phase. More frequent assessments are required in high-risk labors. High-risk fetal status assessments should also occur every 30 minutes during the latent phase, every 15 minutes during active phase, and every 5 minutes in the second stage.

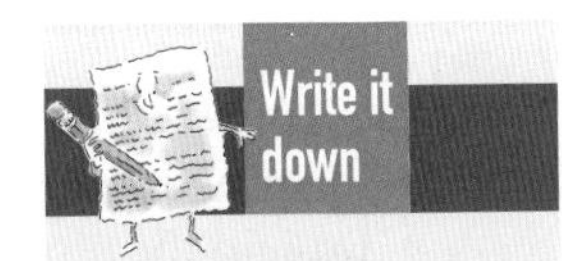

Documenting contraction palpation

In your notes, record:
- frequency, duration, and intensity of contractions
- relaxation time between contractions
- patient's response to contractions.

Practice pointers

- If any contraction lasts longer than 90 seconds and isn't followed by uterine muscle relaxation, or if relaxation period is less than 1 minute between contractions, notify the doctor. This is referred to as tachysystole and may contribute to fetal hypoxia. Tachysystole is more than 5 contractions in 10 minutes, contraction that last longer than 2 minutes, less than 1 minute resting period, or increasing resting tone greater than 20 to 25 mm Hg or peak pressure of greater than 80 mm Hg (with internal monitoring). (See *Documenting contraction palpation*.)

Vaginal examination

During first-stage labor, a vaginal examination may be done to assess cervical dilation and effacement, membrane status, and fetal presentation, position, engagement, and descent. If the patient has excessive vaginal bleeding, which may signal placenta previa, vaginal examination is contraindicated.

What you need

Sterile gloves ✳ sterile water-soluble lubricant or sterile water ✳ mild soap and water or cleaning solution ✳ linen-saver pads ✳ antiseptic solution.

Getting ready

Identify the patient using two patient identifiers per facility policy. Explain the procedure to the patient and have her empty her bladder. Perform hand hygiene. Use Leopold's maneuvers to identify the fetal presenting part and position. Then help the patient into a lithotomy position for the vaginal examination. Place a linen-saver pad under the patient's buttocks and put on sterile gloves.

A vaginal exam works best when the patient is relaxed. Take a moment to help her breathe deeply.

How you do it

- Clean the perineum with mild soap and water or cleaning solution with your independent hand.
- Lubricate the index and middle fingers of your examining hand with sterile water or sterile water-soluble lubricant. If the membranes are ruptured, use an antiseptic solution.

Breathe and release

- Ask the patient to relax by taking several deep breaths and slowly releasing the air. Then insert your lubricated fingers (palmar surface down) into the vagina. Keep your uninserted fingers flexed *to avoid the rectum.*
- Palpate the cervix, noting its consistency. The cervix gradually softens throughout pregnancy, reaching a buttery consistency before labor begins. (See *Cervical effacement and dilation.*)
- After identifying the presenting fetal part and position and evaluating dilation, effacement, engagement, station, and membrane status, gently withdraw your fingers. Help the patient clean her perineum and change the linen-saver pad, as necessary.

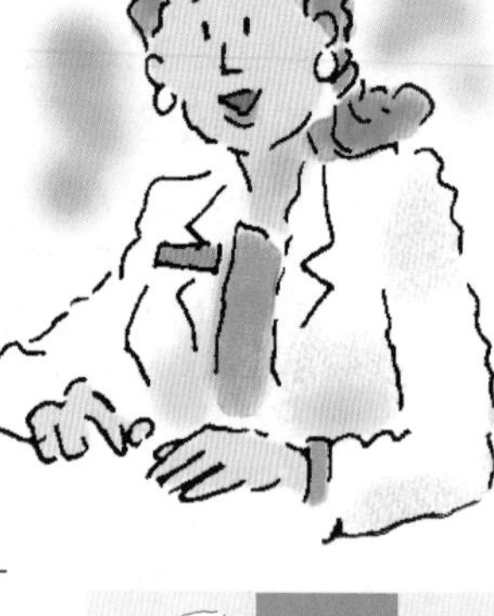

Write it down

Documenting vaginal examination

After each vaginal examination, record:
- percentage of effacement and dilation
- station of the presenting fetal part
- amniotic membrane status
- patient's tolerance of the procedure.

Practice pointers

- In early labor, perform the vaginal examination between contractions, focusing on the extent of cervical dilation and effacement. At the end of first-stage labor, perform the examination during a contraction to focus on assessing fetal descent.

Water, water everywhere

- If the amniotic membrane ruptures during the examination, record the FHR and time and describe the color, odor, and approximate amount of fluid. If FHR becomes unstable, determine fetal station, check for umbilical cord prolapse, and notify the doctor. After the membranes rupture, perform the vaginal examination only when labor changes significantly *to minimize*

Cervical effacement and dilation

As labor advances, so do cervical effacement and dilation, promoting delivery. During effacement, the cervix shortens and its walls become thin, progressing from 0% effacement (palpable and thick) to 100% effacement (fully indistinct, or effaced, and paper thin). Full effacement obliterates the constrictive uterine neck to create a smooth, unobstructed passageway for the fetus.

At the same time, dilation occurs. This progressive widening of the cervical canal—from the upper internal cervical os to the lower external cervical os—advances from 0 to 10 cm. As the cervical canal opens, resistance decreases. This further eases fetal descent.

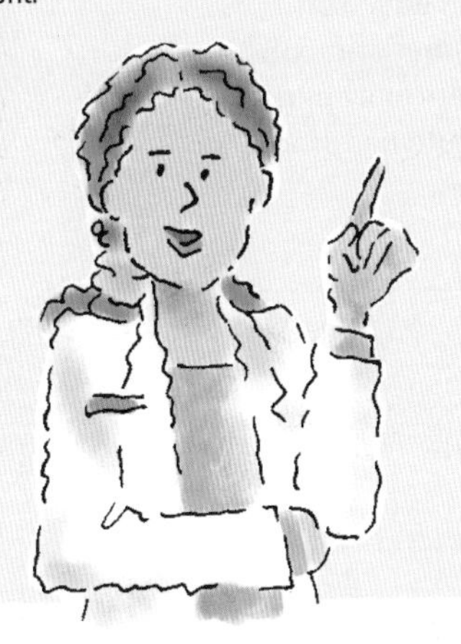

No effacement or dilation

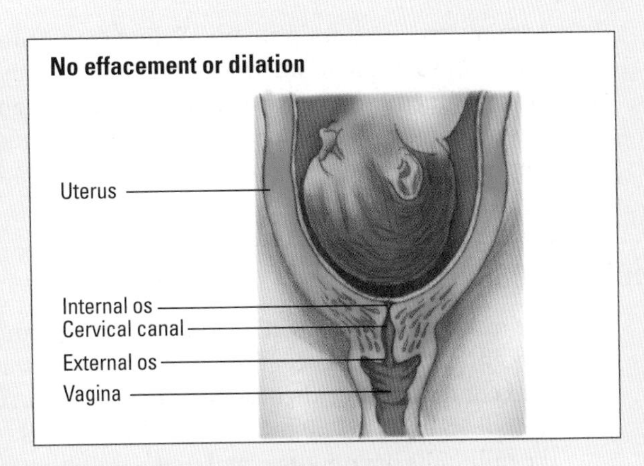

Full effacement and dilation

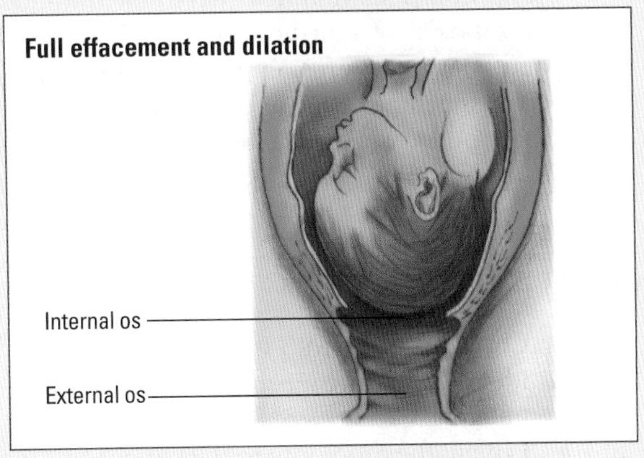

the risk of introducing intrauterine infection. (See *Documenting vaginal examination.*)

Oxytocin administration

Synthetic oxytocin (Pitocin) is used to induce or augment labor. It's also used to control bleeding and enhance uterine contraction after the placenta is delivered.

Oxytocin is always administered I.V. with an infusion pump. It may be used in pregnancy-induced hypertension, prolonged gestation, maternal diabetes, Rh sensitization, premature or prolonged rupture of membranes, incomplete or inevitable abortion, and evaluation of fetal distress after 31 weeks' gestation.

What you need

Administration set for primary I.V. line ✳ infusion pump and tubing ✳ I.V. solution as ordered ✳ external or internal fetal monitoring equipment ✳ oxytocin ✳ 20G 1″ needle ✳ label ✳ venipuncture equipment with an 18G through-the-needle catheter ✳optional: autosyringe.

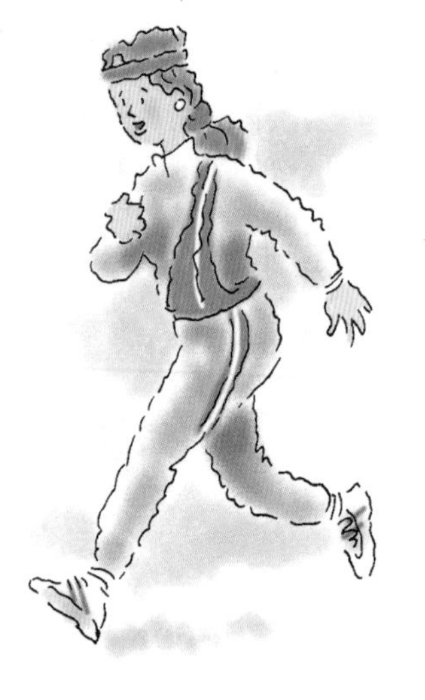
Oxytocin can get labor going in a hurry.

Getting ready

The oxytocin solution will be sent from the pharmacy as a premixed concentration. As a safety precaution, the oxytocin is mixed in a standard concentration either as 30 units in 500 mL of Lactated Ringers (LR) or 15 units in 250 mL of LR. Mixing in this concentration makes the milliunits per minute equal to the milliliters per hour. This reduces the risk of a medication error that could lead to an adverse event. Attach the infusion pump tubing to the I.V. container and connect to the pump. Set up the infusion pump and medication as per facility policy. The patient should have at least a 20-minute baseline FHR monitor strip recorded before the oxytocin is started.

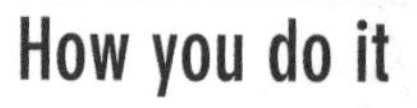

How you do it

- Check the order with the medication.
- Identify the patient using two patient identifiers per the facility policy.
- Explain the procedure to the patient and provide privacy. Perform hand hygiene.

Administering oxytocin during labor and delivery

- Help the patient to a lateral-tilt position and support her hip with a pillow.
- Identify and record the FHR and assess uterine contractions occurring in a 20-minute span.

Piggyback ride

- Start the primary I.V. line using an 18G or 20G catheter and piggyback the oxytocin solution to the primary I.V. line at the Y injection site closest to the patient.
- Begin the oxytocin infusion as ordered. The typical recommended labor-starting dosage is 0.5 to 1.0 milliunit (mU)/minute with the maximum dosage of 20 mU/minute.

And we mean now

- *Because oxytocin begins acting immediately,* be prepared to start monitoring uterine contractions. The nurse should remain in the patient's room to assess the action of the oxytocin.
- Increase the oxytocin dosage as ordered—but never infuse more than 1 to 2 mU/minute once every 30 to 60 minutes. Typically, the dosage continues at a rate that maintains activity closest to normal labor.

Everyone relaxed?

- Before each increase, be sure to assess contractions, maternal vital signs, and fetal heart rhythm and rate. If you're using an external fetal monitor, the uterine activity strip or grid should show contractions occurring every 2 to 3 minutes. The contractions should last for about 60 seconds and be followed by uterine relaxation. If you're using an internal fetal monitor, look for an optimal baseline value ranging from 5 to 15 mm Hg. Your goal is to verify uterine relaxation between contractions. (See "Fetal heart rate monitoring," page 542.)
- Assist with comfort measures, such as repositioning the patient on her other side, as needed.

Too riled up

- Continue assessing maternal and fetal responses to the oxytocin. Review the infusion rate *to prevent uterine hyperstimulation. To manage hyperstimulation,* discontinue the infusion, administer oxygen, and notify the doctor. (See *Complications of oxytocin administration,* page 566.)
- *To reduce uterine irritability,* try to increase uterine blood flow. Do this by changing the patient's position and increasing the infusion rate of the primary I.V. line.
- After hyperstimulation resolves, resume the oxytocin infusion as per your facility's policy for the appropriate method.

Administering oxytocin after delivery

- As ordered, after delivery, administer 10 to 40 units of oxytocin added to 1,000 mL of physiologic electrolyte solution. Infuse at a rate titrated to decrease postpartum bleeding or uterine atony after placental delivery. The oxytocin administered after delivery may remain on an infusion pump or may be administered by gravity in drops per minute.

Documenting oxytocin administration

In your notes, record:
- patient education
- oxytocin infusion rate in milliunits per minute
- fluid intake and output
- FHR
- uterine activity.

On the labor progression chart, record the patient's:
- response to contractions
- blood pressure
- pulse rate and pattern
- respiratory rate and quality.

Practice pointers

- Monitor and record intake and output. Output should be at least 30 mL/hour. Oxytocin has an antidiuretic effect at rates of

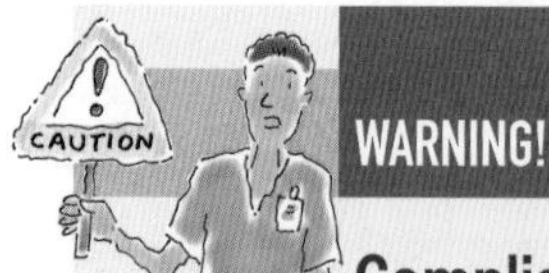

WARNING!

Complications of oxytocin administration

Oxytocin can cause uterine hyperstimulation or tachysystole. This, in turn, may progress to tetanic contractions, which last longer than 2 minutes. Signs of hyperstimulation include contractions less than 2 minutes apart and lasting 90 seconds or longer, uterine pressure that doesn't return to baseline between contractions, and intrauterine pressure that rises over 75 mm Hg.

What else to watch for

Other potential complications include fetal distress, abruptio placentae, and uterine rupture. In addition, watch for signs of oxytocin hypersensitivity such as elevated blood pressure. Rarely, oxytocin leads to maternal seizures or coma from water intoxication.

Stop signs

Contraindications to administering oxytocin include placenta previa, diagnosed cephalopelvic disproportion, fetal distress, prior classic uterine incision or uterine surgery, or active genital herpes. Oxytocin should be administered cautiously to a patient who has an overdistended uterus or a history of cervical surgery, uterine surgery, or grand multiparity.

16 mU/minute and more, so you may need to administer an electrolyte-containing I.V. solution *to maintain electrolyte balance.* (See *Documenting oxytocin administration,* page 565.)

Amniotomy

In amniotomy, the doctor or nurse-midwife uses a sterile amniohook to rupture the amniotic membranes. This prompts amniotic fluid drainage, which enhances the intensity, frequency, and duration of uterine contractions by reducing uterine volume.

Amniotomy is performed to induce or augment labor when the membranes fail to rupture spontaneously, to expedite labor after dilation begins, and to ease insertion of an intrauterine catheter and a spiral electrode for direct fetal monitoring. Amniotomy is contraindicated in high-risk pregnancies, unless more accurate fetal assessment using internal fetal monitoring is necessary. It's also contraindicated when the presenting fetal part is unengaged because of the risk of transverse lie and umbilical cord prolapse.

Because amniotomy can compress the umbilical cord, it's imperative that you keep an eye on fetal heart rate. Umbilical cord prolapse will produce a variable deceleration.

CAUTION

What you need

Povidone-iodine solution ✳ linen-saver pads ✳ bedpan ✳ soap and water ✳ 4″× 4″ gauze pads ✳ external EFM equipment or a fetoscope or Doppler stethoscope ✳ sterile gloves ✳ sterile amniohook.

Getting ready

Assemble the equipment at the patient's bedside.

How you do it

- Verify the order in the medical record.
- Identify the patient using two patient identifiers per facility policy.
- Reinforce explanation of the procedure and answer the patient's questions. Perform hand hygiene and don sterile gloves.
- Clean the perineum with soap and water or 4″ × 4″ gauze pads moistened with povidone-iodine solution and place linen-saver pads under the patient.
- Note the baseline FHR *to evaluate fetal status before and after amniotomy.*
- Open the amniohook package. Using sterile gloves, the doctor or nurse-midwife removes the amniohook from the package.

Pressure point

- If ordered, apply pressure to the uterine fundus as the amniohook is inserted vaginally to the cervical os. Then, while carefully avoiding contact with the fetal presenting part, the amniotic membrane is ruptured at the internal os.
- Evaluate FHR for at least 60 seconds after the membrane ruptures and check for large, variable decelerations in FHR suggesting cord compression. (See *Complications of amniotomy*, page 568.)
- Clean and dry the perineal area and replace the linen-saver pads.

Practice pointers

- During a vaginal examination after amniotomy, maintain strict aseptic technique *to prevent uterine infection.* For the same reason, minimize the number of examinations. (See *Documenting amniotomy.*)

Documenting amniotomy

In your notes, record:
- patient education
- FHR before and at frequent intervals immediately after amniotomy (every 5 minutes for 20 minutes and then every 30 minutes)
- presence of meconium or blood in amniotic fluid
- amount of amniotic fluid
- whether amniotic fluid has an odor
- maternal temperature every 2 hours
- labor progress as appropriate.

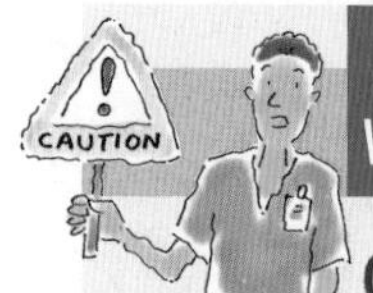

WARNING!

Complications of amniotomy

Umbilical cord prolapse—a life-threatening complication of amniotomy—is an emergency requiring immediate cesarean delivery to prevent fetal death. It occurs when amniotic fluid, gushing from the ruptured sac, sweeps the cord down through the cervix. Prolapse risk is higher if the fetal head isn't engaged in the pelvis before rupture occurs. If an emergency cesarean delivery is needed, prepare the patient and position the patient with her hips higher than her chest to try to relieve pressure off the cord. The nurse may also insert two fingers into the vagina and put pressure on the fetal presenting part to relieve the pressure on the umbilical cord. The knee-chest position can also be used to remove pressure on the umbilical cord.

Another complication, intrauterine infection, can result from failure to use aseptic technique for amniotomy or from prolonged labor after amniotomy.

The nurse's role in epidural anesthesia

Epidural anesthesia is increasing as the choice for pain relief during labor through delivery. Literature supports that three out of every five women in the United States elect to receive an epidural for their pain management during labor and delivery. The nurse assesses the women's pain during labor and educates her about alternatives for the relief of pain.

What you need

1,000 mL of LR ✳ FHR monitor ✳ patent I.V. site ✳ blood pressure monitor for woman ✳ labs collected for complete blood count to check platelet count ✳ epidural preparation cart.

Getting ready

- Identify the patient using two patient identifiers per facility policy.
- Explain the procedure to the patient. Prepare the epidural cart with the epidural set-up. Infuse between 500 and 1,000 mL of LR per physician order.

How you do it

The nurse prepares the patient for the epidural through completion of the following nursing actions.

- Assess the patient's pain level.
- Notify the anesthesiologist when the patient requests an epidural. Have informed consent available for signature after anesthesiologist informs the patients of the risks and benefits of the epidural anesthesia. The consent form must be signed and in the chart.
- Assess the baseline blood pressure, pulse, respiratory rate, and temperature.
- Assess FHR to confirm a normal pattern.
- Request the patient to void.
- Infuse the I.V. bolus per physician orders.
- Verify that the platelet count is above 100,000.
- Conduct the preprocedure verification process and perform the "time out."

Nursing actions during insertion and initial administration of the epidural anesthesia:

- The nurse assists the patient into a sitting or lateral position with head flexed toward chest.

Nursing actions after epidural administration of the epidural:

- Monitor vital signs every 5 minutes for the first 15 minutes and then follow agency protocol. Observe for hypotension, difficulty breathing, maternal tachycardia, tinnitus, dizziness, metallic taste, and loss of consciousness, as these may indicate intravascular injection.
- Assess FHR every 5 minutes after epidural administration.
- Position patient in a side-lying position to avoid supine hypotension.
- Assess pain relief and motor activity in the lower extremities.
- Monitor for pruritus, nausea, vomiting, and urinary retention. Many facilities inset a urinary catheter after the epidural.

Postpartum fundal assessment

After delivery, the uterus gradually shrinks and descends into its prepregnancy position in the pelvis—a process known as involution.

Day by day

You can evaluate involutional progress by palpating and massaging the uterus to identify uterine size, firmness, and descent. Initially, the uterus rises to the umbilicus; after the first postpartum day, it begins returning to the pelvis at a rate of 1 cm or fingerbreadth daily—slightly slower if the patient had a cesarean delivery or uterine overdistension. By the 10th postpartum day, the uterus lies deep in the pelvis, at or below the symphysis pubis.

When the uterus fails to contract or remain firm during involution, uterine bleeding or hemorrhage can result.

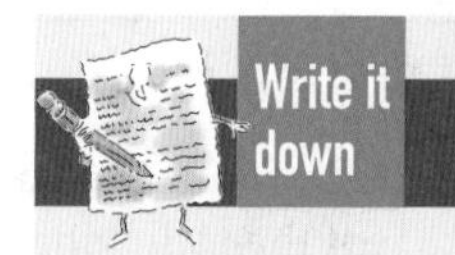

Documenting fundal assessment

In your notes, record:
- patient's vital signs
- patient education
- fundal height in centimeters or fingerbreadths
- fundal position (midline or off-center)
- fundal tone (firm or soft and boggy)
- fundal massage administered
- clot passage
- Excessive bleeding, if present, and your notification of this sign to the doctor or nurse-midwife.

What you need

Gloves ✳ analgesics ✳ perineal pad ✳ optional: urinary catheter.

Getting ready

Identify the patient using two patient identifiers per facility policy. Explain the procedure to the patient and provide privacy. Perform hand hygiene and don gloves. Unless the doctor orders otherwise, schedule fundal assessments every 15 minutes for the first hour after delivery, every 30 minutes for the next 2 to 3 hours, every hour for the next 4 hours, every 4 hours for the rest of the first postpartum day, and every 8 hours until the patient's discharge.

How you do it

- Have the patient urinate. You may need to catheterize the patient if she can't urinate.
- Lower the head of the bed until the patient lies supine or is slightly elevated and expose the abdomen for palpation and the perineum for observation. Watch for bleeding, clots, and tissue expulsion while massaging the fundus.

Two hands are better than one

- Gently compress the uterus between both hands *to evaluate uterine firmness.* (See *Hand placement for fundal palpation and massage.*) Note the level of the fundus above or below the umbilicus in fingerbreadths or centimeters.

Rub for results

- If the uterus seems soft and boggy, gently massage the fundus with a circular motion until it becomes firm. Without digging into the abdomen, gently compress and release, always supporting the lower uterine segment with the other hand. Observe for lochia flow during massage.
- Massage long enough to produce firmness but not discomfort. (See *Complications of fundal palpation.*)

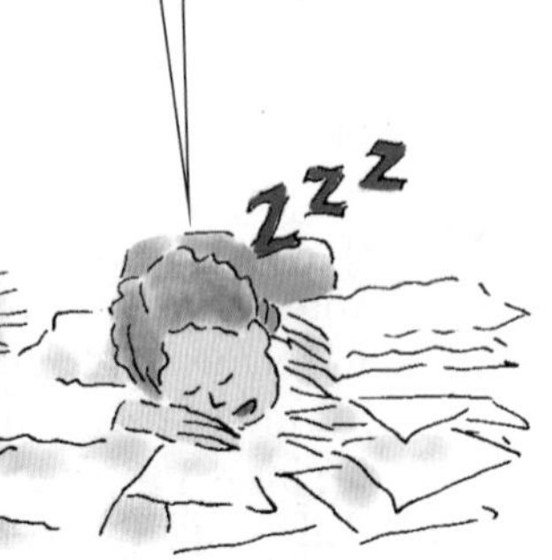
After all this reading, I'm the one who's feeling soft and boggy.
ZZZ

Hand placement for fundal palpation and massage

A full-term pregnancy stretches the ligaments supporting the uterus, placing the uterus at risk for inversion during palpation and massage. To guard against this, place one hand against the patient's abdomen at the symphysis pubis level. This steadies the fundus and prevents downward displacement. Then place the other hand at the top of the fundus, cupping it.

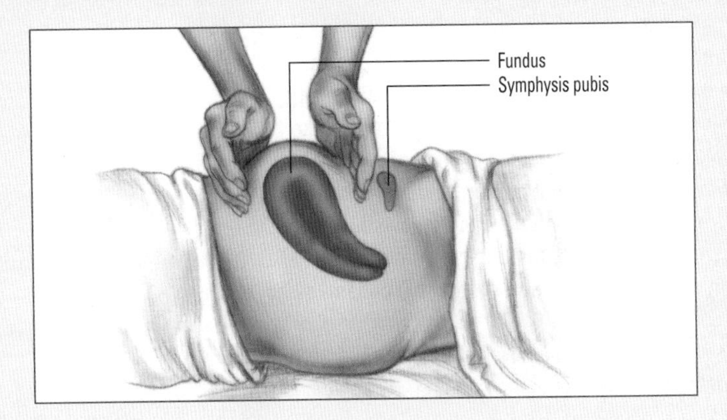

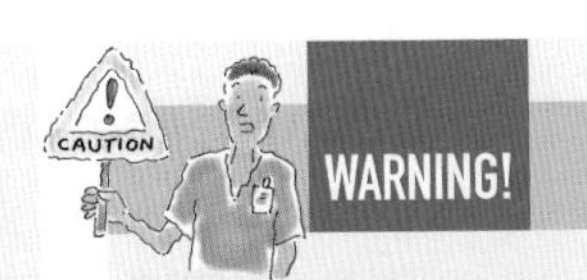

Complications of fundal palpation

Because the uterus and its supporting ligaments usually are tender after delivery, pain is the most common complication of fundal palpation and massage. Excessive massage can stimulate premature uterine contractions, causing undue muscle fatigue and leading to uterine atony or inversion. Only massage the uterus if it is boggy. Palpate first to determine the need for massage.

Lack of lochia may signal a clot blocking the cervical os. Subsequent heavy bleeding may result if a position change dislodges the clot. Take the patient's vital signs to assess for hypovolemic shock.

Cause for concern

- Notify the doctor or nurse-midwife immediately if the uterus fails to contract and if heavy bleeding occurs. If the fundus becomes firm after massage, keep one hand on the lower uterus and press gently toward the pubis *to expel clots.*
- Clean the perineum, apply a clean perineal pad, and help the patient into a comfortable position. (See *Postpartum perineal care*, page 572.)

Practice pointers

- *Because incisional pain makes fundal palpation uncomfortable for the patient who has had a cesarean section,* provide pain medication beforehand as ordered. Palpation from the sides of the uterus is also less painful. (See *Documenting fundal assessment.*)

Apgar scoring

The Apgar score quantifies neonatal heart rate, respiratory effort, muscle tone, reflexes, and color. Each category is assessed 1 minute after birth and again 5 minutes later. Scores in each category range from 0 to 2.

Postpartum perineal care

Vaginal birth (which stretches and sometimes tears the perineal tissues) and episiotomy (which may minimize tissue injury) usually cause perineal edema and tenderness. Postpartum perineal care aims to relieve discomfort, promote healing, and prevent infection.

Cleaning the perineum

- Typically, you'll use a water-jet irrigation system or a peri bottle to clean the perineum. Assist the patient to the bathroom, wash your hands, and put on gloves.
- If you're using a water-jet irrigation system, insert the prefilled cartridge containing antiseptic or medicated solution into the handle and push the disposable nozzle into the handle until you hear it click into place. Instruct the patient to sit on the commode. Next, place the nozzle parallel to the perineum and turn on the unit. Rinse the perineum for at least 2 minutes from front to back, turn off the unit, remove the nozzle, and discard the cartridge. Dry the nozzle and store it appropriately for later use.
- If you're using a peri bottle, fill it with cleaning solution and instruct the patient to pour it over the perineal area.
- Help the patient to stand up and assist her in applying a new perineal pad before returning to bed. Educate the patient not to touch the side of the pad that will be against her perineum and apply it front to back.

Assessing healing progress

- To inspect the perineum, perform hand hygiene, don gloves, ensure adequate lighting, and place the patient in the lateral Sims' position.
- When inspecting the wound area, be alert for such signs of infection as unusual swelling, redness, and foul-smelling drainage.

Even the best don't rate 11

The highest Apgar score is 10—the greatest possible sum of the five categories. The evaluation at 1 minute indicates the neonate's initial adaptation to extrauterine life. The evaluation at 5 minutes gives a clearer picture of overall status.

What you need

Apgar score sheet or neonatal assessment sheet * stethoscope * clock with second hand or Apgar timers * gloves. (See *Recording the Apgar score.*)

Getting ready

If you use Apgar timers, make sure both timers are on at the instant of birth.

Recording the Apgar score

Use this chart to record the neonatal Apgar score at 1 minute and 5 minutes after birth. For each category listed, assign a score of 0 to 2, as shown. A total score of 7 to 10 indicates good condition; 4 to 6, fair condition (the neonate may have moderate central nervous system depression, muscle flaccidity, cyanosis, and poor respirations); 0 to 3, danger (the neonate needs immediate resuscitation, as ordered).

Sign	Apgar score		
	0	1	2
Heart rate	Absent	Less than 100 beats/minute (slow)	More than 100 beats/minute
Respiratory effort	Absent	Slow, irregular	Good crying
Muscle tone	Flaccid	Some flexion and resistance to extension of extremities	Active motion
Reflex irritability	No response	Grimace or weak cry	Vigorous cry
Color	Pallor, cyanosis	Pink body, blue extremities	Completely pink

How you do it

- Note the exact time of delivery. Perform hand hygiene. Don gloves and dry the neonate *to prevent heat loss*.
- Place the neonate in a 15-degree Trendelenburg position *to promote mucus drainage*. Then position his head with the nose slightly tilted upward *to straighten the airway*.

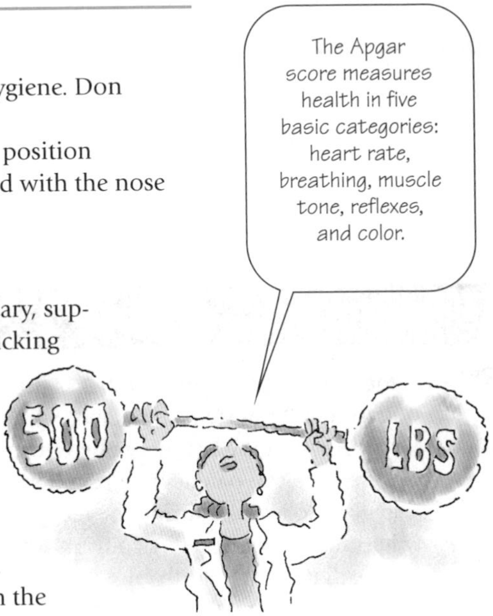

The Apgar score measures health in five basic categories: heart rate, breathing, muscle tone, reflexes, and color.

Jump start

- Assess the neonate's respiratory efforts. If necessary, supply stimulation by rubbing his back or gently flicking his foot.
- If the neonate exhibits abnormal respiratory responses, begin neonatal resuscitation according to the guidelines of the American Heart Association and the American Academy of Pediatrics. Then use the Apgar score to judge the progress and success of resuscitation efforts.
- If the neonate exhibits normal responses, assign the Apgar score at 1 minute after birth.
- Repeat the evaluation at 5 minutes after birth and record the score.

500 LBS

Assessing neonatal heart rate

- Using a stethoscope, listen to the heartbeat for 30 seconds and record the rate. To obtain beats per minute, double the rate.

Assessing respiratory effort

- Count unassisted respirations for 60 seconds, noting quality and regularity (a normal rate is 30 to 60 breaths/minute).

Assessing muscle tone

- Observe the extremities for flexion and resistance to extension. This can be done by extending the limbs and observing their rapid return to flexion—the neonate's normal state.

Assessing reflex irritability

- Observe the neonate's response to nasal suctioning with the bulb syringe or to flicking the sole of his foot.

Assessing color

- Observe skin color, especially at the extremities.
- To assess color in a dark-skinned neonate, inspect the oral mucous membranes and conjunctiva, the lips, the palms, and the soles.

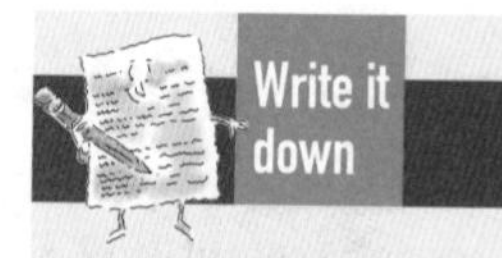

Documenting Apgar scoring

Record the Apgar score on the Apgar score sheet or the neonatal assessment sheet required by your facility. To guide postnatal care, be sure to indicate the total score and the signs for which points were deducted.

Practice pointers

- Closely observe a neonate whose mother has received heavy sedation just before delivery. Even if he has a high Apgar score at birth, he may exhibit secondary effects of sedation in the nursery. Be alert for respiratory depression or unresponsiveness. (See *Documenting Apgar scoring*.)

Measure muscle tone by extending the baby's arm or leg.

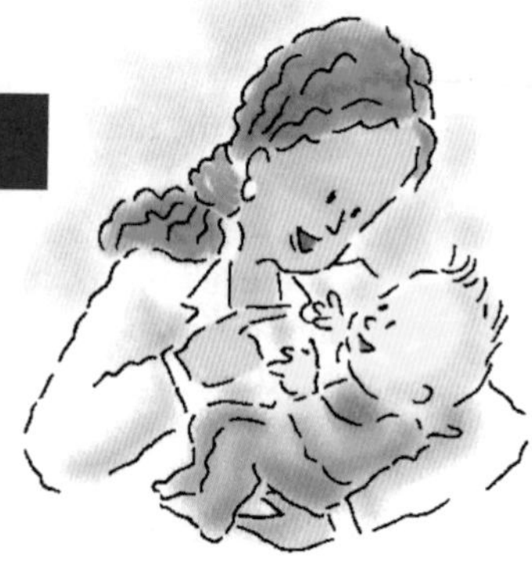

Vital signs

Measuring vital signs establishes the baseline of any neonatal assessment. Vital signs include the respiratory rate, heart rate taken apically, and the first neonatal temperature (this is taken rectally to verify rectal patency). Subsequent temperature readings are axillary to avoid injuring the rectal mucosa. Blood pressure readings may be assessed by sphygmomanometer or by palpation or auscultation. An electronic vital signs monitor may also be used. (See "Temperature," "Measuring a pulse," "Blood pressure," and "Respiration" in chapter 1, Fundamental procedures.)

What you need

Pediatric stethoscope ✱ watch with second hand ✱ gloves ✱ thermometer ✱ water-soluble lubricant ✱ sphygmomanometer with

10 (2.5 cm) cuff ✳ optional: Doppler ultrasound device with conduction gel or an electronic vital signs monitor.

Getting ready

Assemble the equipment beside the infant. If you have an electronic thermometer, apply the cover to the rectal probe. Using water-soluble lubricant, coat the probe cover before taking a rectal temperature.

How you do it

- Perform hand hygiene. Don clean gloves.

Determining respiratory rate

- Observe respirations first, before the neonate becomes active or agitated. Watch and count respiratory movements for 1 minute and record the result. Normal respiratory rate is usually 30 to 60 breaths/minute.
- *To evaluate breath sounds,* auscultate the anterior and posterior lung fields, placing the stethoscope over each lung lobe for at least 5 seconds for a total of 1 minute. Immediately after birth, you may hear a few crackles resulting from retained fetal lung fluid.

Assessing heart rate

- Place the stethoscope over the apical impulse on the fourth or fifth intercostal space at the left midclavicular line over the cardiac apex. Listen to and count the heartbeats for 1 minute. Normal heart rate is 110 to 160 beats/minute.

Taking a rectal temperature

- Wash your hands and put on gloves.
- With the neonate lying supine, place a diaper over the penis and firmly grasp his ankles with your index finger between them and insert the lubricated thermometer no more than ½″ (1.3 cm). Place the palm of your hand on his buttocks and hold the thermometer between your index and middle fingers. If you meet resistance during insertion, withdraw the thermometer and notify the doctor.
- Hold a mercury thermometer in place for 3 minutes and an electronic thermometer in place until the temperature registers. (See "Temperature" in chapter 1, Fundamental procedures.) Remove the thermometer and read the number on the digital display. Record the result.

Taking an axillary temperature

- Dry the axillary skin. Then place the thermometer in the axilla and hold it along the outer aspect of the neonate's chest between the axillary line and the arm. Hold the thermometer in place until the temperature registers. Normal temperature axillary is 97.5° F (36.38° C)—97.6° to 99° F (36.4° to 37.2° C) with rectal readings one degree higher.
- Reassess axillary temperature in 15 to 30 minutes if it registers outside the normal range. If the temperature remains abnormal, notify the doctor.
- Document the temperature.

Determining blood pressure

- Measure blood pressure in a quiet neonate.
- Make sure that the blood pressure cuff is small enough for the patient (cuff width should be about half the circumference of the neonate's arm).
- Wrap the cuff one or two fingerbreadths above the antecubital or popliteal area. The blood pressure should also be taken in the lower extremities. Hold the cuffed extremity firmly *to keep it extended* and use the monitor to measure the infant's blood pressure. Record the result. Systolic readings are 60 to 80 mm Hg, and diastolic readings are 40 to 50 mm Hg.

Documenting vital signs

Record the neonate's vital signs and related measurements in your notes, a neonatal appraisal form, or a flowchart. Include observations about the neonate's condition, such as abnormal breath sounds.

Practice pointers

- You may hear heart murmurs resulting from a delayed closing of fetal blood shunts. If you hear an unorthodox rhythm while assessing heart tones, assess whether the irregularity follows a definite or random pattern.

Get your pen ready

- Excessive neonatal activity—such as restlessness and crying during vital signs assessment—may elevate the heart rate above normal. For this reason, describe the neonate's activity along with measured findings. (See *Documenting vital signs*.)

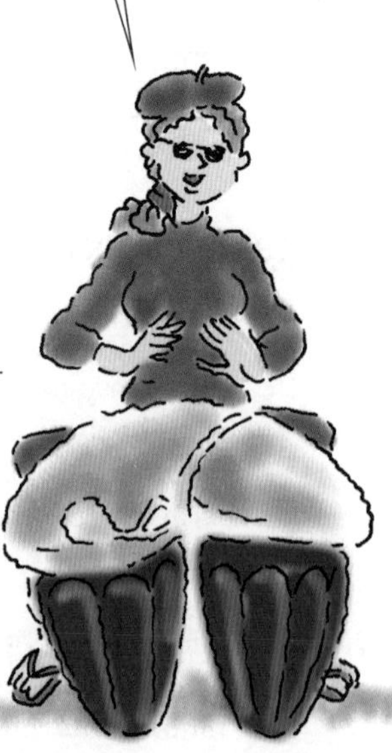
Get hip to the beat. Always check out an unusual heart rhythm.

Size and weight

Size and weight measurements establish the baseline for monitoring normal growth. Size and weight help detect such disorders as failure to thrive, small size for gestational age, and hydrocephalus. Compare the results with previous measurements and with normal values. (See *Average neonatal size and weight.*)

Average neonatal size and weight

Besides weight, anthropometric measurements include head and chest circumferences and head-to-heel length. These measurements serve as a baseline and show whether neonatal size is within normal ranges or whether there may be a significant problem or anomaly—especially if values stray far from the mean.

Average initial anthropometric ranges are:

- head circumference—13″ to 14″ (33 to 35 cm)
- chest circumference—12″ to 13″ (30 to 33 cm)
- head-to-heel—18″ to 21″ (46 to 53 cm)
- weight—5 lb 8 oz to 8 lb 13 oz. (2,500 to 4,000 g).

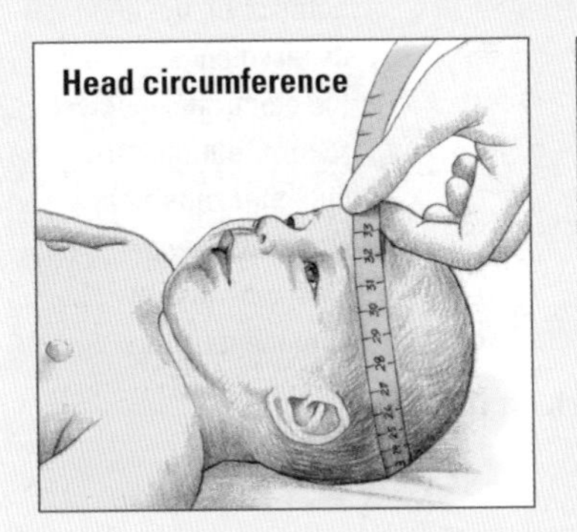
Head circumference

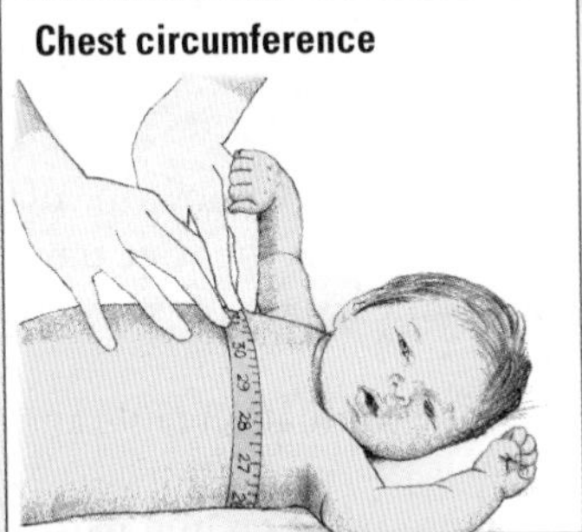
Chest circumference

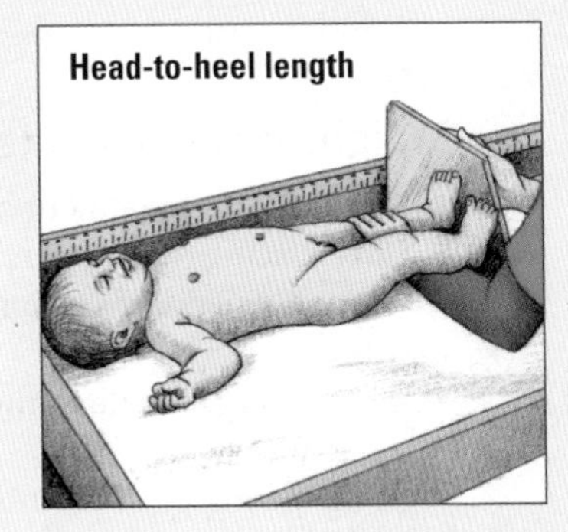
Head-to-heel length

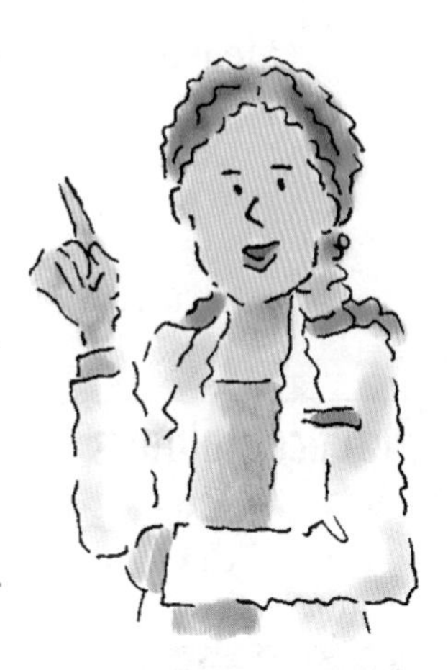

What you need

Crib or examination table with a firm surface ✳ scale with tray ✳ scale paper if necessary ✳ tape measure (disposable) ✳ length board ✳ gloves, if the neonate hasn't been bathed yet.

Getting ready

Clean the scale and place the clean paper on the scale and balance the scale at zero as directed by the manufacturer.

How you do it

- Explain the procedure to the parents if they are present. Perform hand hygiene and don gloves if you haven't bathed the neonate yet.
- To begin, position the neonate supine in the crib or on the examination table. Remove all clothing. Be sure to record all measurements.

Measuring head circumference

- Slide the tape measure under the neonate's head at the occiput and draw the tape around snugly, just above the eyebrows.

Measuring chest circumference

- Place the tape under the back and wrap it snugly around the chest at the nipple line, keeping the back and front of the tape level.
- Take the measurement after the neonate inspires and before he begins to exhale.

Measuring head-to-heel length

- Fully extend the neonate's legs with the toes pointing up. Measure the distance from the heel to the top of the head. A length board may be used, if available. The scale may also have a tape measure on the plastic bed to measure the length.

Weighing the neonate

- Take this measurement before a feeding. Remove the diaper before placing the neonate in the middle of the scale tray.
- Note the neonate's weight. Keep one hand poised over him at all times.
- Return the neonate to the crib or examination table and clean the scale tray.
- If the neonate has clothing or equipment on him (such as an I.V. armband), be sure to record this information.

Measuring abdominal girth

- Place the neonate supine and measure his girth just above the umbilicus.
- When you finish, dress and diaper the neonate, then return him to his crib or to a parent who can hold and comfort him. Always match the baby's armband with the mother's per facility policy.

Documenting size and weight

Record each neonatal weight and dimension measurement in your notes or on the neonatal assessment sheet in the electronic medical record. During routine checkups, share information with the parents, who also may be documenting their child's weight and dimensions.

Practice pointers

- Head swelling or molding after delivery may skew initial head circumference measurements. (See *Documenting size and weight.*)

Apnea monitoring

Apnea monitors signal when the breathing rate falls dangerously low. These monitors may be used for premature infants; those with life-threatening medical emergencies; and those with neurologic, respiratory, or cardiac problems. It is also used in a family history of sudden infant death syndrome or in cases of acute drug withdrawal.

Two types of monitors are used most commonly. The *thoracic impedance monitor* uses chest electrodes to detect conduction changes caused by respirations. Some models have alarm systems and memories that record cardiorespiratory patterns. The *apnea mattress*, or *underpad monitor*, relies on a transducer connected to a pressure-sensitive pad, which detects pressure changes resulting from altered chest movements. The nurse should always assess for the time length of the apnea, oxygen saturation level, and heart rate.

Many facilities will perform a car seat challenge assessment on the baby with apnea before discharge to determine if the baby develops apnea (>20 seconds), bradycardia (<80 beats/minute), or decreased oxygen saturations when sitting in the car seat for 90 to 120 minutes. If the baby passes the car seat challenge, the baby will not necessarily need home apnea monitoring.

Home delivery

Monitoring begins in the hospital (or birthing center) and continues at home, so parents will need to learn how to operate the monitor and what actions to take when the alarm sounds. (See *Using a home apnea monitor.*)

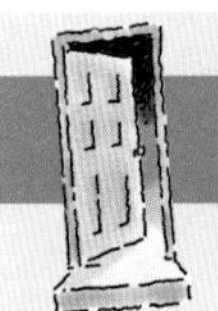

Home care connection

Using a home apnea monitor

If a neonate in your care will require the use of a home apnea monitor, you'll need to prepare his parents to operate the equipment safely, correctly, and confidently. First, review the neonate's breathing problem with his parents. Explain that the monitor will warn them of breathing or heart rate changes.

Teach the parents well

- Advise the parents to prepare their home and family for the equipment by providing a sturdy, flat surface for the monitor and by posting emergency telephone numbers (doctor, nurse, equipment supplier, and ambulance) accessibly.
- Teach other responsible family members how to use the monitor safely. Suggest that older siblings, grandparents, babysitters, and other caregivers learn cardiopulmonary resuscitation (CPR).
- Instruct the parents to notify local service authorities—police, ambulance service, telephone company, and electric company—if their neonate uses an apnea monitor so that alternative power can be supplied if a failure occurs.
- Explain to the parents how a monitor with electrodes works. Advise them to make sure the respirator indicator goes on each time the neonate breathes. If it doesn't, describe troubleshooting techniques such as moving the electrodes slightly. Tell them to try this technique several times.
- Show the parents how to respond to either the apnea or bradycardia alarm. If the neonate doesn't respond, urge them to begin CPR.
- Advise the parents to keep the operator's manual attached to or beside the monitor and to consult it as needed. Explain that an activated loose-lead alarm, for example, may indicate a dirty electrode, a loose electrode patch, a loose belt, or a disconnected or malfunctioning wire or monitor.

What you need

Monitor unit ✳ electrodes ✳ leadwires ✳ electrode belt ✳ electrode gel if needed ✳ pressure transducer pad, if using apnea mattress ✳ stable surface for monitor placement. Prepackaged and pretreated disposable electrodes are available.

Getting ready

Plug the monitor's power cord into a grounded wall outlet. Attach the leadwires to the electrodes and attach the electrodes to the belt. If appropriate, apply conduction gel to the electrodes. (Or apply gel to the neonate's chest, place the electrodes atop the gel, and attach the electrodes to the leadwires. Then secure the belt.)

How you do it

- Explain the procedure to the parents and perform hand hygiene.

Thoracic impedance monitoring

- To hold the electrodes securely in position, wrap the belt snugly around the neonate's chest at the point of greatest movement—optimally at the right and left midaxillary line about ⅘" (2 cm) below the axilla. Be sure to position the leadwires according to the manufacturer's instructions.
- Follow the color code to connect the leadwires to the patient cable. Then connect the cable to the proper jack at the rear of the monitoring unit.

You're so sensitive

- Turn the sensitivity controls to maximum *to facilitate tuning when adjusting the system.*
- Set the alarms according to recommendations so that an apneic period lasting for a specified time activates the signal.
- Turn on the monitor. If the monitor has two alarms—one to signal apnea, one to signal bradycardia—both will sound until you adjust the monitor and reset the alarms according to the manufacturer's instructions.
- Adjust the sensitivity controls until the indicator lights blink with each breath and heartbeat.

Apnea mattress or underpad monitor

- If you use an apnea mattress or underpad monitor, assemble the monitor and pressure transducer pad according to the manufacturer's directions.
- Plug the monitor into a grounded wall outlet and plug the cable of the transducer pad into the monitor.
- Touch the pad to make sure it works. Watch for the monitor's respiration light to blink.

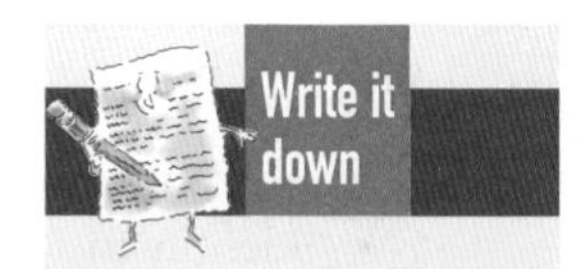

Documenting apnea monitor use

In your notes, record:
- all alarm incidents
- time and duration of the apneic episode
- neonate's color
- stimulation measures implemented
- other pertinent information.

Practice pointers

- Avoid applying lotions, oils, or powders to the neonate's chest, *where they could cause the electrode belt to slip.*
- Periodically, check the alarm by disconnecting the sensor plug. Then listen for the alarm to sound after the preset time delay. (See *Documenting apnea monitor use.*)

Administration of eye treatment

Eye treatment is administered to all newborns to prevent damage and blindness from conjunctivitis caused by *Neisseria gonorrhoeae.* It consists of instilling 1% tetracycline ointment, 0.5% erythromycin ophthalmic ointment, or 1% silver nitrate into the neonate's eyes Tetracycline and erythromycin provide the antimicrobial effects of broad-spectrum antibiotics without the chemical irritation that silver nitrate can cause. Most facilities use 0.5% erythromycin ointment. This is required by law in all 50 states.

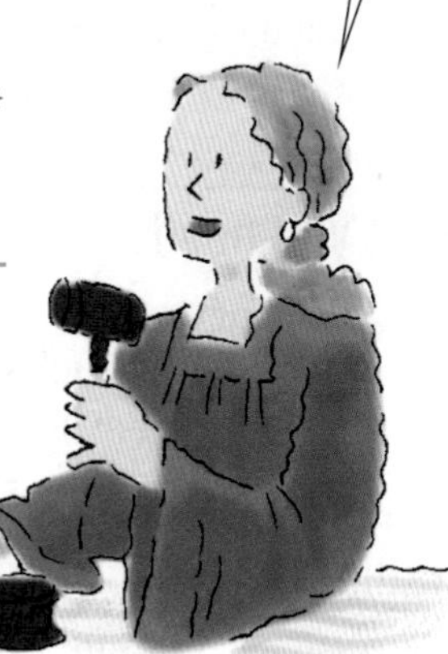
The administration of the antibiotic treatment, an important treatment to prevent neonatal blindness, is required by law in all 50 states.

What you need

Silver nitrate ampule or ophthalmic antibiotic ointment as ordered ✱ sterile needle or pin supplied by silver nitrate manufacturer ✱ gloves.

Getting ready

Puncture one end of the wax silver nitrate ampule with the needle or pin. If you're administering ophthalmic antibiotic ointment, remove the cap from the ointment container. A single-dose ointment tube should be used *to prevent contamination and spread of infection.*

How you do it

- Verify the order in the patient's medical record.
- Identify the patient using two patient identifiers per facility policy.
- If the parents are present for the procedure, explain that state law mandates the antibiotic treatment. Forewarn them that the neonate may cry and that the treatment may irritate his eyes. Reassure them that these are temporary effects.

Supply shade

- Perform hand hygiene and don gloves. *To ensure comfort and effectiveness,* shield the neonate's eyes from direct light, tilt his head slightly to the side of the intended treatment, and instill the medication. (See "Eye medications," in chapter 4, page 194.)
- Close and manipulate the eyelids to spread the medication over the eye.

Documenting the administration of eye treatment

If you perform the eye ointment in the delivery room, record the treatment on the delivery room form. If you perform it in the nursery, document it in your notes. You may wait up to 2 hours to administer the eye ointment so that parents are able to maintain eye-to-eye contact after delivery.

Practice pointers

- If chemical conjunctivitis occurs or if the skin around the neonate's eyes discolors, reassure the parents that these temporary effects will subside within a few days. Especially after silver nitrate instillation, chemical conjunctivitis may cause redness, swelling, and drainage. (See *Documenting the administration of the eye treatment.*)

Vitamin K administration

Vitamin K is administered as prophylaxis to the newborn to prevent bleeding caused by a lack of vitamin K in the newborn. The newborn does not have adequate vitamin K because of the sterile environment in the gastrointestinal (GI) tract. After feedings are introduced, the vitamin K is synthesized and then influences the coagulation factors.

What you need

Vial of vitamin K at 1 mg/0.5 mL * tuberculin syringe with a 25G ½" needle * alcohol wipe * filter needle if the vitamin K is in an ampule * cotton ball or 2 × 2 gauze * gloves * Band-Aid, if needed.

Getting ready

In many facilities, the vitamin K is administered on the left leg in the vastus lateralis muscle. Perform hand hygiene. Don gloves as it is given before the infant is bathed.

How you do it

Locate the thickest part of the vastus lateralis on the anterolateral thigh. Clean the site with an alcohol pad. Wait until it dries. Inject intramuscular (I.M.) at 90 degrees. Do not aspirate, as the size of needle length will unlikely result in injection into the vein. Inject the medication, remove the needle, and slide the safety sheath. Apply gentle pressure with the cotton ball or gauze pad. If needed, apply a Band-Aid.

Practice pointers

Location of the vastus lateralis is important and do not aspirate before injecting the vitamin K.

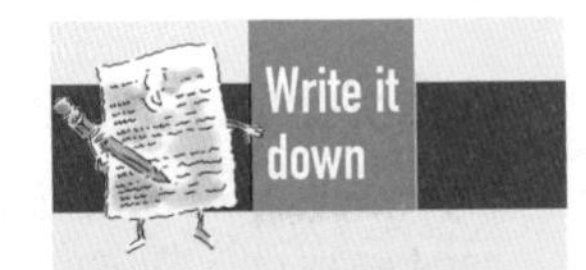

Documenting the administration of vitamin K

Document the injection of vitamin K and the location of the site in the electronic medication administration record.

Thermoregulation

Thermoregulation provides a neutral thermal environment that helps the neonate maintain a normal core temperature of 97.7° F (36.5° C) without expending excess oxygen and calories. Use a radiant warmer or isolette to control environmental temperature until the neonate's temperature stabilizes and he or she can occupy a bassinet. If the temperature doesn't stabilize or if the neonate has a condition that affects thermoregulation, a temperature-controlled incubator/isolette will house him or her. (See *Understanding thermoregulators*, page 584.)

What you need

Radiant warmer or incubator (if necessary) ✳ blankets ✳ washcloths or towels ✳ skin probe ✳ adhesive pad ✳ water-soluble lubricant ✳ thermometer ✳ clothing (including a cap).

Getting ready

Turn on the radiant warmer in the delivery room and set the desired temperature. Warm the blankets, washcloths, or towels under a heat source.

How you do it

- Continue nursing measures to conserve neonatal body warmth until the patient's discharge.

Understanding thermoregulators

Thermoregulators preserve neonatal body warmth in various ways. A radiant warmer maintains the neonate's temperature by *radiation.* An incubator/isolette maintains the neonate's temperature by *conduction* and *convection.*

Temperature settings

Radiant warmers and incubators have two operating modes: *nonservo* and *servo.* The nurse manually sets temperature controls on nonservo equipment; a probe on the neonate's skin controls temperature settings on servo models.

Other features

Most thermoregulators come with alarms. Incubators/isolettes have the added advantage of providing a stable, enclosed environment, which protects the neonate from evaporative heat loss.

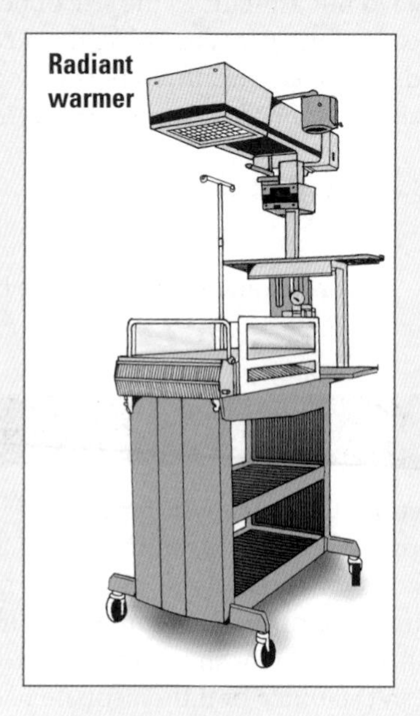
Radiant
warmer

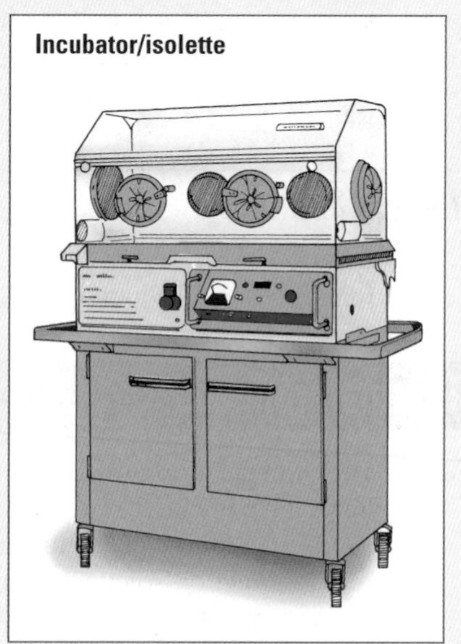
Incubator/isolette

In the delivery room

- Place the neonate under the radiant warmer, dry him with warm washcloths or towels, and then cover his head with a cap *to prevent heat loss.* Caring for the low-birth-weight infant requires the nurse to prewarm the delivery room and place the baby "in a plastic bag up to the neck during delivery room stabilization to prevent heat loss."
- Perform required procedures quickly and wrap him in the warmed blankets. If his condition permits, give him to the parents *to promote bonding.* The infant may also be placed on the mother's lower abdomen and dried so that the mother can touch her infant.
- Transport the neonate to the nursery in the warmed blankets and use a transport incubator as necessary.

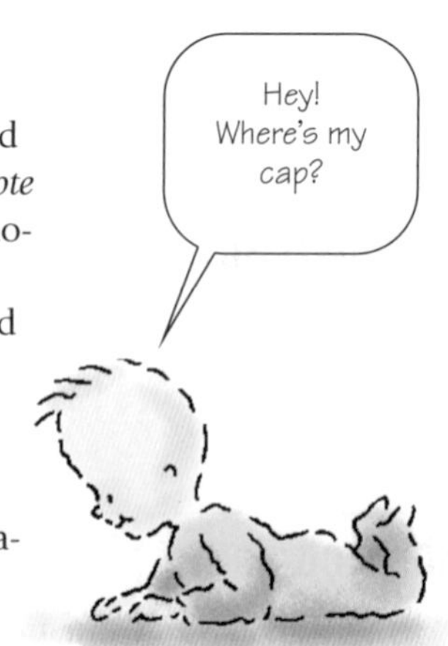
Hey!
Where's my
cap?

In the nursery

- Remove the blankets and cap and place the neonate under the radiant warmer.
- Use the adhesive pad to attach the temperature control probe to his skin in the upper right abdominal quadrant. If the neonate

will lie prone, put the skin probe on his back. Don't cover the device with anything *because this could interfere with the servo control.* Be sure to raise the warmer's side panels *to prevent accidents.*

- Take the neonate's rectal temperature on admission, then take axillary temperatures thereafter every 15 to 30 minutes until the temperature stabilizes, then every 4 hours *to ensure stability.*

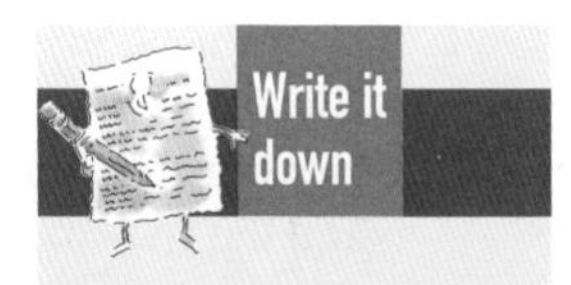

Documenting thermoregulation

In your notes, record:
- name and temperature of the heat source used
- neonate's temperature (when taken)
- Complications resulting from use of thermoregulatory equipment.

Bathing beauty

- Sponge-bathe the neonate under the warmer only after the temperature stabilizes and the glucose level is normal. Leave the baby under the warmer until the temperature remains stable.
- If the temperature doesn't stabilize, place the neonate under a plastic heat shield or in a warmed incubator, as per facility policy. Assess for signs of infection, one of which can be hypothermia.
- Apply a skin probe to the neonate in an incubator as you would for a neonate in a radiant warmer. Move the incubator away from cold walls or objects. Perform all required procedures quickly and close portholes in the hood after completion. If procedures must be performed outside the incubator, do them under a radiant warmer.

On the road

- To leave the facility or to move to a bassinet, a neonate must be weaned from the incubator by slowly reducing the temperature to that of the nursery. Check periodically for hypothermia.
- When the normal neonate's temperature stabilizes, dress him, put him in a bassinet, and cover him with a blanket.

Practice pointers

- *To prevent conductive heat loss,* preheat the radiant warmer bed and linen, warm stethoscopes and other instruments before use, and pad the scale with paper or a preweighed, warmed sheet before weighing the neonate.
- *To avoid convective heat loss,* place the neonate's bed out of direct line with an open window, fan, or an air-conditioning vent.
- *To control evaporative heat loss,* dry the neonate immediately after delivery. When bathing, expose only one body part at a time; wash each part thoroughly, and then dry it immediately. (See *Documenting thermoregulation.*)

Oxygen administration

A neonate with signs and symptoms of respiratory distress requires oxygen. Initially, nasal prongs can be used to supply this oxygen.

If the neonate is less than 32 gestational weeks, the physician may administer surfactant replacement. The administration of the surfactant occurs within 15 minutes after birth after the airway is cleared and the endotracheal tube is inserted. Research document that surfactant therapy decreases the occurrence of respiratory distress syndrome.

O_2 options

If the neonate needs continuous positive airway pressure (CPAP) to prevent alveolar collapse at the end of a breath (as in respiratory distress syndrome), he may receive oxygen through a nasopharyngeal or an endotracheal (ET) tube. (In an emergency, a handheld resuscitation bag and mask are sufficient until an ET tube can be initiated.) If the neonate cannot breathe on his or her own or needs to conserve his or her energy, he or she may receive oxygen through a ventilator. (See chapter 6, Respiratory care, for a discussion of these areas.)

What you need

Oxygen source (wall, cylinder, or liquid unit) ✻ compressed air source ✻ flowmeters ✻ nasal prongs ✻ large- and small-bore oxygen tubing (sterile) ✻ blood gas analyzer ✻ stethoscope ✻ nasogastric (NG) tube.

For handheld resuscitation bag and mask delivery

Specially sized mask with handheld resuscitation bag and pressure-release valve ✻ manometer with connectors.

For nasal prong delivery

Nasal prongs ✻ water-soluble lubricant.

For CPAP delivery

Manometer with connectors ✻ nasopharyngeal or ET tube ✻ water-soluble lubricant ✻ hypoallergenic tape.

For delivery with a ventilator

Ventilator unit with manometer and in-line thermometer ✻ specimen tubes for arterial blood gas (ABG) analyses ✻ ET tube ✻ optional: pulse oximeter.

Getting ready

Perform hand hygiene. Gather and assemble the necessary equipment.

To set up a handheld resuscitation bag and mask, place the assembled resuscitation bag and mask in the crib.

How you do it

- Always perform hand hygiene before working with a neonate *to prevent cross-contamination after handling other neonates.*

Using nasal prongs

- Match the prong size to the neonate's nose. Apply a small amount of water-soluble lubricant to the outside of the prongs. Turn on the oxygen and compressed air, if necessary. Connect the prongs to the oxygen tubing. Insert the prongs into the nose and steady them. Use transparent dressing to hold the nasal prongs in place.
- Be sure to clean the prongs each shift *to ensure patency.*

Using a handheld resuscitation bag and mask

- Turn on the oxygen and compressed air flowmeters and place the mask on the neonate's nose and mouth. Check pressure settings and mask size.
- Have another staff member notify the physician immediately.

Success signs

- The recommended compression-to-ventilation rate is 3:1, using enough pressure to cause a visible rise and fall of the chest. Provide enough oxygen to maintain the oxygen saturation at 92%.
- Continuously watch the neonate's chest movements and listen to breath sounds, avoiding overventilation. If the neonate's heart rate falls below 100 beats/minute, continue to use the handheld resuscitation bag until the heart rate rises to 100 beats/minute or higher.
- Insert an NG tube *to vent air from the neonate's stomach.*

Using CPAP

- Position the neonate on his back with a rolled towel under the neck *to keep the airway open without hyperextending the neck.*
- Assist with ET intubation. (See chapter 6, "Assisting with endotracheal tube intubation," pages 323.) Turn on the oxygen and compressed air source and attach the oxygen delivery system to the tube. Confirm placement and tape the tube in place. Next, insert an NG or orogastric tube *to keep the stomach decompressed,* if ordered. Leave it open unless the neonate is receiving gavage feedings.

Using a ventilator

- Turn on the ventilator and set the controls as ordered.
- Help the physician insert the ET tube, connect it to the ventilator, and tape the tube securely.
- Watch the manometer *to maintain pressure at the prescribed level* and monitor the in-line thermometer *for correct temperature.*

Always assess first

Assessment of heart rate, respiratory rate, and oxygenation determine the initiation of resuscitation efforts. Remember, "Once positive-pressure ventilation or supplementary oxygen administration is begun, assessment should consist of simultaneous evaluation of 3 clinical characteristics: heart rate, respiratory rate, and evaluation of the state of oxygenation. State of oxygenation is optimally determined by a pulse oximeter rather than by simple assessment of color."

Know your ABGs

- Monitor ABG levels every 15 to 20 minutes (or other reasonable interval) after any changes in oxygen concentration or pressure. If ordered, monitor oxygen perfusion with pulse oximetry or mixed venous oxygen saturation monitoring.
- Keep the physician aware of ABG levels *so he can order appropriate changes in oxygen concentration.*
- Auscultate the lungs for crackles, rhonchi, and bilateral breath sounds.

Practice pointers

- When administering oxygen, always take safety precautions *to avoid fire or explosion.* Take measures to keep the neonate warm *because hypothermia impedes respiration.* (See *Hazards of oxygen therapy.*)

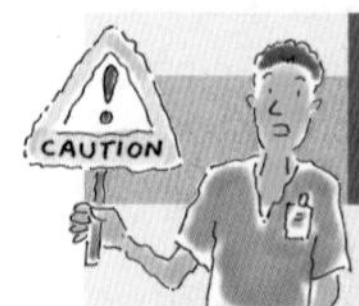

WARNING!

Hazards of oxygen therapy

No matter which system delivers the oxygen, oxygen therapy is potentially hazardous to a neonate. The gas must be warmed and humidified to prevent hypothermia and dehydration. Given in high concentrations over prolonged periods, oxygen can cause retinopathy of prematurity leading to blindness. With low oxygen concentration, hypoxia and central nervous system damage may occur. Also, depending on how it is delivered, oxygen can contribute to bronchopulmonary dysplasia.

Other worries

- Infection or "drowning" can result from overhumidification. This condition, in turn, allows water to collect in tubing, providing a growth medium for bacteria or suffocating the neonate.
- Hypothermia and increased oxygen consumption can result from administering cool oxygen.
- Metabolic and respiratory acidosis may follow inadequate ventilation.

And finally . . .

- Pressure ulcers may develop on the neonate's head, face, and around the nose during prolonged oxygen therapy.
- A pulmonary air leak (pneumothorax, pneumomediastinum, pneumopericardium, interstitial emphysema) may arise spontaneously with respiratory distress or result from forced ventilation.
- Decreased cardiac output may result from excessive CPAP.

- Check ABG or oxygenation saturation levels at least every hour whenever an unstable neonate receives high oxygen concentrations or experiences a clinical change. (See *Documenting oxygen administration*.)

Phototherapy

Phototherapy involves exposing the neonate to high-intensity fluorescent light that breaks down bilirubin (a pigment of red blood cells) for transport to the GI system and excretion. The treatment is commonly given to neonates with hyperbilirubinemia—a symptom of physiologic jaundice, breast-milk jaundice, or hemolytic disease. The bilirubin nomogram is used to determine the need for treatment with phototherapy. The age of the baby and the level of the bilirubin are plotted on the bilirubin nomogram, and the physician follows the levels to determine treatment with phototherapy.

Color correction

Phototherapy continues until bilirubin drops to normal levels because unchecked hyperbilirubinemia can lead to kernicterus (deposits of unconjugated bilirubin in the brain cells), permanent brain damage, and even death.

What you need

Phototherapy unit ✱ photometer ✱ opaque eye mask ✱ thermometer ✱ urinometer ✱ surgical face mask or small diaper ✱ optional: thermistor (if the phototherapy unit is combined with a temperature-controlled radiant heat warmer) or incubator (if the neonate is small for his gestational age); bilimeter. Prepackaged eye coverings are available.

Getting ready

Set up the phototherapy unit about 18″ to 20″ above the neonate's crib and verify placement of the light bulb shield. If the neonate is in an incubator, place the phototherapy unit at least 2″ to 3″ above the incubator and turn on the lights. Place a photometer probe in the middle of the crib *to measure the energy emitted by the lights*; average range is 6 to 8 μw/cm^2/nm.

Documenting oxygen administration

In your notes, record:
- family education
- respiratory distress requiring oxygen administration
- oxygen concentration given
- oxygen delivery method used
- each change in oxygen concentration
- routine checks of oxygen concentration
- neonate's fraction of inspired oxygen (as measured by the oxygen analyzer)
- ABG values, noting the time that each sample was obtained
- each time suctioning is performed
- amount and consistency of mucus
- type of continuous oxygen monitoring, usually pulse oximetry is used
- complications, such as absent or diminished breath sounds
- neonate's condition during oxygen therapy, including respiratory rate (with breath sound descriptions) and signs of additional respiratory distress.

How you do it

- Identify the patient using two patient identifiers per facility policy.
- Explain the procedure to the parents.
- Record the neonate's initial bilirubin level and axillary temperature.
- Place the opaque eye mask over the neonate's closed eyes and fasten securely.

Dress code

- Undress the neonate and place a diaper under him. Cover male genitalia with a surgical mask or a small diaper *to catch urine and to prevent possible testicular damage from the heat and light waves.*
- Take the neonate's axillary temperature every 2 hours and provide additional warmth by adjusting the warming unit's thermostat.
- Monitor elimination and weigh the neonate twice daily. Watch for dehydration signs (dry skin, poor turgor, depressed fontanels) and check urine specific gravity with a urinometer, if ordered, to *gauge hydration status.*

Eye spy

- Take the neonate out of the crib, turn off the phototherapy lights, and unmask his eyes at least every 3 to 4 hours with feedings. Assess his eyes for inflammation or injury.

All-over tan

- Reposition the neonate every 2 hours *to expose all body surfaces to the light and to prevent head molding and skin breakdown from pressure.*
- Check the bilirubin level at least once every 24 hours—more often if levels rise significantly. Turn off the phototherapy unit before drawing venous blood for testing *because the lights may degrade bilirubin in the blood.* Notify the doctor if the bilirubin level nears 20 mg/dl in full-term neonates or 15 mg/dl in premature neonates.

Practice pointers

- Clean the neonate's eyes periodically *to remove drainage and check circulation.*
- If the physician diagnoses breast-feeding jaundice, teach the mother to express milk manually or with a pump. Encourage continued breast-feeding when indicated.
- Monitor for bronze baby syndrome (an idiopathic darkening of the skin, serum, and urine). (See *Documenting phototherapy.*)

Documenting phototherapy

In your notes, record:
- family education
- progress of phototherapy (at least once every 2 hours)
- maintenance of neonatal eye protection
- eye covering changes and eye care given
- times of bilirubin testing (with plotting of test results)
- radiant energy measurement (initially and then every 8 hours)
- neonate's time away from the lights (for example, for feeding or other procedures)
- neonatal fluid intake
- amount of urine and feces eliminated
- changes in skin appearance and characteristics, feeding patterns, and activity level.

Breast-feeding assistance

Breast-feeding is the safest, simplest, and least expensive way to provide complete infant nourishment. Successful and satisfying breast-feeding includes proper breast care, normal milk flow, and a comfortably positioned mother and infant. Breast-feeding is contraindicated for a mother with a severe chronic condition, such as active tuberculosis, human immunodeficiency virus infection, or hepatitis. The Association of Women's Health, Obstetric and Neonatal Nurses support the Healthy People 2020 goal for breast-feeding to include breast-feeding initiation at 81.9%, with continued breast-feeding at 60.6% at 6 months, and 34.1% at 1 year of age.

What you need

Nursing or support bra ✱ pillow ✱ protective cover, such as cloth diaper or small towel ✱ optional: commercially available breast pads without plastic liners, or pads made from sanitary napkins, gauze, cloth diapers, or cotton handkerchiefs; instructional materials.

Getting ready

Explain the procedure and provide privacy. Encourage the mother to drink a beverage before and during or after breast-feeding to *ensure adequate fluid intake and maintain milk production.* Urge her to attend to personal needs and change the infant's diaper before breast-feeding begins *to avoid feeding interruptions.*

How you do it

- Perform hand hygiene and instruct the mother to do the same.
- Help the mother find a comfortable position. (See *Breast-feeding positions,* page 592.) Have her expose one breast and rest the nape of the infant's neck in the crook of her arm, supporting his back with her forearm.

Easy does it

- Encourage the mother to relax.
- Guiding the mother's free hand, have her place her thumb on top of the exposed breast's areola and her first two fingers beneath it, forming a "C" with her hand. Turn the infant so that he faces the breast.

Putting down roots

- Tell the mother to stroke the infant's cheek located nearest her exposed breast or the infant's mouth with the nipple to *stimulate the rooting instinct.*

Breast-feeding positions

A breast-feeding position should be comfortable and efficient. By changing positions periodically, the maternity patient can alter the infant's grasp on the nipple and thereby avoid contact friction on the same area. As appropriate, suggest these typical breast-feeding positions.

Cradle position

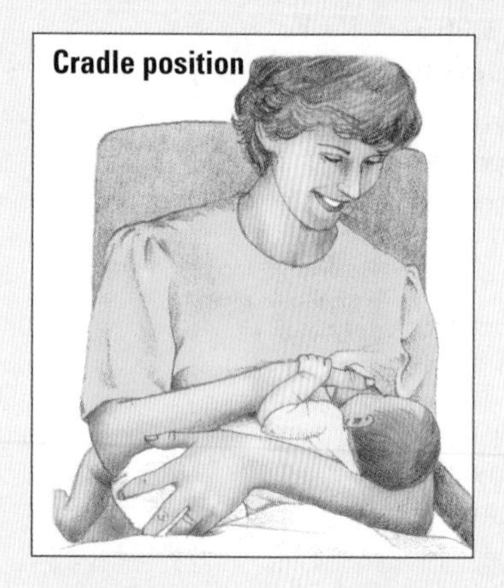

The mother cradles the infant's head in the crook of her arm.

Side-lying position

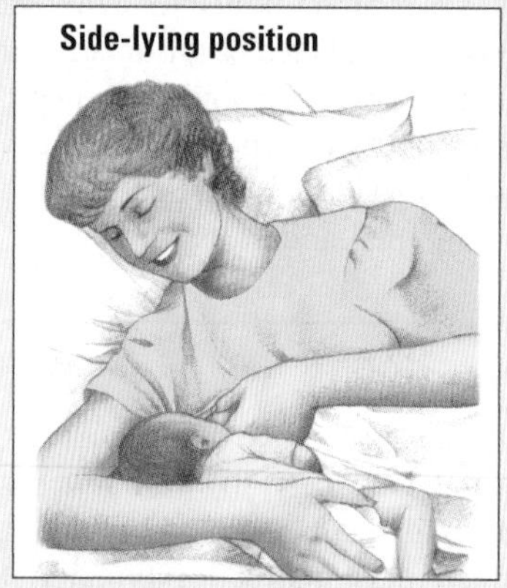

The mother lies on her side with her stomach facing the infant's. As the infant's mouth opens, she pulls him toward the nipple.

Football position

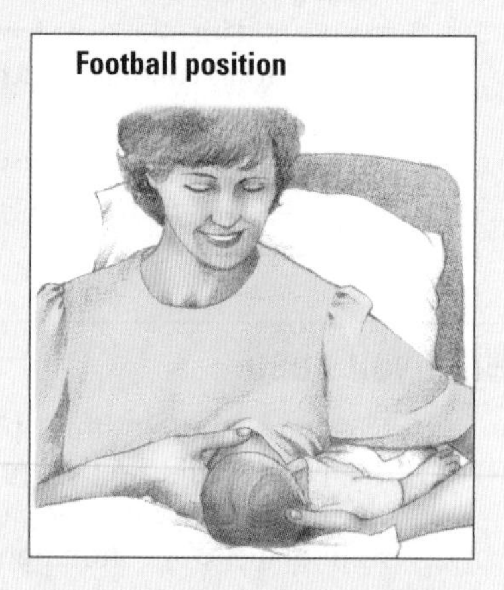

Sitting with a pillow under her arm, the mother places her hand under the infant's head. As the infant's mouth opens, she pulls his head near her breast.

- When the infant opens his mouth, have the mother insert the nipple and as much of the areola as possible into his mouth.
- Check for occlusion of the infant's nostrils by the mother's breast. If this happens, reposition the infant to give him room to breathe.

Here to there

- Suggest that the mother begin nursing the infant for 15 minutes on each breast.
- To alternate breasts, instruct the mother to slip a finger into the side of the infant's mouth *to break the seal* and move him to the other breast.

Excuse me

- *To burp the infant,* have the mother hold the infant in an upright forward-tilting position with one hand supporting his chest and chin. Tell her to gently pat or rub the infant's back *to expel any ingested air.* Help her place a protective cover, such as a cloth diaper, under the infant's chin.

Breast care for new mothers

A mother who plans to breast-feed her infant should prepare her breasts as directed by her doctor. After the infant's birth, she'll need to maintain breast tissue integrity. Although postpartum care varies for breast-feeding and non-breast-feeding mothers, both may benefit from the following guidelines.

For the breast-feeding mother

- Instruct the mother to wash her areolae and nipples with water, without soap or a washcloth, to avoid washing away the natural oils and keratin.
- Advise the mother with sore or irritated nipples to apply ice compresses just before breast-feeding. This numbs and firms the nipples, making them less sensitive and easier for the infant to grasp.
- Suggest that lubricating the nipple with a few drops of expressed breast milk before feeding may help prevent tenderness.
- Recommend placing breast pads over the nipples to collect colostrum or milk, which commonly leaks during the first few breast-feeding weeks. Advise replacing pads often to guard against infection.
- Inform the mother that breast milk comes in 2 to 5 days after delivery and is accompanied by a slight temperature elevation and breast changes—increased size, warmth, and firmness.
- Tell the mother that a well-fitting support bra may help control engorgement.
- Advise the mother with engorged breasts to apply warm compresses, massage the breasts, take a warm shower, or express some milk before feeding. This dilates the milk ducts, promotes letdown, and makes the nipples more pliable.

For the non-breast-feeding mother

- Instruct the mother to clean her breasts using the same technique as the breast-feeding mother. Add that she may use soap.
- Advise her to wear a support bra to help minimize engorgement and to decrease nipple stimulation.
- Advise her to avoid stimulating the nipples or manually expressing her milk to minimize further milk production. Instead, provide pain medication, as ordered, ice packs, or a breast binder.

- When the mother finishes breast-feeding, she should place the infant on his back.
- Instruct the mother to air-dry her nipples for 15 minutes after she finishes feeding and give her additional breast-care instructions as necessary. (See *Breast care for new mothers.*)
- Instruct the mother on signs of complications to report. (See *Breast-feeding complications,* page 594.)

Practice pointers

- Reassure the mother that no standard schedule for breast-feeding exists and that developing a comfortable breast-feeding routine takes time.
- Tell her to expect uterine cramping during breast-feeding until her uterus returns to its original size.

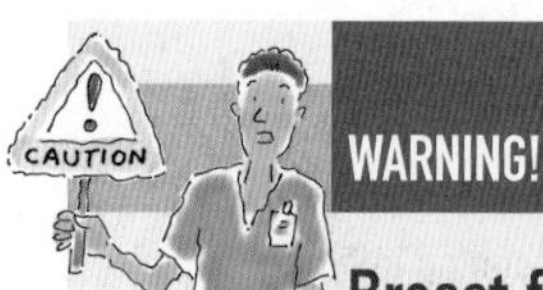

WARNING!

Breast-feeding complications

Breast-feeding may cause complications, such as breast engorgement and mastitis.

Too much milk

Breast engorgement may result from venous and lymphatic stasis and alveolar milk accumulation. Advise the mother to start breast-feeding with the breast she used last at the previous feeding to help avoid breast engorgement. Suggest attaching a safety pin to the bra strap supporting the breast she last used to serve as a reminder.

When sharing is bad

Instruct the mother to report signs of mastitis—a red, tender, or warm breast and fever—that may occur after discharge. Mastitis occurs postpartum in about 1% of mothers. It usually results from a pathogen that passes from the infant's nose or pharynx into breast tissue through a cracked or fissured nipple.

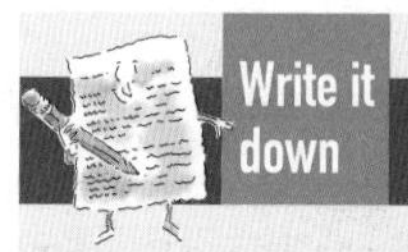

Write it down

Documenting breast-feeding assistance

After helping the mother breast-feed, record:

- patient teaching provided
- topics in which she needs further instruction
- feeding times on each breast
- feeding positions used
- neonate's sucking ability
- difficulty arousing the neonate
- nipple assessment findings.

Learning curve

- If the infant shows little interest in breast-feeding, reassure the mother that he may need several days to learn and to adjust. If the infant is sleepy, advise her to try rubbing the infant's feet, unwrapping his blanket, changing his diaper, changing her position or the infant's position, and manually expressing milk and then allowing the infant to suckle.

Mom needs to eat, too

- Urge the mother to eat balanced meals, to drink at least eight 8-oz glasses of fluid daily, and to nap daily for at least the first 2 weeks after giving birth. Before she goes home, inform her about local breast-feeding and parenting support groups such as La Leche League International. (See *Documenting breast-feeding assistance*.)

Breast pumps

By creating suction, manual and electric breast pumps stimulate lactation. They are used when the mother and her infant are separated or while illness temporarily incapacitates one or the other, or both. A breast pump also can relieve engorgement, collect milk for a premature infant with a weak sucking reflex, reduce pressure on sore or cracked nipples, or to reestablish milk supply if a weaned infant becomes allergic to formula. The mother can also use it to collect milk from inverted nipples or when she cannot express milk by hand.

What you need

Manual cylinder or electric breast pump ✻ sterile collection bag or bottle (to store milk if desired) ✻ optional: warm compresses.

An electric breast pump should come with a sterile, single-use accessory kit, which many pump manufacturers supply. The kit contains shields, milk cups, an overflow bottle, and tubing. These parts can be washed with soap and water and then sterilized for repeated use.

Getting ready

Assemble the breast pump according to the manufacturer's instructions. If milk will be stored or frozen, thoroughly clean any removable parts that the milk will touch.

How you do it

- Explain the procedure, provide privacy, and give the patient time to attend to personal needs, and have her wash her hands.
- Help the patient to assume a comfortable position and to relax. Offer pillows and provide privacy.

Visit to the vending machine

- Instruct the patient to drink a beverage before and after breast pumping.
- If the patient's breasts are engorged, have her apply warm compresses for 5 minutes or take a warm shower.
- *To help trigger the release of milk-producing hormones*, instruct the patient to use her thumb and forefinger to stimulate the nipple and areola for 1 to 2 minutes.

Using a manual cylinder pump

- Instruct the patient to place the flange or shield against her breast with the nipple in the center of the device. Have her pump each breast using a piston-like motion until it is empty.
- If the milk will be stored or frozen, direct the patient to fill a sterile plastic bottle with the milk. If the infant will drink the milk directly, attach a rubber nipple to the cylinder.

Using a battery-powered or electric breast pump

- Unless the pump is battery-powered, make sure the pump has a three-pronged plug to ground it *to prevent electric shock.*
- Instruct the patient to set the suction regulator on low and to hold the collection unit upright while centering the nipple in the shield.
- Direct her to activate the machine and adjust the suction regulator to achieve a comfortable pressure.

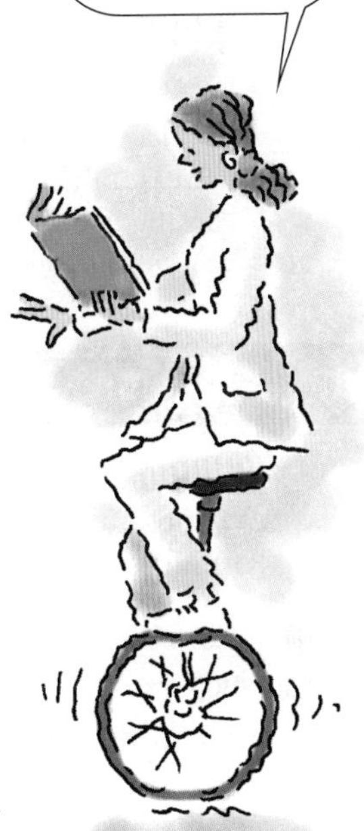

That's interesting. To trigger milk hormones before pumping, rub the nipple and areola for up to 2 minutes.

Start, stop, start

- Instruct her to pump each breast for 5 to 8 minutes or until the spray grows scant. Then pump each breast again for 3 to 5 minutes and then again for 2 to 3 minutes. (Usually, 8 oz can be pumped within 15 to 30 minutes.)
- Tell the patient to remove the shield from the breast by inserting a finger between the breast and the shield while on the low setting, then have her turn off the machine.

Documenting breast pump assistance

Record the duration that the patient pumped each breast, the amount of milk collected, and the patient's tolerance of the procedure.

Now or later

- If the milk will be stored or frozen, pour it from the collection unit into a sterile plastic container. (If it will be frozen, place it in the freezer immediately.)
- If the infant will drink the milk directly, pour it into a sterile plastic bottle.
- Label the collected milk with the date, the time of collection, and the amount. Also, be sure the label contains the infant's name if applicable.

Concluding the procedure

- Instruct the patient to air-dry her nipples for about 15 minutes.
- Instruct her to disassemble the removable parts of the pump and wash them according to the manufacturer's directions.

Practice pointers

- Be sure to use a sterile plastic collection bottle for the milk *because antibodies in the breast milk will adhere to a glass bottle.*
- Breast milk can be stored in the refrigerator for 48 hours and in the freezer at 0° F (−17.8° C) for up to 6 months. (See *Documenting breast pump assistance.*)

Bottle-feeding

When a neonate requires a special diet, or when a mother cannot or chooses not to breast-feed, formula is the next best food source. Formula preparations supply all needed vitamins and nutrients and can be administered by anyone.

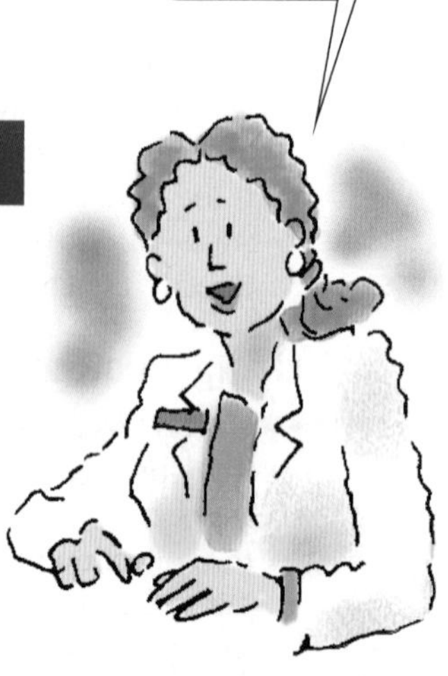
If the mother is not breast-feeding, the neonate can get all the vitamins and minerals he needs from formula.

Packaged food

Most formulas used in hospitals come ready-to-feed in disposable containers. Some formulas and equipment, however, may require advance preparation, such as mixing and sterilization.

What you need

Commercially prepared formula or ingredients ✳ bottle, nipple, and cap ✳ tissue or cloth. Hospitals commonly use disposable bottle and nipple units for neonatal feeding.

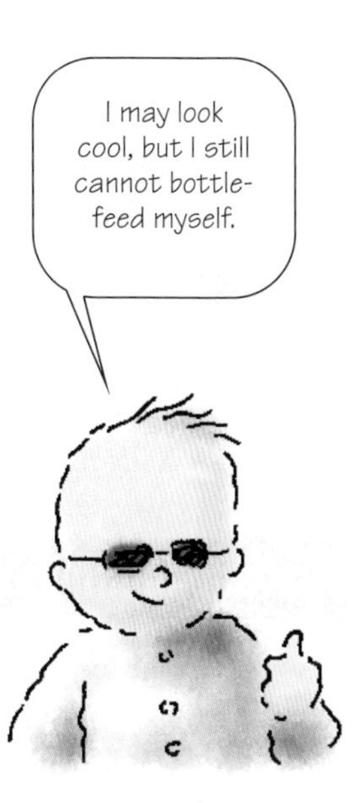
I may look cool, but I still cannot bottle-feed myself.

Getting ready

If you are using commercially prepared formula, uncap the formula bottle and make sure the seal was not previously broken *to ensure sterility and freshness*. Then screw on the nipple and cap. Keep the protective sterile cap over the nipple until the neonate is ready to feed. If you are preparing formula, follow the manufacturer's instructions or the doctor's prescription. Administer the formula at room temperature or slightly warmer.

How you do it

- Perform hand hygiene.

Drip test

- Invert the bottle and shake some formula on your wrist *to test the patency of the nipple hole and the formula's temperature*. The nipple hole should allow formula to drip freely but not to stream out.
- Sit comfortably in a semireclining position and cradle the neonate in one arm to support his head and back. If he cannot be held, sit by him and elevate his head and shoulders slightly.

Tickle the chin

- Place the nipple in the neonate's mouth while making sure the tongue is down. He should begin to suck, pulling in as much nipple as is comfortable. If he doesn't start to suck, stroke him under the chin or on his cheek, or touch his lips with the nipple *to stimulate his sucking reflex*.
- As the neonate feeds, tilt the bottle upward *to keep the nipple filled with formula* and watch for a steady stream of bubbles in the bottle, indicating proper venting and flow.

He does not have to say "excuse me"

- Burp the neonate after each ½ oz of formula.
- After you finish feeding and burping the neonate, place him on his back to prevent aspiration if he regurgitates.
- Discard any remaining formula and dispose of equipment.

Practice pointers

- Always hold the bottle for a neonate. If left to feed for himself, he may aspirate formula.

Try, try again

- If the neonate pushes out the nipple with his tongue, reinsert the nipple. Expelling the nipple is a normal reflex. It does not necessarily mean that the neonate is full. (See *Documenting bottle-feeding*.)

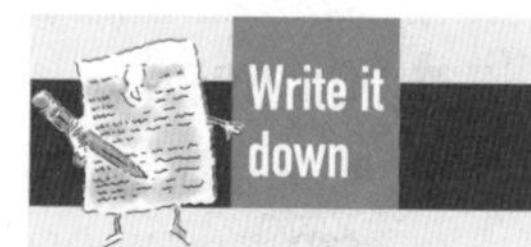

Documenting bottle-feeding

In your notes, record:
- times of feedings
- amount of formula consumed
- how well the neonate fed
- whether the neonate seemed satisfied
- regurgitation or vomiting.

If the mother fed him, observe and describe the mother–child interaction and document patient teaching provided.

Gavage feeding

Gavage feeding involves passing nutrients directly to the neonate's stomach by a tube advanced nasally or orally. If a neonate can't suck (because of prematurity, illness, or congenital deformity) or is at risk for aspiration (because of gastroesophageal reflux, ineffective gag reflex, or easy tiring), gavage feeding supplies nutrients until he is ready to take food by mouth.

What you need

Feeding tube (#3½ to #6 French for NG feeding of premature neonate; #8 French for others) ✳ feeding reservoir or large (20- to 50-mL) syringe ✳ prescribed formula or breast milk ✳ sterile water ✳ tape ✳ stethoscope ✳ gloves ✳ pacifier. A commercial feeding reservoir is available.

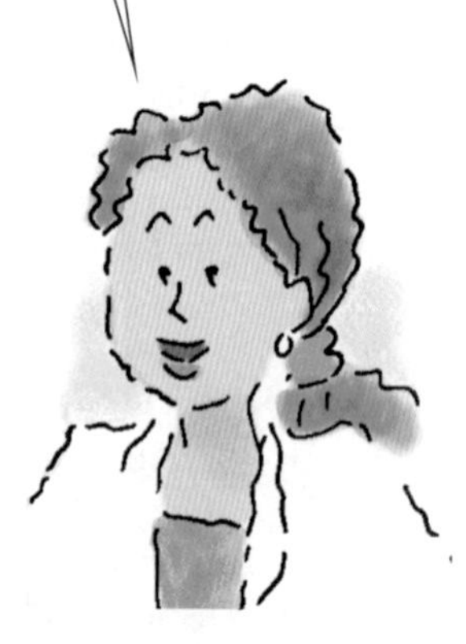
Gavage feeding provides an alternate food route when the newborn cannot suck.

Getting ready

Allow the formula or breast milk to warm to room temperature if necessary. Wash your hands and open the sterile water if it comes in a small-sized disposable container. Remove the syringe or reservoir and the feeding tube from the packaging.

How you do it

- Identify the neonate using two patient identifiers and verify the doctor's orders.
- Position the neonate supine, with the head of his mattress elevated one notch, or tilted slightly to his right with his head and chest slightly elevated.

- Perform hand hygiene and don gloves. Stabilize the neonate's head with one hand and lubricate the feeding tube with sterile water with the other hand.

Didn't I read that?

- Insert the feeding tube as described in "Feeding tube insertion and removal," in chapter 8, Gastrointestinal care.
- Synchronize tube insertion with throat movement if the neonate swallows *to facilitate tube passage into the stomach.* During insertion, watch for choking and cyanosis, signs that a tube has entered the trachea. If these occur, remove the tube and reinsert it. Also watch for bradycardia and apnea resulting from vagal stimulation.
- If the tube will remain in place, tape it flat to the neonate's cheek.

Destination check

- Make sure the tube is in the stomach (and not the lungs) by aspirating residual stomach contents with the syringe and checking the content's pH. Note the volume obtained and then reinject or, as ordered, reduce the feeding volume by the residual amount or prolong the interval between feedings. You can also check placement by injecting 0.5 to 1 cc of air into the tube while listening with the stethoscope for air sounds in the stomach and on each side of the anterior chest.
- When the tube is in place, fill the feeding reservoir or syringe with formula or breast milk. Connect the feeding reservoir or syringe to the top of the tube and start the feeding.
  - Many preterm neonates receive their tube feedings over an extended period of time (30 minutes to 1 hour). The breast milk/formula is placed on an infusion pump to deliver the feeding slowly over the prescribed time period.
- If the neonate is on your lap, hold the container about 4" (10 cm) above his abdomen. If he's lying down, hold it between 6" and 8" (15 and 20 cm) above his head. When using a commercial feeding reservoir, look for air bubbles in the container, an indicator of formula passage.

Just like the bottle

- Regulate flow by raising and lowering the container so the feeding takes 15 to 20 minutes, the average time for a bottle-feeding.
- When the feeding is finished, pinch off the tubing before air enters the neonate's stomach.
- Withdraw the tube smoothly and quickly. If the tube will remain in place, flush it with several milliliters of sterile water if ordered.
- Burp the neonate *to decrease abdominal distention.*
- Place him on his back or right side for 1 hour after feeding.

Practice pointers

- Observe a premature neonate for indications that he is ready to begin bottle- or breast-feeding: strong sucking reflex, coordinated sucking and swallowing, alertness before feeding, and sleep after feeding. These feeding readiness behaviors usually begin about 32 gestational weeks but can vary based on the infant's development.
- Provide the neonate with a pacifier during feeding *to soothe him, to help prevent gagging, and to promote an association between sucking and the full feeling that follows feeding.* (See *Documenting gavage feeding*.)

Documenting gavage feeding

In your notes, record:

- amount of residual fluid
- amount currently taken
- type and amount of any vomitus
- adverse reactions to tube insertion or feeding.

Circumcision

Circumcision is the removal of the penile foreskin. It is thought to promote a clean glans, minimize the risk of phimosis (foreskin tightening) in later life, and reduce the risk of penile cancer and cervical cancer in sexual partners. However, after 40 years of research on the benefits and risks of circumcision, the American Academy of Pediatrics has concluded that it cannot recommend a policy of routine newborn circumcision.

Slice or stretch

One method of circumcision involves removing the foreskin by using a Yellen clamp to stabilize the penis. With this device, a cone fits over the glans, providing a cutting surface and protecting the glans penis. Another technique uses a plastic circumcision bell (Plastibell) over the glans and a suture tied tightly around the base of the foreskin. This method prevents bleeding. The resultant ischemia causes the foreskin to slough off within 5 to 8 days. This method is thought to be painless because it stretches the foreskin, which inhibits sensory conduction.

What you need

Circumcision tray (contents vary but usually include circumcision clamps, various-sized cones, scalpel, probe, scissors, forceps, sterile basin, sterile towel, and sterile drapes) ✳ povidone-iodine solution ✳ restraining board with arm and leg restraints ✳ sterile gloves ✳ petroleum gauze ✳ sterile 4″ × 4″ gauze pads ✳ anesthetic agent ✳ optional: sutures, plastic circumcision bell, antimicrobial ointment, topical anesthetic, and overhead warmer.

Getting ready

Using a Yellen clamp

Assemble the sterile tray and other equipment in the procedure area. Open the sterile tray and pour povidone-iodine solution into the sterile basin. Using aseptic technique, place sterile 4″ × 4″ gauze pads and petroleum gauze on the sterile tray. Arrange the restraining board and direct adequate light on the area.

Using a plastic circumcision bell

You will not need a circumcision tray but do assemble sterile gloves, sutures, restraining board, petroleum gauze and, if ordered, antibiotic ointment. A mohel usually brings his own equipment.

How you do it

- Beforehand, make sure the parents understand the procedure and have signed the proper consent form.
- Withhold feeding for at least 1 hour before the procedure *to reduce the possibility of emesis or aspiration, or both.*
- Perform hand hygiene. Identify the patient using two patient identifiers. Place the neonate on the restraining board and restrain his arms and legs. Don't leave him unattended.
- Assist the physician as necessary throughout the procedure and comfort the neonate as needed.
- Secure oral sucrose, which can be given in small amounts to the baby during the procedure. Oral sucrose has been documented as an effective analgesic for reducing crying time during and after the circumcision.
- After putting on sterile gloves, the physician will clean the penis and scrotum with povidone-iodine, drape the neonate, and administer a local anesthetic.

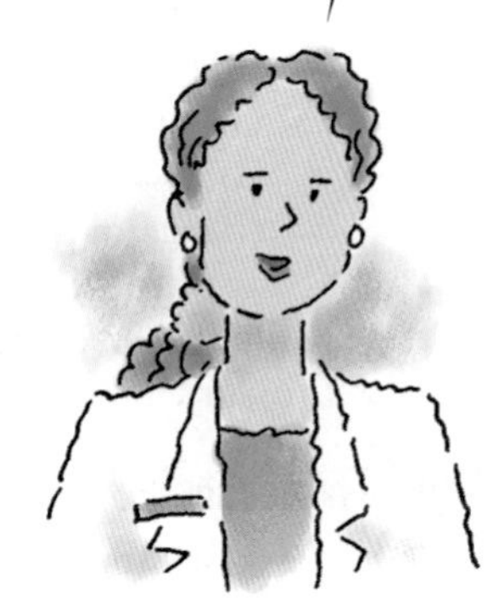
Make sure the newborn has not eaten for at least 1 hour before circumcision.

Using a Yellen clamp

- The physician will apply a Yellen clamp to the penis, loosen the foreskin, insert the cone under it *to provide a cutting surface and to protect the penis,* and remove the foreskin.
- Then he will cover the wound with sterile petroleum gauze *to prevent infection and control bleeding.*

Using a plastic bell

- The doctor will slide the plastic bell device between the foreskin and the glans penis.
- Then the physician will tie a suture tightly around the foreskin at the coronal edge of the glans. The foreskin distal to the suture will become ischemic and then atrophic. After 5 to 8 days, the foreskin will drop off with the plastic bell attached, leaving a clean, well-healed excision. No special care is required but watch for swelling, which may indicate infection or interfere with urination.

Providing aftercare

- Remove the neonate from the restraining board and check for bleeding.
- Place him in a side-lying or supine position, *to minimize pressure on the excisional area.* Leave him diaperless or apply a loose-fitting diaper for 1 to 2 hours *to observe for bleeding and to reduce possible chafing and irritation.*

New dress

- Once you diaper the neonate, change it as soon as he voids. If the dressing falls off, clean the wound with warm water. Don't remove the original dressing until it falls off (usually after the first or second voiding).
- Check for bleeding every 15 minutes for the first hour and then every hour for the next 24 hours. If bleeding occurs, apply pressure with sterile gauze pads. Notify the doctor if bleeding continues. (See *Complications of circumcision.*)
- Loosely diaper the neonate *to prevent irritation.* At each diaper change, apply ordered antimicrobial ointment, petroleum jelly, or petroleum gauze until the wound appears healed. Avoid leaving the neonate under the radiant warmer after placing petroleum gauze on the penis *because the area might burn.*

Natural protection

- Watch for drainage, redness, or swelling. Don't remove the thin, yellow-white exudate that forms over the healing area within 1 to 2 days. *This normal incrustation protects the wound until it heals in 3 to 4 days.*
- Sometimes the discharge of the neonate is held until he has voided. If the baby is discharged, instruct the parents to observe for urination in approximately 4 to 6 hours. Instruct the parents to notify the physician if the baby has not voided in 24 hours.

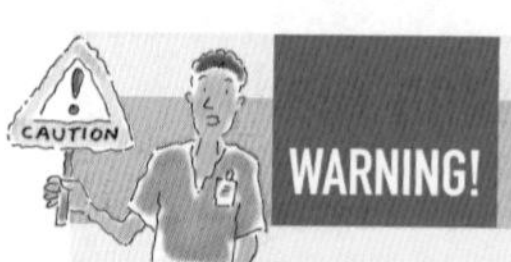

WARNING!

Complications of circumcision

Stay alert for the following complications after circumcision:

- urethral fistulas and edema
- infection or bleeding (if a Yellen clamp was used)
- delayed healing or infection, indicated by pus or bloody discharge
- scarring or fibrous bands, from adherence of penile shaft skin to the glans
- incomplete foreskin amputation, from use of a plastic circumcision bell.

Contraindications

Contraindications to circumcision include:

- illness
- bleeding disorders
- ambiguous genitalia
- congenital penile anomalies, such as hypospadias or epispadias (because the foreskin may be needed for later reconstructive surgery).

Practice pointers

- Always be sure to show parents the circumcision before discharge *so they can ask any questions and so you can teach them how to care for the area.* (See *Documenting circumcision.*)

Documenting circumcision

In your notes, record:
- family education
- circumcision date and time
- parent teaching provided
- excessive bleeding
- time that the infant urinates before discharge.

RhoGAM administration

RhoGAM is a concentrated solution of immune globulin containing $Rh_0(D)$ antibodies. I.M. injection of RhoGAM keeps the Rh-negative mother from producing active antibody responses and forming anti-$Rh_0(D)$ to Rh-positive fetal blood cells and endangering future Rh-positive infants. Maternal isoimmunization to the Rh antigen commonly results from transplacental hemorrhage during gestation or delivery. If unchecked during gestation, incompatible fetal and maternal blood can lead to hemolytic disease in the neonate.

When you give it

RhoGAM is indicated for the Rh-negative mother after abortion, ectopic pregnancy, or delivery of a neonate having $Rh_0(D)$-positive or Du-positive blood and Coombs-negative cord blood, accidental transfusion of Rh-positive blood, amniocentesis, abruptio placentae, or abdominal trauma. A RhoGAM injection should be given within 72 hours after delivery to prevent future maternal sensitization.

Administration of RhoGAM at approximately 28 weeks' gestation can also protect the fetus of the Rh-negative mother, if fetal red blood cells enter the maternal circulatory system.

What you need

3-mL syringe ✳ 22G 1½" needle ✳ RhoGAM vial ✳ alcohol pads ✳ gloves ✳ triplicate form and patient identification (from the blood bank or laboratory).

Getting ready

Identify the patient. Explain RhoGAM administration and obtain a history of allergies and reaction to immunizations.

Two nurses must check the vial's identification numbers and sign the triplicate form that comes with RhoGAM. Complete the form as indicated. Attach the top copy to the patient's chart. Send the remaining two copies, along with the empty RhoGAM vial, to the laboratory or blood bank.

How you do it

- Provide privacy, wash your hands, and put on gloves.
- Withdraw RhoGAM from the vial with the needle and syringe. Clean the gluteal injection site with an alcohol pad and administer RhoGAM I.M.
- Give the patient a card that identifies her Rh-negative status and instruct her to carry it with her or keep it in a convenient location.

Documenting RhoGAM injection

In your notes, record:
- blood type of the mother and baby and the Coombs tests results.
- date, time, and site of RhoGAM injection
- patient's refusal to accept the injection, if applicable
- patient teaching about RhoGAM provided
- whether the patient received a card identifying her Rh-negative status.

Practice pointers

- After the procedure, watch for redness and soreness at the injection site. (See *Documenting RhoGAM injection.*)

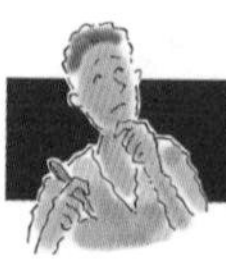

Quick quiz

1. When reading the fetal monitor strip, the nurse notes early decelerations. Which nursing intervention is priority?
   A. Turn the patient onto her left side.
   B. Increase the I.V. fluid rate and administer oxygen.
   C. Assess fetal heart rate and document the frequency of early decelerations.
   D. Contact the physician immediately.

Answer: C. Early decelerations are benign and indicate fetal head compression at a dilation of 4 to 7 cm.

2. The nurse is assessing the fetal heart rate and the mother asks what a normal heart rate is for her baby? What it the nurse's response?
   A. 60 to 90 beats/minute
   B. 90 to 110 beats/minute
   C. 110 to 160 beats/minute
   D. 160 to 180 beats/minute

Answer: C. Normal fetal heart rate ranges from 110 to 160 beats/minute.

3. A neonate has a heart rate of 130 beats/minute, is crying vigorously and regularly, and has pink skin. He's moving all four extremities, which appear blue. What is the Apgar score?
   A. 9
   B. 8
   C. 7
   D. 6

Answer: A. You should assign the neonate 2 points each for a heart rate over 100 beats/minute, respiratory effort, muscle tone, and reflexes. However, you should assign only 1 point for color because the neonate's extremities are blue and his body is pink.

4. A new mother is breast-feeding and has sore nipples. What is the best advice for the nurse to give?
   A. Drink more fluids.
   B. Use ice compresses before breast-feeding.
   C. Wear a well-fitting support bra.
   D. Decrease breast-feeding time.

Answer: B. Ice compresses numb and firm the nipples, making them less sensitive and easier for the infant to grasp.

5. The nurse is providing care during an amniotomy. What is the nurse's priority intervention?
   A. Observe the amount of amniotic fluid.
   B. Help the patient clean up after the amniotomy.
   C. Assess the fetal heart rate.
   D. Reposition the patient on her left side.

Answer: C. The fetal heart rate should be assessed immediately during and after an amniotomy to determine if the cord has been compressed.

Scoring

☆☆☆ If you answered all five items correctly, beautiful! You've got the goods on mom and baby.

☆☆ If you answered four or three items correctly, super! You've done a nice job with neonates.

☆ If you answered fewer than two items correctly, keep cool. A quick review should deliver you to success.

Selected references

American Academy of Pediatrics. (2011). *AAP issues guidelines on phototherapy for neonates*. Retrieved from http://www.medscape.com/viewarticle/750366

American Academy of Pediatrics. (2011). *AAP updates recommendation on car seats*. Retrieved from http://www.aap.org/en-us/about-the-aap/aap-press-room/pages/aap-updates-recommendation-on-car-seats.aspx

American Academy of Pediatrics Subcommittee on Hyperbilirubinemia. (2004). Management of hyperbilirubinemia in the newborn 35 or more weeks of gestation. *Pediatrics, 114*, 294–316.

American Heart Association. (2010). *Highlights of the 2010 American Heart Association guidelines for CPR and ECC*. Retrieved from http://www.heart.org/idc/groups/heart-public/@wcm/@ecc/documents/downloadable/ucm_317350.pdf

Askin, D. (2010). Respiratory distress. In M. Verklan & M. Walden (Eds.), *Core curriculum for neonatal intensive care nursing*. St. Louis, MO: Elsevier Saunders.

Association of Women's Health, Obstetric and Neonatal Nurses. (2007). *Position on breastfeeding*. Retrieved from http://onlinelibrary.wiley.com/enhanced/doi/10.1111/1552-6909.12530/

Association of Women's Health, Obstetric and Neonatal Nurses. (2011). *Nursing care of the woman receiving analgesia/anesthesia in labor. Evidence-based clinical practice guideline* (2nd ed.). Washington, DC: Author.

Bass, J. (2010). The infant car seat challenge: Determining and managing an "abnormal" result. *Pediatrics, 125*(3), 597–598.

Centers for Disease Control and Prevention. (2012). *Vaccine administration*. Retrieved from http://www.cdc.gov/vaccines/pubs/pinkbook/downloads/appendices/D/vacc_admin.pdf

Durham, R., & Chapman, L. (2014). *Maternal-newborn nursing: Critical components of nursing care* (2nd ed.). Philadelphia, PA: F.A. Davis.

Hartfield, L., Chang, K., Bittle, M., et al. (2011). The analgesic properties of intraoral sucrose. An integrative review. *Advances in Neonatal Care, 11*(2), 83–92.

Hensel, E., Morson, G. L., & Preuss, E. A. (2013). Best practices in newborn injections. *MCN, 38*(3), 163–167.

Jones, L. (2012). Oral feeding readiness in the neonatal intensive care unit. *Neonatal Network, 31*(3), 148–154.

Lewis, S., Dirksen, S. R., Heitkemper, M., et al. (2010). *Medical-surgical nursing: Assessment and management of clinical problems* (8th ed.). St Louis, MO: Mosby Elsevier

Lyndon, A., & Ali, L. U. (Eds.). (2009). *Fetal heart monitoring: Principles and practice* (4th ed.). Dubuque, IA: Kendal/Hunt.

Macones, G., Hankins, G., Spong, C., et al. (2008). The 2008 National Institute of Child Health and Human Development workshop report on electronic fetal monitoring: Update on definitions, interpretations, and research guidelines. *Journal of Obstetric, Gynecologic, & Neonatal Nursing, 37*, 510–515.

Osterman, M. J. K., & Martin, J. A. (2011). Epidurals and spinal anesthesia use during labor: 27-State reporting area, 2008. *National Vital Statistics Reports, 59*(5), 1–13.

Potter, P. A., Perry, A. G., Stockert, P., et al. (2013). *Fundamentals of nursing* (8th ed.). St. Louis, MO: Elsevier.

U.S. Department of Health and Human Services. (2020). *Healthy people 2020*. Retrieved from http://www.healthypeople.gov/2020/topicsobjectives/topic/maternal-infant-and-child-health/objectives

Chapter 13

Pediatric care

Just the facts

In this chapter, you'll learn:

- about pediatric care procedures and how to perform them
- what child care and family teaching are associated with each procedure
- how to manage complications associated with each procedure
- about essential documentation for each procedure.

Urine collection

As with an adult child, a urine specimen collected from a pediatric child allows screening for urinary tract infection and renal disorders, helps evaluate treatment, and helps detect systemic and metabolic disorders.

The pediatric urine collection bag provides a simple, effective alternative for a child without bladder control, who cannot provide a clean-catch midstream urine specimen. The bag offers minimal risk of specimen contamination without resorting to catheterization. Because the collection bag is secured with adhesive flaps, its use is contraindicated in children with extremely sensitive or excoriated perineal skin.

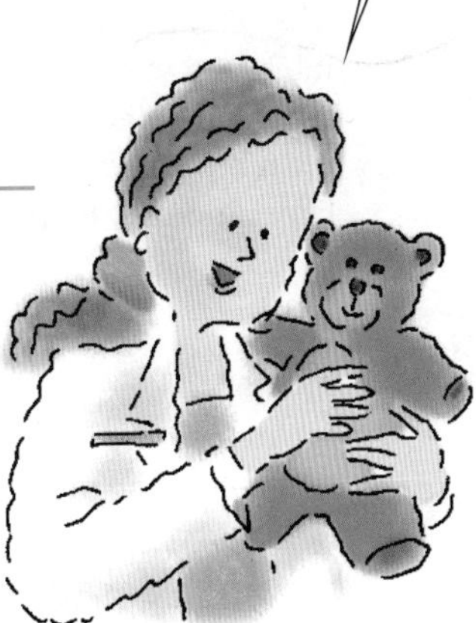
You have read about most of these procedures already, but this chapter gives helpful hints for adapting them to children.

What you need

For a random specimen

Pediatric urine collection bag (individually packaged) ✳ urine specimen container ✳ label ✳ laboratory request form ✳ two disposable diapers of appropriate size ✳ washcloth ✳ soap ✳ water ✳ towel ✳ bowl ✳ linen-saver pad.

For a culture and sensitivity specimen

Sterile pediatric urine collection bag * sterile urine specimen container * label * laboratory request form * two disposable diapers of appropriate size * scissors * gloves * sterile bowl * sterile or distilled water * sterile 4″ × 4″ gauze pads * antiseptic skin cleaner * alcohol pad * 3-mL syringe with needle * linen-saver pad.

For a timed specimen

24-hour pediatric urine collection bag with evacuation tubing * 24-hour urine specimen container * label * laboratory request form * scissors * two disposable diapers of appropriate size * gloves * washcloth * soap and water * bowl * towel * sterile 4″ × 4″ gauze pads * compound benzoin tincture * small medicine cup * 35-mL luer-lock syringe or urinometer * tubing stopper U specimen preservative such as formaldehyde solution * linen-saver pad.

Kits containing sterile supplies for clean-catch collections are commercially available and may be used to obtain a culture and sensitivity specimen.

Getting ready

Check the doctor's order for the type of specimen needed and assemble the appropriate equipment. Check the child's chart for allergies to iodine. Complete the laboratory requisition and verify it with the order. Perform hand hygiene.

With scissors, make a 2″ (5-cm) slit in one diaper. Pour water into the bowl, using sterile water and a sterile bowl if you need a culture and sensitivity. Check the expiration date on sterile packages and inspect for tears. Put on gloves and open several packages of sterile 4″ × 4″ gauze pads. Pour benzoin into the medicine cup. Cut the tubing on the urine collection bag so that only 6″ (15 cm) remain attached and discard the excess. Place the stopper in the severed end of the tubing. If you are going to use a urinometer for the child who voids large amounts, do not cut the tubing but simply attach the device.

How you do it

- Identify the patient using two patient identifiers.
- Explain the procedure and provide privacy.

Collecting a random specimen

- Perform hand hygiene and place the child on a linen-saver pad.
- Clean the perineal area gently with soap, water, and a washcloth, working from the urinary meatus outward. Separate the labia of

the female child and retract the foreskin of the uncircumcised male child *to expose the urinary meatus*. Thoroughly rinse the area with clear water and dry with a towel.

Jeremiah was a . . .

- Place the child in the frog position, with his legs separated and knees flexed. If necessary, have another nurse hold the child while you apply the collection bag. The parent can provide distraction for the child.
- Remove the protective coverings from the collection bag's adhesive flaps. For the female child, first separate the labia and gently press the bag's lower rim to the perineum. Then, working upward toward the pubis, attach the rest of the adhesive rim inside the labia majora. For the male child, place the bag over the penis and scrotum and press the adhesive rim to the skin.
- Gently pull the attached bag through the slit in the diaper and fasten the diaper on the child.

It's in the bag

- Guidelines support that a specimen from a sterile urine bag attached to the perineal site has a false-positive rate so it cannot be used alone to diagnosis a urinary tract infection. If the culture is negative from the sterile urine bag, there is strong evidence that there is not a urinary tract infection.
- When urine appears in the bag, put on gloves and gently remove the diaper and the bag. Hold the bag's bottom port over the collection container, remove the tab from the port, and let the urine flow into the container.
- Measure the output if necessary.
- Label the specimen and verify the labels match the requisition and the medical record, attach the laboratory requisition, and send it directly to the laboratory. Remove and discard gloves.
- Put the second diaper on the child.
- Perform hand hygiene.

Collecting a culture and sensitivity specimen

Follow the procedure for collecting a random specimen, with these modifications:

- Using gloves, clean the urinary meatus wiping outward with antiseptic skin cleaner and sterile 4″ × 4″ gauze pad, wiping once with each pad then discarding it.
- After the child urinates, remove the bag and use an alcohol pad to clean a small area of the bag's surface. Puncture the clean area with the needle, aspirate urine into the syringe, and inject it into the sterile specimen container. Remove and discard your gloves. Perform hand hygiene.

Collecting a timed specimen

- Check the doctor's order for the duration of the collection and the indication for the procedure. Prepare the child, don gloves, and clean the perineum as for random specimen collection.

Sticky issues

- If getting the bag to adhere is difficult, apply compound benzoin tincture to the perineal skin area with a gauze pad or spray, if ordered; cover the genitalia with a gauze pad before spraying.
- Allow the benzoin to dry. Then apply the collection bag, pull the bottom of the bag and the tubing through the slit in the diaper, and fasten the diaper. Remove and discard your gloves. Perform hand hygiene.
- Check the collection bag and tubing to ensure a proper seal.
- When urine appears in the bag, perform hand hygiene, don gloves, and remove the stopper in the bag's tubing. Then attach the syringe to the end of the tubing and aspirate the urine. Remove the syringe and insert the stopper into the tubing.
- Discard the specimen and begin timing the collection. Perform hand hygiene.

Visit the fridge

- When the next urine specimen is obtained, add the preservative to the 24-hour specimen container along with the specimen and refrigerate it, if ordered.
- Each time you remove urine, add it to the specimen container; then use the syringe to inject a small amount of air into the collection bag *to prevent a vacuum, which can block urine drainage.*
- When the prescribed collection period has elapsed, stop the collection and send the total accumulated specimen to the laboratory. Label the container and verify that the information on the label matches the medical record and the information on the requisition.
- Perform hand hygiene. Don gloves and wash the perineal area thoroughly with soap and water; then put the second diaper on the child.

Practice pointers

- To collect a urine specimen from an infant or a young child with extremely sensitive or excoriated perineal skin, cotton balls may be placed in the perineal area of the diaper to absorb urine. After he has voided, remove the diaper and squeeze urine from the cotton balls into a specimen cup. (See *Documenting urine collection*.)

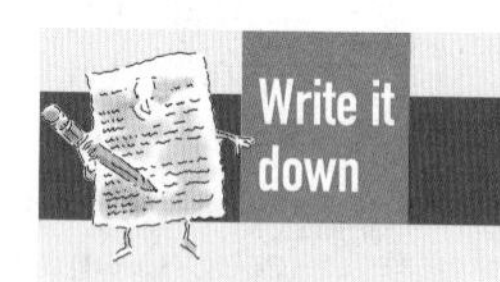

Documenting urine collection

In your notes, record:

- date, time, and method of urine collection
- amount of urine collected (if necessary)
- name of the ordered test
- time of specimen transport to the laboratory
- use of restraints, if applicable
- complications
- child's tolerance of the procedure
- child's and family's responses to teaching.

Drug administration

A child responds more rapidly and unpredictably to drugs than does an adult. Factors such as age, weight, body surface area, and drug form and route all play a part. Certain disorders can also affect a child's response to medication. For example, gastroenteritis increases gastric motility, which in turn impairs absorption of certain oral medications. Liver or kidney disorders can hinder the metabolism of some medications.

Make the adjustment

You may need to adjust usual drug administration techniques to account for the child's age, size, and developmental level. For example, the thin epithelium of a neonate or infant can absorb topical medications much faster than an older child. In addition, the injection site and needle size varies depending on the child's age and physical development.

What you need

For oral medications

Prescribed medication ✳ disposable plastic syringe, plastic medicine dropper, or spoon ✳ medication cup ✳ water, syrup, or jelly (for tablets) ✳ optional: fruit juice.

For injectable medications

Prescribed medication ✳ appropriately sized syringe and needle ✳ alcohol pads or povidone-iodine solution ✳ gloves ✳ gauze pads ✳ cold compresses ✳ adhesive bandage.

Getting ready

Check the doctor's order for the prescribed drug, dosage, and route. Compare the order with the drug label, checking the expiration date. Review for allergies.

When one isn't enough

Calculate the dosage to ensure proper milligram per kilogram amount, if necessary, and have another nurse verify it. Check your hospital's policy *to learn which drugs must be calculated and checked by two nurses.*

Centers for Disease Control and Prevention recommendations for intramuscular injections

Age	Preferred site	Needle gauge	Needle length
Neonate (first 28 days of life) and preterm	Anterolateral thigh	22G to 25G	⅝″
Infant (<12 months)	Anterolateral thigh	22G to 25G	1″
Toddlers (12 months to 2 years)	Anterolateral thigh or deltoid if enough muscle mass	22G to 25G	1″
Children through adolescents (3 to 18 years)	Deltoid	22G to 25G	⅝″ to 1¼″*

*Smaller children use a ⅝″.

For giving an intramuscular injection, select the appropriate needle. (See *Centers for Disease Control and Prevention recommendations for intramuscular injections.*)

For subcutaneous injections, select a 23G to 25G ⅝″ needle and for intradermal medications, a 27G ½″ needle. To administer viscous medications, select a larger gauge needle.

How you do it

- Identify the child using two patient identifiers per facility policy validated with the medication administration record (MAR). If using the electronic MAR, scan the child's identification band and the medication to verify accuracy. If the child can talk and respond, ask him his name.
- Explain the procedure and provide privacy.
- Teach the patient/family about the medication, action, and side effects.
- Perform hand hygiene.

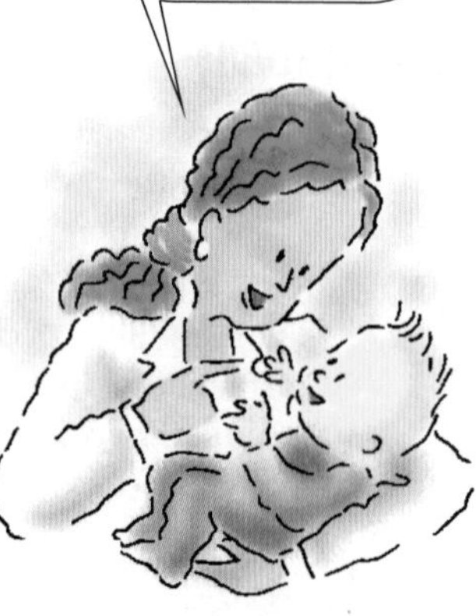
With an infant, you need to put the medicine dropper right in the side of the mouth . . .

Giving oral medication to an infant

- Use either a plastic syringe without a needle or a drug-specific medicine dropper to measure the dose. If the medication comes in tablet form, first crush the tablet (if appropriate) and mix it with water or syrup. Then draw the mixture into the syringe or dropper.

- Pick up the infant, raising his head and shoulders or turning his head to one side, holding him close to your body.

Press down and slide

- Using your thumb, press down on the infant's chin and slide the syringe or medicine dropper into the infant's mouth alongside his tongue and let the medication slowly flow into the pocket between the cheek and gum.
- Place the infant on his side or back or allow an active infant to assume a position that is comfortable for him.

Giving oral medication to a toddler

- Use a disposable plastic syringe or plastic medicine dropper to measure liquid medication then transfer the fluid to a medication cup.
- Elevate the toddler's head and shoulders.

Want to help?

- The child may help hold the cup *to enlist his cooperation*. Otherwise, hold the cup to his lips or use a syringe or a spoon to administer the liquid. Make sure that the toddler ingests all of the medication.
- If the medication is in tablet form, first crush the tablet, if appropriate, and mix it with water, syrup, or jelly. Use a spoon, syringe, or dropper to administer the medication. You may also offer a favorite drink to give after taking the medication.

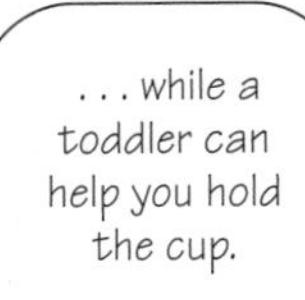
. . . while a toddler can help you hold the cup.

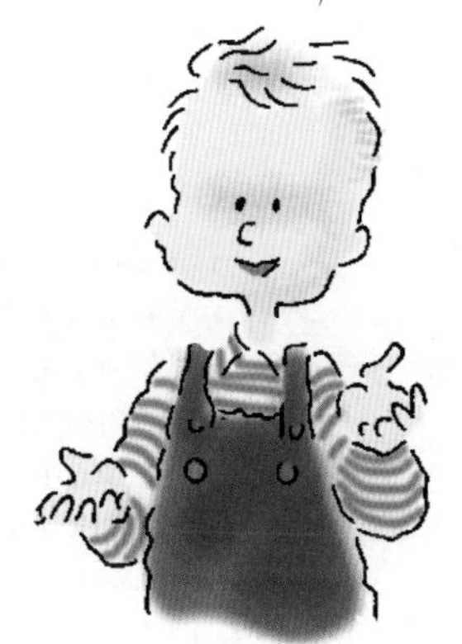

Giving oral medication to an older child

- If possible, let the child choose both the liquid medication mixer and a beverage to drink after taking the medication. If appropriate, allow him to choose where he will take the medication; for example, sitting in bed or sitting on a parent's lap.

Just checking

- A child between ages 4 and 6 may swallow solid medication, such as tablet or capsule form, by having him place it on the back of his tongue and swallow it immediately with water or juice. Look inside the child's mouth *to confirm that he swallowed the pill*.
- If the child can't swallow the pill whole, crush it (if appropriate) and mix it with water, syrup, or jelly. Or, after checking with the child's doctor, order the medication in liquid form.

Giving an I.M. injection

- Choose an injection site that's appropriate for the child's age and muscle mass. (See *Centers for Disease Control and Prevention recommendations for intramuscular injections*.)

Location notation

- Position the child appropriately for the site chosen and locate key landmarks, for example, the posterior superior iliac spine and the greater trochanter. Have someone help you restrain an infant; seek an older child's cooperation before enlisting assistance.
- Perform hand hygiene and don gloves. Clean the injection site with an alcohol or povidone-iodine pad, wiping outward from the center with a spiral motion. If the child is older than 6 months, consider using topical anesthetic such as EMLA. Note that EMLA should be applied 1 hour before the intramuscular (I.M.) injection.

Grasp and dart

- Grasp the tissue surrounding the site between your index finger and thumb and insert the needle quickly, using a darting motion at a 90-degree angle. If you're using the ventrogluteal site, insert the needle at a 45-degree angle toward the knee.
- Aspirate the plunger to ensure that the needle is not in a blood vessel. If no blood appears, inject the medication slowly at 10 seconds/mL. Wait 10 seconds for the medication to absorb and withdraw the needle. To reduce injection site discomfort, there is no longer a need to aspirate after the needle is inserted when administering vaccines per the Centers for Disease Control and Prevention. Follow facility policy regarding aspirating after injecting the needle.
- Withdraw the needle and gently massage the area with a gauze pad.
- Provide comfort and praise.

Giving a subcutaneous injection

- The middle third of the upper outer arm, the middle third of the upper outer thigh, or the abdomen may be used. You may apply a cold compress to the injection site *to minimize pain.*
- Perform hand hygiene and don gloves. Prepare the injection site with alcohol or povidone-iodine solution.
- Pinch the tissue surrounding the site between your index finger and thumb and hold the needle at a 45-degree angle. Quickly insert it into the tissue, release your grasp on the tissue, and slowly inject the medication. Remove the needle quickly and, unless contraindicated, gently massage the area.

Giving an intradermal injection

- Put on gloves and pull the child's skin taut at the inner aspect of the forearm.
- Insert the needle, bevel up, at a 10- to 15-degree angle just beneath the outer skin layer and slowly inject the medication, watching for a bleb to appear. Quickly remove the needle and

draw a circle around the bleb, if required (such as in allergy testing). Avoid massaging the area.

Practice pointers

- Allow the child choices, if possible, such as choosing from the appropriate sites for an injection. You can also allow the child to play with a medication cup or syringe and to pretend to give medication to a doll.

It's the best policy

- When giving medication to an older child, be honest. Reassure him that distaste or discomfort will be brief. Emphasize that he must remain still and that an assistant will help him to remain still if necessary. Keep your explanations brief and simple.
- Certain medications are considered "high-alert medications" and should be double checked for accurate dosages with another nurse. Check the facility policy for high-alert medications. These include: digoxin, heparin, insulin, narcotics such as morphine, potassium and calcium, epidural medications, chemotherapy, sedation and anesthesia, and intravenous (I.V.) medications greater than 20% glucose.

Medal of honor

- *To divert the child's attention,* have him start counting just before the injection and challenge him to try to reach 10 before you finish the injection. If the child cries, do not scold him or allow the parents to scold him. After the injection, have one of the parents hold a younger child and praise him for allowing you to give him the injection. You can also apply an adhesive bandage to the injection site *as a form of reward or badge. Allow the child to select the Band-Aid he wants.*
- Return to the room in 15 to 20 minutes to check if there is any pain, burning, numbness, or tingling at the injection site.
- Teach the parents about the proper dosage and administration of all prescribed medications. Use written materials to reinforce your teaching. (See *Documenting drug administration.*)

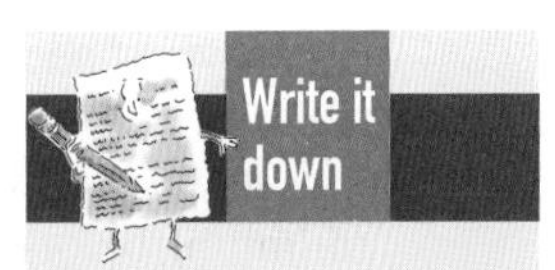

Documenting drug administration

In your notes or other appropriate form, record:

- drug name, form, and dosage
- administration date, time, route, and site
- drug effect
- child's tolerance of the procedure
- complications and nursing actions taken
- drug-related child and parent teaching provided.

Iontophoresis

Iontophoresis is a technique for delivering dermal analgesia quickly (in 10 to 20 minutes) with minimal discomfort and without distorting the tissue. The Numby 900 iontophoretic drug-delivery system is a handheld device with two electrodes. It uses a mild electric current to deliver charged ions of lidocaine 2% and epinephrine 1:100,000 solution into the skin. The device is powered by a 9-volt battery.

Because iontophoresis acts quickly, it is an excellent choice for numbing before an I.V. injection site, especially in children.

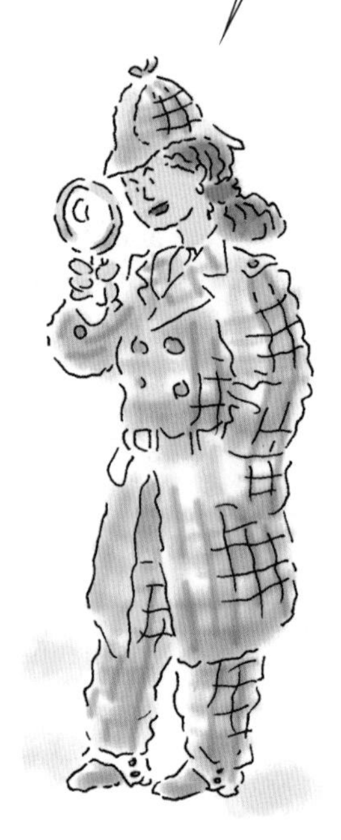
ION is the key part of iontophoresis—mild electricity sends ions of numbing medication right through the skin. It's elementary!

What you need

Dose-control device with battery ✳ drug-delivery electrode kit ✳ lidocaine 2% with epinephrine 1:100,000 solution ✳ alcohol pads ✳ syringe with needle ✳ gloves ✳ tongue blade.

How you do it

- Ask the parents if the child has any allergies or sensitivity to any medications. Avoid using iontophoresis in patients with implanted devices such as a pacemaker.
- Identify the patient using two patient identifiers per facility policy and verify with the medical record.
- Perform hand hygiene.
- Explain the procedure to the child and tell him that he may feel tingling or warmth under the electrode pads while they are on the skin.

On the muscle

- Assess the patient for appropriate electrode placement. You will place a drug-delivery electrode over the intended I.V. insertion site. The second electrode, which drives drug ions into the skin, must be applied over a muscle 4″ to 6″ (10 to 15 cm) away.
- Don gloves. Examine the child's skin and select intact electrode placement sites, avoiding areas with pimples, unhealed wounds, or ingrown hairs. With alcohol pads, briskly rub an area slightly larger than the electrode at each site.
- Remove the paper flap from the back of the drug-delivery electrode.

Splash down

- Draw up the lidocaine with epinephrine in a syringe out of the child's view to reduce anxiety. Remove the needle from the syringe and saturate the medication pad with the amount of lidocaine and epinephrine solution indicated on the electrode pad. (See photo at top of next page.) The amount of lidocaine and epinephrine solution required to saturate the pad varies with pad size: for a standard-sized pad, use about 1 mL; for a large pad, use about 2.5 mL.
- Remove the remaining backing from the drug-delivery pad and apply the pad to the selected site. Remove the backing from the grounding electrode and apply it to the second prepared site.

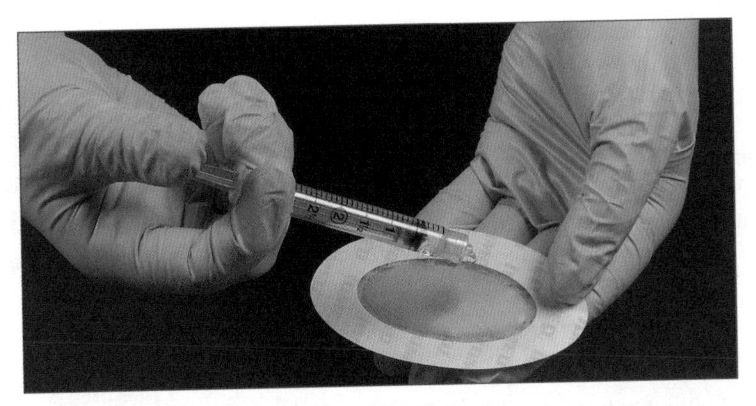

- Connect the lead clips: red (positive charge) to the drug-delivery electrode and black (negative charge) to the grounding electrode.
- Turn on the device. (See photo below.)

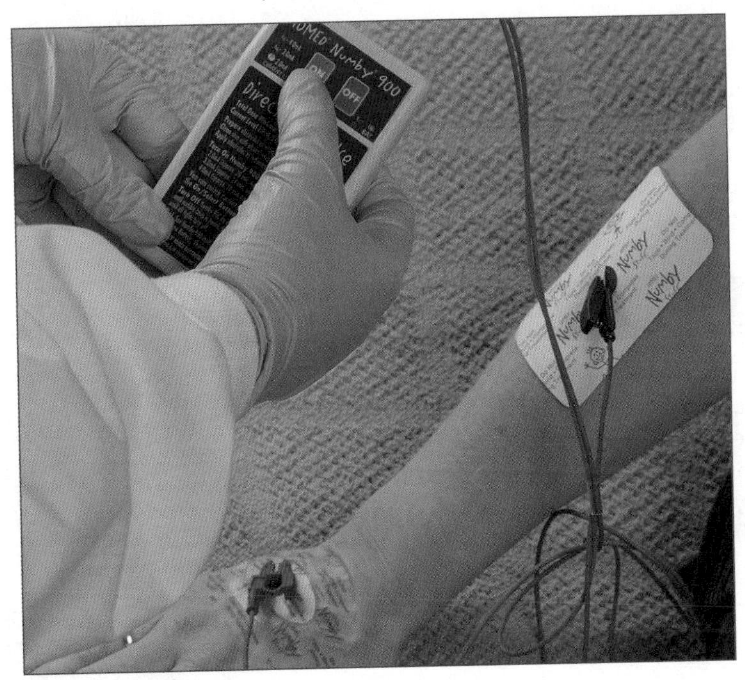

Automatic stop

- As indicated by the green light, the device will automatically operate at the lowest current, 2 milliamperes (mA), unless you increase the level to 3 mA or 4 mA by pressing the ON button. If your child has discomfort at a higher setting, reduce the current by pushing the ON button until the appropriate light indicates the desired level. The device will stop automatically after delivering 40 mA-minutes. If the setting remains at 4 mA, treatment is completed in 10 minutes. However, if you decrease the setting because

the child has discomfort, the device will automatically adjust to a longer treatment time to deliver the entire dose.
- After the dose has been delivered, remove the electrodes. Assess the skin at the drug-delivery site for numbness by touching it with a blunt object such as a tongue blade.
- Promptly prepare the site and perform the venipuncture because the numbness may last only a few minutes.
- Discard gloves and perform hand hygiene.

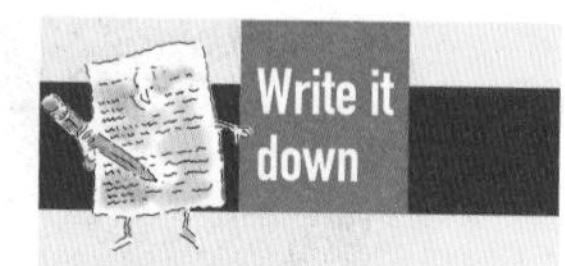

Documenting iontophoresis

In your notes, record:
- patient/family education
- treatment given
- sites used
- whether analgesia was achieved
- allergic responses, if any.

Practice pointers

- To avoid interfering with energy emission, do not tape or compress the electrodes.

Press and hold

- If you need to stop the treatment for any reason, press the OFF button and hold it. The lights will indicate decreasing current levels and then the device will beep and turn off. Do not disconnect the lead clips or the electrodes until all signals have stopped *because the device is still transmitting energy until it turns off.*
- Allergic reaction may occur in children sensitive to lidocaine or epinephrine. (See *Documenting iontophoresis.*)

I.V. therapy

In children, I.V. therapy may be used to administer medications or to correct a fluid deficit, improve serum electrolyte balance, or provide nourishment. You need to correlate the I.V. site and equipment with the reason for therapy and the child's age, size, and activity level. During I.V. therapy, you must continually assess the child and the infusion to prevent fluid overload and other complications.

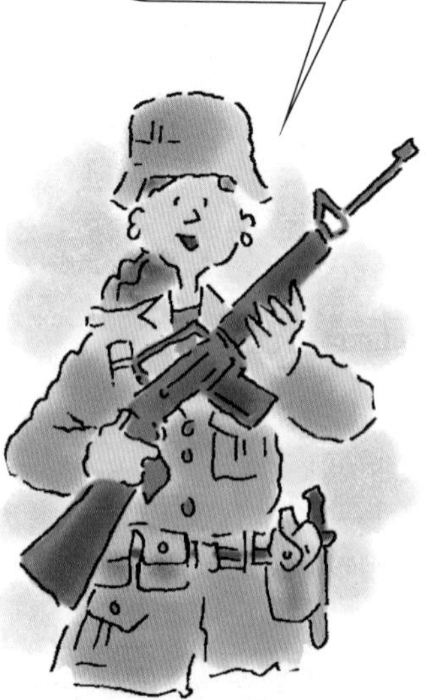
Do not let your guard down with I.V. therapy. Fluid overload can sneak right up on you.

What you need

Prescribed I.V. fluid ✱ volume-control set with microdrip tubing ✱ infusion pump ✱ I.V. pole ✱ normal saline solution or sterile dextrose 5% in water (D_5W) for injection ✱ povidone-iodine solution ✱ alcohol pads ✱ child-sized butterfly needle or I.V. catheter ✱ tourniquet ✱ ½″ or 1″ tape ✱ gloves ✱ optional: arm board.

Comfort counts

Whenever possible, use a catheter instead of a needle. *To promote compliance and reduce discomfort,* consider using a transdermal anesthetic cream.

Getting ready

Gather the I.V. equipment. Check the expiration date on the I.V. fluid and then inspect the I.V. container for leakage and I.V. tubing for defects or cracks. Perform hand hygiene. Set up the I.V. fluid, tubings, and pumps as described in chapter 4, Drug administration and I.V. therapy. Prime tubing and pumps according to the manufacturer's instructions.

Cut as many strips of ½″ or 1″ tape as you will need to secure the I.V. line. Prepare a syringe with 3 mL of flush solution—either the normal saline solution or D_5W.

How you do it

- Use two patient identifiers and validate with the MAR or scan the name on the patient's wristband with the name on the doctor's order (or on the medication card). Check for allergies, then explain the reason for the I.V. therapy, and enlist a staff member to assist you.
- Perform hand hygiene, don gloves, and select the insertion site. (See *Common pediatric I.V. sites*, page 620.) Choose the most distal site, avoiding the dominant arm, child's preference in thumb-sucking, or areas of flexion.

Head hunting

- To locate an appropriate scalp vein, avoid sites of arterial pulsations. Before inserting the I.V. line, prepare the selected site. To find an appropriate peripheral site, apply a tourniquet to the arm or leg and palpate a suitable vein.
- Clean the insertion site with povidone-iodine solution or an alcohol pad. Then insert the I.V. needle into the vein, watching for blood return, as outlined in chapter 4, Drug administration and I.V. therapy.
- Loosen the tourniquet, attach the I.V. tubing, and begin the infusion.

Batten the hatches

- Secure the device by applying a piece of ½″ tape over the hub. Next, place a piece of tape, adhesive side up, underneath and perpendicular to the device. Lift the ends of the tape and crisscross them over the device. (For more information, see *Taping a venous access site* in chapter 4, page 240.) Further secure and protect the I.V. line as needed. (See *Protecting an I.V. site*, page 621.)
- Adjust the I.V. flow, as ordered, and add solution hourly (or as needed) from the I.V. bag to the volume-control set.

Common pediatric I.V. sites

Here are the most common sites for I.V. therapy in infants and children. Typically, peripheral hand, wrist, or foot veins are used with older children, whereas scalp veins are used with infants. If the child is walking, do not use a vein in the foot, as it will interfere in walking.

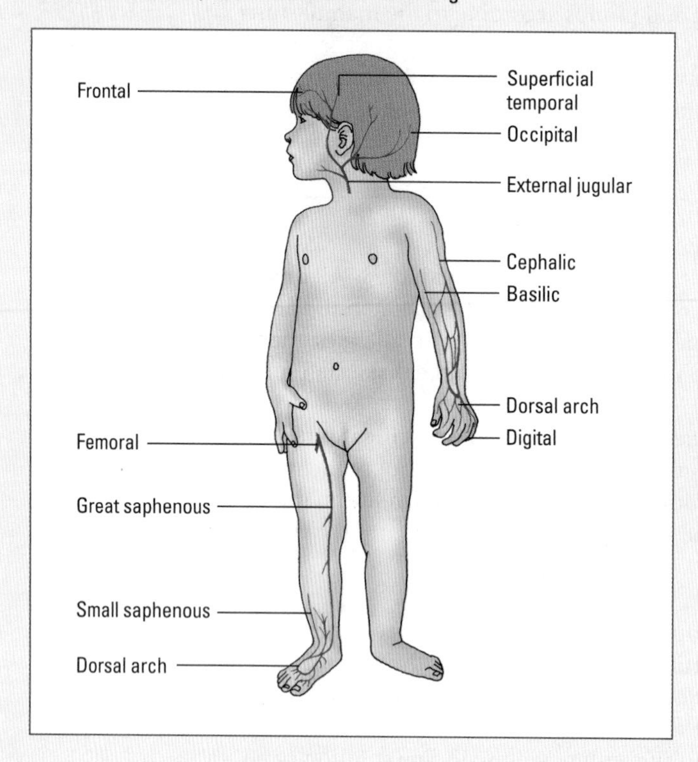

Frequent checkups

- Assess the I.V. site frequently for signs of infiltration and check the I.V. bottle or bag for the amount of solution infused. In infants and young children, the I.V. site should be assessed every hour and in older children, assess the site every 2 hours. (See *Complications of I.V. therapy*.)
- Change the I.V. dressing and solution every 24 hours or as needed, I.V. tubing every 48 to 72 hours, and I.V. insertion site every 72 hours or according to facility policy. Label the I.V. solution, tubing, and volume-control set with the time and date of change.

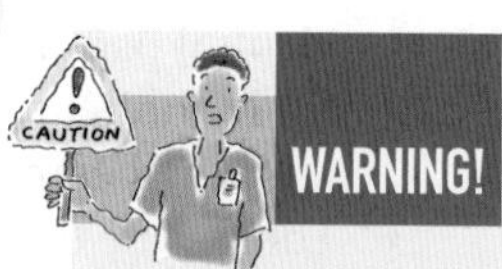

Complications of I.V. therapy

A child receiving I.V. therapy is at risk for such complications as infection, fluid overload, electrolyte imbalance, infiltration, and circulatory impairment.

Protecting an I.V. site

Protecting a child's I.V. site can be a challenge. An active child can easily dislodge an I.V. line. Besides possibly injuring the child, dislodgment necessitates reinsertion, causing the child further discomfort.

To prevent a child from dislodging an I.V. line, secure the needle or catheter carefully. Tape the I.V. site as you would for an adult, so the skin over the tip of the venipuncture device is easily visible. Avoid over taping the site because it will be harder to inspect.

If the child is old enough to understand, warn him not to play with or jostle the equipment and teach him how to walk with an I.V. pole to minimize tension on the line. If necessary, restrain the extremity.

Also, create a protective barrier between the I.V. site and the environment by using one of the following methods:

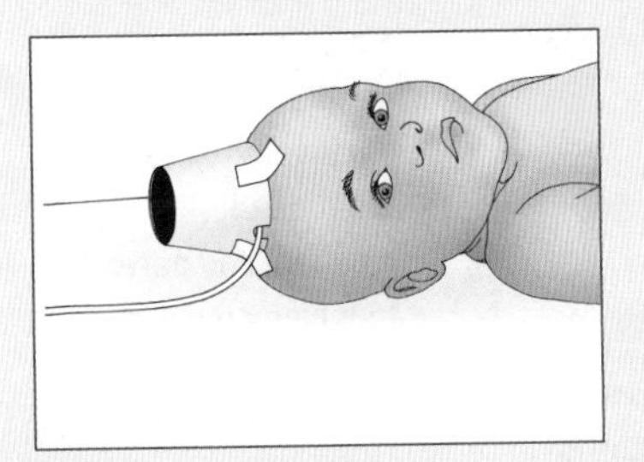

Paper cup

You can use a small paper cup to protect a scalp site. First, cut off the cup's bottom, making sure there are no sharp edges, and cut a small slot through the top rim to accommodate the I.V. tubing. Place the cup upside down over the insertion site, so the I.V. tubing extends through the slot. Then secure the cup with strips of tape (as shown). The opening you cut in the cup lets you examine the site.

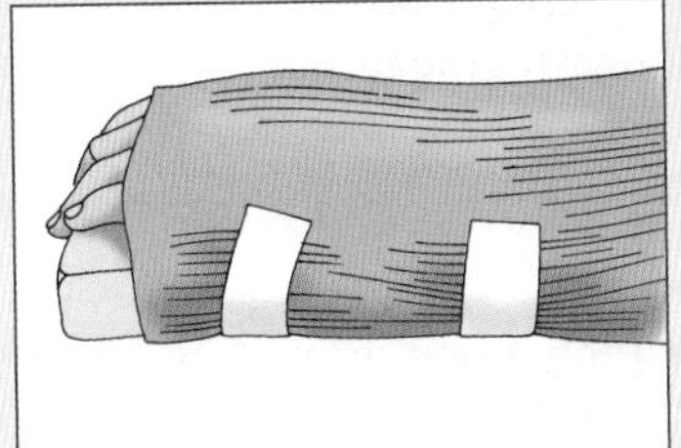

Stockinette

Cut a piece of 4" (10 cm) stockinette the same length as the child's arm. Slip the stockinette over the child's arm and lay the arm on an arm board. Then grasp the stockinette at both sides of the arm and stretch it under the arm board. Securely tape the stockinette beneath the arm board (as shown). You also may protect a scalp site by placing a stockinette on the patient's head, leaving a hole to allow access to the site.

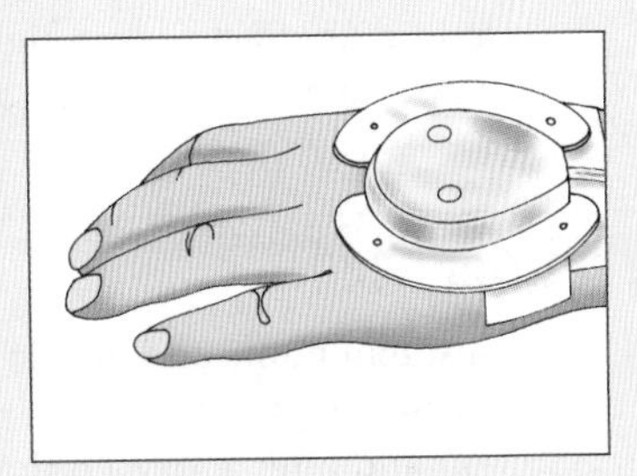

I.V. shield

Peel off the strips covering the adhesive backing on the bottom of the shield. Position the shield over the site so the I.V. tubing runs through one of the shield's two slots. Then firmly press the shield's adhesive backing against the patient's skin. The shield's clear plastic composition allows you to see the I.V. site clearly.

Practice pointers

- Forewarn parents if you will start the I.V. infusion in a scalp vein. Also tell them that you may have to shave hair from a small section of the infant's head.

Free to move about the cabin

- Evaluate the need for restraints and apply them only if necessary. Assess the skin integrity, provide hourly skin care, remove the restraints at frequent intervals, and encourage the parents to hold and comfort the child.

- Teach the parents and family about I.V. therapy and prepare them if therapy is to continue in the home environment. (See *Documenting I.V. therapy*.)

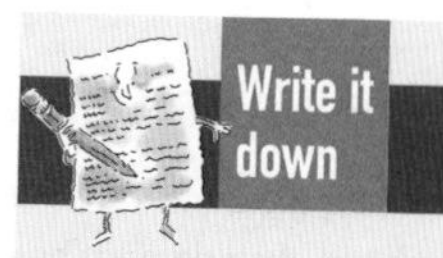

Documenting I.V. therapy

In your notes, record:

- date and time of the I.V. infusion
- I.V. insertion site
- type and size of I.V. needle or catheter used
- patient's tolerance of the procedure
- patient and parent teaching provided
- condition of the I.V. site according to facility policy. If infiltration occurs, document the site's condition at every shift change until the condition resolves.

Mist tent therapy

Also known as a croupette (for infants) or a cool-humidity tent (for children), a mist tent houses a nebulizer that transforms distilled water into mist. Mist tent therapy benefits the patient by providing a cool, moist environment that eases breathing and helps to decrease respiratory tract edema, liquefy secretions, and reduce fever. Oxygen may also be administered along with the mist.

What you need

Mist tent frame and plastic tenting ✱ bed sheets ✱ plastic sheet or linen-saver pad ✱ two bath blankets ✱ nebulizer with water reservoir and filter ✱ oxygen flowmeter and oxygen analyzer, if ordered ✱ sterile distilled water ✱ optional: stockinette cap or booties, infant seat.

Getting ready

Perform hand hygiene and place the tent frame and plastic tenting at the head of the crib or bed. Cover the mattress first with a bed sheet, then a plastic sheet or linen-saver pad tucked under the mattress, and finally a bath blanket. Next, fill the reservoir with sterile distilled water, making sure the inlet for air contains a clean filter.

If the child will have oxygen in the tent, make sure that the flowmeter is set at the desired setting and percentage of oxygen is analyzed. Wait 2 minutes after mist begins filling the tent before placing the child in it.

How you do it

- Check the order in the medical record. Identify the patient using two patient identifiers per facility policy.
- Explain the purpose of the therapy.
- Elevate the head of the bed to enhance the child's comfort. If the patient is an infant, you can place him in an infant seat. If the child will be in the room alone, position him on his side.

Booties and blanket

- Use a stockinette cap, booties, and bath blanket *to keep the child from becoming chilled.* Change the child's bed sheets and clothing if damp.
- Elevate the rails and monitor him frequently for a change in condition, keeping in mind that the mist may make observation difficult.

Family camping

- Encourage parents to stay with the child. If he grows irritable and uncooperative, take him out and let his parents comfort him, then return him to the tent when he calms down.
- If secretions coat the inside of the tent, wipe it down with a hospital-approved cleaner. Clean the reservoir with sterile water *to prevent bacterial growth.*

Practice pointers

- Allow the child to have toys in the mist tent or mobiles as age appropriate but avoid cloth or stuffed toys.

Bells are ringing

- *To prevent a fire,* forbid toys or games that may spark or trigger an electric shock (such as battery-operated toys) and remove the electric call light. Give older children a hand bell to use. If the child is receiving oxygen, analyze the percentage at least every 4 hours.
- For bathing, remove the child from the tent *to prevent hypothermia.*
- If the mist tent will be used at home, show the parents how to set up, use, and clean the tent properly. (See *Documenting mist tent therapy.*)

Documenting mist tent therapy

In your notes, record:
- patient and family education
- date and time of the child's placement in the tent
- child's vital signs and respiratory status (including breath sounds, sputum production, and perfusion)
- percentage of oxygen delivered
- child's oxygen saturation
- dates and times of all analyses
- date and time of the child's removal from the tent.

Hip spica cast care

After orthopedic surgery to correct a fracture or deformity, a child may need a hip spica cast to immobilize both legs. Occasionally, the doctor may apply a hip spica cast to treat an orthopedic deformity that does not require surgery. Infants usually adapt more easily to the cast than do older children but need encouragement, support, and diversionary activity during their prolonged immobilization.

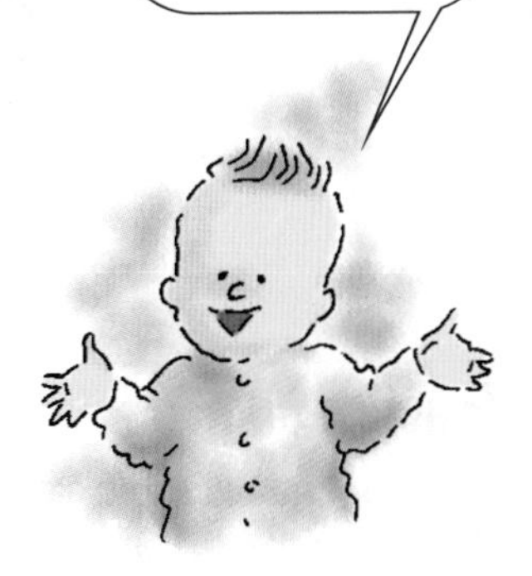
Infants adapt better to hip spica casts than older children.

What you need

Waterproof adhesive tape ✳ moleskin or plastic petals ✳ cast cutter or saw ✳ scissors ✳ nonabrasive cleaner ✳ hair dryer ✳ optional: disposable diaper or perineal pad.

Getting ready

- Identify the patient using two patient identifiers per facility policy.
- Before the physician applies the cast, describe the procedure to the child and his parents.

How you do it

- When the physician constructs the cast, keep it uncovered, draping a small cover over the perineal opening. Turn the child every 1 to 2 hours toward his unaffected side using your palms. Do not use the stabilizer bar between his legs for leverage.

Soften the edges

- After the cast dries, cut several petal-shaped pieces of moleskin and place them around the open edges of the cast. Use waterproof adhesive tape around the perineal area.
- Give the child a sponge bath *to remove any cast fragments from his skin.*
- Assess the child's legs for coldness, swelling, cyanosis, or mottling. Also assess pulse strength, toe movement, sensation (numbness, tingling, or burning), and capillary refill. Perform these circulatory assessments every 1 to 2 hours while the cast is wet and every 2 to 4 hours after the cast dries.
- Check the child's exposed skin for redness or irritation, and observe the child for pain or discomfort caused by hot spots (pressure-sensitive areas under the cast). Also, be alert for a foul odor.

Salon-style care

- *To relieve itching,* blow cool air from a handheld hair dryer under the cast. Warn the child and his parents not to insert any object into the cast to relieve itching by scratching.
- Encourage the child's family to visit and participate in his care and recreation and be sure to teach them home care techniques. (See *Hip spica cast care.*)

Practice pointers

- Tuck a folded disposable diaper or perineal pad around the perineal edges of the cast to protect from soiling. Then apply a second

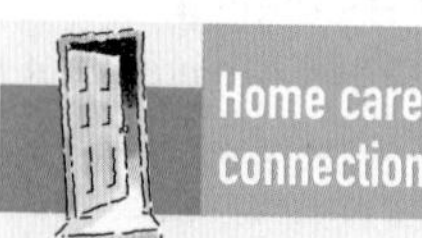

Hip spica cast care

Before discharge, teach the parents how to care for the cast and have them demonstrate their understanding. Include instructions for checking circulatory status, recognizing signs of circulatory impairment, and notifying the doctor. Also demonstrate how to turn the child, apply moleskin, clean the cast, and ensure adequate nourishment.

diaper to the child, over the top of the cast, to hold the first diaper in place. Plastic petals can be tucked into the cast *to channel urine and feces into a bedpan.* If the cast still becomes soiled, wipe it with a nonabrasive cleaner and a damp sponge or cloth. Then air-dry it with a hair dryer set on "cool."
- Keep a cast cutter or saw available at all times.
- During mealtimes, position older children on their abdomens *to promote safer eating and swallowing.* (See *Documenting hip spica cast care.*)

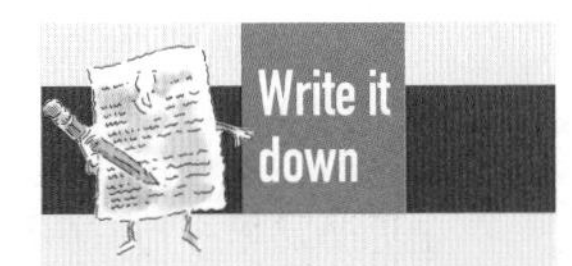

Documenting hip spica cast care

In your notes, record:
- date and time of cast care
- circulatory status in the child's legs
- measurements of bleeding or drainage
- condition of the cast and the child's skin
- all skin care given
- bowel and bladder assessment findings
- child and family tolerance of the cast
- child and family teaching provided.

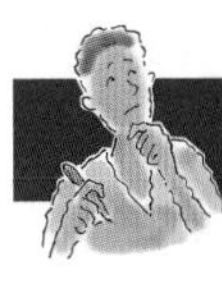

Quick quiz

1. To administer a capsule to an older child, what is the best technique for the nurse to use?

A. Crush the medicine and mix it in water.
B. Have the medicine changed to liquid form.
C. Have him drink enough water to swallow the pill.
D. Pour the granules into a glass of juice.

Answer: C. An older child can place the capsule at the back of his tongue and then drink water or juice.

2. Which site is recommended for an I.M. injection in a 12-month-old child?

A. Vastus lateralis
B. Dorsogluteal
C. Deltoid
D. Ventrogluteal

Answer: A. The vastus lateralis or rectus femoris is used for a child under age 3.

3. Which technique can be used to reduce the pain of I.V. insertion in a toddler?

A. Play therapy
B. EMLA cream
C. Cold compresses
D. Oral pain medication

Answer: B. EMLA, an anesthetic cream, can be applied to reduce the discomfort of I.V. insertion.

4. Before initiating mist tent therapy, which step must the nurse take?

A. Use sterile distilled water.
B. Check the temperature in the tent.
C. Wait 20 minutes before placing the child in the tent.
D. Request the mother to sit in the mist tent with the child.

Answer: A. You must pour sterile distilled water into the reservoir of the nebulizer before initiating mist tent therapy.

5. What cleansing solution is recommended for skin preparation for a central line insertion?
   A. Alcohol
   B. Betadine
   C. Chlorhexidine gluconate
   D. Sterile water

Answer: C. Chlorhexidine gluconate is the cleansing solution recommended by Association of Women's Health, Obstetric and Neonatal Nurses and National Association of Neonatal Nurses.

Scoring

☆☆☆ If you answered all five items correctly, cool! You're all caught up on caring for kids.

☆☆ If you answered four items correctly, great! You have passed this pediatric pop quiz.

☆ If you answered fewer than three items correctly, stay positive. Just peek through the chapter again and give this quiz another try.

Selected References

American Academy of Pediatrics & Canadian Paediatric Society. (2010). *Prevention and management of pain in the neonate: An update policy statement.* Retrieved from http://pediatrics.aappublications.org/content/118/5/2231.full.pdf

Ball, J. W., Bindler, R. C., & Cowen, K. (2012). *Principles of pediatric nursing: Caring for children* (5th ed.). Upper Saddle River, NJ: Pearson Education.

Knobel, R., & Holditch-Davis, D. (2010). Thermoregulation and heat loss prevention after birth and during neonatal intensive-care unit stabilization of extremely low-birthweight infants. *Advances in Neonatal Care, 10*(Suppl. 5), S7–S14.

Linnard-Palmer, L. (2010). *Peds notes: Nurse's clinical pocket guide.* Philadelphia, PA: F.A. Davis.

London, M. L., Ladewig, P. W., Ball, J. W., et al. (2011). *Maternal & child nursing care* (3rd ed.). Upper Saddle River, NJ: Prentice Hall.

Roberts, K. B. (2011). Urinary tract infection: Clinical practice guideline for the diagnosis and management of the initial UTI in febrile infants and children 2 to 24 months. *Pediatrics, 128*(3), 595–610.

Stevens, B., Johnston, C., Taddio, A., et al. (2010). The Premature Infant Pain Profile: Evaluation 13 years after development. *The Clinical Journal of Pain, 26*(9), 813–830.

The Joint Commission. (2010). *Approaches to pain management: An essential guide for clinical learners* (2nd ed.). Retrieved from http://www.jcrinc.com/approaches-to-pain-management-an-essential-guide-for-clinical-leaders-second-edition/

Index

Note: i refers to an illustration; t refers to a table.

C

Note: i refers to an illustration; t refers to a table.

Note: i refers to an illustration; t refers to a table.

Note: i refers to an illustration; t refers to a table.

Note: i refers to an illustration; t refers to a table.

Note: i refers to an illustration; t refers to a table.

Note: i refers to an illustration; t refers to a table.

Note: i refers to an illustration; t refers to a table.

Note: i refers to an illustration; t refers to a table.

U

Note: i refers to an illustration; t refers to a table.

Note: i refers to an illustration; t refers to a table.